Mosby's
Review of practical nursing

Mosby's Review of practical nursing

Mary Elizabeth Faircloth, R.N., B.A., M.S.
Eva Wilson Caldwell, R.N., M.S.N.
Margaret Aenchbacher Callaway, R.N., M.S.N.
Freddie Shaw Hepner, R.N., M.S.N.
Carole Moylan Massey, R.N., M.S.N.
Robert Emory Stephenson, R.Ph., M.S.
Claudia Turner Welch, R.N., M.S.N.

EIGHTH EDITION
Illustrated

The C. V. Mosby Company

ST. LOUIS • TORONTO • LONDON 1982

MOSBY

A TRADITION OF PUBLISHING EXCELLENCE

Editor: Alison Miller
Assistant editor: Susan R. Epstein
Manuscript editor: Terry Young
Design: Diane Beasley
Production: Jeanne A. Gulledge

EIGHTH EDITION

Printed in the United States of America

The C.V. Mosby Company
11830 Westline Industrial Drive, St. Louis, Missouri 63141

Library of Congress Cataloging in Publication Data

Mosby (C.V.) Company.
Mosby's review of practical nursing.

Includes bibliographies.
Includes index.
1. Practical nursing—Outlines, syllabi, etc.
2. Practical nursing—Examinations, questions, etc. I. Title. II. Title: Review of practical nursing. [DNLM: 1. Nursing, Practical—Examination questions. WY 18 M8945]
RT62.M6 1982 610.73'076 81-14105
ISBN 0-8016-3538-1 AACR2

C/D/D 9 8 7 6 5 4 3 2 1 03/B/323

Contributors

Eva Wilson Caldwell, R.N., M.S.N.
Director, Department of Education,
Memorial Medical Center,
Savannah, Georgia

Margaret Aenchbacher Callaway, R.N., M.S.N.
Assistant Professor,
Department of Associate Degree Nursing,
Armstrong State College,
Savannah, Georgia

Mary Elizabeth Faircloth, R.N., B.A., M.S.
President, Organizational Resource Development,
A Division of Career Management of Savannah, Inc.,
Savannah, Georgia

Freddie Shaw Hepner, R.N., M.S.N.
Instructor,
Department of Associate Degree Nursing,
Armstrong State College,
Savannah, Georgia

Carole Moylan Massey, R.N., M.S.N.
Assistant Professor,
Department of Baccalaureate Nursing,
Armstrong State College,
Savannah, Georgia

Robert Emory Stephenson, R.Ph., M.S.
Associate Director, Pharmacy Service,
Memorial Medical Center,
Savannah, Georgia

Claudia Turner Welch, R.N., M.S.N.
Instructor, Staff Development,
Saint Joseph Hospital,
Savannah, Georgia

Preface

This book is designed to serve as a tool to use constantly during your educational experience in practical nursing and particularly as you prepare for success on your licensure examination. The authors, all of whom are experienced teachers of practical nursing subjects, have given careful thought to the revision of this book. In an easily followed outline form, it reflects the rapidly expanding body of medical technology as well as an updated version of essential nursing knowledge needed in your chosen field.

The central theme of this review book is the nursing process, which provides a natural order for the presentation of nursing content areas. A patient care plan format is utilized that emphasizes assessment, planning, implementation, and evaluation, enabling you to use the text readily in classroom and clinical settings.

The four aspects of the nursing process and the ability to function in the role of an LPN/LVN as a member of the profession are highlighted in accord with the National League for Nursing competency expectations for graduates of PN/VN education programs.

The final examination has been completely rewritten. It is presented in four sections and was developed around multiple problem situations that require decision-making skills and application of scientific principles to arrive at the correct answer. Every effort has been made to provoke critical thinking.

Finally, another new feature of this edition of the review book is the index, which will enhance the book's value to you as a ready reference and review tool.

We wish you every success in your quest for knowledge, in your pursuit of licensure, and in the practice of nursing. We offer the following story* for your consideration before you begin to study.

In a small eastern country there lived a sage venerated as the "Wisest of All Men." No one had ever been able to confound him. He answered all questions correctly and was able to propose the most successful solutions for seemingly insoluble problems.

In that same country lived a brilliant and ambitious youth. The lad had won all philosophic competitions he had entered within his own country and beyond its borders. At last there was only one challenge left to him. Somehow he must ask an unanswerable question or pose an insoluble problem to the Wisest of All Men and thus win the title for himself. He planned carefully and requested an audience with the sage.

On the appointed day, the youth stood in the presence of the world's greatest scholars before the Wisest of All Men. He extended his clasped hands and said, "I hold a small bird between my hands. Is it alive or dead?"

The sage realized that the lad had complete control over the fate of the small bird. If this wise man answered, "Dead," the boy could open his hands and let the bird fly away. If he answered "Alive," the boy had only to crush the bird before opening his hands to show the bird was dead.

The sage paused, then quietly and gently said to the youth, "The answer to that question is in your hands."

The answer to your effective use of this review, like the little bird in the fable, lies in your hands.

Mary Elizabeth Faircloth

*Adapted from Baughman, M.D., editor: Teacher's treasury of stories for every occasion, Englewood Cliffs, N.J., 1958, Prentice-Hall, Inc., p. 335.

Contents

1 INTRODUCTION

REFERENCES

Spaney, E., and Jennings, J.A.: The art of studying, Philadelphia, 1958, J.B. Lippincott Co.

Staton, T.F.: How to study, ed. 5, Montgomery, Ala., 1968, T.F. Staton.

Wrenn, C.G., and Larsen, R.P.: Studying effectively, ed. 2, Stanford, Calif., 1966, Stanford University Press.

HOW TO USE THIS BOOK

This book is designed to reinforce your knowledge, develop your self-confidence, and help you diagnose your own learning needs, either in content or in your test-taking ability. Intelligent use of this book will lead you to spend your study time in the most productive way.

As a review book

Your preparation for the licensure examination is as important to you as successful completion of your practical/vocational nursing program. It is reasonable to expect that you have been exposed, as you pursued your course of studies, to all of the information you need to allow you to perform safely and successfully. However, you may need help in organizing the material, in relating it to "situation" type questions, and in improving your ability to take objective tests.

As you prepare for your licensure examination, use good study habits. At a desk, in an armchair, or wherever you feel comfortable; in a quiet atmosphere or with your choice of music as a background, settle down to review the content outline until you feel reasonably certain you know the material.

As soon as you can, take the test covering the content you have just reviewed.

Using the answer section, grade your test after you have completed it. If the results of this testing show marked weakness in one specific area, review the subject and the related materials in your text or reference books in the library and retake the test. Repeat the process until you feel confident you know the necessary content before moving on to the next area. When you have reviewed and tested yourself in each of the separate areas to your satisfaction, you are ready for the final examination. Follow the grading of this examination with review of the rationale for the content missed or omitted, and retest yourself. If time permits, it would be an excellent plan to put studying and testing aside for several days and then retest yourself to determine how well you have retained the material.

There is no way for you to cover in one study period all the material you spent approximately a year in school learning. Give yourself a good chance for success by allowing sufficient time for review and testing. Pace yourself.

Licensure examinations are *timed* tests. Avoid rushing and fatigue in the early period of your preparation for licensure. Gradually increase pressure on yourself by lengthening the study and testing periods and by setting your alarm clock as a means of limiting the time you allow yourself for any one test. By the time you take the final examination in this book, you should be allowing yourself approximately 1/2 minute per question.

As a workbook

You, the student practical/vocational nurse, will find it useful to read the outlined content of a specific area before the first class session in that subject. This practice will provide an overview of the total subject and help you to recognize important areas for deeper study as the course progresses. New vocabulary can be identified and definitions found in the glossary of this book, in your assigned textbook, or in a dictionary. As each part of the content is covered in class, use the review outline as a basis for note taking. Such a practice will help you to organize, for easy review, notes taken in class. Use the test questions for study in preparation for quizzes and examinations. Review all material in the areas of weakness revealed by your missed or omitted test items. Retest until you are satisfied that you have learned the material.

HOW TO TAKE EXAMINATIONS

Taking examinations is a science that should be learned by every student. The rules for test taking are specific and relate to the kind of test being taken. Because licensure examinations use only one kind of test, the information presented here pertains only to objective tests and in particular to objective, multiple choice tests.

Understanding the objective test

Generally, on licensure examinations, a situation is presented from which several different related questions have been developed. For each question, four or five answers are proposed. You must select the *one best answer* from those listed under the question. Answers are not recorded on the test booklet, but on an answer sheet that will be graded by a machine. For each question, there can be only *one* mark on the answer sheet. The one mark, which is the answer you give, must be placed by the *number* that corresponds to the number of the *question* you are answering. (Question 5 in the test booklet must be answered in the space beside 5 on the answer sheet.) Read carefully and follow directions exactly.

To help you be successful, we offer the following paragraphs as a guide to taking your licensure examination.

Begin with a positive attitude. Licensure examinations are not prepared to trick you or determine what you do not know. Rather, they are designed to determine what you do know. You probably know a great deal more than will be asked for in the examination. Objective, multiple choice questions do not ask for total recall. They ask you to recognize the *one best answer*. The answer is already there! All you have to do is recognize it, select it, and place a mark in the correct place on the answer sheet. Believe in yourself, and approach the test as a contestant determined to win a prize.

Read what is there to be read. Avoid scanning; each word in the question and its answers is as important as any other word, so read them all. Avoid reading into questions more than is there to be read. Accept questions and answers at face value.

Follow directions completely. Read directions carefully; skipping them may be costly. Many errors on objective tests are the result of failure to follow instructions. Questions scored *wrong* may have been answered *right* in the mind of the test taker. The pencil mark on the answer sheet, however, may have been the result of not following directions. The grading machine cannot read your mind.

Believe your first impulse. Read the question and all the answers carefully. In many instances you will recognize the one best answer immediately. Accept that you know that one, and make the mark in the correct space on the answer sheet. In some instances you will "feel" one answer is the best one. What you feel is probably subconscious recognition of the one best answer. For each of these two examples, there is established proof that the first impulse answer is more apt to be correct than a changed answer.

If you do not consciously recognize or feel that one answer is best, eliminate those answers you know or feel are incorrect. Reread the remaining answers to determine if you then know or feel which is the best.

• • •

Avoid spending too much time deliberating over one question. That one question could cost you several right answers toward the end of the examination because you did not get to the questions in the allotted time.

Do not guess. It is improbable that guessing will improve your score. As a means of correcting for pure guessing, a certain percentage of wrong answers are subtracted from the number of right answers. Omitted answers do not contain wrong answers, but guessed ones might. Skip the questions in which you would have to guess the answer, and proceed to the next question. You may pick up a clue as you progress through the test, and you will have a better chance to finish all the questions and return to restudy the ones you have skipped.

Beware of limiting or key words and phrases. Be alert to key words and phrases, such as never, always, only, all, none, at all times, at no time, and under any or all circumstances. Few nursing situations and problem solutions are without exceptions. Answers containing these words are frequently wrong answers. Please note we did not say "always wrong" because there are also exceptions to the preceding statement.

As a general rule, test writers tend to write questions

and answers that agree in grammatical construction. In other words, do the question and selected answer make sense and agree in tense and number? For example, if the question is in the past tense, the right answer will also be in the past tense. If the question contains a plural subject, the correct answer will contain a plural verb.

Answer with care. Regardless of the amount of your knowledge and preparation for the licensure examination, there will be excitement and a certain amount of nervousness. The resultant tension and the awareness that time is limited may cause you to become careless unless you guard carefully against it. As cautioned in the directions, avoid extra pencil marks on the answer sheet. Take the time to be certain that the question number in the test booklet and the number beside which you mark your chosen number on the answer sheet are the same. This is extremely important when you skip a question or questions. Marking the answer for question number 12 on the answer sheet in the space allotted for question number 11 may cause all subsequent questions to be answered in the wrong space and result in what is called a ''bad take.'' The scoring machine cannot know you selected the correct answer but marked the incorrect space.

• • •

A few additional hints and words of caution before you begin the practice questions. The correct answer is frequently the longest answer, because the test writer usually writes the correct answer first. Principles of good test construction caution writers to avoid developing any kind of pattern for test answers. Therefore, you may find several questions in a row that have the same correct answer number. Do not be concerned about this or spend valuable time trying to break a code or find a pattern.

Being skilled in taking objective tests is not enough—you must have sufficient knowledge of the subject matter. Follow the suggestions for review, and practice your test-taking skills using this book. You will then be able to approach the licensure examination with confidence as a competitor for a prize—your license. We wish you success.

PRACTICE TEST QUESTIONS

To measure your test-taking skill, we present you with a situation followed by 10 related questions. Read everything carefully—the situation, each question, and all possible answers. When you have decide which answer is **best** for the question under consideration, blacken the corresponding space on the answ There is only **one** best answer for each question.

Situation: Larry P. Noble is a student vocational nurse who plans to graduate in about 6 weeks. Larry has begun to study for his licensure examination. He has made rather good grades in all his courses, but his principal problem remains in the area of test taking. Larry has been aware that he has usually known a great deal more about the subject on which he was being tested than his grades showed. He decided to use *Mosby's Review of Practical Nursing* for his review. He believes that a consistent, planned study pattern will help to ensure his success on the licensure examination.

1 Larry is using the good study habits recommended in *Mosby's Review*. Before taking a test he
1. Rereads his textbook until he knows the content
2. Reviews all of his lecture notes thoroughly
3. Studies the subject for at least 2 days
4. Gets comfortable and reviews the content outline until he feels he knows it

2 Larry was surprised to find out that taking tests is
1. Often difficult because of the demand for total recall
2. A science that every student should learn
3. Not nearly as difficult as he had thought
4. Easier for one who is older

3 One of the important things Larry learned was that he should
1. Look for a pattern in the answers
2. Begin with a positive attitude
3. Scan the questions before answering
4. Take plenty of time deliberating over each question

4 Some additional things to remember when taking objective tests are
(A) Answer with care
(B) Read what is there to be read
(C) Believe your first impulse
(D) Guessing will improve your score
1. A and B
2. B, C, and D
3. C and D
4. A, B, and C

5 Some limiting or key words and phrases Larry was warned to beware of were
1. Sometimes, almost, few, some
2. Almost, occasionally, few, seldom
3. Rarely, frequently, generally, as a rule
4. All, none, at no time, always

6 As he practiced taking tests Larry came to appreciate the admonition to "answer with care." He skipped a question and from that point forward his answers were wrong because he placed his answer marks in the wrong spaces. This kind of carelessness can result in
1. No skill on tests
2. Anxiety
3. A "bad take"
4. Broken machinery

7 Larry read that when you take objective test
1. It is not necessary to know the material
2. You will be asked for total recall
3. You should always answer every question
4. You can usually trust your first impulse

8 Larry told his friend, John, that *Mosby's Review* can be used as a
(A) Workbook during the school year
(B) Textbook
(C) Review book to prepare for the licensure examination
(D) Substitute for studying
1. A and C
2. A, C, and D
3. A, B, and C
4. B and D

9 Larry followed the suggestion that he avoid rushing in the beginning and gradually increase his speed. When he took the final examination, he set his clock and allowed himself
1. ½ minute per question
2. 1 minute per question
3. ½ hour per section
4. 1 hour per section

10 Larry passed his licensure examination with ease. He agreed that *Mosby's Review* helped him by
1. Teaching him all the answers
2. Helping him gain speed and catch trick questions
3. Making him self-conscious but test-wise
4. Reinforcing his knowledge and developing his self-confidence

ANSWERS AND RATIONALES

1. (4) A simple multiple choice question. Note that the correct answer is the longest one. A chair or desk where you are comfortable, with or without background music, is recommended. You should review the content outline until you are reasonably sure you know the material. Such a procedure will help ensure a positive, successful experience in test taking.
2. (2) Taking tests is a science that students should learn early in their educational life.
3. (2) Beginning with a positive attitude is extremely important. The answer is there before you. You just have to recognize it.
4. (4) This is a more complex type of multiple choice question. There is still only *one* correct answer. Guessing is not likely to improve your score. Omitted answers do not contain wrong answers. Guessed answers might.
5. (4) Avoid answers that do not allow for exceptions for few situations and problem solutions are without exception.
6. (3) A "bad take" usually is the result of misplacing an answer early in a test. Only (3) reads smoothly and is grammatically correct.
7. (4) Your first impulse is usually a form of "recognition." Your subconscious recognizes the one best answer.
8. (1) This is more practice for you in the more complicated multiple choice questions. While the material in this book is accurate and helpful, this book is not a substitute for a textbook or studying.
9. (1) If you pace yourself and gradually increase pressure on yourself, you should be allowing yourself no more than ½ minute per question.
10. (4) Through reinforcement of the knowledge you have and an increase in your self-confidence, you, too, can be successful at taking objective tests.

How well did you do? Continue working through this book with a positive attitude. Read what is there to read, and follow directions completely. Believe your first impulse, but *do not guess*. Beware of limiting or key words and phrases. Be careful!

2 THE PRACTICAL NURSE

REFERENCES

Deloughery, J.K.: History and trends of professional nursing, ed. 8, St. Louis, 1977, The C.V. Mosby Co.

DeYoung, L.: The foundations of nursing: as conceived, learned, and practiced in professional nursing, ed. 3, St. Louis, 1976, The C.V. Mosby Co.

Heckel, R.V., and Jordan, R.M.: Psychology: the nurse and the patient, ed. 2, St. Louis, 1967, The C.V. Mosby Co.

Kron, T.: Communications for nurses, ed. 2, Philadelphia, 1972, W.B. Saunders Co.

Lockerby, F.K.: Communication for nurses, ed. 3, St. Louis, 1968, The C.V. Mosby Co.

Matheney, R.V., Noland, B.T., Hogan, A.E., and Griffin, G.J.: Fundamentals of patient-centered nursing, ed. 3, St. Louis, 1972, The C.V. Mosby Co.

National League for Nursing: Competencies of educational programs in practical nursing, New York, 1979, The League.

Notter, L.E., and Spalding, E.K.: Professional nursing, ed. 9, Philadelphia, 1976, J.B. Lippincott Co.

Nursing homes: their patients and their care, Public Health Monograph No. 46, U.S. Department of Health, Education and Welfare, Washington, D.C., 1957, U.S. Government Printing Office.

Programs and services, U.S. Department of Health, Education and Welfare, Washington, D.C., 1966, U.S. Government Printing Office.

Spaney, E., and Jennings, J.A.: The art of studying, Philadelphia, 1958, J.B. Lippincott Co.

Thompson, L.F., Miller, M.H., and Bigler, H.F.: Sociology: nurses and their patients in a modern society, ed. 9, St. Louis, 1975, The C.V. Mosby Co.

Wood, L.A., and Rambo, B.J.: Nursing skills for allied health services, ed. 2, Philadelphia, 1977, W.B. Saunders Co.

NURSING

A. Definition—a practice discipline that uses the nursing process to assist the patient in achieving and maintaining his maximum level of wellness. Supportive, nurturative, and ministrative skills of the nurse are used, as well as active participation by individual patients in the planning, implementing, and evaluation of their care

B. The nursing process—a method of problem solving used in nursing that consists of
   1. Assessing—identifying patient problems or needs, strengths, and coping mechanisms
   2. Planning—setting goals and identifying methods to solve problems and meet patient needs
   3. Implementing—carrying out the designated methods to achieve established goals
   4. Evaluating—assessing the patient's response to his plan of care in terms of goal attainment

Nurses

A. Professional nurses
   1. Complete prescribed course in professional school of nursing
      a. Two-year associate degree program
      b. Three-year diploma program
      c. Four-year baccalaureate degree program
   2. Pass state board examination as basis for becoming licensed by state
   3. Use title, RN (registered nurse)
   4. May specialize in many fields through postgraduate education

B. Practical/vocational nurses
   1. Complete prescribed course in state-approved vocational education facility
   2. Pass state board examination as basis for becoming licensed by state
   3. Use title, LVN (licensed vocational nurse) or LPN (licensed practical nurse)
   4. Practice nursing under the supervision of a registered nurse or physician
   5. Have role legally defined by states (see individual state laws)

6. May specialize in many fields through postgraduate education

C. History of nursing
   1. During ancient times, women took care of the sick and invalids
   2. Hippocrates, father of modern medicine, removed superstition from medicine by relating scientific principles to diagnosing and testing
   3. The Hebrews established "sick houses" and outlined principles for sanitation and personal hygiene
   4. In the Christian era, nursing came about as an expression of charity
   5. Three nursing organizations developed during the Middle Ages: military, religious, and secular orders
   6. During the Protestant Reformation, hospitals were run by the state out of need, not charity
   7. Florence Nightingale, founder of modern nursing, established the concept of health maintenance and caring for the sick.
   8. Practical nursing evolved to meet the increasing need for health care workers
   9. The first school of practical nursing was the Ballard School, established in 1893
   10. Modern training programs for practical nurses must meet state requirements and are usually 12 months in length
   11. Role of practical nurse is being reevaluated continually because of changing health care needs and technologic advances
   12. Schools of high standards may apply for accreditation by the National League for Nurses or the National Association of Practical Nurse Education and Service

Health team concept

A. The health team consists of members of all health disciplines who work together with the patient to achieve established goals

B. Members of the health team vary depending on patient needs; however, the physician and the nursing staff are constant members

C. The disciplines are interdependent with overlapping skills and shared responsibilities

D. Practical nurses function under immediate direction and supervision of the registered nurse or physician

E. Practical nurses may be responsible for the supervision of other auxiliary personnel

Nursing care delivery systems

A. Case method—assignment made for a specific nurse to one patient

B. Functional method—assignments are made according to functions (TPRs, medicines, treatments)

C. Team method—a group of patients is cared for by a team consisting of professional nurse, practical nurses, and hospital aides
   1. Professional nurse is team leader and makes assignments to all team members
   2. Practical nurses go to team leader for instruction and help in carrying out patient care

D. Primary care method—a specified professional nurse assumes 24-hour responsibility for care of the patient, with assistance of other nurses and health team members

PERSONAL ATTRIBUTES AND VOCATIONAL RESPONSIBILITIES

Personal

A. Usually are 18 to 55 years old (varies in different states)

B. Have high school diploma or equivalent

C. Usually have U.S. citizenship (most states require)

D. Have good physical and mental health

E. Assume responsibility for health maintenance and well-being

F. Have good personal appearance in uniform
   1. Are neat and clean with no extremes in cosmetics and hair fashions
   2. Follow dress code of employing agency

Vocational

A. Focus energies on the patient and meet his needs

B. Demonstrate loyalty to patient, institution, and other health personnel

C. Maintain code of ethics (code of acceptable behavior)

D. Adjust constructively to new situations and working conditions

E. Demonstrate interest in continued learning

F. Maintain satisfactory interpersonal relationships

NATIONAL LEAGUE FOR NURSING—COMPETENCIES

Graduates of practical nursing educational programs can be expected to have the following competencies

A. Assessing
   1. Contribute to the identification of basic physical,

emotional, and cultural needs of the health care client
2. Identify basic communication techniques in a structured care setting
3. Interview health care clients to obtain specified information
4. Identify overt learning needs of the health care client
5. Make significant observations of the health care client and communicate these to the health team
6. Identify appropriate resources in some other agencies within the health care delivery system.

B. Planning
   1. Contribute to the development of basic nursing care plans in an institutional setting
   2. Contribute, with assistance, to the development of health plans for health care clients and/or families

C. Implementing
   1. Safely perform basic therapeutic and preventative nursing procedures, incorporating fundamental biologic and psychologic principles in giving individualized care
   2. Show respect for the dignity of individuals
   3. Apply basic communication techniques in a structured care setting
   4. Demonstrate the ability to do incidental teaching during routine care
   5. Assume shared responsibility for the health care delivery system in structured situations

D. Evaluating
   1. Seek guidance as needed in evaluating the care given and making necessary adjustments
   2. Identify own strengths and weaknesses and seek assistance for improvement of performance

E. Assuming role as members within the profession of nursing
   1. Recognize own roles as LPN/LVN in the health care delivery system.
   2. Seek out and take advantage of learning situations and opportunities for continuing their education

FIELDS OF EMPLOYMENT

A. Clinical specialties
B. Community health nursing
C. Military nursing
D. Industrial nursing
E. Physician's office
F. Ambulatory care facilities
G. Extended care facilities
H. Private duty agencies
I. Home health care agencies

HOSPITALS AND OTHER INSTITUTIONS CARING FOR PATIENTS

Hospitals

May be classified in terms of function, size, or the way in which they are supported

A. Functions
   1. Expand medical knowledge and research
   2. Invent technical equipment
   3. Provide clinical facilities for education of physicians, nurses, and other health care personnel
   4. Diagnose, treat, and prevent diseases
   5. Give specialized care in pediatrics and obstetrics and in treatment of communicable diseases, tuberculosis, mental illness, and chronic illness
   6. Provide clinical facilities for learning
   7. Promote public health through outpatient clinics

B. Classification of hospitals
   1. Public (nonvoluntary)
      a. Supported by city, county, state, or federal taxes
      b. Provide wide range of services and medical and nursing education
      c. Usually care for patients who cannot afford private hospital care or patients who have chronic or long-term illnesses
   2. Private (voluntary)
      a. Supported by patients through direct payment, insurance, community funds, or gifts and endowments
      b. Usually offer wide range of services because of needs of education and research
   3. Proprietary
      a. Designed to make a profit for stockholders as business establishments
      b. May not include as many services as voluntary and nonvoluntary hospitals
      c. Usually have patients with less acute illnesses

C. Standards
   1. City and state requirements
   2. Joint Commission on Accreditation of Hospitals (JCAH) provides standards for better hospital care regardless of type of hospital; usually federal funding is dependent on JCAH accreditation
   3. Accrediting agencies, such as American Hospital Association and American College of Surgeons, examine hospitals

4. Regardless of governmental or nongovernmental regulations, hospitals are increasingly under the control of standard-enforcing agencies that ensure proper criteria for patient care
5. Audit committees establish criteria for evaluation of patient care according to recognized standards of care
6. Professional Standards Review Organizations (PSROs), a federally mandated program, ensure appropriate utilization of hospital facilities and set standards of care

D. Organization and administration
   1. Hospital departments are generally organized under the direction of a hospital administrator
   2. Hospital policies and budget allocation are usually controlled by a governing board
   3. Hospitals are highly specialized into departments such as laboratory, dietary, medical, and nursing
   4. A professional nurse is usually the director of nursing service and is responsible for staffing and direction of all patient care areas
   5. Practical nurse is usually responsible (line of authority) directly to
      a. Charge nurse or team leader or both
      b. Head nurse
      c. Floor supervisor
      d. Director of nursing service (indirectly)

Community agencies

A. Classified according to means of support (tax or private)
B. Governmental or official agencies are supported by local, state, and federal taxes
C. Administration of federal programs relating to health, education, and welfare is under the jurisdiction of the Department of Health and Human Services

Federal government (tax supported)

A. Department of Health and Human Services (HHS)
   1. National Institutes of Health
      a. Bureau of Health Professions and Manpower Training
      b. National Cancer Institute
      c. National Heart Institute
      d. National Institute on Aging
      e. National Institute of Allergy and Infectious Diseases
      f. National Institute of Arthritis and Metabolic Diseases
      g. National Institute of Child Health and Human Development
      h. National Institute of Dental Research
      i. National Institute of General Medical Sciences
      j. National Institute of Neurological Disease and Stroke
      k. National Eye Institute
      l. National Institute of Environmental Health Services
      m. National Library of Medicine
      n. Fogarty International Center
   2. Consumer Protection and Environmental Health Service
      a. Environmental Control Administration
      b. Food and Drug Administration
      c. National Air Pollution Control Administration
   3. Health Services and Mental Health Administration
      a. National Center for Health Services Research and Development
      b. National Center for Health Statistics
      c. National Communicable Diseases Center
      d. National Institute of Mental Health
      e. Health Facilities Planning and Construction Services
      f. Community Health Services
      g. Regional Medical Programs Service
      h. Indian Health Service
      i. Federal Health Programs Service

B. Other departments
   1. Office of Education
      a. Elementary and secondary education
      b. Higher education
      c. Education for the handicapped
      d. Adult and vocational education
      e. Educational personnel development
      f. Educational research
   2. Social and Rehabilitation Service
   3. Social Security Administration

State and local departments of health and welfare (tax supported)

A. Set standards to meet local needs
B. Provide for sanitation; water, milk, and food inspection; and garbage collection
C. Inspect restaurants, factories, and other institutions in order to protect the health and welfare of the public

D. License various personnel, such as physicians, nurses (professional and practical), barbers, and beauticians
E. Set standards for hospitals and institutions caring for the sick and socially dependent
F. Provide laboratory services for diagnosis of disease
G. Provide consultant services in matters of health and welfare
H. Maintain hospitals, clinics, and institutions for needy sick and other people with health and welfare problems
I. Keep record of vital statistics—numeric record of marriages, births, deaths, and diseases

Voluntary agencies

Supported by private funds, donations, United Fund, or other agencies interested in health and welfare, such as American Cancer Society, National Foundation–March of Dimes, American Heart Association, and American Red Cross

International programs

Following World War II and the organization of the United Nations, the World Health Organization (WHO) was established. It is concerned with the scope of and appropriate international action in the field of public health

THE PRACTICAL NURSE REVIEW QUESTIONS

Read each question carefully and consider all possible answers. When you have decided which answer is **best,** blacken in the corresponding space on the answer sheet. There is only **one** best answer for each question.

1 The practical nurse
(A) Must pass a state board examination
(B) Be at least 21 years of age
(C) Practices under the supervision of a registered nurse
(D) Functions as a professional nurse
1. A and C
2. A, C, and D
3. A and B
4. A, B, and C

2 Functioning of the health care team is necessary because it
1. Allows more time for nurses to care for a greater number of patients
2. Allows for better scheduling of patient assignments
3. Meets the Joint Commission on Accreditation of Hospitals (JCAH) requirements for licensure of hospitals
4. Allows goals to be set by the patient and all those involved in his care

3 The government protects the health of its citizens by establishing
(A) Communicable disease regulations
(B) Agencies to enforce the Pure Food and Drug Act
(C) Standards for hospital buildings
(D) Marriage laws
(E) Child labor laws
1. A, B, and C
2. B, C, and D
3. A, B, D, and E
4. B, C, D, and E

4 The modern hospital has the following functions
(A) Treatment of disease
(B) Research
(C) Rehabilitation
(D) Custodial care of the aged
(E) Education of personnel
1. A, C, and D
2. A, C, and E
3. A, B, C, and E
4. A, B, C, and D

5 Qualifications for the LPN must include
(A) Good health
(B) Emotional maturity
(C) Graduation from a National League for Nursing–approved school
(D) Adherence to a code of ethics
(E) Maintenance of satisfactory interpersonal relationships
1. A, B, and C
2. A, B, and D
3. A, B, D, and E
4. A, C, D, and E

6 Licensing of practical nurses is
1. Regulated by individual state nurse practice acts
2. Not required by all states
3. Regulated by the National League for Nursing
4. Regulated by the federal government

7 The tax-supported divisions of HHS sponsors are which of the following?
(A) Social and Rehabilitation Service
(B) Social Security Administration
(C) National Institutes of Health
(D) Consumer Protection and Environmental Health Service
1. A, C, and D
2. A, B, and C
3. C and D
4. B, C, and D

8 The nursing process is a method
1. Of problem solving used in nursing
2. Of assigning patient care
3. Of obtaining licensure
4. By which nursing evolved as a practice discipline

9 If a friend asks you to recommend a physician, you would
1. Advise which physician you would choose
2. Give the friend a list of several physicians and allow him to choose
3. Call the local Practical Nurse Association
4. Call the nurses' registry

10 Mandatory licensing of practical nurses means that
1. Only nurses in hospitals need to be licensed
2. The practical nurse can decide when to obtain the license
3. The practical nurse can register by waiver
4. All practical nurses are required by law to be licensed

11 Hospitals may be financially supported by
(A) Taxes
(B) Endowments
(C) United Fund
(D) Legacies
(E) State grants
1. A, B, C, and E
2. A, B, C, and D
3. A, B, and C
4. A, B, C, D, and E

12 When employed by a hospital, practical nurses are directly responsible for their work to the
1. Administrator of the hospital
2. Director of personnel
3. Director of nurses
4. Head nurse, charge nurse, or team leader

13 The components of the nursing process are used in the following order
1. Assessing, planning, implementing, and evaluating
2. Planning, assessing, implementing, and evaluating
3. Evaluating, planning, assessing, and implementing
4. Implementing, assessing, evaluating, and planning

14 Examples of the assessment component of the nursing process that should be demonstrated by graduates of LPN programs are
(A) Identify overt learning needs
(B) Interview patients on admission
(C) Initiate plan of care
(D) Perform basic preventive and therapeutic nursing procedures
1. A and B
2. B and C
3. B and D
4. C and D

15 The numeric record of births, deaths, marriages, and disease is called
1. Mortality statistics
2. Morbidity statistics
3. Vital statistics
4. State records

16 A code of behavior is called
1. Hospital regulations
2. Personnel policies
3. Ethics
4. Licensure

17 Good nursing is dependent on qualities other than clinical knowledge and technical skill; some such qualities are
(A) Satisfactory interpersonal relationships
(B) Effective communication
(C) Interest in continued learning
(D) Chronological age of nurse
1. A, B, and D
2. A, B, and C
3. A, C, and D
4. B, C, and D

18 A federally mandated program to ensure appropriate use of hospital facilities and set standards of care is known as
1. Professional Standards Review Organization (PSRO)
2. Audit
3. Joint Commission on Accreditation of Hospitals (JCAH)
4. Health, Education and Welfare (HEW)

19 In many hospitals, practical nurses work under the leadership of professional nurses in caring for groups of patients; this is called
1. Case study method
2. Functional assignment
3. Team nursing
4. Comprehensive care

20 A system whereby a specified professional nurse assumes 24-hour responsibility for care of the patient with the assistance of other nurses and health team members is known as
1. Primary care nursing
2. Case method
3. Team nursing
4. Functional nursing

21 Federal Aid to Families with Dependent Children is provided by the
1. State Department
2. Department of Agriculture
3. Department of Health and Human Services
4. Department of Pensions

22 Setting goals to solve patient problems or meet their needs occurs in which stage of the nursing process?
1. Assessing
2. Planning
3. Implementing
4. Evaluating

23 Schools of practical nursing may be accredited by
(A) State boards of nursing
(B) National Federation of LPNs
(C) National Association of Practical Nurses Education and Services
(D) National League for Nursing
1. A, C, and D
2. C and D
3. A
4. A, B, and C

24 The length of most practical nursing programs is
1. 18 months
2. 9 months
3. 24 months
4. 12 months

25 The term most commonly applied to the practical nurse who has passed the state board examination is
1. Vocational Nurse
2. Practical Nurse
3. Licensed Practical Nurse
4. Trained Practical Nurse

26 The nurse can stay abreast of latest developments by
1. Reading current professional magazines and newspapers
2. Attending refresher classes
3. Participating in inservice programs
4. Joining and participating in professional organizations

27 The practical nurse who has successfully passed the state board examination would sign his or her name followed by which of the following titles?
1. RN
2. BSN
3. LPN
4. ADN

Items 28 through 30 relate to the four methods often used to plan nursing care.

28 The method that assigns staff by tasks is known as
1. Case method
2. Team nursing
3. Functional method
4. Primary care

29 The method that uses a planned grouped approach is known as
1. Case method
2. Team nursing
3. Functional method
4. Primary care

30 The method that is most often used by private duty agencies is known as
1. Case method
2. Team nursing
3. Functional method
4. Primary care

---

31 The founder of modern nursing was
1. Florence Nightingale
2. Frances Bolton
3. Dorothea Dix
4. Linda Richards

32 The first school of practical nursing was established in 1893 and was called the
1. Bellvice Hospital School
2. Kaisenworth Institute
3. Ballard School
4. Charity Hospital School

33 Setting goals and identifying methods to solve problems and meet patient needs occurs in which of the following steps of the nursing process?
1. Assessing
2. Planning
3. Implementing
4. Evaluating

34 Hospital accrediting agencies establish standards for
1. Budget allocation
2. Hospital policies
3. Nursing education
4. Quality patient care

35 Identifying problems or needs of the patient occurs in which of the following steps of the nursing process?
1. Assessing
2. Planning
3. Implementing
4. Evaluating

3 BASIC SCIENCE

REFERENCES

Anthony, C.P., and Thibodeau, G.A.: Textbook of anatomy and physiology, ed. 10, St. Louis, 1979, The C.V. Mosby Co.

Arnow, L.E.: Introduction to physiological and pathological chemistry, ed. 9, St. Louis, 1976, The C.V. Mosby Co.

Brooks, S.M., and Paynton-Brooks, N.: The human body: structure and function in health and disease, ed. 2, St. Louis, 1980, The C.V. Mosby Co.

Flitter, H.H.: An introduction to physics in nursing, ed. 7, St. Louis, 1976, The C.V. Mosby Co.

Francis, C.C., and Martin, A.H.: Introduction to human anatomy, ed. 7, St. Louis, 1975, The C.V. Mosby Co.

Frobisher, M., and Fuerst, R.: Microbiology in health and disease, ed. 14, Philadelphia, 1978, W.B. Saunders Co.

Hahn, A.B., Barkin, R.S. and Oestreich, S.J.K.: Pharmacology in nursing, ed. 15, St. Louis, 1982, The C.V. Mosby Co.

Jacob, S.W., and Francone, C.A.: Structure and function in man, ed. 4, Philadelphia, 1978, W.B. Saunders Co.

Kerschner, V.L.: Nutrition and diet therapy for practical nurses, ed. 2, Philadelphia, 1976, F.A. Davis Co.

Laughlin, A.: Roe's principles of chemistry, ed. 12, St. Louis, 1976, The C.V. Mosby Co.

Robinson, C.H.: Basic nutrition and diet therapy, ed. 4, New York, 1980, Macmillan Publishing Co., Inc.

Sackheim, G.I., and Schultz, R.M.: Chemistry for the health sciences, ed. 3, New York, 1977, Macmillan Publishing Co., Inc.

Shackelton, A.D., and Poleman, C.L.: Practical nurse nutrition education, ed. 4, Philadelphia, 1978, W.B. Saunders Co.

Smith, A.L.: Microbiology and pathology, ed. 12, St. Louis, 1980, The C.V. Mosby Co.

Williams, S.R.: Nutrition and diet therapy, ed. 4, St. Louis, 1981, The C.V. Mosby Co.

Introduction

A. Biologic and physical sciences are a necessary part of nurse's preparation in order to understand
   1. Body functions
   2. Underlying principles of nursing care
   3. How to be a health teacher for patients

B. Subject matter includes physics, chemistry, microbiology, anatomy and physiology, nutrition, and basic pharmacology. They are briefly covered in following material; some are integrated with body structure and function

Principles of physics

GENERAL

Classifications (types) of measurement

A. British imperial system—primarily used in the United States (inches, pint, pound)

B. Metric, or international, system—used in most of world and in science and is based on multiples of 10 (meter, liter, gram)

Mass

A. Mass is a quantity of matter

B. Matter is anything that occupies space

C. State of matter may be solid, liquid, or gas, depending on the temperature, given pressure at a given moment, and type of matter

D. All matter is composed of molecules

E. Law of conservation of mass states that under ordinary conditions, matter is neither created nor destroyed

Energy

A. Energy is capacity to do work; work is overcoming resistance and can be measured
B. Types of energy are
   1. Kinetic—energy of motion
   2. Potential—energy of position; energy exists but is not in use
   3. Radiant—is transmitted in space (radiowaves, x rays)
C. Changes of energy are physical, chemical, or both
D. Theory of conservation of energy states that under ordinary conditions, energy cannot be lost

Density

A. Density means weight per unit of volume; expressed in grams per cubic centimeter
B. Water at a given temperature is taken as a standard measurement for densities of solids and liquids
C. Common air at set temperatures serves as standard for comparison of densities of gases
D. Specific gravity is density of a substance divided by density of equal volume of water. Specific gravity of liquids is measured by an instrument called a hydrometer
E. Applications to nursing are
   1. A body displaces equal volume of water, for example, a foot placed in tub of water
   2. Density of particle in urine is denoted by specific gravity

Surface tension

A. Surface tension is the ability of the surface of a liquid in contact with a gas or another liquid to contract to the smallest possible area
B. Surfactant is agent that has ability to lower surface tension (emulsifiers, detergents, germicides)
C. Capillary action is rise of liquid on surface that it wets (means by which cotton and gauze absorb drainage)

Solution

A. Solution is a homogeneous mixture of two or more substances
B. Properties of solution are related to the concentration of solute
C. Colligative properties are freezing point, boiling point, and osmotic pressure
D. Milligrams per 100 ml is expression of concentration of solution

Diffusion

Movement of molecules from an area of greater concentration to area of lower concentration

Osmosis

A. Osmosis is movement of water, or other solvent, through semipermeable membranes with flow principally being from the less concentrated to the more concentrated, until a state of dynamic equilibrium is obtained
B. Osmotic pressure is amount of pressure that is applied to the solution to prevent osmosis across a semipermeable membrane separating the solute from the pure solvent
C. The greater the solute concentration, the greater the osmotic pressure

Gravity and pressure

A. Gravity is the force that causes a body to fall toward the center of the eaarth
B. Pressure is stress or strain using compression, expansion, pull, or thrust
   1. Center of gravity is center of the mass of the object
   2. Gravity causes liquids to flow
   3. The smaller the surface, the greater the pressure
   4. Fluids move from an area of greater pressure to an area of lesser pressure
   5. Atmospheric pressure is pressure exerted by air above the earth—14.7 pounds per square inch
   6. Applications in nursing are
      a. Factors affecting fluid flow (important in administering intravenous fluids, hypodermics, enemas) are
         (1) Height of solution (pressure)
         (2) Length of tubing
         (3) Diameter of tubing
         (4) Viscosity of fluid
      b. Elevating the foot of the bed facilitates circulation of blood to the heart
      c. Secretions can be drained from mouth by gravity
      d. Lowering the head of a person who is faint will increase blood flow to brain

Friction

A. Friction is resistance met by one body moving over another
B. Static friction exists between two bodies standing still

C. Sliding friction exists between one surface moving on another
D. Friction is greater for rough than for smooth, lubricated surfaces
E. Presence of wind and water increases friction
F. Applications in nursing are
   1. Powder is used in back rubs to reduce friction
   2. Lubricants are used in inserting tubes to reduce friction
   3. Rubbing on skin surfaces produces heat and dilates blood vessels
   4. Friction is important in cleansing
   5. Pills are swallowed more easily with water as lubricant

Motion

A. Motion is act indicating change of place or position
B. Lever is simple machine used to produce motion
C. Levers involve power (P), fulcrum (F), and weight (W)
   1. First class—power and weight act on opposite sides of fulcrum (scissors)
   2. Second class—power and weight act on same side of fulcrum with weight nearer fulcrum
   3. Third class—power and weight act on same side of fulcrum with weight near fulcrum (tissue forceps)
D. Muscles, bones, and cartilage function on principles of mechanical levers
E. Applications in nursing care are
   1. Wide base enables more steady and less tiring maintenance of position (nurse keeps feet at least 18 inches apart)
   2. Support to knees and back prevents strain
   3. Tray carried in front of nurse and close to body helps prevent strain
   4. Support to head and back of patient when sitting prevents strain

SOUND

A. Is waves of vibrating motion
B. Travels faster in solids than in liquids
C. Travels faster in liquids than in gases

LIGHT

A. Light is the sensation produced by electromagnetic radiation that falls on the retina
B. Light rays are narrow beams of light diverging from a common center
C. Types of light rays are
   1. Infrared
   2. Ultraviolet
   3. Radiation
   4. X rays
D. Applications in nursing are
   1. Glare causes eye fatigue and strain
   2. Ultraviolet rays do not penetrate clothing
   3. Infrared rays will penetrate normal clothing

HEAT

A. Heat is the energy produced by the motion of molecules
B. Calorie is amount of heat needed to raise temperature of 1 g water 1°C
C. In most cases, materials expand when their temperature is raised and shrink when their temperature is lowered
D. The common mercury thermometer makes use of the expansion and contraction of liquid mercury to measure heat
E. Transfer of heat takes different forms
   1. Conduction is rapidly moving hot molecules colliding with cooler molecules (hot water bottle)
   2. Convection is passage of heat by circulation of heated parts of liquids and gases (air conditioning to cool environment and therefore patient)
   3. Radiation is the transfer of heat in the form of waves (perineal lamp)
F. Vaporization is changing of liquids and solids to gases and vapors
   1. Liquids at ordinary temperatures vaporize at slow rate (evaporation)
   2. Heat causes faster vaporization
   3. Pressure causes faster vaporization
G. Applications in nursing are
   1. Water warmer than body temperature prevents chilling
   2. Water and alcohol evaporate, causing cooling of skin
   3. Mercury expands with heat

Principles of chemistry

DEFINITIONS

A. Atom—the smallest unit of element, composed of neutrons, protons, and electrons

B. Element—basic form of matter; classified as metal or nonmetal
C. Molecule—structural form of matter
D. Physical change—one in which no new substance is produced but there is a change in state or color
E. Chemical change—one in which a new substance is produced
F. Catalyst—a substance that facilitates a chemical reaction without changing its own form

OXYGEN

A. Occurs in air, water, earth's crust, foods, and body
B. Is heavier than air, transparent, colorless, odorless, and tasteless
C. Is soluble in water
D. Forms oxides with other elements
E. Is used
   1. By living animals for metabolism
   2. As disinfectant
   3. As bleaching agent

WATER

A. Is composed of hydrogen and oxygen
B. Is most abundant compound in all living things
C. Is universal solvent; colorless, odorless, tasteless, stable liquid that reacts with metals and nonmetals
D. Is used as treatment in form of hydrotherapy, steam, and ice packs

ACIDS, BASES, AND SALTS

Acids

A. Furnish hydrogen ions
B. Produce a sour taste and exhibit a pH of less than 7
C. Most commonly used include hydrochloric (HCl), sulfuric (H_2SO_4), nitric (HNO_3), and acetic (CH_3COOH)

Bases

A. Furnish hydroxyl (OH) ions
B. Produce a bitter taste and exhibit a pH of greater than 7
C. Neutralize salts to form salts and water
D. Include ammonium hydroxide (NH_4OH), potassium hydroxide (KOH), and sodium hydroxide (NaOH)

Salts

A. A chemical compound, usually crystalline, resulting from the interaction of an acid and a base. An example is sodium (base) chloride (acid) (NaCl)
B. Salts may exhibit a neutral pH (7) when mixed with water if the acid and base are both strong
C. If the acid is strong, an acidic solution (pH less than 7) will result when the salt is combined with water. If the base is strong, a basic solution (pH greater than 7) will result

IONIZATION

A. Ionization is the dissociation of compounds, acids, bases, or salts into their constituent ions
B. An ion is a free-floating particle carrying an electrical charge. It may carry positive charge (cation) or negative charge (anion)
C. An electrolyte is a compound that conducts a current when in solution

NUCLEAR CHEMISTRY

A. The discovery of x rays by Roentgen in 1895 stimulated other scientists to look for similar mysterious radiations
B. Elements that emit energy rays are said to be radioactive. Examples are radium and uranium
C. Radioactive elements emit three types of rays
   1. Alpha rays are completely absorbed by a thin sheet of paper and possess powerful photographic properties
   2. Beta rays are absorbed by 1 mm of lead or equivalent
   3. Gamma rays have a high power of penetration and are the most powerful of the three types of rays
D. During the breakdown of radioactive elements, enormous quantities of heat are liberated

ORGANIC CHEMISTRY

A. Organic chemistry is the study of carbon compounds found in plants and animals
B. Carbohydrates, fats, and proteins are organic compounds used in the body for metabolism
C. Metabolism is the sum total of all chemical activity in the cell
   1. Catabolism—breakdown of complex substances into simpler forms to release energy and heat (digestion)
   2. Anabolism—process by which cell obtains substances from the blood required for growth and repair
D. Enzyme is an organic catalyst that facilitates a chemical reaction without changing its own form

SOME APPLICATIONS TO NURSING

A. Perspiration is colorless liquid, slightly acidic in action, and composed of sodium chloride and other materials
B. Muscle tissue is composed of three-fourths water and one-fourth solid
C. Active muscle is acid; resting muscle is alkaline; lack of oxygen causes fatigue by forming sarcolactic acid
D. Heat speeds metabolism of body
E. Alcohol combines with protein of skin forming hard substance that toughens skin
F. Alkalinity of soaps removes protective oils of skin and can cause irritation
G. Powder keeps skin dry and acts as astringent
H. Heat in body is produced by oxidation of food
I. Benzene is solvent for adhesive but also irritating to skin if not washed off after application
J. Urine, in decomposing, produces substance irritating to skin
K. Color of feces is caused by undigested foods, metallic substances, and bile
L. Heat coagulates protein (blood, urine); rinse soiled equipment with cold water first
M. Sodium bicarbonate neutralizes acid of stomach
N. Weak acids and bases used as antidotes for each other

Table 1 □ *Elements in the human body*

Element	Symbol	Percentage
Oxygen	O	65
Carbon	C	18
Hydrogen	H	10
Nitrogen	N	3
Calcium	Ca	2
Phosphorus	P	1
Potassium	K	0.35
Sulfur	S	0.25
Sodium	Na	0.15
Chlorine	Cl	0.15
Magnesium	Mg	0.05
Iron	Fe	0.004

Principles of microbiology

GENERAL

A. Microbiology is study of microorganisms, some of which are visible only with microscope and others visible only by electron microscope
B. Microorganisms include groups of plants and animals
C. Study of microbiology necessary because
   1. Knowledge will ensure correct procedures to maintain medical and surgical asepsis
   2. Knowledge of microorganisms and immunity will help in teaching and practicing prevention of disease
D. Nursing procedures based on principles of microbiology prevent spread of disease and promote recovery
E. Antonj van Leeuwenhoek, father of microbiology, was first person to see and describe microorganisms
F. There are seven principal groups of microorganisms
   1. Algae cause no disease
   2. Protozoa cause amebic dysentery and malaria
   3. Fungi (yeasts) do more good than harm; they ferment sugar, producing carbon dioxide, and are essential in baking. Some are disease producing, such as those causing ringworm or tinea
   4. Fungi (molds) do more good than harm; they are used to flavor cheese and to manufacture antibacterial drugs such as penicillin; some are disease producing and cause food to spoil
   5. Bacteria cause tuberculosis and staphylococcic infection
   6. Rickettsiae cause Rocky Mountain spotted fever
   7. Viruses cause measles, chickenpox, poliomyelitis, and influenza
G. For survival, microorganisms need moisture, nutrients, favorable temperature, favorable osmotic pressure, neutral or slightly alkaline fluid, and no sunlight. Some need oxygen (aerobes) and some do not (anaerobes)
H. In laboratory study of microorganisms, certain microorganisms take certain stains and are classified according to stain (gram-negative [red or brown] and gram-positive [violet])
I. Microorganisms are also classified as pathogenic (harmful to humans) and nonpathogenic (not harmful to humans but may be to animals and plants)
J. Many bacteria have been identified; only a small percentage cause disease in humans

K. Microorganisms, through the process of decomposition of organic matter, function in
   1. Purification of air, water, and sewage
   2. Food processing
   3. Industry
   4. Manufacture of some medications
L. Pathogenic microorganisms must be destroyed, removed, or inhibited
M. Definitions
   1. Disinfection is process that kills pathogenic organisms (pasteurization)
   2. Sterilization is process that destroys all microorganisms (autoclaving)
   3. Antisepsis is process that prevents or combats infection or sepsis by killing or inhibiting bacteria (chemicals)
N. Problems encountered in inhibiting and destroying microorganisms are
   1. All microorganisms consist of protoplasm, which is protein
   2. Some microorganisms have protective protein coats (tuberculosis bacillus)
   3. Some can adapt to adverse environments and develop resistant forms (spores)
O. Factors influencing inhibition and destruction of microorganisms are
   1. Physical—temperature, light, radiation, contact, and time
   2. Chemical—antiseptics, germicides, antibiotics, and pH of environment

---

Anatomy and physiology (body structure and function)

ORGANIZATION OF THE HUMAN BODY

Anatomic reference systems

A. Anatomic position—body is erect, facing forward with the arms at the side and the palms toward the front (All descriptions of location or position assume the body to be in this position)
B. Directions (see Glossary)
   1. Superior
   2. Inferior
   3. Anterior
   4. Posterior
   5. Medial
   6. Lateral
   7. Proximal
   8. Distal
C. Planes (see Glossary)
   1. Midsagittal
   2. Sagittal
   3. Transverse
   4. Frontal
D. Cavities
   1. Ventral (front or anterior) cavity
      a. Thoracic cavity
         (1) Pleural cavities contain lungs
         (2) Pericardial cavity contains heart
         (3) Mediastinum contains great blood vessels, nerves, thymus, trachea, esophagus, and lymphatic vessels
      b. Abdominal and pelvic cavities
         (1) Abdominal portion contains abdominal organs
         (2) Pelvic portion contains pelvic organs
   2. Dorsal (back or posterior) cavity
      a. Cranial cavity contains brain
      b. Spinal cavity (vertebral portion) contains spinal cord

Structural units

A. Cell is simplest unit of structure and function
B. Tissue consists of groups of like cells having like function (muscle or nerve)
C. Organ consists of groups of several kinds of tissues having special function (stomach)
D. System consists of group of organs put together to perform particular function (cardiovascular system)
E. All function as an integrated whole

INTRODUCTION TO GENERAL BODY PHYSIOLOGY

Basic life processes

Metabolism—sum total of all body chemical reactions
A. Anabolism—construction of complex molecules from simple molecules with the subsequent storage of energy
B. Catabolism—breakdown of complex molecules into simple molecules with the subsequent release of energy

Compounds in living matter and their functions

A. Water is universal solvent
B. Proteins build and repair tissues and supply energy
C. Carbohydrates supply energy

D. Fats are source of energy
E. Inorganic salts regulate body fluids and maintain fluid balance
F. Enzymes act as catalysts to speed chemical reactions
G. Hormones help to regulate growth and activity of body

INTEGUMENTARY SYSTEM

Functions

A. Excretes waste in perspiration
B. Regulates body temperature
C. Relays sensations
D. Protects underlying tissues

Layers of skin

A. Epidermis is thick outer layer
B. Dermis contains blood vessels, nerve endings, hair follicles, and sweat glands
C. Subcutaneous layer attaches dermis to underlying structures

Appendages of skin

A. Glands
   1. Sebaceous—arise from walls of hair follicles and produce oil (sebum) for skin lubrication
   2. Sweat—simple tubular glands, found in most parts of the skin, that aid in control of body temperature
B. Hair
C. Nails

SKELETAL SYSTEM

Bone

A. Bone is type of connective tissue hardened by deposits of calcium and phosphorus salts. There are 206 in body
B. Compact or solid bone is dense and strong; it forms shape of long bones and outside of flat bones
C. Spongy bone is light and porous; it forms ends of long bones and inside of most flat bones

Growth and development of bone

A. Cartilage skeleton is completely formed by 3 months' gestation; ossification and growth occur in remaining months
B. Bone cells absorb calcium from blood; calcium salts give bone its hardness
C. Vitamin D facilitates absorption of calcium and phosphorus necessary for growth
D. Growth of bone occurs at epiphyseal plate

Functions of bone

A. Gives shape to body
B. Provides attachment for muscles
C. Forms cavities that protect delicate organs
D. Manufactures red and white blood cells

Types of bones

A. Long bones consist of shaft, diaphysis, and epiphysis (humerus or femur)
B. Short bones consist of core of spongy bone surrounded by compact bone (carpus or tarsus)
C. Flat bones consist of two plates with spongy bone between (patella or cranial bones)
D. Irregular bones are similar to short bones but are not symmetrical (vertebrae or vomer)

Divisions of skeletal system (Fig. 1)

A. Head or skull
   1. Cranial bones (flat bones)
      a. Parietal—two
      b. Temporal—two
      c. Frontal—one
      d. Occipital—one
      e. Ethmoid—one
      f. Sphenoid—one
   2. Facial bones (irregular bones)
      a. Zygomatic is cheek bone
      b. Vomer separates nostrils
      c. Turbinates are small bones in nose
      d. Palate is roof of mouth
      e. Hyoid is a horseshoe-shaped bone just above Adam's apple, which attaches tongue muscle. It is only bone in body that does not attach to another bone
      f. Nasal is bridge of nose
      g. Maxilla is upper jawbone
      h. Mandible is lower jawbone
B. Trunk
   1. There are 24 ribs in the body
      a. True—seven attached to sternum anteriorly and vertebral column posteriorly
      b. False—five on each side; attached to cartilage of superior rib
      c. Floating—two ribs attached only to vertebral column

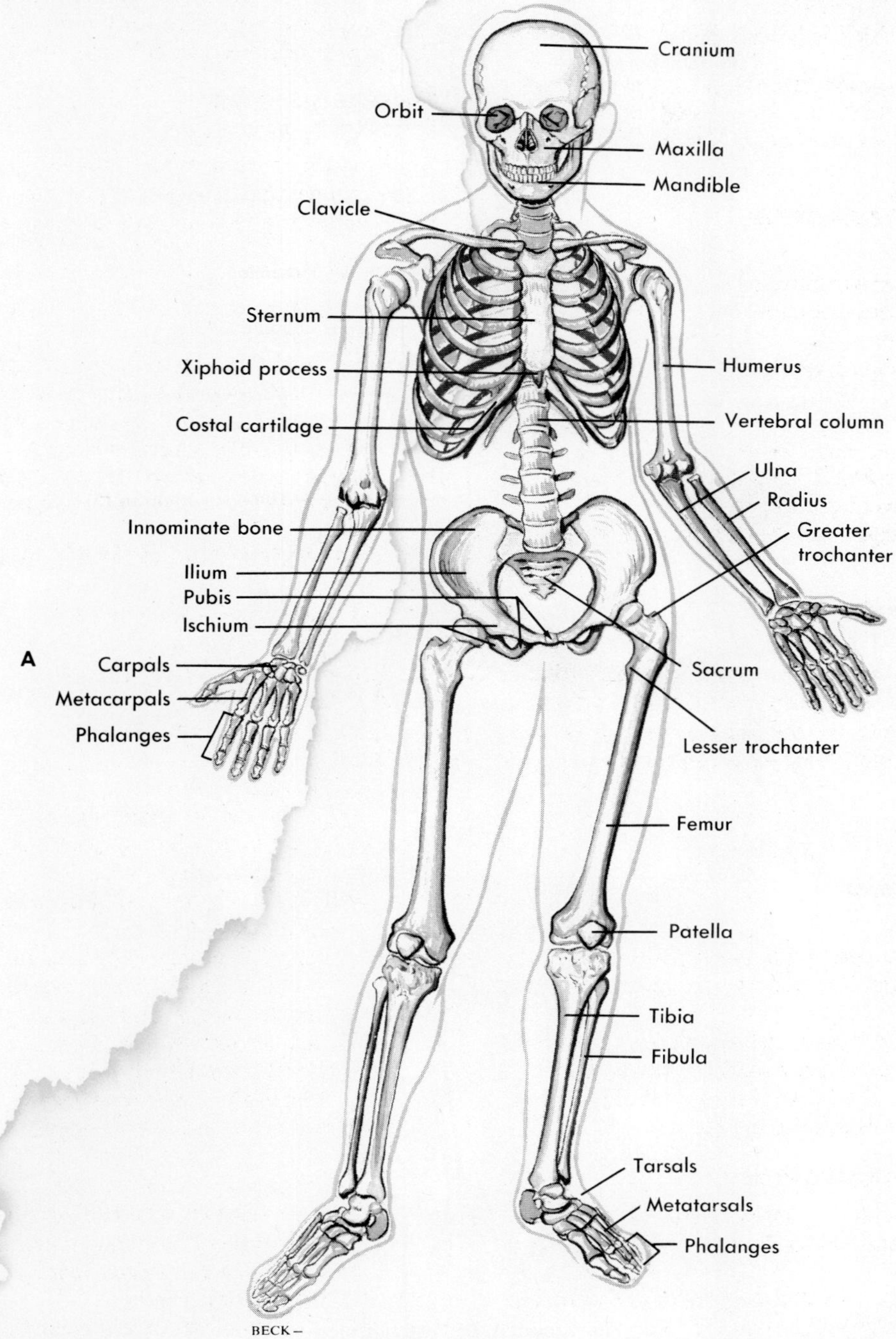

Fig. 1. Skeleton. **A,** Anterior view. (From Anthony, C.P., and Kolthoff, N.J.: Textbook of anatomy and physiology, ed. 9, St. Louis, 1975, The C.V. Mosby Co.) *Continued.*

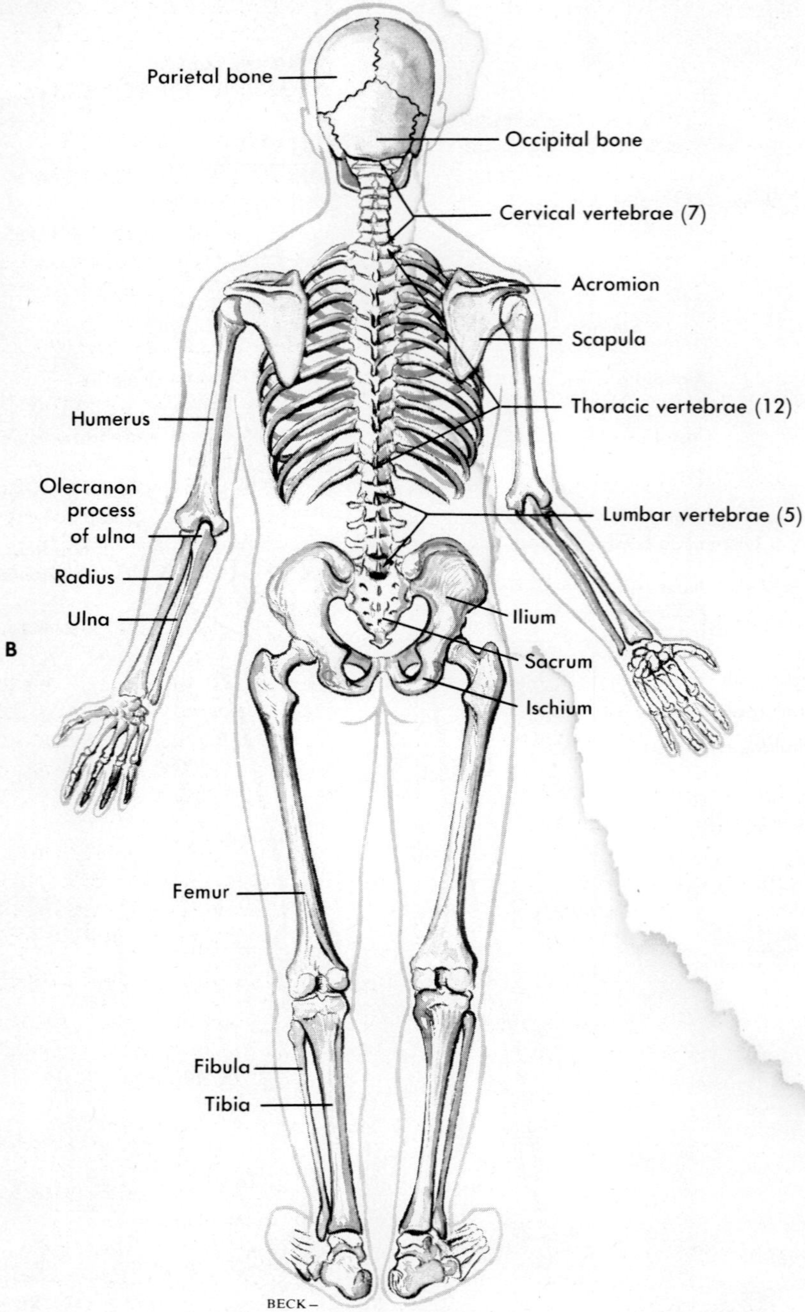

Fig. 1, cont'd. B, Posterior view.

2. The flat bone in the midline of chest is divided into three parts
   a. Manubrium
   b. Sternum
   c. Xiphoid process
3. The vertebral column is composed of 26 bones
   a. Cervical—seven bones form back of neck
   b. Thoracic—12 bones of chest to which ribs are attached
   c. Lumbar—five thick and heavy bones in lower back
   d. Sacral—five fused bones forming the sacrum
   e. Coccygeal—fusion of four tiny bones into the coccyx
   f. Primary curves—present in body at birth
      (1) Thoracic
      (2) Pelvic
   g. Secondary curves—formed later in life
      (1) Cervical forms as child holds up head
      (2) Lumbar forms as child learns to walk

C. Upper extremities
   1. Shoulder girdle
      a. Clavicle, or collarbone
      b. Scapula, or shoulder blade
   2. Arm
      a. Humerus is large bone of upper arm
      b. Ulna is larger of two bones in forearm forming elbow
      c. Radius is shorter and smaller of two bones in forearm. It is located on the thumb side
   3. Hand
      a. Carpals are eight wrist bones
      b. Metacarpals are five bones in palm of hand
      c. Phalanges are 14 finger bones attached to metacarpals

D. Pelvic girdle
   1. Forms protection for pelvic organs and lower digestive system. Composed of six bones
      a. Ilium—two
      b. Ischium—two
      c. Pubis—two
   2. The six bones unite to form two innominate bones

E. Lower extremities
   1. Femur is large bone in upper leg
   2. Tibia is shin bone; it extends from knee to ankle and is larger weight-bearing bone
   3. Fibula is parallel to tibia
   4. Patella is kneecap
   5. Tarsus is composed of seven ankle bones
   6. Metatarsus is composed of five bones forming arch of foot
   7. Phalanges are 14 bones of toes

Attachments of skeleton

A. Ligaments attach bone to bone
B. Cartilage pads bone
C. Tendons attach muscle to bone
D. Joints are the point of union between two bones
   1. Immovable joints—synarthroses (cranial sutures)
   2. Slightly movable joints—amphiarthroses (vertebrae and symphysis pubis)
   3. Freely movable or universal joints—diarthroses (There are different types of universal joints in body)
      a. Ball-and-socket joint (shoulder joint)
      b. Hinge joint (joints of elbow)
      c. Gliding joint (wrist)
      d. Pivot joint (between skull and first two vertebrae)
      e. Condyloid joint (wrist joint at radius and carpal bones)
      f. Saddle joint (joints of thumb)
      g. Types of movement—diarthrotic joints
         (1) Angular movements, such as flexion, extension, abduction, and adduction
         (2) Circumduction
         (3) Rotation
         (4) Special movements, such as supination, pronation, inversion, and eversion
   4. Bursae or sacs (synovial joint) filled with fluid act as cushions; they are located at joints

Male and female skeletal differences

A. Female skeleton lighter and smaller
B. Female pelvis broad and shallow with flaring pubic arch (an aid to childbirth)

Skeletal development

A. Longitudinal growth continues systematically until approximately age 15 years in the female and 16 years in the male
B. Maturation and remodeling continue until age 21 years in both the male and female
C. Bones become more brittle with age

MUSCULAR SYSTEM

Functions of muscle

A. Controls locomotion and movement
B. Keeps body erect and gives it shape
C. Produces heat and energy

Three types of muscle tissue

A. Skeletal or striated—voluntary muscles that function to move bones
B. Visceral or smooth—nonstriated, involuntary muscles that form walls of all organs including blood vessels
C. Cardiac—striated, involuntary muscles of heart

Nervous control of muscle

A. Skeletal muscle is only type supplied with nerves for voluntary movement
B. Visceral and cardiac muscle contract automatically by way of autonomic nervous system

Blood supply of muscle

Consists of capillaries surrounding and lying between muscle fibers

Physiology of muscle tissues

A. Characteristics are
 1. Contractility makes muscle shorter and thicker
 2. Irritability (excitability) causes response to stimuli
 3. Extensibility enables muscle to stretch
 4. Elasticity enables muscle to resume original length
 5. Tonus is state of continuous partial contraction
B. Muscle activity produces heat, energy, and waste products
C. Fatigue is reduced activity as result of accumulated waste products; it is relieved by rest, food, and oxygen

Muscles of head

A. Epicranius located across head
B. Orbicularis oculi located around eye
C. Orbicularis oris located around mouth
D. Masseter located at sides of jaw
E. Buccinator located horizontally at sides of jaw

Muscles of back (Fig. 2)

A. Trapezius located back of shoulder
B. Latissimus dorsi located across back

Muscles of chest

A. Intercostals are located between ribs
B. Pectoralis major and minor are located in anterior chest
C. Diaphragm separates chest cavity from abdominal cavity

Muscles of abdomen

All these muscles have fibers running in four different directions to add support
A. Transversalis abdominis
B. External oblique
C. Internal oblique
D. Rectus abdominis

Muscles of lower extremities

A. Buttocks, or gluteus maximus, medius, and minimus
B. Thigh
 1. Hamstring groups (including biceps femoris) located at back of legs
 2. Rectus femoris located at front of legs
 3. Quadriceps femoris (including rectus femoris and vasti) located at front of legs
C. Lower leg
 1. Gastrocnemius is calf muscle
 2. Tibialis anterior is located at front of lower part of lower extremity
 3. Soleus helps form calf muscle

Muscles of upper extremities

A. Tricpes brachii is located at back of upper arm
B. Biceps brachii is located at front of upper arm
C. Deltoid provides shoulder padding

NERVOUS SYSTEM

Functions

A. Is center of all mental processes
B. Controls communication between different parts of body
C. Integrates activities of body systems
D. Controls consciousness
E. Maintains homeostasis

Physiology

Neuron—basic unit of nervous impulse
A. Neurons conduct electrical impulse from one part of body to another
B. There are three types
 1. Motor—conduct impulses away from brain and spinal cord

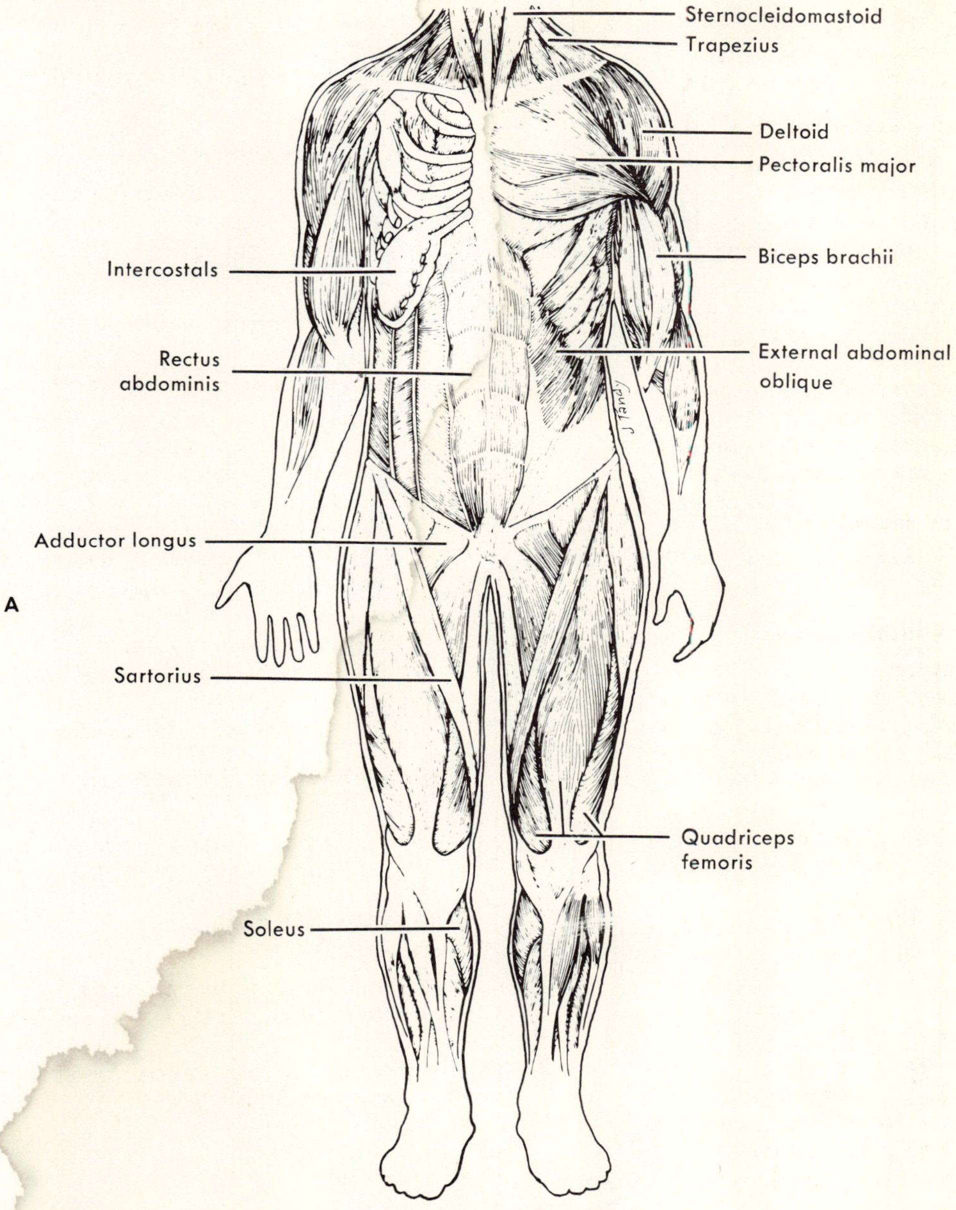

Fig. 2. Muscles of the body. **A,** Anterior view. (From Radcliff, R.K., and Ogden, S.J.: Nursing and medical terminology: a workbook, St. Louis, 1977, The C.V. Mosby Co.) *Continued.*

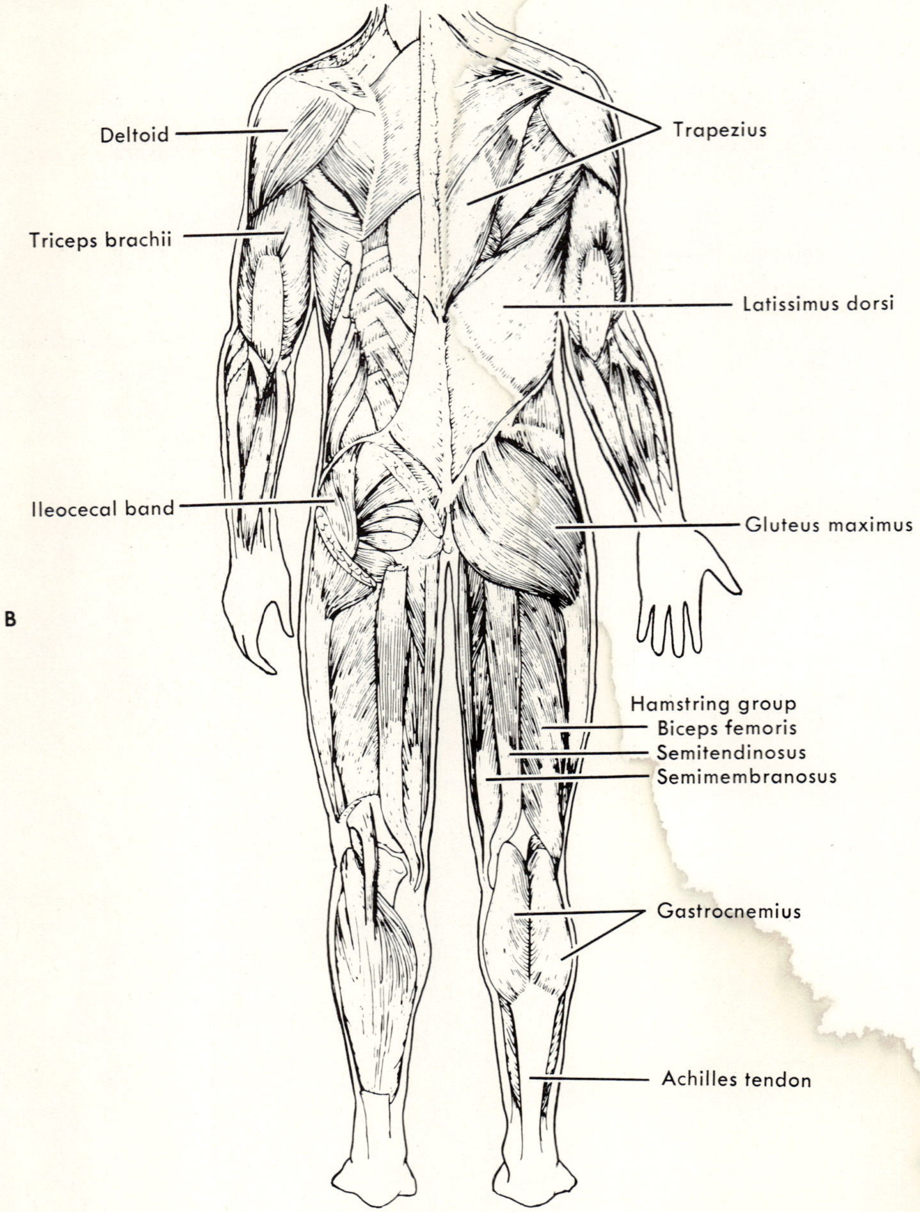

Fig. 2, cont'd. B, Posterior view.

2. Sensory—conduct impulses toward brain and spinal cord
3. Reflex—link motor and sensory

Characteristics of nervous tissue

A. Irritability (excitability) causes response of nerve to stimuli
B. Conductivity is transmission of impulses
C. All-or-none principle means nerve fibers will not transmit impulses below level of sensation

Central nervous system

Brain and spinal cord (Fig. 3)

A. Cerebrum
   1. It consists of two hemispheres and is the brain's largest part
   2. Location is in upper part of cranium
   3. Functions are thinking, memory, emotions, judgment, consciousness, and control over reflexes

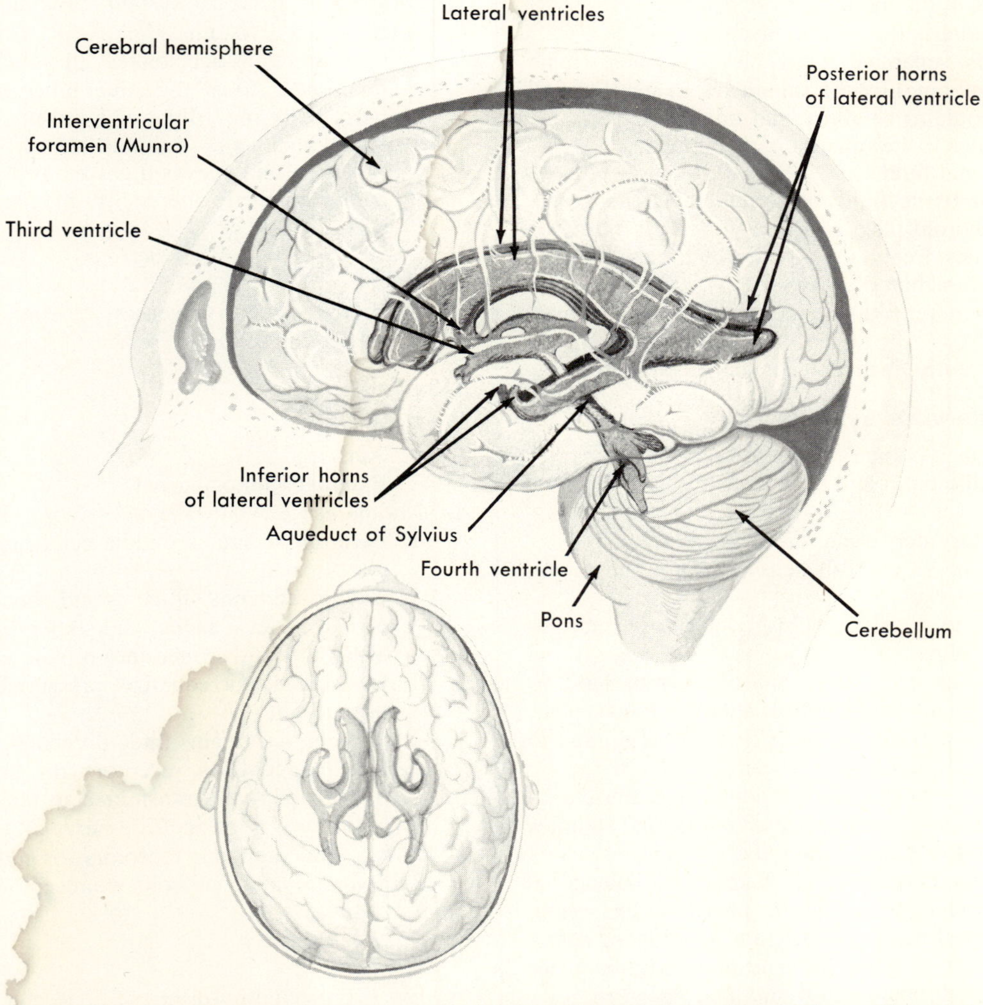

Fig. 3. The cerebral ventricles projected on the lateral surface of the cerebrum. The smaller drawing shows the ventricles from above. (From Anthony, C.P., and Thibodeau, G.A.: Textbook of anatomy and physiology, ed. 10, St. Louis, 1979, The C.V. Mosby Co.)

B. Cerebellum
   1. Location is below and at back of cerebrum
   2. Functions are control of body balance and muscle rhythm
C. Medulla oblongata connects with spinal cord and contains respiratory and cardiac centers
D. Midbrain is seat of third cranial nerve (oculomotor)
E. Spinal cord functions to conduct messages to and from brain
F. Meninges are three membranes that cover the brain and spinal cord
   1. Dura mater is the outermost layer
   2. Arachnoid is the middle layer
      a. It is separated from the pia mater (inner membrane) by the subarachnoid space
      b. It contains cerebrospinal fluid
   3. Pia mater is the innermost membrane
G. Cerebrospinal fluid
   1. Is clear tissue fluid manufactured in the ventricles (choroid plexuses)
   2. Circulates freely within the ventricles of brain and subarachnoid space
   3. Serves to protect and nourish brain and spinal cord
   4. Is frequently examined for diagnostic purposes

Peripheral nervous system

Craniospinal or voluntary—nerves and branches located outside the brain and spinal cord

A. Cranial nerves—12 pairs
   1. Olfactory nerve controls sense of smell
   2. Optic nerve controls sense of sight and movement of eyes
   3. Oculomotor nerve helps control eye muscles and eyelids
   4. Trochlear nerve helps control eye muscles
   5. Trigeminal nerve controls sense of touch, pain, heat, and cold to skin of face and scalp and to mucous membranes of head
   6. Abducent nerve helps to control eye muscle
   7. Facial nerve controls sense of taste and supplies muscles of facial expression
   8. Acoustic nerve controls hearing and balance
   9. Glossopharyngeal nerve provides for reflex control of heart and taste and swallowing reflex
   10. Vagus nerve provides sensation and movement to most structures in thorax and abdomen
   11. Accessory nerve provides movement for palate and neck muscles
   12. Hypoglossal nerve provides movement to inferior surface of tongue
B. Spinal nerves—31 pairs
   1. Cervical—eight
   2. Thoracic—12
   3. Lumbar—five
   4. Sacral—five
   5. Coccygeal—one
   6. Anterior sets—supply anterior body and extremities
   7. Posterior sets—supply muscles of back
C. Autonomic nervous system (involuntary or visceral)—two divisions
   1. Sympathetic—accelerates all involuntary body functions, slows digestive processes, and prepares body for "flight or fight"
   2. Parasympathetic—inhibits all involuntary body functions and speeds digestive processes; largest parasympathetic nerve is the vagus (cranial nerve X)

SPECIAL SENSES

Often referred to as five senses: hearing, sight, smell, taste, and feeling

Hearing

A. External ear
   1. Auricle
   2. External auditory canal
B. Middle ear
   1. Eardrum separates middle ear from external auditory canal
   2. Cavity contains three small bones (ossicles) called malleus, incus, and stapes
   3. Mastoid sinuses open into middle ear
   4. Eustachian tube equalizes pressure on either side of eardrum
C. Internal ear—contains three divisions
   1. Cochlea contains receptors for hearing sensations, which are transmitted to temporal part of brain by way of acoustic nerve
   2. Vestibule contains receptors for equilibrium
   3. Semicircular canal contains receptors for equilibrium

Vision

A. Eye—protected by orbit
B. Layers of eyeball
   1. Sclera—fibrous, white outer layer

2. Cornea—transparent anterior portion of sclera
3. Choroid—middle, vascular layer
4. Ciliary body and iris—anterior structures, continuous with choroid, which aid in the refraction of light rays
5. Retina—inner nervous layer, continuous with optic nerve, which transmits impulses to occipital lobe of brain

C. Chambers of eye
1. Anterior chamber contains aqueous humor
2. Posterior chamber contains vitreous humor

D. Muscles of eye
1. Intrinsic muscles (involuntary) control the ciliary body and iris
2. Extrinsic muscles (voluntary) connect eyeball to orbital cavity and control rotary eye movements

E. Refraction
1. Refraction is bending of light rays to focus on retina
2. Refractory media include cornea, aqueous humor, crystalline lens, and vitreous humor

F. Accessory structures of eye
1. Eyebrows and lashes
2. Eyelids
3. Lacrimal apparatus

Smell

A. Smell is sensed by way of olfactory nerve to temporal lobe
B. Olfactory nerve cells in mucous membrane are sensitive to gases
C. Olfactory nerves tire easily

Taste

A. Taste is sensed by way of seventh and ninth cranial nerves to parietal lobes
B. Nerves of taste are in tastebuds on tongue, epiglottis, pharynx, and roof of mouth
1. Foods in solution are tasted
2. Taste is sweet, sour, bitter, or salty; other tastes are blends

Cutaneous sense

By way of spinal nerves to spinal cord

A. Skin and mucous membrane sensations
1. Nerves from spinal column
2. Sensations of heat, cold, pain, touch, and pressure

B. Tendon and joint sensations
C. Muscle, or kinesthetic, sense

CIRCULATORY SYSTEM

Consists of heart, arteries, capillaries, veins, and lymphatics

Functions

A. Transports substances, such as oxygen, carbon dioxide, hormones, salts, and antibodies, from one part of body to another
B. Protects from invading organism
C. Assists in heat regulation
D. Assists in fluid balance
E. Maintains homeostasis in internal cellular environment

Heart (Fig. 4)

A. Is hollow, muscular organ about size of fist
B. Is located slightly to left in thorax between lungs in mediastinum
C. Is composed of
1. Pericardium—outer covering in two portions—one outer fibrous (fibrosum) and the other inner serous (serosum)
2. Myocardium—heart muscle or middle layer
3. Endocardium—membranous sac lining heart; also continuous with valves

D. Has four chambers
1. Atria—two upper (left and right)
2. Ventricles—two lower (left and right)

E. Has four valves—close to prevent back flow of blood
1. Bicuspid valve located between left atrium and left ventricle
2. Tricuspid valve located between right atrium and right ventricle
3. Pulmonary semilunar valve located between right ventricle and pulmonary artery
4. Aortic semilunar valve located between left ventricle and aorta

F. Has cardiac cycle
1. Contraction (systole) heard through stethoscope as ''lubb'' sound
2. Relaxation (diastole) caused by closing of valves between heart and aorta; heard through stethoscope as ''dup'' sound
3. Period of rest

G. Has conduction system
1. Network of nervous tissue located in myocardium, which has the ability to initiate and conduct an electrical impulse resulting in cardiac cycle

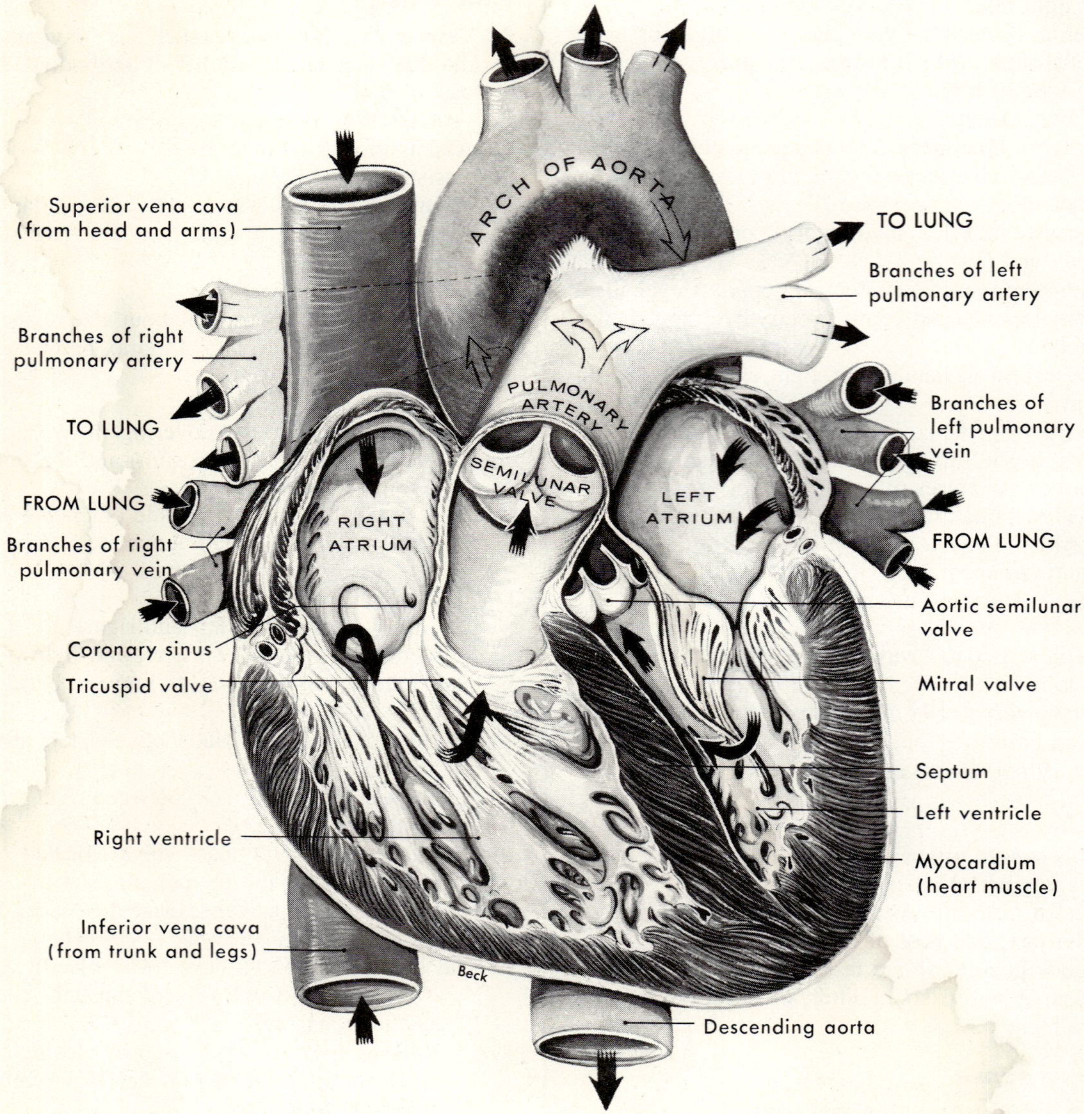

Fig. 4. Cross-section of the front section of the heart showing the four chambers, the valves, the openings, and the major vessels. Arrows indicate the direction of blood flow. The two branches of the right pulmonary vein extend from the right lung behind the heart to enter the left atrium. (From Anthony, C.P., and Kolthoff, N.J.: Textbook of anatomy and physiology, ed. 9, St. Louis, 1975, The C.V. Mosby Co.)

2. Composed of
   a. SA node (primary pacemaker)—junction of right atrium and superior vena cava
   b. Atrioventricular node (secondary pacemaker)—junction of right atrium and right ventricle
   c. Bundle of His—septum of right and left ventricle
   d. Bundle branches—either side of right and left ventricle
   e. Purkinje fibers—ventricular muscular wall

H. Has heart rate—controlled by autonomic nervous sytem; may be affected by
   1. Chemicals, carbon dioxide in blood, epinephrine and drugs
   2. Changes in hormones
   3. Physical activity
   4. Emotional excitement
   5. Extremes of hot or cold

Arteries (Fig. 5)

A. Arteries are firm, elastic, muscular tubes
B. They carry blood from heart
C. They carry oxygenated blood, except for pulmonary artery, which carries blood from heart to lungs, and umbilical artery in fetal circulation
D. Aorta arises from left ventricle; it is largest artery in body
E. Pulse is regular alternate contractions and expansions of artery at same time as heartbeat
   1. Caused by periodic thrusts felt over artery
   2. Usually counted at radial artery in wrist; may also be counted at carotid artery or other areas where artery is near surface
F. Blood pressure is pressure exerted on walls of arteries by blood
   1. Systole or systolic blood pressure
   2. Diastole or diastolic blood pressure
G. Pulse pressure is the difference between systole and diastole

Capillaries

A. Are smallest of blood vessels—microscopic
B. Link arteries and veins
C. Carry oxygen and nutrients to tissues
D. Collect wastes from tissues and transport to veins

Veins

A. Carry blood from capillaries to heart
B. Have thinner, less elastic walls than arteries
C. Have valves on inner surfaces to assist return of blood

Circulation

Consists of pulmonary, systemic, and portal circulation

A. Pulmonary circulation takes venous blood from right side of heart through lungs and back to left side of heart
B. Systemic circulation takes arterial blood through left side of heart through body and back to right side of heart
C. Portal circulation takes blood from veins of stomach, small intestine, spleen, pancreas, gallbladder, colon, and rectum to liver, inferior vena cava, and right atrium of heart

Blood

A. Plasma, or liquid part—about 92% water and 8% protein
B. Solid materials or cells
   1. Red blood cells (erythrocytes), numbering from 4.5 to 5 million per milliliter of blood, carry hemoglobin, give blood its red color, and are manufactured by red bone marrow
   2. Platelets (thrombocytes), numbering 250,000 to 350,000 per milliliter of blood, aid in clotting
   3. White blood cells (granulocytes and agranulocytes), numbering 5000 to 10,000 per milliliter of blood, are colorless and help in fighting infection and building tissue
C. Amount in body—8 to 12 pints
D. Functions
   1. Carries oxygen, nutrients, mineral salts, and hormones to tissues for nourishment, repair, and growth
   2. Removes waste materials from tissues
E. Blood clotting
   1. Clotting elements in blood are fibrinogen to fibrin and prothrombin to thrombin
   2. Clotting is nature's way of preventing hemorrhage
   3. Bleeding time (when an incision stops bleeding) is 1 to 3 minutes
   4. Coagulation time is length of time blood takes to clot—3 to 5 minutes in small tube and 5 to 15 minutes in large tube
   5. Vitamin K is necessary for prothrombin formation in liver

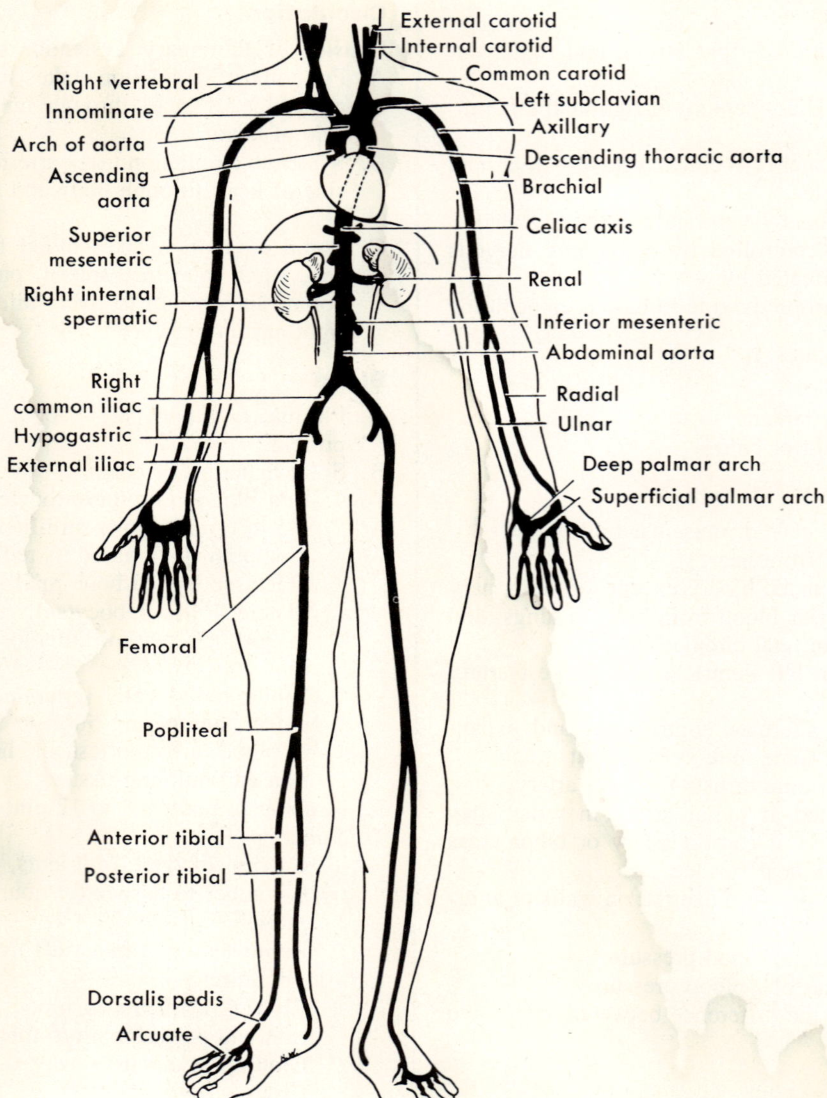

Fig. 5. Main arteries of the body. (Adapted from Anthony, C.P., and Thibodeau, G.A.: Textbook of anatomy and physiology, ed. 10, St. Louis, 1979, The C.V. Mosby Co.)

6. Blood types are A, B, AB, and O; Rh+ and Rh−
   a. Universal donor is O−
   b. Universal recipient is AB+

Lymphatic system

A. System includes lymphatic capillaries, vessels, and lymph nodes or glands
B. Lymph is transparent fluid found in lymph vessels and tissue spaces
C. All lymph empties into the venous circulation
D. Functions of system are to
   1. Return vital substances, chiefly proteins, to the blood
   2. Provide drainage channels for transportation of toxic or malignant substances
   3. Assume an important role in the absorption of digested fats
E. Lymphatic vessels
   1. Start in tissue spaces
   2. Are similar to veins in structure
   3. Are distributed throughout body
   4. Come together into right lymphatic duct draining right upper portion of body, including head and neck; and thoracic duct draining lower portion of body and left upper part, including head and neck
   5. Drain into veins leading to heart
F. Lymph nodes or glands
   1. Lymph carried to nodes or glands by lymphatic vessels
   2. Injurious substances filtered out
   3. Lymphocytes are manufactured
   4. Important lymph nodes are
      a. Submaxillary—in floor of mouth
      b. Cervical—in neck
      c. Cubital—in elbow
      d. Axillary—in armpit
      e. Inguinal—in groin
G. Organs related to lymphatic system
   1. Spleen
      a. Is located in upper left abdominal cavity
      b. Is similar to lymph node in structure
      c. Releases stored blood when circulating blood is needed
      d. Destroys worn-out red blood cells (erythrocytes)
      e. Manufactures lymphocytes
      f. Carries on phagocytic process in which certain cells destroy or remove bacteria and other injurious substances (body's defense against infection)
   2. Tonsils
      a. Three sets form ring of lymphatic tissue
      b. Tonsils guard the entrance of the alimentary and respiratory tracts from bacterial invasion
   3. Thymus
      a. Located in the mediastinal cavity anterior to and above heart
      b. Relatively large in infancy; increases in size until puberty and then begins to atrophy
      c. Believed to be involved in development of body's immunologic system

RESPIRATORY SYSTEM

Function

Exchange of gases between blood and air
A. Inspiration—inhaling air that contains oxygen
B. Expiration—exhaling carbon dioxide

Organs of respiration

Nose, pharynx, larynx, trachea, bronchi, and lungs
A. Nose
   1. Consists of external and internal portion
   2. Is divided into right and left and external and internal nares
   3. Is lined with ciliated mucosa
   4. Is drained into by frontal, maxillary, sphenoid, and ethmoid sinuses
   5. Functions
      a. Filters warms, and moistens air
      b. Contains organs of smell
B. Pharynx
   1. Is muscular tube with mucous lining
   2. Is divided into three parts—behind nose (nasopharynx), mouth (oropharynx), and larynx (laryngopharynx)
   3. Connects nasal passages with trachea and esophagus
   4. Maintains communication with middle ear through eustachian tube
   5. Contains tonsils and adenoids
   6. Serves as passageway for air and food and aids in speaking
C. Larynx (voice box)
   1. Larynx is located at base of tongue at upper end of trachea

2. Larynx is composed of nine pieces of cartilage, largest being thyroid cartilage (Adam's apple)
3. Epiglottis covers the entrance to the larynx and prevents food from getting into the airway during swallowing
4. Vocal cords are formed by bands stretched across larynx, which produce voice as air causes cords to vibrate

D. Trachea
1. Is composed of cartilage in C-shaped rings
2. Is lined with ciliated mucosa
3. Extends from larynx to bronchi
4. Serves as air passageway to and from lungs

E. Bronchi
1. Trachea divides into two tubes to form right and left bronchus
2. Each bronchus divides and subdivides many times when it enters lung
3. Bronchi serve as passageways for air to lungs
4. Bronchi aid in exchange of gases between blood and air

F. Lungs
1. Lungs are cone-shaped organs filling pleural cavity with their bases resting on diaphragm
2. Right lung is divided into three lobes
3. Left lung is divided into two lobes
4. Lungs are covered with moist membrane called pleura
5. Lungs are composed of light spongy, porous material, blood vessles, and nerves
6. Lung airways are the two bronchi and numerous bronchioles
7. Alveoli (air sacs) are functional units of the lungs; gas exchange between blood and air occurs only in alveoli

G. Respiration, or breathing
1. External respiration is exchange of oxygen and carbon dioxide between lungs and circulatory system
2. Internal respiration is exchange of oxygen and carbon dioxide between blood and tissue cells
3. Respiration is controlled by respiratory center in medulla
4. Respiration is affected by certain drugs and by change in carbon dioxide content in blood
5. Muscles of respiration are
   a. Diaphragm—dome-shaped muscular partition separating thoracic and abdominal cavity
   b. Intercostal—muscles between ribs that elevate the rib cage during inspiration

DIGESTIVE SYSTEM

Functions

A. Prepares food for absorption and metabolism by mechanical and chemical changes
B. Eliminates waste products

Digestion

A. Mechanical digestion consists of all processes by which food is broken into smaller particles and moved along in alimentary tract
1. Chewing (mastication)
2. Swallowing (deglutition)
3. Peristalsis
4. Defecation

B. Chemical digestion consists of all processes by which food is changed in composition and prepared for absorption
1. Saliva containing ptyalin in mouth moistens food and changes simple starches to sugars
2. Gastric juices (pepsinogen, hydrochloric acid, and mucus) in stomach act on proteins, preparing them for digestion; they curdle milk and emulsify fats
3. Intestinal juices (maltase, lactase, sucrase, and others) in small intestines complete digestive process of proteins and sugars and aid in absorption
4. Pancreatic juice (amylase, trypsin, lipase, and others) helps in digestion of proteins, carbohydrates, and fats; endocrine secretion if islands of Langerhans in pancreas is called insulin and is essential in control of carbohydrate metabolism
5. Bile manufactured in liver and stored in gallbladder empties into small intestine to emulsify fats

C. Time required for digestive process varies
1. With amount and type of foods eaten
2. With conditions, both chemical and mechanical, in digestive system
3. Normally from 3 to 5 hours in stomach, 3 to 6 hours in small intestine, and 24 to 30 hours in large intestine for a total of 30 to 40 hours after eating

Organs of digestion

A. Four coats of layers
1. Mucous lining secretes digestive juices
2. Submucous lining holds other layers together
3. Muscular coat moves food by peristaltic waves

4. Fibroserous coat is strong, moist membrane that is part of peritoneum

B. Mouth—consists of cheeks, hard palate, soft palate, tongue, teeth, and salivary glands

C. Pharynx—transports food to esophagus

D. Esophagus
1. Is located posteriorly to trachea and heart
2. Connects pharynx to stomach, transporting food to stomach

E. Stomach
1. Is elongated, bean-shaped pouch located in abdominal cavity
2. Varies in size depending on contents
3. Has two openings
   a. Esophagus into stomach protected by cardiac sphincter
   b. Pylorus (lower part) into intestine protected by pyloric sphincter
4. Contains glands that secrete mucus, hydrochloric acid, and enzymes that act on proteins

F. Small intestine
1. Is approximately 20 feet long and 1 inch in diameter
2. Is divided into duodenum (8 to 10 inches long), jejunum (8 feet long), and ileum (12 feet long)
3. Secretes intestinal juice and receives pancreatic juice and bile to complete digestion
4. Controls absorption of digested material
5. Controls peristaltic movement so that digested material is not passed along too rapidly and can be absorbed

G. Large intestine
1. Large intestine is approximately 5 or 6 feet in length and about $2^1/_2$ inches in diameter
2. Large intestine is divided into cecum and colon (ascending, transverse, descending, and sigmoid)
3. Rectum consists of last 5 inches of large intestine
4. Anus
   a. Is last $1^1/_2$ inch of rectum
   b. Is controlled by two round muscles—internal and external sphincters
   c. Controls defecation

H. Liver
1. Is largest organ in body
2. Is situated in right side of epigastrium under diaphragm
3. Manufactures bile stored in gallbaldder
4. Changes glucose to glycogen; stores and releases it when necessary
5. Stores iron and vitamins A, D, E, K, and B_{12}
6. Manufactures fibrinogen and prothrombin necessary for blood clotting
7. Helps in formation of red blood cells and production of plasma proteins

I. Pancreas
1. Is posterior to stomach
2. Secretes pancreatic juice necessary for digestion
3. Secretes insulin, hormone necessary in body utilization of glucose, from islands of Langerhans

J. Gallbladder
1. Is attached to interior surface of liver
2. Is hollow, pear-shaped sac
3. Stores bile
4. Concentrates bile
5. Discharges bile into small intestine by way of cystic and common ducts during digestive process

K. Appendix
1. Blind-end tube off cecum 3 to 6 inches long
2. Located in lower right abdominal quadrant
3. Same structure as intestines
4. No apparent function

URINARY SYSTEM (Fig. 6)

Functions

A. Manufactures urine from waste products of cell metabolism

B. Eliminates urine from body (voiding, urination)

Excretory organs

A. Kidneys—two
1. Kidneys are bean shaped, about $4^1/_2$ inches by 2 inches by 1 inch, and are located against posterior abdominal wall behind peritoneum
2. External structure consists of hilusand capsule
3. Internal structure consists of
   a. Cortex—outer rim of kidney
   b. Glomeruli—clusters of capillaries through which blood flows to kidneys
   c. Pelvis—sac in center to which ureters attach
4. Excess water, liquid wastes, and salt are filtered out of blood and passed on as waste (urine)

B. Ureters—two
1. Lie behind peritoneum and extend from kidneys to bladder
2. Convey urine from kidney to bladder by way of peristaltic action

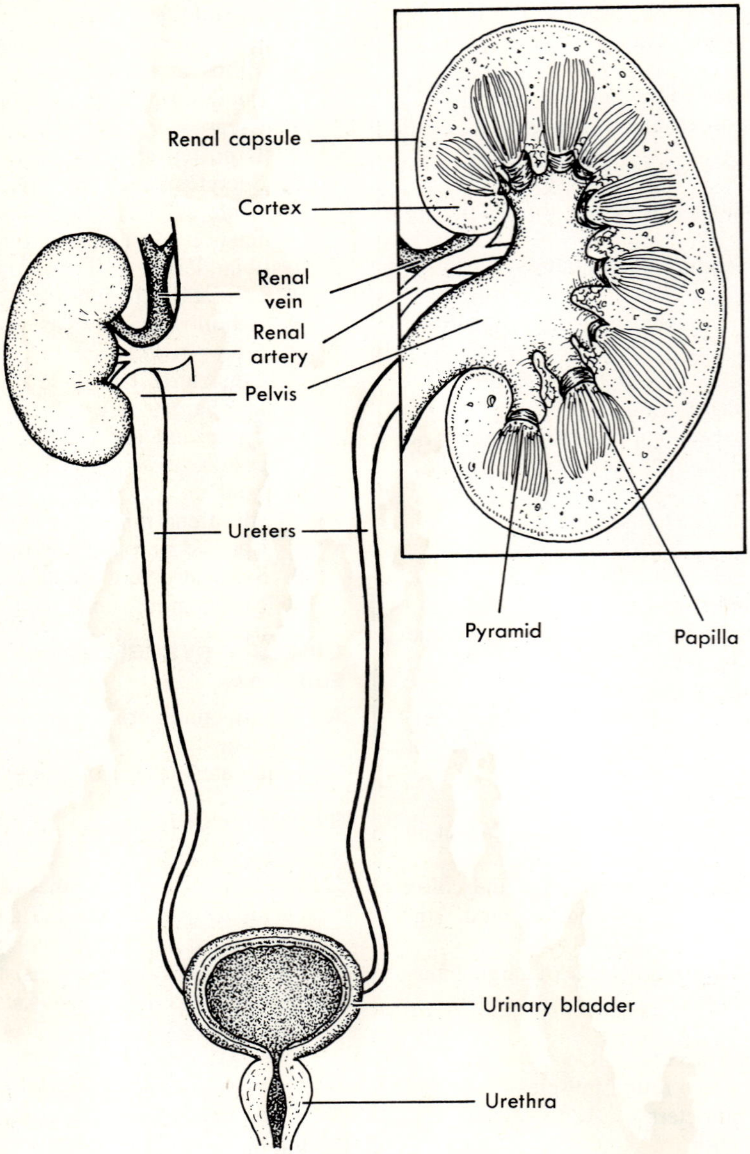

Fig. 6. Urinary system. (Illustration by Dan W. Massey.)

C. Urinary bladder
   1. Is located behind symphysis pubis below parietal peritoneum
   2. Is expandable sac
   3. Serves as reservoir for urine and helps to expel urine to exterior
D. Urethra
   1. Located behind symphysis pubis and in front of vagina in female; extends through prostate in male
   2. Passageway to exterior; excretes urine in female and urine and semen in male

Urine

A. Physical characteristics are amber color, clear, characteristic odor, and specific gravity of 1.010 to 1.025
B. Chemical composition is 95% water and 5% solids; uric acid, creatinine, ammonia, and urea make up about one half of the solid material; urine also contains sodium chloride, sulfates, phosphates of sodium, potassium, magnesium, and calcium
C. Average amount eliminated in 24 hours is 1500 ml

REPRODUCTIVE SYSTEM

Functions

A. Reproduction
B. Production of hormones
   1. Testosterone in male
   2. Estrogen and progesterone in female

Male reproductive system

A. Organs
   1. Testes are paired gonads located in the scrotum
   2. Ducts are epididymis, seminal or vas deferens, and ejaculatory
   3. Accessory glands are paired seminal vesicles, one prostate, and paired bulbourethral glands
   4. Supporting structures are paired spermatic cords (internal), scrotum, and penis (external)
   5. Perineum is area between anus and scrotum
B. Functions
   1. To manufacture and mature spermatozoa
   2. To secrete semen
   3. To manufacture male hormone (testosterone)
   4. To deposit spermatozoa in female reproductive system
   5. To serve as a passageway for urine and semen containing sperm by way of the urethra located in the penis

Female reproductive system

A. Ovaries
   1. Are female gonads located behind and below uterine tubes and anchored to uterus and broad ligaments
   2. Have the shape of large almonds
   3. Manufacture and mature ova within the ovary (ovarian follicle) and expel them into pelvis to be picked up by the uterine tubes
   4. Are the site where, following ovulation, a small yellow body (corpus luteum) develops within the ruptured ovarian follicle to secrete progesterone and some estrogen. In the absence of pregnancy the corpus luteum will degenerate
   5. Manufacture estrogen and progesterone, which, along with pituitary hormones, regulate menstruation, appearance of secondary sex characteristics, and preparation of uterus for pregnancy
B. Uterine tubes (fallopian tubes)
   1. Are attached to upper outer angles of uterus
   2. Have three coats and fimbriated ends opened at outer edges
   3. Pick up and conduct ova to uterus
   4. Are site of fertilization, which normally occurs when the ovum is approximately one third of the way down the tube
C. Uterus
   1. Is pear shaped, about 3 inches by 2 inches by 1 inch in virginal state
   2. Consists of body and cervix
   3. Is located in pelvic cavity between bladder and rectum
   4. Is supported and held in place by two broad ligaments, two uterosacral ligaments, one posterior ligament, one anterior ligament, and two round ligaments
   5. Is composed of
      a. Myometrium (smooth muscle)
      b. Endometrium (lining)
      c. Parietal peritoneum (covering of upper surface)
   6. Has generous supply of blood vessels
   7. Functions in menstruation, pregnancy, and labor
D. Vagina
   1. Is located between rectum and urethra
   2. Is collapsible tube, capable of distention
   3. Receives semen from male, constitutes lower part of birth canal, and serves as discharge passage for menstrual flow

E. Vulva—consists of structures composing external genitals
   1. Mons veneris—pad of hair, skin-covered fat over symphysis
   2. Labia minora—small inner folds covered with modified skin
   3. Labia majora—hairy skin-covered out folds
   4. Clitoris—small mound of erectile tissue at junction of two labia minora
   5. Urinary meatus—orifice located just below clitoris, opening into urethra
   6. Vaginal orifice—opening located below urinary meatus, partially covered by folds of mucous membrane called hymen
   7. Bartholin's glands—glands located one on each side of vaginal opening at base of labia minora
F. Perineum
   1. Is region between vaginal orifice and anus
   2. Contains perineal body (mass of fibromuscular tissue important in childbirth)
G. Breasts (mammary glands)
   1. Breasts are located anterior to pectoral muscles, just under the skin
   2. Each breast has 15 to 20 lobes arranged radially and embedded in fat and connective tissue
   3. Each lobe empties into a duct, which discharges through a separate orifice on the surface of the nipple
   4. Size depends on disposition of adipose (fatty) tissue influenced by heredity, nutrition, and hormone level
   5. Main function is lactation

Menstruation

A. Menstruation is sloughing of endometrium to rid the uterus of lining built up for expected pregnancy
B. Menstruation is controlled by interaction of ovarian and pituitary hormones
C. Menarche is the first menstrual period; it occurs at approximately 13 years of age
D. Menopause, or climacteric, is cessation of menstrual periods; it occurs at approximately 45 years of age
E. Menstrual cycle occurs every $3^1/_2$ to 5 weeks
   1. Menstrual phase lasts from 1 to 5 days; endometerial lining is destroyed and sloughed when fertilization has not occurred
   2. Proliferative phase is approximately from fifth day to fourteenth day; endometrium thickens as estrogen level increases
   3. Ovulation occurs during middle of cycle (approximately fourteenth day) and is initiated by drop in estrogen level before rise in progesterone level; female is considered fertile at this time
   4. Secretory phase is approximately from fifteenth day to the onset of menses; endometrium differentiates into tissue appropriate for implantation

ENDOCRINE SYSTEM (DUCTLESS GLANDS)

Definition

Glands whose secretions are discharged into bloodstream or lymph; secretions are called hormones

General functions

A. Integrating mechanisms of body to ensure
   1. Normal growth and development
   2. Reproduction
   3. Metabolism
   4. Nervous and mental activity
   5. Cardiovascular activity
   6. Digestion

Pituitary

A. Located in sella turcica of sphenoid bone and attached to undersurface of cerebrum
B. Often referred to as "master gland" because it influences other glands
C. Divided into two divisions
   1. Anterior lobe (adenohypophysis) secretes somatotropin (STH), which regulates growth; adrenocorticotropin (ACTH), which regulates adrenal cortex; thyrotropin (TSH), which regulates thyroid gland; follicle-stimulating hormone (FSH), which stimulates estrogen production and graafian follicle in female and sperm production in male; luteinizing hormone (LH), which controls testosterone production in male and progesterone production in female; and melanocyte-stimulating hormone (MSH), which together with ACTH produces increased pigmentation of the skin
   2. Posterior lobe (neurohypophysis) stores two hormones, antidiuretic hormone (ADH), which enhances reabsorption of water in kidneys, and oxytocin, which stimulates uterus to contract during childbirth and stimulates breasts to release milk

Thyroid

A. Is located just below larynx, at sides of trachea
B. Secretes hormone called thyroxine
C. Influences metabolism and rate at which food is burned in tissues

Parathyroids

A. Are attached to posterior surface of lateral lobes of thyroid
B. Secrete hormone called parathormone, which regulates calcium-phosphorus metabolism

Gonads

A. Male testes
   1. Secrete testosterone
   2. Influence development of secondary sex characteristics
B. Female ovaries
   1. Secrete estrogen, which controls menstrual cycle
   2. Secrete progesterone, which controls changes in uterus preparing for pregnancy

Adrenals

A. Adrenals are superior to each kidney
B. Central part (medulla) secretes epinephrine (adrenalin), which maintains blood pressure, heart rate, and muscle tone
C. Cortex (outer part) secretes
   1. Glucocorticoids, which influence protein, carbohydrate, and fat metabolism
   2. Mineralocorticoids, which influence water and electrolyte metabolism
   3. Androgens, which influence sexual development

Islands of Langerhans

A. Are located in pancreas
B. Consist of three types of cells
   1. Alpha cells produce glucagon, which stimulates liver to release glucose into the blood
   2. Beta cells produce insulin, which regulates the cellular uptake of glucose and the blood sugar level
   3. Delta cells' function is unknown

Pineal body

A. Pineal body is present in central part of brain
B. Although function is not clearly understood, current research reveals the gland may regulate sexuality in mammals and the timing of menstrual cycle in human beings

FLUID AND ELECTROLYTES

Introduction

A. Body cells are bathed in tissue fluid kept constant in composition
B. Major ingredients in tissue fluid are water and certain electrolytes
C. Fluids and electrolytes are compartmentalized
   1. Extracellular—outside cell membrane
   2. Intracellular—within cell membrane

Water

A. Water is largest single constituent of human body
B. Total body weight is 45% to 70% water
C. Water replacement occurs through ingestion of liquids and through metabolism
D. Water leaves body through kidneys, lungs, skin, and gastrointestinal (GI) tract
E. Weight change of 2.2 pounds equals fluid loss or gain of 1000 ml
F. The kidneys, influenced by ADH (antidiuretic hormone), withhold or excrete water according to body needs

Electrolytes

A. Electrolytes are chemical compounds that break up into their ions in water
B. Concentration of electrolytes in the intracellular and extracellular spaces is maintained within very narrow range
C. Compartmental shifts in electrolytes are of great significance in the treatment of disease
D. Common electrolytes are sodium and potassium
   1. Sodium (Na^+) is found primarily in extracellular space; it promotes fluid and acid-base balance in the body
   2. Potassium (K^+) is principal element in intracellular space; it is essential for synthesis of protein, enzyme functioning within the cell, and maintenance of fluid balance
E. Other electrolytes that are found in the body are calcium, magnesium, chloride, phosphates, and bicarbonates

ACID-BASE BALANCE

Introduction

A. Body is kept at a pH of 7.35 to 7.45 (slightly alkaline)
B. Acidosis is a condition in which body's pH is 7 to 7.2
C. Alkalosis is a condition in which body's pH is above 7.5

Regulation

A. Lungs assist in regulation through the elimination of carbonic acid in the form of carbon dioxide
B. Minerals function in buffer salts and react with and neutralize strong acids or bases
C. Excessively acidic or basic substances are eliminated by way of kidneys
D. Diseases of the regulating mechanisms (lungs and kidneys) may result in acidosis or alkalosis

Principles of nutrition

DEFINITION

Combination of processes by which the living organism receives and utilizes food for the maintenance of its functions and for the growth and regeneration of its parts

EVIDENCE OF GOOD NUTRITION

A. Body is well developed for age; weight is in proportion to height
B. Appetite, digestion, and elimination are within normal limits
C. Muscles are developed and firm; skin is smooth, clear, and moist
D. Facial expression is alert but relaxed; eyes are clear with no dark circles around them
E. Hair is smooth and glossy
F. Posture is good
G. Sleep is regular and uninterrupted
H. Energy is abundant

NUTRIENTS

Carbohydrates

A. Function is to provide energy
B. Sources are cereals, starches, sugars, fruits, and vegetables
C. Digestion of carbohydrates is simple process that starts in mouth; changes starch to dextrin to simple sugars
D. Metabolism of carbohydrates yields waste products, carbon dioxide, and water
E. Simple sugars like glucose, fructose, and galactose are ready for absorption in the digestive tract
F. Double sugar (sucrose) must be changed to simple sugar for absorption
G. Complex sugar (starches) requires two steps in digestion (to simple sugars) for absorption in the intestinal tract
H. Cellulose is indigestible carbohydrate found in plants
I. Storage occurs when more is eaten than is needed for energy
   1. Small portion is stored as glycogen in liver and muscle tissue
   2. Greater portion is stored as adipose tissue (fat)
J. One gram carbohydrate yields 4 calories

Proteins

A. Functions are to
   1. Supply energy and heat to body
   2. Build and repair; proteins are necessary for growth of new tissue
   3. Aid in maintaining water balance
   4. Provide immunity
B. Sources are
   1. Complete—contain all essential amino acids (milk, meat, fish, poultry, eggs, and soybeans—only member of vegetable kingdom to provide complete protein)
   2. Incomplete (gelatin, cereals, legumes, lentils, and nuts)
C. Digestion starts in stomach; end products are amino acids
D. Metabolism yields waste products, such as hydrogen, oxygen, nitrogen, water, uric acid, and urea; last two are normally eliminated through kidneys
E. Amino acids cannot be stored for later use in building and repairing tissue; therefore, it is important that complete proteins be eaten daily
F. One gram protein yields 4 calories

Fats

A. Functions are to provide
   1. Energy
   2. Lubrication of GI tract
   3. Insulation for body heat (subcutaneous fat)
   4. Carrying mechanism for fat-soluble vitamins A, D, E, and K
B. Sources are
   1. Animal (cream, butter, whole milk, whole milk cheeses, egg yolk, meat, fish, and poultry)
   2. Vegetable (avocado, chocolate, corn oil, cottonseed oil, coconut, nuts, and olives)

C. Digestion takes place in small intestine
   1. Fats that become liquid at room temperature are more easily digested
   2. Digestion is slow
   3. Bile salts and pancreatic juice are necessary
   4. Fats are digested to fatty acids and glycerol for use by body
D. Metabolism results in waste products such as fatty acids, carbon dioxide, and water
E. Excess fats in diet are stored as adipose tissue
F. Chemical composition of fat substances is
   1. Saturated fat—this fat contains all hydrogen possible in its molecule and is solid at room temperature
   2. Unsaturated fats—this fat can take on more hydrogen under certain conditions and is soft or liquid at room temperature
   3. Cholesterol—fatty acid that is essential in blood is sometimes found in deposits inside blood vessels; source is animal
   4. False fats—hydrocarbons of no nutritional value, such as mineral oil; frequent intake inhibits absorption of fat-soluble vitamins
   5. Margarine—a saturated fat resulting from hydrogenation
G. One gram fat yields 9 calories

Minerals

A. Functions
   1. Compose necessary part of all cells and body fluids
   2. Compose the structural framework of the body
   3. Regulate vital processes, such as acid-base balance
B. Best known minerals, functions, and sources
   1. Calcium (Ca) and phosphorus (P)
      a. Calcium and phosphorus function to develop and maintain bones and teeth, clotting of blood, normal heart action, iron utilization, and healthy nerves and muscles
      b. Calcium and phosphorus must have acid environment (GI tract) and vitamin D for proper absorption
      c. Deficiency symptoms are rickets, poor tooth formation, slow clotting of blood, porous bones, and retarded growth
      d. Best sources are milk, cheese, yogurt, green vegetables, fish, egg yolks, nuts, and whole grain cereal
   2. Iron (Fe)
      a. Iron functions as essential element in formation of hemoglobin in red blood cells (hemoglobin carries oxygen to tissue)
      b. Deficiency results in nutritional anemia with symptoms of pallor, weakness, dizziness, weight loss, and gastric disturbance
      c. Best sources are red meat (especially liver) eggs, legumes, and green vegetables
   3. Iodine (I)
      a. Function is to aid in the synthesis of the thyroid hormone
      b. Deficiency symptom is simple goiter
      c. Best sources are kelp, seafood, and iodized salt
   4. Sodium chloride (NaCl)
      a. Function is regulation of water balance of muscles, nerves, and other tissues
      b. Deficiency symptom is dehydration
      c. Best sources are salt, carrots, spinach, and asparagus

Vitamins

A. Functions
   1. Promote normal growth and development
   2. Protect body from infection
   3. Prevent deficiency diseases
B. Fat-soluble vitamins
   1. Are absorbed along with dietary fats
   2. Are stored in liver
   3. Include vitamins A, D, E, and K
   4. Are stable to ordinary cooking and processing procedures
   5. Are derived from
      a. Vitamin A—dark green, leafy vegetables, deep yellow vegetables, orange fruits, and milk
      b. Vitamin D—milk, egg yolk, and liver
      c. Vitamin E—dark green, leafy vegetables, vegetable oil, cereals, and wheat germ oil
      d. Vitamin K—green, leafy vegetables and pork liver
   6. Deficiencies can cause
      a. Night blindness (vitamin A)
      b. Rickets (vitamin D)
      c. Anemia and sterility—not yet positively determined in humans (vitamin E)
      d. Poor blood clotting (vitamin K)

C. Water-soluble vitamins
   1. Are readily absorbed
   2. Must be provided daily; body does not store
   3. Are easily destroyed by heat and alkalinity and by being dissolved in liquid
   4. Include vitamin B complex and vitamin C
   5. Are derived from
      a. Vitamin B complex—liver, meat, and milk
      b. Vitamin C—citrus fruits, cabbage, tomatoes, strawberries, and cantaloupe
   6. Deficiency can cause
      a. Beriberi, poor wound healing, anemia, and sprue (vitamin B complex)
      b. Scurvy (vitamin C)

Water

A. Amount—two thirds of body weight
B. Functions—necessary for
   1. Digestion
   2. Absorption
   3. Metabolism
   4. Elimination
C. Sources
   1. Water in foods (milk, fruits, juice, vegetables)
   2. Water we drink (six to eight glasses per day)
   3. Water formed by metabolism of foods within body

Bulk

A. Function is to help mass of food move along gastrointestinal tract
B. Source is cellulose from vegetables and fruits and bran layer (outside) of grain
C. Cellulose is not digested or metabolized by human body

NUTRITIONAL REQUIREMENTS

A. Requirements are determined by consideration of age, sex, size and activity (sedentary, moderately active, very active)
B. Four basic food groups and recommended daily requirements
   1. Milk group (milk, cheese, ice cream)
      a. Adults, two servings
      b. Children, three to four servings
      c. Pregnant women, four servings
      d. Nursing mothers, six servings
   2. Meat group (meat, fish, poultry, eggs, dried beans, peas, nuts), two servings
   3. Vegetable and fruit group (citrus fruits, green, leafy, and yellow vegetables), four servings
      a. Vitamin C group, one serving
      b. Vitamin A group, one serving
   4. Bread and cereal group (cereals—whole grain or enriched), four servings

MENU PLANNING AND MARKETING

Marketing to fit income

A. Factors to consider in buying food
   1. Cost per serving, not cost per pound

1 package frozen peas (12 oz)	Serves four
1 pound (16 oz) fresh peas in pod	Serves two
1 pound standing rib roast	Serves two
1 pound hamburger (ground chuck)	Serves four

   2. Economy versus luxury

Economy

Vegetables and fruits	In season
Meats	Grade good
Eggs	Medium and small
Fats	Margarine
Milk	Dry and evaporated

Luxury

Vegetables	Out of season
Meats	Grade choice and prime
Eggs	Large and extra large
Fats	Butter
Milk	Bottle

B. Sample dinner menu (served in January)

Economy

Chuck roast (grade good)
Mashed potatoes
Peas and carrots
Grapefruit with cottage cheese
Bread and margarine
Pound cake with custard sauce

Luxury

Standing rib (grade prime)
Creamed new potatoes
Broccoli, fresh
Grapefruit, avocado, and cream cheese
Blueberry muffins and butter
Angel cake with frozen strawberries and whipped cream

Basic normal diet

A. Follow diet as ordered by physician when patient is on special diet; otherwise, plan menu to contain "Basic Four" foods
B. Consider likes and dislikes of individual patient
C. Have contrast in foods in each meal
   1. In color (sample menu)
      Not: Creamed chicken, mashed potatoes, and cauliflower
      Rather: Creamed chicken, baked potato, and string beans
   2. In texture (sample menu)
      Not: Meat loaf, mashed potato, mashed squash, and cottage cheese
      Rather: Meat loaf, whole potatoes, peas, and lettuce with peaches and cottage cheese
   3. In flavor (sample menu)
      Not: Barbecued ribs, french fried onions, pickled beets, garlic bread, and mince pie
      Rather: Barbecued ribs, mashed potato, carrots and peas, hard rolls, and baked apples
D. Have hot foods *hot* and cold foods *cold*
E. When planning a patient's menu, use family or hospital menus whenever possible
F. The following are patterns for simple menu planning

Breakfast

Fruit or fruit juice
Cereal or egg or both
Breakfast meat occasionally
Bread or rolls and butter
Milk, tea, or coffee

Lunch or supper

Main dish
Vegetable or fruit or both
Dessert (optional)—dessert usually should be fresh, frozen or cooked fruit
Bread and butter
Milk, tea, or coffee

Dinner

Meat dish (meat, fish, poultry, or combination dishes)
Potato or substitute
Vegetable (green or yellow)
Salad (fruit or vegetable)
Bread and butter
Dessert (optional)—dessert usually should be fresh, frozen, or cooked fruit
Milk, tea, or coffee

FOOD PREPARATION

Cereals, breads, and flour

A. Sources
   1. Whole grains are cereals with bran (whole grain flour and whole kernel corn)
   2. Refined grains are cereals without bran (polished rice and white flour)
B. Storage—store flour and cereals in sealed containers and bread in well-ventilated box or refrigerator
C. Cooking—softens cellulose, aids in digestion, and improves flavor; processed cereals (dry) are already cooked
D. Purchasing—cereals to be cooked are cheapest; individual servings of dry cereal are most expensive

Eggs

A. Are good source of protein, iron, phosphorus, and vitamins (A, D, B_1, niacin)
B. Should be purchased for quality; carton shows grade, size, and date of grading (buy only refrigerated eggs)
   1. Sizes are extra large, at least 27 oz per dozen; large, 24 oz; medium, 21 oz; small, 18 oz
   2. Grades are in terms of soundness and cleanliness of shell, size of air cells, and condition of yolk and white
      a. AA and A—top quality
      b. B and C—satisfactory for cooking
C. Should never be washed before storage
   1. Place in covered container at temperature below 40°F
   2. Store egg whites up to 10 days in refrigerator in sealed container
   3. Store egg yolks covered with water two to three days in refrigerator
D. Should be cooked at low temperature—poaching, soft boiling, hard boiling, scrambling, and custard; also eggs may be used in recipes

Milk

A. Nutrition
   1. Good source of protein, minerals (calcium and phosphorus), and vitamins (A, B_1, riboflavin)
   2. Poor source of vitamin C, iron, niacin, and bulk
B. Purchasing
   1. Grades A, B, and C—grading depends on bacterial count; only grade A should be used without cooking

2. Types of milk
   a. Certified milk is clean, unprocessed milk of uniform composition, from healthy cows, with bacterial count of less than 10,000 per milliliter
   b. Raw milk is fresh from cow with no processing
   c. Pasteurized milk is heated to at least 143°F and held at this temperature for 30 minutes then cooled rapidly to destroy disease-producing bacteria (*Note:* Many health departments recommend that only pasteurized milk be used for drinking)
   d. Evaporated milk has part of water removed ($^1/_2$ cup water plus $^1/_2$ cup evaporated milk equals 1 cup whole milk)
   e. Condensed milk is evaporated milk plus added sugar
   f. Dried milk is whole or skim milk with all water removed; dried skim milk is good source of protein and minerals; cheapest form of milk
   g. Homogenized milk has fat globules broken down so that cream does not rise; whole milk has 3.9% butterfat; 2% homogenized has only 2% butterfat; skim milk has no butterfat
   h. Whole milk is 87% water, 0.7% minerals, 3.5% protein, 4.9% carbohydrates, and 3.9% butterfat
   i. Vitamin D milk has vitamin D added either by fortification (addition of crystalline vitamin D) or irradiation (passage of milk through ultraviolet light)
   j. Buttermilk (cultured) is whole or skim (fat-free) milk soured by addition of bacteria
   k. Sodium-free skim milk (Lonalac) has sodium removed

Cheese

A. Nutrition—varies with type of milk used (goat, cow, whole, or skim)
B. Purchasing—there are over 400 varieties; the most common are
   1. Very hard—Parmesan
   2. Hard—cheddar and Swiss
   3. Semisoft—Roquefort (mold), Muenster, and brick (bacteria)
   4. Soft—cottage, cream, Neufchâtel (unripened), Brie, Camembert (mold), Liederkranz, and Limburger (bacteria)
   5. Processed cheese—blended with an emulsifying agent and pasteurized; most common example is American
C. Storage
   1. Soft cheeses must be refrigerated
   2. Hard cheeses may be refrigerated or wrapped tightly or kept under glass in cool place
D. Cooking—provides economical substitute for meat; cook at low temperature

Meat, fish, and poultry

A. Nutrition—good source of protein and has ''satiety value''; lean meat has high source of minerals and B vitamins; port is especially high in B_1; red meats are high in iron, and liver is high in iron and vitamin A
B. Selection
   1. Grades of meat
      a. Beef grades
         (1) Prime is highest grade; it is lean, firm, bright red, and fine textured with marbling of fat
         (2) Choice is highest grade usually found in markets; fat is marbled and smooth
         (3) Good is most popular grade; it is not quite so juicy and tender
         (4) Standard includes young animals formerly in commercial grade
         (5) Commercial includes older animals; fat covering is very thin, and there is no marbling
         (6) Utility includes older animals; it lacks tenderness and juiciness
         (7) Cutter and canners are two lowest grades, which seldom appear in retail market; they are used for canning, sausage, and dried beef
      b. Veal grades—choice, good, commercial, utility, and cull
      c. Pork grades—choice, medium, and cull
      d. Mutton and lamb grades—choice, good, commercial, utility, and cull
      e. Poultry grades—A, B, and C
   2. Standards to judge quality of meat
      a. Beef should be bright red and fine grained, with creamy, white, firm fat
      b. Veal (calves 3 to 12 weeks old) should be grayish pink, fine grained, and smooth, with pinkish white, brittle fat

c. Lamb (8 to 12 months old) should be reddish pink, fine grained, and smooth to touch, with firm fat, and red, spongy bones
d. Mutton should be light to dark red, with firm fat
e. Pork should be grayish pink, with white, firm fat
f. Poultry should have plump, compact legs and breastbone that can be bent at lower end; stewing chicken has hard breastbone
g. Fish should have bright, clear eyes, reddish pink gills, no slime, scales that are tight to skin, fresh odor, and bright, shiny, firm, elastic flesh

C. Cooking
1. Pork, wild game, poultry, and any other meat you are not sure has been graded correctly must be well cooked to destroy trichinae present
2. Methods of cooking are
a. Roasting (dry)—cooking at medium-low temperature, 250° to 300°F, for long time, with no lid and no added liquid (tender cuts)
b. Broiling and pan broiling—cooking at high temperature under or over direct heat for short time (tender cuts)
d. Braising—browning meat on both sides in small amount of fat, then cooking it slowly in small amount of liquid in covered kettle (less tender cuts)
e. Simmering—cooking in liquid just below boiling point (less tender cuts)
f. Stewing—cooking in liquid at boiling temperature or under pressure (less tender cuts)
g. Microwave—cooking in specially designed ovens that use high-frequency waves to penetrate food; waves turn to heat energy that cooks all food (all cuts)

D. Storage
1. Fresh meat must be refrigerated
2. Freezing, canning, salting, smoking, and drying are used if meat is to be kept long time

E. Purchasing
1. Price depends on
a. Grade of animal
b. Cut of meat (higher the price, more tender the raw meat)
2. Best piece of meat to purchase depends on
a. Method used for cooking
b. Servings per pound

Vegetables

A. Nutrition—are 2% to 40% carbohydrate, have no protein except legumes, but are good source of vitamins and cellulose and some minerals

B. Purchasing
1. Fresh—choose quality first (fresh, firm, and free from bruises); if uniform size and shape, there is less waste; buy by weight when possible
2. Frozen—never refreeze
3. Dried and canned—most economical when vegetable is not in season

C. Cooking
1. Cook vegetables whole or in large pieces, with skin nutrients saved
2. Start in boiling water (no water for greens)
3. Cook *only* until tender
4. Stir as little as possible; *do not boil violently*
5. Serve as soon as possible after cooking
6. Use usual methods of cooking, baking, steaming, steaming under pressure, broiling, pan frying, or deep fat frying

D. Storage
1. Fresh—store roots and tubers (onions, potatoes, squash, turnips) in cool, dark, dry room; clean and place other vegetables in hydrator or wrap in paper and store in refrigerator
2. Frozen—never thaw before cooking
3. Dried—keep in tightly closed container

Fruits

A. Nutrition—are 3% to 25% carbohydrate, have no protein or fat except olives and avocado, and are high in minerals, vitamins, and cellulose

B. Purchasing
1. Fresh—choose firm, ripe fruit; purchase by weight if possible; fruit is cheapest in season
2. Frozen, canned, and dried

C. Storage
1. Fresh
a. Refrigerated, covered or uncovered—apples, very mellow apricots, avocados, berries (unwashed), cherries, grapes, nectarines, peaches, pears, and plums
b. Room temperature—grapefruit, lemons, limes, oranges, and pineapple
c. Cool room temperature (60° to 70°F)—apples, firm bananas, firm peaches
2. Frozen—never thaw until ready to use; never refreeze
3. Dried—keep in covered container at room temperature

Beverages

A. Common ones are used for stimulation, fluids, and sociability
B. Use in diet is to add fluids and nourishment

Basic pharmacology

DEFINITION AND SCOPE

A. Pharmacology is the study of drugs, dealing with their characteristics, actions, and effects on the body
B. A drug is any substance used to diagnose, treat the symptoms of, cure, or prevent a disease
C. Therapeutics, which usually involves drug therapy, consists of any treatment used to restore the body to its normal condition. The therapeutic effect of a drug is its desired effect
D. Toxicology is that branch of pharmacology that involves the treatment of poisoning, including drug overdosage

DRUG NOMENCLATURE

Most drugs are assigned to at least three names
A. The *chemical name* describes the chemical makeup or molecular structure
B. The *official name,* also called the *generic name,* is a nonproprietary name recognized in official literature. Use of official names is increasing in institutional settings
C. The *trade name* or *brand name* is a registered trademark belonging to a particular manufacturer. It should be capitalized and is often followed by the superscript ®. A drug may be marketed under several brand names
D. An example is
Chemical name—acetylsalicylic acid
Official name—aspirin
Brand name—A.S.A.®

SOURCES OF DRUG INFORMATION

The United States Pharmacopeia (USP) and the National Formulary (NF)

A. These books are known as the official reference books; published in a single volume
B. They set forth legally binding standards to which drugs must conform
C. Clinically useful information is found in the USP Dispensing Information supplement
D. They are revised every 5 years with interim supplements
E. "USP" or "NF" following an official drug name means that drug conforms to standards set forth therein

The package insert

Pamphlet accompanying a drug product, giving information about that product, must be approved by the Food and Drug Administration (FDA)

The Physician's Desk Reference (PDR)

A. Contains information supplied by drug manufacturers, usually identical to that of the package insert
B. Is most useful for looking up drugs according to their brand names
C. Is published annually with interim supplements
D. Contains a pictorial products identification section

The American Hospital Formulary Service (AHFS)

A. Contains extensive, unbiased drug information kept current by periodic supplements
B. Arranges drugs into therapeutic or pharmacologic classes according to official names

Facts and Comparisons

A. Arranges drugs into therapeutic classes for easy comparison with similar agents
B. Contains basic information for each class of drugs
C. Is useful for determining official or brand names when one names is known

DRUG LEGISLATION

Food, Drug, and Cosmetic Act

A. Act contains detailed regulations to ensure that drugs meet standards of safety and effectiveness
B. Legend drugs require physician's prescription for purchase
C. Nonlegend drugs (nonprescription, over-the-counter [OTC] drugs) available without prescription
D. Regulations administered by the Food And Drug Administration

Controlled Substances Act

A. Regulates drugs that have a potential for abuse or addiction, including narcotics, stimulants, and depressants
B. Requires special records and distribution procedures

C. Classifies drugs subject to act into Schedules I through V, with drugs in lower schedules having a greater abuse potential and more stringent controls. Schedule I drugs have no accepted medical usage and are available investigationally only
D. Is administered by the Drug Enforcement Administration (DEA)

SOURCES OF DRUGS

A. Animals (insulin, heparin)
B. Plants (quinine, digitalis)
C. Microorganisms (antibiotics)
D. Synthetic chemical substances (aspirin)
E. Food substances (vitamins)

DOSAGE FORMS

A. Tablet—solid dosage unit made by compression of a powdered drug
   1. Sugar-coated tablet has smooth coating
   2. Enteric-coated tablet disintegrates in small intestine to prevent stomach upset
   3. Sublingual or buccal tablet dissolves under tongue or between cheek and gum respectively
   4. Chewable tablet is soft and pleasantly flavored
   5. Hypodermic tablet dissolves in water for injection (obsolete)
   6. Troche or lozenge dissolves in mouth over a long period of time
B. Capsule—drug contained in gelatin shell, which quickly dissolves in stomach
   1. Hard gelatin capsule is used for powdered drugs
   2. Soft gelatin capsule, usually oval, contains a semisolid or liquid
C. Pill (obsolete)
   1. Hard oval mass made by hand
   2. Slang term for tablet or capsule
D. Solution—liquid that consists of a drug (the solute) completely dissolved in a solvent
   1. Syrup—solution containing a large amount of sugar
   2. Elixir—a sweetened, clear, hydroalcoholic solution that serves as the vehicle for a drug
   3. Tincture—alcoholic or hydroalcoholic solution of a drug
E. Suspension—liquid preparation containing finely divided insoluble drug particles, which must always be shaken vigorously before use
   1. Emulsion—type of suspension usually containing microscopic oil particles dispersed throughout an aqueous medium
   2. Lotion—a suspension for external application
F. Suppository—mass containing a drug, which melts or dissolves after insertion through a body orifice; various sizes and shapes are manufactured for rectal, vaginal, or urethral use
G. Ointment—semisolid mixture of a drug with an oleaginous, occlusive base, which is rubbed onto the skin
H. Cream—semisolid mixture of a drug in a thick emulsion, which is rubbed onto the skin; water miscible
I. Injections (parenterals)
   1. Sterile solutions or suspensions
   2. Sterile powders that form a solution or suspension when mixed with sterile water or other suitable diluent
   3. Sterile emulsions
   4. Sterile pellets for implantation beneath the skin
J. Sustained release medications (sustained action, prolonged action, repeat action)—have long duration of effect
   1. Sustained release tablets (Repetabs, Extentabs)
   2. Sustained release capsules (Spansule)
   3. Long-acting injections usually in the form of a suspension or pellet

FACTORS INFLUENCING DRUG ACTIVITY

Dosage of drug

A. Therapeutic dose produces desired effect with minimal side effects
B. Maximum dose is largest dose recommended for therapeutic effect
C. Toxic dose produces severe side effects, while lethal dose causes death

Route of administration

A. Intravenous administration produces most rapid effect
B. Oral administration has least rapid action
C. Intramuscular or subcutaneous administration produces more rapid effect than oral administration but is slower than intravenous administration

Age

Infants, children, and geriatric patients often respond differently to drugs, thereby requiring dosage adjustment

Weight

Dosage is often based on body weight or size. Ideal body weight may be considered for determining dosage of certain drugs if the patient is obese

Blood serum levels

Dosage of some drugs, e.g., digoxin, is regulated based on serum levels as determined by laboratory analysis

Metabolism and excretion

A. Liver and kidney are responsible for metabolism and excretion respectively
B. Disease of liver or kidney may prevent elimination of drug, resulting in increased drug serum levels that can produce toxicities; dosage alteration is then required

Tolerance

Resistance to effects of drug; larger dose required for desired effect if patient is resistant

Allergy

Hypersensitivity reactions may develop in certain patients

Time of administration

A. Interval between doses
B. Relationship of dose to meals, sleep, and other activities
   1. Oral administration on empty stomach speeds absorption of drug
   2. Oral administration on full stomach decreases chance of stomach upset but slows absorption

Pregnancy

Many drugs should be avoided because of toxic effects on fetus

Drug interactions

Drugs may increase or decrease effect of another drug. Foods may interact with certain drugs; e.g., the absorption of tetracycline is inhibited by milk

BASIC PHARMACOLOGIC AND THERAPEUTIC DRUG CLASSIFICATIONS

A. Analgesics, such as aspirin, relieve pain
B. Local anesthetics, such as lidocaine, cause loss of sensation in a small area, while general anesthetics, such as halothane, produce profound sleep and loss of all sensations
C. Antacids, such as Maalox, neutralize excess gastric acidity
D. Anthelmintics, such as thiabendazole (Mintezol), destroy worm infestations of the GI tract
E. Antiarrhythmics, such as quinidine, control cardiac rhythm
F. Antibacterials, such as sulfisoxazole (Gantrisin), kill or inhibit the growth of microorganisms
G. Antibiotics, such as penicillin, are substances produced by living microorganisms, which kill or inhibit the growth of other microorganisms
H. Anticholinergics, such as belladonna, block the actions controlled by the parasympathetic nervous system
I. Anticoagulants, such as heparin, prevent or delay blood clotting
J. Anticonvulsants, such as phenytoin (Dilantin), prevent or relieve convulsions
K. Antidepressants, such as amitriptyline (Elavil), elevate mood
L. An antidote neutralizes or counteracts the toxic effects of a poison or overdose
M. Antiemetics, such as prochlorperazine (Compazine), prevent or relieve nausea and vomiting
N. An antifungal, such as nystatin (Mycostatin), controls fungus infections
O. An antihistamine, such as diphenhydramine (Benadryl), blocks the actions of histamine to relieve allergy symptoms
P. Antihypertensive, or hypotensive, agents, such as reserpine, lower blood pressure
Q. Antineoplastic agents, such as 5-fluorouracil, prevent the growth of cancerous tumors
R. An antipruritic, such as trimeprazine (Temaril), relieves itching
S. Antipyretics, such as acetaminophen (Tylenol), reduce fever
T. Antiseptics, such as alcohol, restrict the growth of bacteria
U. Antispasmodics, such as atropine, relieve smooth muscle spasm
V. Antitoxins, such as tetanus antitoxin, neutralize a specific bacterial toxin
W. Antitubercular drugs, such as isoniazid, are used to treat tuberculosis
X. Astringents, such as alum, constrict skin or mucous membranes, arresting discharges
Y. Bactericides kill bacteria; certain antibiotics are bactericidal

Z. Bacteriostatic agents inhibit multiplication of bacteria; certain antibiotics are bacteriostatic

AA. Bronchodilators, such as aminophylline, relieve bronchial constriction and are used in the treatment of asthmatic conditions

BB. Cathartics, laxatives, and purgatives produce evacuation of the bowel; they vary in method of action and potency

CC. Caustics, such as glacial acetic acid, destroy tissue by local application

DD. A counterirritant, such as camphor, produces an irritation that is intended to relieve some other irritation

EE. Decongestants, such as phenylephrine (Neo-Synephrine), relieve nasal and sinus congestion by shrinkage of mucous membranes

FF. Disinfectants, such as povidone iodine (Betadine), destroy pathogenic microorganisms

GG. Diuretics, such as furosemide (Lasix), increase the volume of urine produced by the kidneys

HH. Emetics, such as syrup of ipecac, induce vomiting for removal of stomach contents

II. Emollients, such as cold cream, soften and soothe the skin

JJ. Expectorants, such as potassium iodide, may promote expulsion of mucus from the respiratory tract by productive cough

KK. Hematinics, such as ferrous sulfate, are drugs used in the treatment of anemia

LL. Hemostatic agents (coagulants), such as vitamin K, promote the clotting of blood to prevent or control hemorrhage

MM. Hormones, such as insulin, are extracts of endocrine glands, given as replacement therapy

NN. Hypertensive agents, such as dopamine (Intropin), increase blood pressure

OO. Hypnotics, such as flurazepam (Dalmane), induce sleep

PP. Miotics, such as pilocarpine, constrict the pupil of the eye

QQ. Mydriatics, such as atropine, dilate the pupil of the eye

RR. A placebo is a therapeutically inactive drug given for its psychologic effect

SS. A sedative, such as phenobarbital, relieves anxiety or excitement

TT. A tranquilizer, such as diazepam (Valium), is used to relieve anxiety and uncomfortable emotional feelings. The more potent major tranquilizers, such as chlorpromazine (Thorazine), are used as antipsychotic agents

UU. Vasoconstrictors, such as epinephrine, produce a narrowing of blood vessels

VV. Vasodilators, such as nitroglycerin, produce dilation of blood vessels

WW. Vitamins are complex chemical substances obtained from foods or synthesized from nonfood sources, needed by the body to carry out normal physiologic processes

PRESERVATION AND STORAGE OF DRUGS

A. Medications should be stored in accordance with any special requirements on the label

B. The stability of drug products may be adversely affected by temperature, light, moisture, air, or microbial contamination

C. Drugs requiring refrigeration should be kept at 36° to 46°F. Drugs requiring freezing should be kept at −4° to 14°F. Drugs requiring a cool place should be stored at 46° to 59°F. Most drugs are stable at room temperature (59° to 86°F)

D. Drugs are protected from light by amber glass or boxes. Intravenous solutions of a light-sensitive drug, such as amphotericin B, should be covered with a paper bag or wrapped in aluminum foil

E. Containers should be tightly sealed to prevent contact between the drug and moisture or air

F. Before administration, drugs should be checked for signs of deterioration, such as color change, formation of a precipitate, change in hardness or appearance of tablets, sticking of capsules, evolution of a gas, foul odor, and softening of suppositories

G. A deteriorated drug should not be administered; it should be returned to the pharmacy for exchange

H. The expiration date of a drug should be checked before administration. Do not use a drug after its expiration date

CALCULATION OF DOSAGE

A. It is the responsibility of the practical nurse to work within the guidelines of the hospital or other institution
   1. Make sure dosage calculations are exact before preparation and administration of drug
   2. Check calculations with knowledgeable person, such as registered nurse, pharmacist, or physician
   3. Measure dosages exactly in accordance with physician's orders

B. The metric system is the universal system of weights and measures based on the number 10. Most medications are labeled and ordered in metric units. Therefore calculations should usually be done within the metric system since conversions to other systems of measurement frequently introduce errors
   1. Metric units of length: meter (m), centimeter (cm), and millimeter (mm)
   2. Metric units of volume: liter (L) and milliliter (ml). One milliliter is equivalent to a cubic centimeter (cc)
   3. Units of weight: kilogram (kg), gram (g or gm), milligram (mg), and microgram (μg or mcg)

C. The apothecary system is an older system. Doses of older medications, such as aspirin and nitroglycerin, are sometimes expressed in apothecary units
   1. Units of weight: grain (gr), dram (ʒ), and ounce (℥)
   2. Units of volume: minim (♏), fluiddram (*f*ʒ), fluidounce (*f*℥), pint (O or pt), quart (qt), and gallon (C or gal)

D. The household system of measurement is useful for patients at home. Household measurements are easily converted to metric or apothecary measurements. Commonly used units of volume are the teaspoonful (tsp), dessertspoonful, and tablespoonful (tbsp)

E. The practical nurse should become familiar with these systems of measurement and be able to make conversions between systems when required (see Appendix)

F. Methods of calculating dosages are
   1. The dose for oral tablets and capsules may be calculated by ratio and proportion using the following method:

   Labeled dose : 1 tablet (or capsule) = Ordered dose : x tablets (or capsules)

      a. EXAMPLE: Give 500 mg of ampicillin using capsules containing 250 mg

$$250 \text{ mg} : 1 \text{ capsule} = 500 \text{ mg} : x \text{ capsules}$$
$$250\,x = 500$$
$$x = \frac{500}{250} = 2 \text{ capsules}$$

      Administer two of the 250 mg capsules

      b. EXAMPLE: Give 15 gr of aspirin using tablets containing 5 gr of aspirin per tablet

$$5 \text{ gr} : 1 \text{ tablet} = 15 \text{ gr} : x \text{ tablets}$$
$$5\,x = 15$$
$$x = \frac{15}{5} = 3 \text{ tablets}$$

      Administer three of the 5 gr tablets

   2. The dosage of an oral liquid preparation or solution for injection may be calculated using ratio and proportion as follows:

$$\text{Available dose} : \text{Volume of solution containing available dose} = \text{Desired dose} : \text{Volume of solution containing desired dose}$$

      a. EXAMPLE: A penicillin suspension contains 125 mg of penicillin per 5 ml; give a dose of 250 mg

$$125 \text{ mg} : 5 \text{ ml} = 250 \text{ mg} : x \text{ ml}$$
$$125\,x = 1250$$
$$x = \frac{1250}{125} = 10 \text{ ml}$$

      Administer 10 ml, which will contain 250 mg of penicillin

      b. EXAMPLE: Gentamicin (Garamycin) injection contains 40 mg per ml; give a dose of 60 mg

$$40 \text{ mg} : 1 \text{ ml} = 60 \text{ mg} : x \text{ ml}$$
$$40\,x = 60$$
$$x = \frac{60}{40} = 1.5 \text{ ml}$$

      Administer 1.5 ml, which will contain 60 mg of gentamicin

PREPARATION OF SOLUTIONS

A. Percentage solutions are expressed as percent weight to volume (W/V) if the drug is a solid dissolved in a liquid. If the pure drug is a liquid, the concentration of the solution is expressed as percent volume to volume (V/V). Calculations may be performed using ratio and proportion if the percentage desired is expressed as a ratio.
   1. EXAMPLE: Prepare 1 L (1000 ml) of a 0.9% W/V sodium chloride solution. In this case there would be 0.9 g of sodium chloride dissolved in each 100 ml of solution. Determine the amount of sodium chloride that would be in 1000 ml of this solution

$$0.9\ g : 100\ ml = x\ g : 1000\ ml$$
$$100\,x = 900$$
$$x = \frac{900}{100} = 9\ g$$

Place 9 g of sodium chloride in a container, and dissolve it in enough water to make a total volume of 1 L

2. EXAMPLE: Prepare 60 ml of a 50% V/V solution of glycerin. The desired solution would contain 50 ml of pure glycerin in each 100 ml of the solution. Determine how much pure glycerin would be contained in 60 ml of the 50% solution

$$50\ ml\ glycerin : 100\ ml\ sol. = x\ ml\ glycerin : 60\ ml\ sol.$$
$$100\,x = 3000$$
$$x = \frac{3000}{100} = 30\ ml$$

Place 30 ml pure glycerin in a graduate and mix with enough water to make a total volume of 60 ml

B. The concentration of a solution may be expressed as ratio strength. Thus in a 1:100 solution, in which a solid drug is dissolved in a liquid, there would be 1 g of pure drug dissolved in each 100 ml of the solution

EXAMPLE: Prepare 500 ml of a 1:1000 solution of neomycin to be used for irrigation

The ratio strength (1:1000) means that there would be 1 g of neomycin dissolved in 1000 ml of the solution. Determine the amount of neomycin needed to prepare 500 ml of solution

$$1\ g\ neomycin : 1000\ ml = x\ g\ neomycin : 500\ ml$$
$$1000\,x = 500$$
$$x = \frac{500}{1000} = 0.5\ g$$

Dissolve 0.5 g neomycin in 500 ml of sterile water for irrigation

CALCULATION OF THE DRIP RATE FOR AN INTRAVENOUS SOLUTION

A. The *volume of solution* to be administered, the *length of time* over which this volume is to be infused, and the *number of drops per milliliter* delivered by the administration set being used must be known

B. The drip rate may be determined as follows:

1. Find the volume of fluid to be administered per hour

$$\frac{\text{ml of fluid to be infused}}{\text{Number of hours fluid is to run}} = \text{ml of fluid/hour}$$

2. Find volume of fluid to be administered per minute

$$\frac{\text{ml of fluid/hour}}{\text{60 min/hour}} = \text{ml to run/min}$$

3. Multiply the milliliters of fluid to run per minute by the number of drops per milliliter delivered by the intravenous set. This gives the number of drops that should fall in the drip chamber per minute

$$\text{ml/min} \times \text{drops/ml} = \text{drops/min}$$

C. If the administration rate has been ordered as milliliters per hour, step 1 is omitted

D. The following formula may also be used to calculate the drip rate:

$$\frac{\text{ml to administer} \times \text{drops/ml}}{\text{Hours to run} \times \text{60 min/hour}} = \text{drops/min}$$

EXAMPLE: Administer 1000 ml of an intravenous solution over 8 hours using an adult intravenous administration set that delivers 10 drops per milliliter

$$\frac{1000}{\text{8 hours}} = \text{125 ml/hour}$$
$$\frac{\text{125 ml/hour}}{\text{60 min/hour}} = \text{2.1 ml/min}$$
$$\text{2.1 ml/min} \times \text{10 drops/min} = \text{21 drops/min}$$

Using the formula,

$$\frac{\text{1000 ml} \times \text{10 drops/ml}}{\text{8 hours} \times \text{60 min/hour}} = \text{21 drops/min}$$

E. Adjust the flow rate to the number of drops per minute calculated above. Check the fluid volume at hourly intervals to see that the fluid is actually being administered at the desired rate. Note that the calculated drip rate is only a good approximation of the actual flow rate. Flow rates may be affected by factors such as the type of solution, additives, position of the patient, and volume of fluid in the container

SELECTED MEDICATIONS USED IN GENERAL CARE OF PATIENTS

Nonnarcotic analgesics and antipyretics

A. Aspirin (acetylsalicylic acid, ASA)
  1. Aspirin controls minor aches, pains, and fever
  2. It is usually administered orally but may be given as rectal suppository
  3. It frequently causes GI upset, which may be prevented by giving after meals or with antacids. Hypersensitivity reactions or GI ulceration may occur
  4. Overdose produces poisoning called salicylism, characterized by tinnitus, GI upset, visual disturbances, and sweating. Severe overdose may produce coma, respiratory failure, and death
  5. Usual adult dose for pain or fever is 10 gr (650 mg). Larger doses, 3 to 6 g per day, are used for antiinflammatory effects

B. Sodium salicylate—similar to aspirin

C. Acetaminophen (Tylenol)
  1. Acetaminophen is a nonsalicylate analgesic/antipyretic of about the same potency as aspirin but lacks antiinflammatory action. Used in patients who cannot tolerate aspirin because of GI problems or concurrent use of anticoagulants
  2. It is less irritating than aspirin to the stomach and is generally considered safer than aspirin for children
  3. It is administered orally as tablet or liquid or rectally as suppository
  4. Usual adult dose is 650 mg

D. APC (aspirin, phenacetin, and caffeine)
  1. Phenacetin is analgesic similar to acetaminophen; caffeine is mild central nervous system stimulant
  2. Has no advantages over aspirin. Long-term use of high doses may cause renal damage
  3. Usual adult dose is two tablets, administered orally

E. Propoxyphene (Darvon) and propoxyphene napsylate (Darvon-N)
  1. Analgesic potency is said to approach that of codeine but has no antipyretic action unless given in combination with aspirin (Darvon with ASA), APC (Darvon Compound), or acetaminophen (Darvocet-N)
  2. Side effects are gastrointestinal upset, dizziness, and drowsiness
  3. Overdose may produce respiratory depression
  4. Usual oral adult doses are
     a. Propoxyphene—32 to 65 mg
     b. Propoxyphene napsylate—100 mg
  5. Psychic and/or physical drug dependence and tolerance may develop. Alcohol, tranquilizers, and other central nervous system depressants should be avoided as additive depressant effects frequently occur

Narcotic analgesics

A. General characteristics and precautions
  1. Narcotic drugs are derivatives of opium or synthetic substitutes used primarily for their analgesic properties. Narcotics may produce addiction and dependency
  2. Narcotic drugs produce state of euphoria that dulls perception of and reaction to pain. Large doses relieve anxiety and produce sleep
  3. Side effects are nausea, vomiting, constipation, lightheadedness, confusion, and urticaria. Large doses may produce respiratory depression, constriction of the pupils, coma, and death
  4. Narcotic drugs must be withheld and a physician contacted for instructions if respiratory rate falls below 12 per minute or respiration becomes shallow
  5. Narcotic drugs must be used with extreme caution in patients with asthma or emphysema
  6. All doses of narcotics must be recorded in the narcotic administration record

B. Morphine sulfate
  1. Morphine is potent narcotic analgesic used to control severe pain
  2. Usual adult dose is 5 to 20 mg subcutaneously or intramuscularly and 2.5 to 15 mg intravenously; oral administration is not recommended

C. Codeine
  1. Codeine is much less potent than morphine
  2. It is used to control less severe pain and suppress cough
  3. Usual adult dose is 15 to 60 mg subcutaneously or orally
  4. Codeine is often given in combination with other nonnarcotic analgesics such as aspirin or acetaminophen

D. Meperidine (Demerol)
  1. Meperidine is synthetic narcotic used as alternative to morphine

2. Usual adult dose is 50 to 150 mg orally, intramuscularly, or subcutaneously (not recommended)

E. Narcotic antagonists—reverse narcotic-induced respiratory depression. Principal narcotic antagonists are
1. Naloxone (Narcan)
2. Levallorphan (Lorfan)

Sedatives, hypnotics, and tranquilizers

A. Sedatives and hypnotics depress central nervous system to produce sedation or sleep depending on dose administered. The potential for abuse or addiction is associated with use of these agents

B. The barbiturates are the largest group of sedative-hypnotic drugs
1. Principal agents are thiopental (Pentothal), secobarbital (Seconal), pentobarbital (Nembutal), butabarbital (Butisol Sodium), amobarbital (Amytal), and phenobarbital (Luminal)
2. Side effects include allergic reactions, gastrointestinal upset, grogginess, and mental disturbances
3. Overdosage may produce respiratory depression, coma, and death
4. Usual dosage range is 15 to 100 mg

C. Nonbarbiturate sedatives and hypnotics include chloral hydrate (Noctec), methaqualone (Quaalude), flurazepam (Dalmane), ethchlorvynol (Placidyl), and paraldehyde

D. Minor tranquilizers control simple nervousness and anxiety. Examples are diazepam (Valium), chlordiazepoxide (Librium), hydroxyzine (Vistaril), and meprobamate (Equanil)

E. The consumption of alcohol with sedatives, hypnotics, and tranquilizers should be avoided because of enhanced depressant activity

Antibiotics

A. General information
1. Broad spectrum antibiotics are effective against many classes of microorganisms; narrow spectrum antibiotics are effective against only a few classes of microorganisms. Antibiotics are ineffective against viruses
2. General side effects from antibiotics are allergic reactions (rash, itching, hives, possible anaphylactic shock), and secondary infections by microorganisms resistant to the antibiotic being used
3. Choice of antibiotic is based on physician's diagnosis and results of culture and sensitivity tests

B. Penicillins
1. Various types of penicillins include potassium penicillin G, procaine penicillin G, benzathine penicillin (Bicillin), ampicillin, amoxicillin (Larotid), cyclacillin (Cyclapen), carbenicillin (Geopen), ticarcillin (Ticar), oxacillin (Prostaphlin), cloxacillin (Tegopen), dicloxacillin (Dynapen), methicillin (Staphcillin), and nafcillin (Unipen)
2. A patient who is allergic to one type of penicillin is allergic to all forms of penicillin
3. Products are made for oral, intramuscular, or intravenous use
4. The dose may be ordered in milligrams or units (250 mg = 400,000 units); there is wide dosage range

C. Tetracycline antibiotics
1. Tetracycline antibiotics are broad spectrum antibiotics
2. They may cause permanent brown discoloration of teeth in children if given when teeth are forming or if given to mothers during pregnancy. Avoid use in these patients
3. Examples of tetracycline products are tetracycline (Achromycin/V), oxytetracycline (Terramycin), and doxycycline (Vibramycin)
4. Products are available for oral, intramuscular, or intravenous use
5. Oral tetracyclines should not be given with milk, antacids, or iron since these substances inhibit absorption of the tetracycline

D. Cephalosporin antibiotics
1. Cephalosporin antibiotics are broad spectrum antibiotics
2. Examples of products are cephalothin (Keflin), cefazolin (Kefzol, Ancef), cephalexin (Keflex), cefamandole nafate (Mandole), and cefoxitin (Mefoxin)
3. Products are available for oral, intramuscular, or intravenous use
4. For patients allergic to penicillin, there is a small chance of cross-allergenicity to cephalosporins. Observe patients carefully

E. Aminoglycoside antibiotics
1. Aminoglycoside antibiotics are potent broad spectrum antibiotics for treatment of serious infections

2. Examples are streptomycin, kanamycin (Kantrex), gentamicin (Garamycin), tobramycin (Nebcin), and amikacin (Amikin)
3. They may cause damage to the ear (tinnitus, hearing loss, dizziness) and kidney (renal failure)
4. These products are usually administered intramuscularly or intravenously

F. Chloramphenicol (Chloromycetin)
1. Chloramphenicol is broad spectrum antibiotic
2. Use is limited because serious, irreversible blood disorders, such as aplastic anemia, may result
3. This product is administered orally or intravenously

G. Erythromycin (Erythrocin, Ilosone)
1. Alternative to penicillin used frequently in patients allergic to penicillin
2. Usually administered orally

H. Antifungal agents
1. Nystatin (Mycostatin) is used for *Candida albicans* (monilia) infections
2. Griseofulvin (Fulvicin) is given orally for topical fungal infections of the skin and nails
3. Amphotericin B (Fungizone) is given intravenously for systemic fungal infections such as histoplasmosis

Sulfonamides ("sulfa" drugs)

A. Sulfonamides are useful for variety of infections; used frequently for urinary tract infections
B. Side effects include GI upset, allergic reactions, headache, and jaundice
C. Examples of products are sulfadiazine, sulfisoxazole (Gantrisin), sulfamethoxazole (Gantanol), and trimethoprim with sulfamethoxazole (Bactrim, Septra)
D. Patients should increase fluid intake to prevent possible sulfonamide crystallization in the kidneys (crystalluri)
E. Products are usually administered orally

Laxatives

A. Used to treat constipation, to prepare bowel for x-ray examination, to prevent straining at stool, and to treat some types of poisoning
B. Bulk-producing laxatives, such as Metamucil or Effersylium, increase the mass of fecal material; used when there is insufficient bulk in diet
C. Lubricant laxatives, such as mineral oil, lubricate large intestine to facilitate passage of fecal material
D. Irritant laxatives, such as phenolphthalein, cascara, castor oil, bisacodyl (Dulcolax), and danthron (Modane), stimulate peristaltic movements of the intestine
E. Saline cathartics retain water in the colon to soften feces and stimulate peristalsis. They act rapidly. Examples are milk of magnesia, magnesium sulfate (Epsom salts), and magnesium citrate solution
F. Stool softeners, such as dioctyl sodium sulfosuccinate (Colace), are detergents that allow water to penetrate and soften the fecal material; they are useful in patients with hemorrhoids or with a recent myocardial infarction where straining at stool could be detrimental

DRUG DISTRIBUTION SYSTEMS

A. These are the methods and procedures by which hospitals and other institutions deliver drugs to their patients
B. In each drug distribution system, the physician must first order the drug for the patient on the physician's order form. The order should include the name of the drug, the dose, the route of administration, and the frequency of administration
C. In the *complete floor stock system,* medications are kept at the nursing station in bulk. The nurse interprets the medication order, prepares the medication card and medication profile (Kardex), prepares the medication tray, and administers the drugs
D. In the *individual patient prescription system,* the nurse interprets the physician's order, prepares the medication card, enters the drug on the Kardex, and requisitions the drug from the pharmacy. The pharmacy dispenses a supply of medication for the individual patient, and the nurse prepares the medication tray and administers the drug
E. Some institutions use a combination of the floor stock system and the individual patient prescription system. Inexpensive, frequently used drugs are kept in the nursing station, and other medications are dispensed by the pharmacy for individual patients
F. In a *unit dose drug distribution system,* a carbon copy of the original physician's order is sent to the pharmacy. The pharmacist interprets the order and keeps a medication profile for each patient. Individually packaged single dosage units of medications are placed into a medication cart that is delivered to the nursing station at predetermined times. Medications are administered by the nurse. This system is

designed to save nursing time and involve the pharmacist to a greater degree. It is used by an increasing number of institutions.

MEDICATIONS AND THE PRACTICAL NURSE

A. Regulations of the hospital or other institution designate which medications, if any, may be administered by the practical nurse. The practical nurse should know this policy
B. The practical nurse should be familiar with each drug he or she administers (desired effect, side effects, dose, precautions, special observations or nursing care required)
C. The practical nurse should be able to calculate and measure doses accurately
D. The five ''rights'' of medication administration are right drug, right patient, right dose, right time, and right route of administration
E. The practical nurse should know hospital procedures for ordering and charting medications
F. No medication may be administered unless ordered by a physician.
G. No medication may be left at the patient's bedside unless specified by a physician

COMMON SYMPTOMS OF DRUG OVERDOSAGE

A. Nausea and vomiting
B. Diarrhea or constipation
C. Changes in respiration
   1. Respiratory rate increase or decrease
   2. Deep or shallow respirations
   3. Dyspnea
D. Cardiovascular changes
   1. Fast or slow pulse rate
   2. Irregular pulse
   3. Blood pressure changes
E. Disorientation or delirium
F. Mental depression or excitement
G. Convulsions
H. Skin changes
   1. Cyanosis or bluish discoloration
   2. Flushing
   3. Pallor
   4. Rash, itching, or hives
   5. Sweating
I. Pupil size changes
J. Fever or subnormal temperature
K. Urinary changes

BASIC SCIENCE REVIEW QUESTIONS

Read each question carefully and consider all possible answers. When you have decided which answer is **best,** blacken in the corresponding space on the answer sheet. There is only **one** best answer for each question.

Physics

1 A basin used for a hand or foot soak should not be filled more than two thirds because of the principle
   1. Molecules of one substance distribute themselves uniformly in another
   2. A body displaces an equal volume of water
   3. The force between two parts of the same substance holds them together
   4. A substance is divided by equal volume of water

2 The exchange of oxygen and carbon dioxide in respiration depends primarily on the principle involving
   1. Adhesion
   2. Cohesion
   3. Density
   4. Diffusion

3 Kinetic energy is energy of
   1. Motion
   2. Position
   3. Function
   4. Distance

4 The principle of gravity is important in all of the following *except*
   1. Blood pressure
   2. Fowler's position for drainage
   3. Elevating an extremity
   4. Capillary action

5 The principle of levers is used in
   (A) Lifting patients
   (B) Carrying trays
   (C) Positioning patients
   (D) Lubricating tubes for insertion

1. A and B
2. B and C
3. B, C, and D
4. A, B, and C

6 The principles of pressure are used in nursing in
1. Stimulation for voiding
2. Use of lubricants on tubes for insertion
3. Cleaning equipment
4. Use of powder for backrub

7 The principles of light are used in
(A) Radiation
(B) X-ray examination
(C) Ultraviolet
(D) Identifying the choroid coat of the eye
1. A and B
2. B and C
3. B, C, and D
4. A, B, and C

8 A calorie is a form of
1. Light
2. Heat
3. Sound
4. Food

9 One of the principles of ventilation is that warm air rises; this depends on
1. Density
2. Cohesion
3. Diffusion
4. Osmosis

10 The rate of flow of blood in the vessels depends on all of the following *except*
1. Pressure
2. Size of the tube
3. Viscosity
4. Amount of surfactant

11 The instrument used to measure specific gravity is
1. Sphygmomanometer
2. Hydrometer
3. Stethoscope
4. Dip stick

Chemistry

12 Oxygen is
1. Slightly acid
2. Insoluble in water
3. Lighter than air
4. Odorless

13 The universal solvent is
1. Oxygen
2. Water
3. Gasoline
4. Carbon dioxide

14 Carbon dioxide is a
1. Respiratory stimulant
2. Respiratory depressant
3. Cough depressant
4. Cough expectorant

15 Since oxygen supports combustion, it is important that
1. The tank is closed tightly when in use
2. All cigarettes and matches are removed from the room
3. Oil is used sparingly
4. Patients get oil rubs rather than alcohol rubs

16 Osmosis is
1. The force that causes the surface of a liquid to contract
2. Insoluble substances suspended in a liquid
3. The flow of a solvent through a semipermeable membrane
4. A solute uniformly distributed into all parts of the solution

17 The presence of blood in the urine is called
1. Hematuria
2. Hematoma
3. Uremia
4. Proteinuria

Microbiology

18 Poliomyelitis is caused by
1. Bacteria
2. Protozoa
3. Virus
4. Rickettsiae

19 Pathogenic organisms are
1. Used in the pasteurization process
2. More plentiful than any other type of organism
3. Important to industry
4. Harmful to humans

20 Autoclaving, a means of sterilization, will destroy
1. All microorganisms
2. Pathogenic microorganisms
3. Nonpathogenic microorganisms
4. Just yeasts and molds

21 All microorganisms
1. Form spores
2. Have a waxy coating
3. Are protoplasm consisting of protein
4. Adapt to adverse environment

22 Factors influencing inhibition of growth and destruction of microorganisms include
(A) Temperature and contact
(B) Absence of organic material
(C) Time
(D) Spore formation
1. B, C, and D
2. A, B, and D
3. A, C, and D
4. A, B, and C

Anatomy and physiology

23 Groups of several kinds of tissues having a special function are called
1. Systems
2. Cavities
3. Organs
4. Muscles

24 The functions of the skeletal system are to
(A) Give shape to the body
(B) Provide attachment for muscles
(C) Protect delicate organs
(D) Manufacture red blood cells
(E) Excrete hormones
1. B, C, and E
2. A, B, C, and E
3. A, B, C, and D
4. A, B, and D

25 The covering of bones is called
1. Endometrium
2. Myocardium
3. Periosteum
4. Pericardium

26 The bone above the knee is the
1. Tibia
2. Femur
3. Fibula
4. Patella

27 The shin bone is the
1. Tibia
2. Fibula
3. Femur
4. Patella

28 The flat bone forming the anterior part of the thoracic cavity is the
1. Scapula
2. Sternum
3. Clavicle
4. Humerus

29 The knee joint is an example of a
1. Ball-and-socket joint
2. Hinge joint
3. Pivot joint
4. Gliding joint

30 The pelvic girdle is formed by the
(A) Ileum
(B) Ischium
(C) Pubis
(D) Femur
(E) Patella
1. A, B, C, and D
2. A, C, and D
3. A, B, and C
4. B, C, D, and E

31 The radius is located
1. In the upper part of the arm
2. On the thumb side of the lower arm
3. On the little finger side of the lower arm
4. At the shoulder joint

32 Paranasal (or head) sinuses are located in the following bones
(A) Frontal bone
(B) Mandible
(C) Maxilla
(D) Nasal bones
(E) Temporal bones
1. A and C
2. A, C, and D
3. A, C, D, and E
4. B, C, and E

33 The lines of junctions of immovable bones are called
1. Neurons
2. Sutures
3. Joints
4. Sinuses

34 The functions of the muscular system are to
(A) Give movement
(B) Keep body erect
(C) Give body shape
(D) Produce heat
(E) Produce red blood cells
1. A, B, D, and E
2. A, B, and D
3. A, B, C, and E
4. A, B, C, and D

35 Muscles are attached to bones by
1. Ligaments
2. Bursae
3. Tendons
4. Neurons

36 The type of muscle found in the visceral organs and blood vessels is called
1. Voluntary
2. Cardiac
3. Myocardium
4. Involuntary

37 The dome-shaped muscle between the chest and abdomen is called the
1. Pericardium
2. Peritoneum
3. Diaphragm
4. Deltoid

38 The large calf muscle is known as
1. Quadriceps femoris
2. Gluteus maximus
3. Hamstring group
4. Gastrocnemius

39 The region of the upper arm into which hypodermics are given is known as the
1. Quadriceps
2. Deltoid
3. Gluteus maximus
4. Triceps

40 The functions of the nervous system are to
(A) Provide communication between parts of the body
(B) Control body systems
(C) Integrate body activities
(D) Be the center of mental processes
(E) Aid in metabolism of fats
1. A, B, D, and E
2. A, B, C, and D
3. A, C, and E
4. B, C, and D

41 The covering of the brain and spinal cord is called
1. Cortex
2. Cerebrum
3. Cerebellum
4. Meninges

42 The cerebellum functions to
(A) Regulate temperature
(B) Maintain body balance
(C) Coordinate working of muscles
(D) Control metabolism
(E) Regulate voluntary movements
1. A, B, C, and E
2. A, B, C, and D
3. B and C
4. B and E

43 The functions of the cerebrospinal fluid are to
(A) Nourish brain and spinal cord
(B) Transmit messages to and from brain
(C) Control consciousness
(D) Protect brain and spinal cord from pressure
(E) Separate brain from spinal cord
1. A and D
2. B and C
3. A, C, and D
4. B, D, and E

44 The following activities are centered in the cerebrum
(A) Thinking
(B) Memory
(C) Consciousness
(D) Judgment
(E) Balance and coordination
1. A, B, and D
2. B, D, and E
3. A, B, D, and E
4. A, B, C, and D

45 The largest parasympathetic nerve in the human body is the
1. Vagus
2. Trochlear
3. Optic
4. Intrinsic

46 In the complex sense of vision the image of an object is focused on the retina and is transmitted to the brain by the
1. Cornea
2. Optic nerve
3. Lens
4. Iris

47 The first coat of the eyeball that covers the anterior portion of the eye is called the
1. Cornea
2. Choroid
3. Sclera
4. Retina

48 The accessory structures of the eye are
(A) Eyelashes
(B) Lens
(C) Eyebrows
(D) Lacrimal apparatus
(E) Cornea
1. A, C, and D
2. A, B, C, and D
3. A, B, and C
4. B, D, and E

49 The organ of hearing is in the part of the ear called the
1. Auditory canal
2. Eustachian tube
3. Semicircular canal
4. Cochlea

50 The functions of the circulatory system are
(A) Transportation
(B) Protection
(C) Coordination
(D) Heat regulation
(E) Metabolism
1. A, B, C, and D
2. A, B, and D
3. B, C, and E
4. C, D, and E

51 The membrane covering the heart is called the
1. Pericardium
2. Myocardium
3. Ventricle
4. Perineum

52 The heartbeat changes under certain conditions and influences. Some of these are
(A) Clotting time
(B) Chemical conditions in blood
(C) Certain drugs

(D) Temperature changes
(E) Exercise
1. A, B, C, and E
2. A, B, and D
3. B, C, and E
4. B, C, D, and E

53 The amount of blood in the average adult human is
1. 9 to 15 pints
2. 10 to 20 pints
3. 8 to 12 pints
4. 2 to 6 pints

54 The blood consists of
(A) Plasma
(B) Insulin
(C) Red blood cells
(D) White blood cells
(E) Platelets
1. A, B, and D
2. B, C, and E
3. B, C, D, and E
4. A, C, D, and E

55 Inflammation of the heart muscle is called
1. Pericarditis
2. Peritonitis
3. Endocarditis
4. Myocarditis

56 The white blood cells are important for health because they
(A) Aid in combating infection
(B) Contain the Rh factor
(C) Combat foreign bodies
(D) Repair tissue
(E) Regulate metabolism
1. A, B, D, and E
2. A, B, C, and D
3. A, C, and D
4. B, C, and E

57 The cells of the blood that aid in blood clotting are called
1. Leukocytes
2. Platelets
3. Lymphocytes
4. Monocytes

58 Into which part of the heart does the blood return from the lungs?
1. Left ventricle
2. Left atrium
3. Right ventricle
4. Right atrium

59 Lymph vessels are in the
1. Arteries
2. Veins
3. Tissue spaces
4. Arterioles

60 Lymph nodes are located in the
(A) Submaxillary
(B) Cervical
(C) Cubital
(D) Spinal canal
(E) Inguinal
(F) Mesentery
1. B, D, and E
2. A, C, and F
3. A, B, C, D, and E
4. A, B, C, E, and F

61 The system that serves to exchange gases between the air and the blood is known as the
1. Cardiovascular system
2. Respiratory system
3. Genitourinary system
4. Excretory system

62 The anatomic name for the ''voice box'' is
1. Pharynx
2. Trachea
3. Bronchi
4. Larynx

63 The lungs function to replace the carbon dioxide with oxygen as blood passes through them; this is called
1. Arterial circulation
2. Venous circulation
3. Pulmonary circulation
4. Bronchial circulation

64 Many children with tonsillitis develop ear infection; this is because the ear and throat are connected by the
1. Larynx
2. Eustachian tube
3. Epiglottis
4. Esophagus

65 The respiratory center is located in the part of the brain called the
1. Medulla
2. Thalamus
3. Midbrain
4. Cerebellum

66 The digestive system has the following functions
(A) Prepares food for metabolism
(B) Prepares food for absorption
(C) Eliminates carbon dioxide
(D) Eliminates waste products
(E) Protects against microorganisms
1. A, B, and D
2. B, C, and E
3. B, C, D, and E
4. A, B, C, and D

67 The *principal* organs of digestion are
(A) Teeth
(B) Mouth
(C) Stomach
(D) Small intestine
(E) Large intestine
1. B, C, D, and E
2. A, B, C, and D
3. A, B, and D
4. B, C, and E

68 *Accessory* organs of digestion are
(A) Teeth
(B) Tongue
(C) Esophagus
(D) Salivary glands
(E) Appendix
1. A, B, D, and E
2. A, B, C, and D
3. A, C, and D
4. A, B, and D

69 During swallowing, food is stopped from entering the larynx by the
1. Esophagus
2. Pharynx
3. Eustachian tube
4. Epiglottis

70 Bile is secreted by the
1. Pancreas
2. Spleen
3. Gallbladder
4. Liver

71 In the walls of the stomach are glands that secrete substances that aid in digestion; these substances include
(A) Saliva
(B) Mucus
(C) Vitamins
(D) Hydrochloric acid
(E) Enzymes
1. A, B, D, and E
2. B, D, and E
3. B, C, and D
4. A, C, D, and E

72 The appendix is attached to the
1. Duodenum
2. Rectum
3. Cecum
4. Ileum

73 The four different kinds of teeth are
(A) Incisors
(B) Canines
(C) Alveolars
(D) Bicuspids
(E) Molars
1. B, C, D, and E
2. A, B, D, and E
3. A, B, C, and E
4. A, B, C, and D

74 Teeth are composed of the following parts
(A) Enamel
(B) Pulp cavity
(C) Nerve
(D) Dentin
(E) Gum
1. A, B, and D
2. A, B, D, and E
3. A, B, C, and E
4. A, C, and E

75 The openings of the parotid glands are situated
1. Behind the sternum
2. In the pancreas
3. Below the cerebrum
4. In the mouth

76 Secretions that chemically aid in digestion are
1. Enzymes
2. Vitamins
3. Osterones
4. Hormones

77 The small intestine is composed of the
(A) Rectum
(B) Duodenum
(C) Cecum
(D) Jejunum
(E) Ileum
1. A, B, and D
2. A, C, and E
3. B, D, and E
4. A, B, and E

78 One of the most important glands in the body, often referred to as the "master gland," is the
1. Thyroid
2. Thymus
3. Adrenal
4. Pituitary

79 The hormone secreted by the male sex glands is called
1. Estrogen
2. Progesterone
3. Insulin
4. Testosterone

80 A ductless gland that decreases at puberty is called the
1. Adrenal
2. Pituitary
3. Thyroid
4. Thymus

81 The skin is essential to health; its functions are to
(A) Protect tissues from injury and infection
(B) Regulate temperature
(C) Aid in elimination
(D) Aid in digestion
(E) Provide nerve endings for senses of pain and touch
1. B, C, and E
2. A, B, C, and E
3. A, B, C, and D
4. A, B, and C

82 Types of glands found in the skin are
(A) Sebaceous
(B) Sweat
(C) Adrenal
(D) Thyroid
(E) Ceruminous, or wax
1. B, C, and D
2. A, B, C, and E
3. A, B, C, and D
4. A, B, and E

83 The lining of the uterus is called the
1. Peritoneum
2. Endometrium
3. Perineum
4. Myometrium

84 Menstruation depends primarily on the
1. Circulating blood
2. Hormone action
3. Digestion
4. Intake of fluids

85 Menarche may be defined as the
1. Climacteric
2. Cessation of menses
3. Onset of menstruation
4. Fertilization of the ovum

86 The sperm of the male as the general rule unites with the ovum or egg of the female in the
1. Ovary
2. Fallopian tube
3. Uterus
4. Cervix

87 The urinary system is lined with
1. Muscle
2. Serous membrane
3. Skin
4. Mucous membrane

88 The urinary system is composed of the following organs
(A) Bladder
(B) Ureter
(C) Vagina
(D) Uterus
(E) Urethra
(F) Anus
1. A, B, C, D, and E
2. A, B, and E
3. A, B, E, and F
4. C, D, and E

89 In the body there are
1. 206 bones
2. 256 bones
3. 215 bones
4. 201 bones

90 The body is divided into two cavities; they are
(A) Dorsal
(B) Trunk
(C) Lumbar
(D) Ventral
(E) Sacral
1. A and D
2. A and B
3. B and C
4. C and E

91 The fibrous tissue connecting bone to bone is called
1. Cartilage
2. Tendon
3. Muscle
4. Ligament

92 The mastoid sinuses open into the
1. Inner ear
2. Middle ear
3. Outer ear
4. Semicircular canal

93 Weak spots in the abdominal wall are the
(A) Umbilicus
(B) Inguinal ring
(C) Femoral ring
(D) Appendix
1. A, B, and D
2. A, B, and C
3. A, C, and D

94 True tastes include all *except*
1. Sweet
2. Sour
3. Bitter
4. Blends

95 The pancreas secretes
1. Insulin
2. Adrenaline
3. Gastric juice
4. Estrogen

96 Most of the digested food is absorbed in the
1. Esophagus
2. Stomach
3. Small intestine
4. Large intestine

97 Water is mostly absorbed from the digestive tract in the
1. Esophagus
2. Stomach
3. Small intestine
4. Large intestine

98 The hormone secreted by the female is
1. Estrogen
2. Progesterone
3. Insulin
4. Testosterone

99 Thyroid is effective only in the presence of
1. Calcium
2. Iodine
3. Potassium
4. Sodium chloride

100 The largest single constituent of the human body is
1. Sodium
2. Water
3. Fat
4. Protein

101 Water leaves the body through
(A) Kidneys
(B) Lungs
(C) Skin
(D) Inspiration
1. A and B
2. A and D
3. C and D
4. A, B, and C

102 Weight change of 2.2 pounds represents a fluid loss or gain of
1. 1000 ml
2. 1100 ml
3. 1050 ml
4. 1200 ml

103 The normal pH for body fluids is
1. 9.1 to 9.6
2. 7.35 to 7.45
3. 4.4 to 5.4
4. 7 to 7.1

104 The major acid produced in the body is carbonic acid, which is eliminated by the
1. Kidneys in the form of urine
2. Skin in the form of urea
3. Lungs in the form of carbon dioxide
4. Gastrointestinal tract in the form of feces

Nutrition

105 The functions of food in the body are to
(A) Give energy
(B) Build and repair body tissue
(C) Regulate the sexes
(D) Regulate body processes
1. A, B, and C
2. B, C, and D
3. A, C, and D
4. A, B, and D

106 In purchasing eggs it is best to buy only eggs that are
(A) Fresh and washed
(B) Grade A or AA
(C) Large or extra large
(D) Refrigerated
1. A and B
2. D
3. A, B, and C
4. C and D

107 Many health departments recommend that only pasteurized milk be used for drinking because
(A) Bacteria will not grow in pasteurized milk
(B) Disease-producing bacteria have been destroyed
(C) Raw milk tastes peculiar
(D) It is not as expensive as raw milk
1. A and B
2. B
3. A and C
4. B and D

108 If followed, the Basic Four food plan will ensure the family against
1. Communicable diseases
2. Obesity
3. Spending too much money for food
4. Malnutrition

109 An adequate diet should include
(A) Fat
(B) Minerals
(C) Vitamins
(D) Carbohydrates
(E) Proteins
1. A, D, and E
2. A, C, and D
3. A, C, D, and E
4. A, B, C, D, and E

110 The caloric value of 1 g of carbohydrate, protein, and fat is as follows
(A) 1 g of carbohydrate provides 4 calories
(B) 1 g of carbohydrate provides 6 calories
(C) 1 g of protein provides 9 calories
(D) 1 g of protein provides 4 calories
(E) 1 g of fat provides 4 calories
(F) 1 g of fat provides 9 calories
1. A, D, and F
2. A, C, and E
3. B, C, and F
4. B, D, and E

111 The main function of protein in the diet is to
1. Supply energy
2. Carry vitamins to all parts of the body
3. Supply material for growth and tissue repair
4. Utilize fluids

112 Substances in the diet that supply energy to the body are
(A) Fat
(B) Minerals
(C) Vitamins
(D) Water
(E) Carbohydrates
1. A and D
2. B and C
3. C and E
4. A and E

113 In order to preserve the vitamin content of food in cooking
(A) Use as little water as possible
(B) Always start cooking in cold water
(C) Cover pan tightly
(D) Add vegetables to boiling water
(E) Cook as short a time as possible
1. A and B
2. A, B, and D
3. A, C, D, and E
4. A, B, C, and D

114 Eggs contribute the following to the diet
(A) Carbohydrate
(B) Vitamins
(C) Iron and protein
(D) Calcium
1. A and C
2. C
3. A and B
4. B and C

115 Meat contributes the following to the diet
1. Carbohydrate and fat
2. Fluid
3. Vitamin B complex and protein
4. Vitamin D

116 Cooking food by dry heat is done by
1. Boiling
2. Steaming
3. Broiling
4. Stewing

117 Good substitutes for meat are
(A) Cheese
(B) Rice and spaghetti
(C) Eggs
(D) Avocados
1. A and B
2. A and C
3. C and D
4. A, B, and C

118 Vitamin C is destroyed by contact with air; therefore, orange juice should
(A) Never be canned
(B) Always be frozen
(C) Be used when freshly squeezed or opened
(D) Be kept in tightly closed container
1. A
2. B
3. C and D
4. A and D

Pharmacology

119 Aspirin is the same as
1. Paraaminobenzoic acid
2. Hydrochloric acid
3. Paraaminosalicylic acid
4. Acetylsalicylic acid

120 Penicillin is known as
1. An antiseptic
2. An antibiotic
3. A sulfonamide
4. An anesthetic

121 Atropine sulfate
1. Dilates the pupils
2. Constricts the pupils
3. Has no effect on pupils

122 One of the tranquilizing drugs is
1. Coramine
2. Adrenalin
3. Digitalis
4. Thorazine

123 Darvon is used as
1. A local anesthetic
2. An antipyretic
3. A sedative
4. An analgesic

124 In giving morphine, a narcotic, the nurse would
1. Count pulse
2. Count respirations
3. Check blood pressure
4. Check color

125 Atropine sulfate is given for one of the following reasons, as
1. An antispasmodic
2. A respiratory depressant
3. A blood stimulant
4. A cough stimulant

126 An antiemetic is given to
1. Prevent nausea and vomiting
2. Stimulate nausea and vomiting
3. Depress a cough
4. Stimulate coughing

127 Phenytoin is used primarily as
1. A hypnotic
2. An anticonvulsant
3. An analgesic
4. An anesthetic

128 Penicillin is made from
1. Bacteria
2. Yeast
3. Mold
4. None of these

129 Toxicology is the branch of pharmacology dealing with the
1. Interactions of drugs
2. Treatment of poisonings
3. Medical treatment of disease
4. Allergic reactions to drugs

130 The official drug reference books are
1. The *Physician's Desk Reference* and the *American Hospital Formulary Service*
2. The *United States Pharmacopeia* and the *Physician's Desk Reference*
3. The *United States Pharmacopeia* and the *National Formulary*
4. The *National Formulary* and *Facts and Comparisons*

131 The current law specifically regulating narcotics and other addictive substances is the
1. Controlled Substances Act
2. Harrison Narcotic Act
3. Food, Drug, and Cosmetic Act

132 A tablet placed under the tongue is called a
1. Chewable tablet
2. Buccal tablet
3. Hypodermic
4. Sublingual tablet

133 An enteric-coated tablet disintegrates in the
1. Mouth
2. Stomach
3. Intestine
4. Rectum

134 Before administering a drug in the form of a suspension, the nurse should always
1. Shake it well
2. Warm it to body temperature
3. Pour off any water at the top
4. Dilute it with water

135 A Spansule is a
1. Type of suppository
2. Pellet for implantation under the skin
3. Sustained-release tablet
4. Sustained-release capsule

136 A drug produces its effect most rapidly when administered by the following route
1. Intramuscular
2. Intravenous
3. Oral
4. Subcutaneous

137 Some oral medications may upset the stomach and should be given
1. After meals on a full stomach
2. Before meals on an empty stomach
3. During the night

138 An anthelmintic is a drug that
1. Neutralizes stomach acid
2. Prevents convulsions
3. Produces bowel movements
4. Destroys worms in the GI tract

139 Drugs used to lower blood pressure in patients with hypertension are called
1. Antihypertensives
2. Antihistamines
3. Hypertensives
4. Antihypotensives

140 Drugs used to reduce fever are called
1. Analgesics
2. Antipruritics
3. Anticholinergics
4. Antipyretics

141 An expectorant is a drug used to
1. Prevent anxiety
2. Prevent nausea
3. Treat nasal congestion
4. Promote expulsion of mucus from the respiratory tract

142 A drug requiring refrigeration should be kept in the following temperature range
1. $-4°$ to 14°F
2. 36° to 46°F
3. 46° to 59°F
4. 59° to 86°F

143 A dose of 0.5 g of erythromycin is to be given using 250 mg tablets. The nurse should administer
1. $^1/_2$ tablet
2. 4 tablets
3. $^1/_5$ tablet
4. 2 tablets

144 Phenobarbital elixir contains 20 mg per 5 ml. For a dose of 30 mg one should administer
1. 5.5 ml
2. 3.3 ml
3. 7.5 ml
4. 10 ml

145 The amount of a pure drug used to prepare a 500 ml of a 10% W/V solution is
1. 10 g
2. 50 g
3. 50 ml
4. 0.5 g

146 The analgesic-antipyretic drug usually given to patients who cannot tolerate aspirin is
1. Tylenol
2. APC
3. Darvon Compound
4. Sodium salicylate

147 Nephrotoxicity and autotoxicity are potential side effects of
1. Erythromycin
2. Propoxyphene
3. Gentamicin
4. Meperidine

148 Narcan is classified as a
1. Narcotic analgesic
2. Cough suppressant
3. Tranquilizer
4. Narcotic antagonist

149 Barbiturates are used mainly as
1. Sedatives and hypnotics
2. Tranquilizers
3. Analgesics
4. Antipyretics

150 Valium is an example of
1. A narcotic
2. An analgesic
3. A tranquilizer
4. A barbiturate

151 Broad spectrum antibiotics are effective against
1. Many varieties of bacteria
2. Most bacteria and viruses
3. A few varieties of bacteria
4. Viruses

152 A patient allergic to one type of penicillin will be allergic to
1. Erythromycin
2. Tetracycline
3. Chloromycetin
4. Other types of penicillin

153 Colace is a member of the
1. Bulk-producing laxatives
2. Lubricant laxatives
3. Stool softener (detergent) laxatives
4. Stimulant (irritant) laxatives

154 When the pharmacist reviews a direct copy of the physician's order and dispenses medications in single dose packages, the drug distribution system is called the
1. Individual patient prescription system
2. Unit dose system
3. Complete floor stock system

4 FUNDAMENTALS OF NURSING

REFERENCES

American National Red Cross: Cardiopulmonary resuscitation, 1980.

American National Red Cross: Standard first aid and personal safety, ed. 2, New York, 1979, Doubleday & Co., Inc.

American National Red Cross: First aid for foreign body obstruction of the airway, 1978.

American National Red Cross: American National Red Cross guidelines and procedures: providing health services in disaster, 1976.

Bower, F.L.: The process of planning nursing care: a theoretical model, ed. 3, St. Louis, 1981, The C.V. Mosby Co.

Dison, N.: Clinical nursing techniques, ed. 4, St. Louis, 1979, The C.V. Mosby Co.

Elhart, D., and others: Scientific principles in nursing, ed. 8, St. Louis, 1978, The C.V. Mosby Co.

French, R.M.: Nurse's guide to diagnostic procedures, ed. 4, New York, 1975, McGraw-Hill Book Co.

Heimlich, H.J.: A life-saving maneuver to prevent food choking, J.A.M.A. **234**(44):398-401, 1975.

Henderson, J.: Emergency medical guide, New York, 1978, McGraw-Hill Book Co.

Holdsworth, V.E.: Fundamentals of bedside nursing, New York, 1968, Macmillan Publishing Co., Inc.

Hood, G.T., and Dincher, J.R.: Total patient care: foundations and practice, ed. 5, St. Louis, 1980, The C.V. Mosby Co.

Hornemann, G.V.: Basic nursing procedures, Albany, N.Y., 1972, Delmar Publishers.

Kozier, B., and Erb, G.L.: Fundamentals of nursing: concepts and procedures, Reading, Mass., 1979, Addison-Wesley Publishing Co., Inc.

Lamonica, E.L.: The nursing process: a humanistic approach, Reading, Mass., 1979, Addison-Wesley Publishing Co., Inc.

McInnes, M.E.: Essentials of communicable disease, ed. 2, St. Louis, 1975, The C.V. Mosby Co.

Meeks, D.R., and others: Practical nursing: a textbook for students and graduates, ed. 5, St. Louis, 1974, The C.V. Mosby Co.

Olsen, J.L., and others: Medical dosage calculations, ed. 2, Meadow Park, Calif., 1978, Benjamin-Cummings Publishing Co.

Scott, L.P.: Self-instruction and review in nursing, vol. 1, ed. 2, New York, 1979, Macmillan Publishing Co., Inc.

Strand, M.M., and Elmer, L.A.: Clinical laboratory tests: a manual for nurses, ed. 2, St. Louis, 1980, The C.V. Mosby Co.

Tucker, S.M., and others: Patient care standards, ed. 2, St. Louis, 1980, The C.V. Mosby Co.

Ulisse, G.C.: POMR: application to nursing records, Reading, Mass., 1978, Addison-Wesley Publishing Co., Inc.

U.S. Department of Health, Education and Welfare, Public Health Service: The role of the licensed practical nurse in national disaster, Health Mobilization Series, Washington, D.C., 1967, U.S. Government Printing Office.

Vaughan-Wrobel, B.C., and Henderson, B.: The problem-oriented system in nursing: a workbook, St. Louis, 1976, The C.V. Mosby Co.

Wood, L.A., and Rambo, B.: Nursing skills for allied health services, vols. 1, 2, and 3, ed. 2, Philadelphia, 1977, W.B. Saunders Co.

ENVIRONMENTAL FACTORS AFFECTING HEALTH

Health defined

A. Health is a dynamic state that is individually perceived and defined. The state of health is defined as the individual's optimal capacity and ability to function normally

B. The World Health Organization (WHO) defines health as "a state of complete physical, mental and social well-being and not merely an absence of disease or infirmity"

Illness defined

A. Illness is defined by the individual and is based on cultural differences and expectations

B. Illness is a state of disturbance in the biologic, psychologic, or sociologic functioning of the human individual

Environmental factors

A. Family
  1. Types of families include the following
    a. Nuclear family consists of parents and natural or adopted children
    b. Extended family consists of nuclear unit and grandparents or other relatives
    c. Single parent family consists of one parent (either sex) and children
  2. The level of fulfillment of family functions and responsibilities may have a relationship to individual health
    a. Providing emotional and financial security for children and other members
    b. Providing physical environment for health and welfare
    c. Setting standards for moral and ethical values for children
    d. Providing religious training
B. Socioeconomics
  1. Usually the health status of the family or individuals is directly related to their economic level
  2. Social or economic stresses are considered to have a relationship to illness
C. Physical environment
  1. Kind of neighborhood. This is determined by economic and social level, ethnic affiliations of residents, and location (rural or urban)
  2. Home. This may or may not be adequate for family needs
  3. Facilities in the neighborhood for recreation, education, and medical care. Availability of these will affect health
  4. Potential environmental hazards. These may include water, air, noise, waste disposal, and radiation. The adequacy of environmental protection affects present and future status of health
D. Religion
  1. Religion is an individual's interpretation or belief in a divine power
  2. One never attempts to force religion on another
  3. Major faiths are
    a. Catholic—Roman Catholic, Western Catholic but non-Roman, Eastern Orthodox, nonorthodox Eastern
    b. Protestant—Methodist, Baptist, Presbyterian, Episcopalian, Congregationalist, Lutheran, Moravian, Reformed, others
    c. Jewish—Orthodox, Conservative, Reformed
    d. Other denominations—Friend or Quaker, Jehovah's Witness, Seventh-Day Adventist, others
    e. Eastern religions—Buddhist, Hindu, Islamic

PATIENT AND FAMILY DURING ILLNESS

A. Patient is concerned with illness as it affects roles and responsibilities within the family
B. Problems may be
  1. Economic—any illness is expensive; how can family meet expenses
  2. Social
    a. Patient may have to leave neighborhood friends
    b. Cultural, educational, vocational, and recreational interests may inhibit adjustment
  3. Religious
    a. Family may have strong religious ties
    b. During illness, family may depend totally on religion
  4. Emotional
    a. Fear of the unknown
    b. Fear of outcome of illness
    c. Fear of what may become of the patient's family and home life

ASSESSMENT OF FACTORS AFFECTING HEALTH

A. Patient's reaction to his illness; patient may be emotionally upset, may be worried, or may refuse treatment
B. Economic aspects of illness
  1. Patient's loss of work permanently or temporarily
  2. Cost of hospital and medical care
  3. Ways of meeting cost (insurance)
C. Physical handicaps resulting from permanent or temporary illness
D. Prevention of future illnesses, handicaps, or accidents that interfere with health and normal activity
E. Social and emotional aspects of illness
  1. Interference with accustomed mode of life, work, recreation, and education
  2. Threat to patient's position in family, at work, and in social groups

F. Family's reaction to patient's illness
   1. Overprotection
   2. Resentment
   3. Constructive help
   4. Guilt

COMMUNICATION

Definition

Process of exchange of thoughts, information, directions, or emotions between two or more persons

A. May be oral, written, or expressed through body actions
B. Must involve sender and recipient

Tools

A. Observation (perception)
B. Body language (nonverbal)
C. Language
   1. Verbal
   2. Written

Principles of communication in nursing

A. Listening
   1. Verifying
   2. Interpreting
B. Reporting
   1. Observing
   2. Understanding observation
   3. Expressing observation to someone else
C. Recording
   1. Observing
   2. Interpreting observation
   3. Writing observation for someone else to interpret
D. Verbal and nonverbal communicating—may accomplish
   1. Diversion
   2. Reassurance
   3. Teaching
   4. Basis for planning better nursing care

Therapeutic communication

A. Definition—language that is purposeful and directed toward goals that benefit the patient
B. Nurses' role
   1. Establish confidence by competent delivery of patient care
   2. Identify and understand patient's needs
   3. Exhibit appropriate appearance, manner, and attitude
   4. Present nonjudgmental approach to patient's needs

ENVIRONMENT OF THE HOSPITALIZED PATIENT

Definition

Sum of immediate and distant external surroundings, which affects people and is in turn affected by them

A. Pleasant environment enhances feelings of safety and comfort
B. Physical environment affects patient recovery

Physical factors

A. Lighting
   1. Lighting should be indirect except for reading or procedures
   2. General lighting should be diffused
   3. Sunlight promotes healing and feeling of well-being
   4. Certain conditions may require decreased light
   5. Night light should be subdued
B. Waste disposal—trash, human excretion, and soiled dressings should be discarded according to institution's procedure
C. Purified water supply

Esthetic factors

A. Sound
   1. Music therapy promotes rest and relaxation
   2. Noise causes fatigue and anxiety
B. Decor
   1. Pastel colors (yellow, pink) are soothing and relaxing
   2. Harsh colors (red, black) overstimulate senses
   3. Flowers and pictures enhance environment
C. Odors
   1. Foul or strong odors should be eliminated by means of room deodorizer or removal of causative factor
   2. Mild, fragrant odors reduce antiseptic smell and patient embarrassment
D. Privacy—curtains, screens, and proper draping should be used as indicated to reduce embarrassment and protect patient's dignity

Atmospheric factors

A. Temperature of room—depends on
   1. Condition of patient
   2. Amount of ventilation
   3. Time of year
   4. Patient's comfort—68° to 74°F is comfortable to most individuals
B. Humidity of room
   1. Ideal humidity is 30% to 60%
   2. High humidity with low or high temperature is uncomfortable because perspiration does not evaporate and heat and cold intensify
   3. Low humidity causes chilliness through rapid evaporation of perspiration
   4. Humidity can be raised by a humidifier
C. Ventilation or movement of air
   1. Is important to supply fresh air free of large numbers of bacteria and dust particles
   2. Aids in evaporation of perspiration and in maintenance of proper humidity
   3. Necessitates care to avoid drafts
D. Air conditioning—helps to maintain proper temperature, humidity, and movement of air; thus windows are not opened

Safety factors

A. Proper care of hospital equipment
   1. Equipment should be stored properly
   2. All apparatus, equipment, and furnishings should be kept in good repair
   3. All equipment, apparatus, and furnishings should be correctly used
B. Prevention of fire
   1. Proper care and use of electrical equipment
   2. Minimization of smoking in bed
   3. Adequate care of oxygen equipment
C. Prevention of accidents
   1. Keep floor dry and clean
   2. Place rubber tips on crutches, canes, and walkers
   3. Dispose of dressings and needles properly
   4. Use siderails and safety straps
   5. Have frequent fire drills
   6. Lock wheels on beds, stretchers, and wheelchairs
   7. Maintain good lighting
D. Protection from germs and pests
   1. Proper disinfection and sterilization
   2. Hand washing
E. Use of restraints
   1. Restraints are used to prevent self-inflicted injury by patient
   2. Nurse should explain purpose to patient and family
   3. Restraints should be removed periodically to prevent tissue injury
   4. Nurse should obtain physician's order (if required by institution)
   5. Types of restraints are
      a. Limb restraint
      b. Jacket or vest
      c. Safety belt
   6. Precautions that must be taken are
      a. Nurse should check for circulation and skin irritation
      b. Restraints should be tied with square knot, which can be easily removed in case of emergency
      c. Placement should allow limited range of motion

Care of environment

A. Responsibilities of hospital housekeeping and ancillary services (central supply, maintenance)
   1. Daily damp dusting and straightening
   2. Scrubbing, disinfecting, sterilizing, and storing of equipment following patient transfer, discharge, or death
   3. Repairing or replacing defective equipment or furnishing
B. Responsibilities of the nurse
   1. Bedside table with call bell, phone, and personal articles is within reach
   2. Bedside unit is straightened and damp dusted (includes removal of dead flowers)
   3. Patient belongings (clothing, valuables, glasses, dentures, prosthesis) are cared for
   4. Cross-infection between patients is prevented

ASEPSIS

Medical

A. Medical asepsis is defined as free from infection (clean) or disease-causing organism (contaminated)
B. Applications to nursing call for
   1. Good hand-washing technique
   2. Proper handling of linen (do not shake linen or hold against clothes)
   3. Disinfection of contaminated items
   4. Cleansing from clean to contaminated area

C. Terminal disinfection is complete disinfection of room and all equipment after patient leaves
D. Isolation unit
   1. Gown, gloves, masks, and hand washing are required, as specified by institutional procedures
   2. Types of isolation include
      a. Respiratory—indicated when bacteria are spread by droplets (requires mask); example: tuberculosis
      b. Enteric—indicated when bacteria are transmitted in feces, throat secretions, or vomitus (requires gown and gloves); example: *Salmonella*
      c. Wound and skin—indicated when bacteria are found in wounds (requires gown, gloves, and mask during dressing change); example: *Staphylococcus*
      d. Blood—indicated when specific bacteria are found in blood (requires careful disinfection of equipment that comes in contact with patient's blood); example: hepatitis
      e. Strict—indicated when bacteria can be spread by contact and air (requires gown, gloves, and mask); example: *Staphylococcus*
      f. Protective or reverse—indicated when patients with lowered resistance to infection require protection from harmful bacteria in the environment (requires gown, gloves, and mask); example: burns
   3. Instructions given by institution for disinfection of linens, dishes, and all equipment used for isolated patients must be followed meticulously

Surgical

A. Surgical asepsis means sterilization of everything coming in contact with operative field or wound
B. Sterile items become contaminated (nonsterile) when touched by nonsterile items
C. Sterile objects falling below waist or table level are considered contaminated
D. Surgical field, once moist, is considerated contaminated

CARE OF PATIENT

Bed making

A. Purpose—to provide area of comfort and rest for patient; bed making should be functional to patient, physicians, and nurses
B. Equipment and linens as found in institutions
   1. Mattress protected with mattress pad and waterproof drawsheet or commercially waterproofed mattress
   2. Two sheets and one drawsheet for each bed
   3. Washable spread
   4. Pillows
      a. Should have protective waterproof case under cotton pillowcase
      b. Disposable pillows are available for single patient use
C. Care of soiled linens
   1. Always placed on a surface above floor or in individual laundry bags
   2. Deposited in linen receptacles provided in hospital (disposable "linens" are available and are used especially for patients with communicable diseases)
D. Types of bed making
   1. Closed bed is made in preparation for new patient
   2. Open bed is occupied, but patient is out of bed
   3. Occupied bed is made while patient is in it
   4. Fracture or orthopedic bed is made from head to foot
   5. Postanesthetic or recovery bed is made for patient while he is in surgery
E. Bed positions
   1. Low Fowler's—head is raised 18 to 20 inches above bed level
   2. Semi-Fowler's—head is raised 45 degrees and knee is raised (gatched) 15 degrees
   3. Trendelenburg's—head is lower than the level of the feet (mattress remains straight)
   4. Reverse Trendelenburg's—feet are lower than the head level (mattress remains straight)
   5. High Fowler's—head of bed is raised to a 90 degree angle

Personal hygiene of patient

A. Daily bath
   1. Bed bath—given to patient restricted to bed
   2. Tub bath or shower—for patient who may be up
B. Care of mouth
   1. Routine mouth care—use of toothbrush, mouthwash, or substitutes
   2. Special mouth care—routine care plus glycerin and lemon swabs or hydrogen peroxide as ordered

3. Care of dentures—important because dentures absorb odors easily
   a. Clean dentures over basin of water to reduce chance of breakage if dropped
   b. Provide privacy for cleaning dentures
   c. Dip dentures in cold water to help prevent friction and to make insertion easier; hot water may distort shape
   d. Keep dentures in denture cup while out of patient's mouth

C. Care of fingernails and toenails—daily and as indicated; must secure a physician's order before cutting fingernails or toenails; extreme care must be taken with those patients who have diabetes or circulatory problems
   1. Cut nails even with tips of fingers and toes
   2. Scrub fingernails and toenails as needed
   3. Round fingernails to curve with fingertips
   4. Cut toenails straight across

D. Care of back
   1. Cleanse thoroughly with soap and water
   2. Dry well
   3. Massage with lotion in long circular motions

E. Decubitus ulcer (bedsore or pressure sore)—watch especially areas over all bony prominences, such as base of spine, heels, elbows, and shoulder blades and along sides of casts or braces
   1. Causes
      a. Crumbs or food particles
      b. Moisture
      c. Wrinkles in sheet
      d. Lying in one position
      e. Poor circulation
      f. Poor nutritional state
   2. Treatment
      a. Care may include special cleansing and dressings as ordered by physician
      b. Ulcer should be prevented if possible by frequent bathing and massage to pressure areas and frequent changes of position
      c. Nurse should report any sign of redness or skin break and initiate proper care
      d. Sheepskin pads, air mattress, or water bed may be used
      e. Use of waterproof pads should be avoided

F. Care of hair
   1. Comb with each bath; groom as desired
   2. If tangled
      a. Use 95% alcohol for oily hair
      b. Use mineral oil for dry hair
      c. Start at end and work toward scalp
      d. Hold hair close to head to prevent pulling
   3. Braid long hair if patient does not object
   4. Shampoo as often as necessary and if patient's condition permits
   5. Give pediculosis treatment as ordered by physician
      a. Vinegar is used to loosen nits, which are then combed out with fine-toothed comb
      b. Patient with pediculosis may be isolated to avoid spread

G. Afternoon or evening (PM) care
   1. Prepares patient for supper and sleep
   2. Consists of
      a. Performing oral hygiene
      b. Washing face, hands, and back
      c. Rubbing back
      d. Tightening bed covers
      e. Straightening unit

H. Patient's comfort—both mental and physical comfort are desired
   1. Maintaining comfortable position in bed or chair
      a. Bed should be firm and smooth; bottom sheets should be tight, clean
      b. Pillows should be provided for support and comfort
      c. Bedside table, light, call bell, and personal belongings should be within reach of patient
      d. Affected limbs should be supported and position of function maintained
      e. Gatch bed or Fowler's position should be used if desired or ordered
      f. Backrest should be used
   2. Moving and turning patient
      a. Change patient's position at least every 2 hours; encourage patient to move if allowed
      b. Encourage passive and active exercise according to individual needs
      c. Get help when moving patient to wheelchair or stretcher if patient is helpless or heavy, and use Hoyer lift if needed
      d. Use Davis roller to assist in moving heavy patients in lying position

I. Care of incontinent patient—may be incontinence of urine or feces or both
   1. Condition is temporary during acute illness and permanent in some types of paralysis or senility
   2. Patient is often embarrassed by condition; help to relieve patient's anxiety by calm manner and

by teaching patient to care for self as soon as possible
3. Nurse should encourage patient to use bedpan or go to toilet at regular intervals (after meals and at bedtime)
4. Absorbent diaper or thick pad with moisture-proof covering is used
5. Nurse should protect mattress and bed covers
6. Skin care includes frequent bathing with mild soap and water, drying thoroughly, and gentle massaging with lotion
7. Personal and room deodorizers should be used

PATIENT'S CHART

Definition

Collection of important data about patients that is kept by nurse and other health team members responsible for any part of diagnosis or therapy of patient while under treatment in hospital, clinic, or home

A. Legal document
B. Complete record of patient's therapy, reactions and progress, and recommendations pertaining to illness and future treatment

Purposes

A. To aid physician in diagnosis and treatment
B. To help in study and research and planning of patient care
C. To keep all workers caring for patient informed

Data recorded by the nurse

A. Physical appearance
B. Mental and emotional state
C. Levels of consciousness
D. State of senses
E. Vital signs
F. Nursing intervention

General principles

A. Charting is always in ink since it is permanent record
B. Wording is short, clear, and specific to avoid confusion
C. Content of all charts is confidential to avoid harming or embarrassing patient
D. Nothing is erased or eradicated from chart; if error is made, line is drawn through error, and word "error" is printed above it in ink
E. Charting is uniform and legible, with each item put in its proper place
F. All signatures are to be written as full names with titles
G. Factual statements employing proper descriptive terminology, rather than complete sentences, are used
H. In most sentences subject is understood; avoid using word "patient" since chart concerns patient
I. Use of abbreviations and symbols is limited to accepted ones

Techniques of charting

A. Problem-oriented medical record (POMR)—organized system of charting and systematic approach to problem solving
B. Standard—symptomatic approach including observations and nursing intervention in time sequence
C. Chronologic—method in which all members of the health team contribute observations and intervention on a single progress note

Charting and nurse

A. Different hospitals and different departments within hospital vary concerning responsibility of practical nurse for charting
B. Nurse should be familiar with information on charts of patients under his or her care
C. It is important to keep chart when caring for patient in home; chart may be only record of patient's progress for physician

ASSESSMENT OF PATIENT

Introduction

A. Systematic assessment of health-illness status derived from patient history, subjective and objective observations, examinations, laboratory data, and patient's response to environment used to formulate an ongoing plan of care
B. Available resources for making the assessment
   1. Patient
   2. Family
   3. Health team members
   4. Records

Physical examination

A. Purposes
   1. To find out type and extent of disease
   2. To check healthy persons at regular intervals for early signs of disease

B. Preparation of patient mentally and physically
   1. Explain procedures to patient
   2. Drape patient to provide comfort, warmth, and privacy
   3. Assist physician
C. Equipment necessary—depends on type of examination, technique, wishes of examining physician, and routine of hospital or clinic
D. Methods used by most physicians
   1. Inspection—looking at patient with trained eye; carefully inspecting entire body, skin, nails, eyes, ears, and muscles
   2. Palpation—feeling certain parts
   3. Percussion—tapping, especially over certain body cavities
   4. Auscultation—listening with ear or stethoscope to certain body sounds, especially from lungs and heart
E. Positions
   1. Supine (flat on back)—position is used for most of basic physical examinations (also called dorsal decubitus); usually only one pillow is used
   2. Prone (on abdomen)—position is used for examination of back
   3. Fowler's position (head of bed raised)—pillow or support is placed under knees as on Gatch frame; position may be high or low
   4. Knee-chest (genupectoral)—patient lies on chest and knees with face turned to one side; position is used for vaginal or rectal examinations or as exercise after childbirth
   5. Lithotomy—patient lies on back on special examining table with buttocks at edge of table and feet in stirrups; position is used for examination and treatment of vagina, bladder, or rectum
   6. Dorsal recumbent—patient lies on back with knees bent and feet flat on bed; position is used for vaginal examination
   7. Modified Trendelenburg's—patient lies on back with bed or table at 45 degree angle so that head is lower than body; knees may be bent over section of table; position is used for certain abdominal operations and if patient is in shock; reverse Trendelenburg's is just the opposite, with head elevated
   8. Sims's, or side-lying, position—patient lies on left side and chest with right knee and thigh drawn up; position is used for pelvic and rectal examinations and enemas

Vital signs

A. Temperature, pulse, respirations, and blood pressure are sometimes called vital signs or cardinal symptoms
B. Knowledge of normal ranges of temperature, pulse, and respirations (TPR) is essential; normal varies according to age, sex, size, and condition of patient
C. Variations are indicative of disease, reaction to therapy, or onset of complications
D. Vital signs are taken every 4 hours unless otherwise ordered; patient should not be awakened unless ordered by physician
E. Temperature
   1. Definition—measurement of balance between heat produced and lost in the body; temperature may be expressed in centigrade (C) or Fahrenheit (F)
   2. Instruments
      a. Clinical thermometer
      b. Electronic thermometer
      c. Heat sensitive paper
   3. Oral temperature—normal is 98.6°F or 37°C
      a. Place thermometer sublingually with lips closed until it registers in 3 to 5 minutes
      b. Cleanse thermometer with cotton or alcohol wipe before and after use unless disposable
      c. Do not take temperature after patient has been smoking, drinking hot or cold drinks, or eating or while patient is chewing gum; wait at least 10 minutes after patient discontinues these activities
      d. Repeat procedure if reading is abnormal
      e. If oxygen mask in use, take rectal temperature unless contraindicated
   4. Rectal temperature—normal is 99.6°F or 37.5°C; this method is contraindicated in rectal or perineal surgery, diarrhea, and other diseases of the rectum
      a. Lubricate tip of thermometer before insertion
      b. Insert thermometer $1\frac{1}{2}$ inches into rectum and hold in place 3 to 5 minutes
      c. Wait at least 30 minutes following an enema
   5. Axillary temperature—normal is 97.6°F or 36.4°C
      a. Dry axilla without causing friction, and put thermometer in place with stem upward
      b. Leave thermometer in place until it registers—approximately 10 minutes

F. Pulse
  1. Pulse is defined as rhythmic dilation of arteries produced by contraction of left ventricle forcing blood out of heart
  2. Nurse notes rate of pulse (number of beats per minute), regularity or rhythm, and general strength and character
  3. Rate varies with age and sex; normal for adults is 60 to 80 beats per minute; in infants and children pulse is more rapid; in aged persons pulse may be slower
  4. Methods and instruments are as follows
    a. Pulse is measured by applying digital pressure at any point where an artery can be compressed on bone, using index and third fingers
      (1) Radial
      (2) Carotid
      (3) Facial
      (4) Temporal
      (5) Femoral
      (6) Dorsal pedis
    b. Apical-radial pulse requires two people
      (1) The heartbeat is counted by placing a stethoscope over the apex of the heart and at the same time taking the radial pulse
      (2) The difference between the heart rate (apical pulse) and the radial pulse is called the pulse deficit
    c. Electronic devices may be used

G. Respiration
  1. Normal—15 to 20 per minute; rate varies with age
  2. Types
    a. Apnea is absence of respiration
    b. Dyspnea is difficult respiration
    c. Orthopnea requires sitting position for breathing
    d. Kussmaul's respiration is paroxysms of breathing preceding diabetic coma
    e. Stertorous respiration is accompanied by abnormal sounds resembling snores
    f. Cheyne-Stokes respiration is rhythmic, repeated cycle characterized by shallow respiration increasing in depth and sound and then stopping for few seconds
  3. Method of taking
    a. Ensure patient's cooperation by taking respiration without patient's knowledge
    b. Count either inspiration or expiration—not both
    c. Place patient's hand across chest when taking pulse to facilitate taking of respiration

H. Blood pressure
  1. Definition—force exerted by blood against walls of arteries
  2. Terms used to describe blood pressure
    a. Systolic pressure is highest degree of force; it is exerted as left ventricle contracts
    b. Diastolic pressure is lowest degree of force; it is exerted as heart rests
    c. Pulse pressure is difference between systolic and diastolic pressure
    d. Hypertension is high blood pressure
    e. Hypotension is low blood pressure
  3. Methods of taking arterial pressure
    a. Auscultatory method uses sphygmomanometer and stethoscope—first sound heard is systolic reading; last sound heard is diastolic reading
    b. Palpatory method uses sphygmomanometer and fingers
    c. Electronic device may be used

Weight

A. Patient should be weighed before breakfast or at same time every day

B. All excess clothing should be removed; approximately same amount of clothing should be worn each time

Laboratory tests

A. Introduction
  1. Purpose is to supplement physical examination in finding out what is wrong with patient
  2. Frequent examinations usually include examination of urine, feces, blood, sputum, and cerebrospinal fluid
  3. In certain cases tests also include gastric analysis, lumbar puncture, kidney and gallbladder analysis, and cultures and smears of discharges from eyes, nose, throat, and vagina
  4. Certain body functions, such as heart and metabolism, may be tested
  5. Practical nurse is often responsible for collection and care of specimens and for helping physician
  6. Patient instruction should be given before any procedure

7. Nurse is to follow procedure routine in accord with institution's policy

B. Collection and handling of specimens
   1. Specimen is sample of something collected for examination and testing
   2. Hospital's or physician's routine should be followed in regard to collecting, labeling, care, recording, and disposal
   3. Specimen is always collected in a clean or (if ordered) a sterile container with tight-fitting cover
   4. All specimens are labeled with patient's name, number, physician's name, specimen, test to be done, and date and time collected
   5. Strict medical asepsis should be followed in handling of specimens

C. Urinalysis (examination of urine)
   1. Single voided specimen (if female menstruating, note on label) is often routine on admission, otherwise specimen is taken from first voiding in morning
   2. Twenty-four-hour specimen is all urine voided in a 24-hour period, collected and measured, starting and ending with an empty bladder
   3. Clean-catch, midstream specimen is taken as follows: the urinary meatus is cleansed; the patient voids and is asked to interrupt voiding; the remaining specimen is caught in a sterile container
   4. Catheterized specimen is collected in sterile jar for sterile specimen
   5. Practical nurse may be responsible for testing urine for sugar and acetone when caring for diabetic patient. Examples of testing kits include Clinitest, Keto-diastix, and Tes-tape
   6. When obtaining sterile specimen from indwelling catheter, nurse should maintain a close drainage system by using a needle and syringe

D. Kidney function tests
   1. Practical nurse may be responsible for collecting specimens and labeling them accurately as ordered; nurse may need to force or restrict fluids as ordered
   2. For special tests, nurse should consult ward manual or laboratory or both

E. Collection of sputum
   1. Sputum is usually collected before breakfast
   2. Patient rinses mouth with clear water (mouthwash may destroy the microorganisms)
   3. Patient instructed to deep breathe, cough, and expectorate into appropriate container to bring up secretions from deep in throat or bronchi
   4. Mouth care is given after sputum collection

F. Examination of gastrointestinal (GI) tract
   1. Vomitus
      a. Vomitus should be saved for physician's inspection if it contains blood or anything unusual
      b. It may be sent to laboratory
      c. Mouth care is done after emesis
   2. Gastric specimen
      a. Gastric specimen is used for examination of contents of stomach
      b. Practical nurse may be responsible for giving test meal or medication as ordered and for preparing patient
   3. X-ray examination of GI tract
      a. Food and fluids are withheld before examination
      b. Following procedure, patient should be observed for evacuation of contrast media
   4. Gallbladder examination
      a. Patient is given dye, by mouth or intravenously, so that gallstones or other abnormalities are seen in x-ray examination
      b. Patient usually fasts before and during test but may be instructed to have high-fat diet before last x-ray examination
   5. Stool (feces)
      a. Patient voids first
      b. Suppository or tap water enema may be given
      c. Feces are collected in clean bedpan
      d. With wooden spatula, small portion of feces is put in container provided and covered immediately
      e. Specimen should be kept warm if it is to be examined for parasites

G. Cultures and smears from mucous membranes or any body opening—made by using aseptic precautions

H. Blood examinations
   1. Test is usually done by technician or physician
   2. Small amount of blood is taken from finger or lobe of ear for cell count, hemoglobin, or coagulation time
   3. For blood chemistry, sedimentation rate, and Wassermann test, blood is taken from vein (venipuncture)

I. Biopsy
   1. Specimen of tissue is taken for microscopic examination
   2. Biopsy is usually done when cancer is suspected
   3. Patient should be observed closely for bleeding following biopsy
J. Lumbar puncture
   1. Lumbar puncture is performed to obtain spinal fluid for examination; sometimes it is done to relieve pressure
   2. Nurse may help prepare patient and get equipment ordered ready for physician
   3. Patient lies on side with head almost touching knees so vertebrae are separated
   4. Physician inserts lumbar puncture needle between third and fourth lumbar vertebrae, and fluid is collected in sterile tubes
   5. Patient is kept quiet and flat in bed after test as ordered by physician
   6. Nurse is responsible for charting, recording, and observation of patient
   7. Specimen containers are labeled and numbered, according to order obtained before sending to laboratory

METHODS IN ADMINISTRATION OF MEDICINES

General principles

A. Nurse is responsible for knowledge of
   1. Nature of the drug
   2. Ranges of dosage
   3. Methods of administration
   4. Use, side effects, and contraindications
   5. Patient's allergies or sensitivities to drugs
B. Drugs may be withheld before laboratory tests or in case of unknown reactions
C. Patient is positioned properly to administer medication
D. Nurse will inform patient of any anticipated alterations in normal body function (drowsiness, urine discoloration, nausea)
E. Physician's order is checked before administration of any medication
F. Nurse gives all medications at time ordered
G. Controlled drugs are stored in a locked cabinet. Some drugs are kept at patient's bedside as ordered
H. Questions regarding medication order or abnormal reactions or both are reported to the physician immediately
I. Nurse carefully checks mathematics of dosage; if in doubt, equation is checked with head nurse or pharmacy
J. Poured medications are kept in a graduated container placed on a flat surface and read at eye level. Nurse measures liquids at bottom of meniscus
K. Nurse must crush large tablets to facilitate administration to children and certain adults
L. Any drug harmful to teeth (liquid ferrous sulfate) is given through straw
M. Oral medications are followed by liberal amounts of water unless contraindicated
N. Juices may be ordered to reduce unpleasant tastes

Routes of administration

A. Oral administration is simplest and most common route
B. Rectal administration of medications is by rectal tube, suppository, or enema
C. Inhalation administration is done by having patient breath in medication given by nebulizer or in steam
D. Inunction (topical) is administered by rubbing drug into clean, dry area of skin
E. Sublingual medications are administered by dissolving drug under tongue
F. Hypodermic administration is injection given under skin into subcutaneous tissue or into muscle as ordered, using sterile solutions with sterile syringe and needle
   1. Intradermal (directly under epidermis into dermis)
      a. A 1 or 2 ml syringe with 25-gauge needle is used
      b. Area of skin 2 inches in diameter is cleansed with disinfectant
      c. Injection is given almost parallel with or at 15 degree angle to skin on thinner portions of skin, such as inner part of lower arm
      d. Only few minims are given; area is not massaged after injection
   2. Subcutaneous (into subcutaneous layer of skin)
      a. A 2 ml syringe with 23- or 25-gauge needle is used because never more than 2 ml is given in one area
      b. Skin is cleansed with disinfectant
      c. Injection is given at 45 to 60 degree angle to skin, depending on size of patient; aspirate before injecting medication except before heparin administration

d. Injection is given mostly into arm, leg, or abdomen, where subcutaneous tissue is most abundant
e. Area is massaged after injection except following the administration of heparin
3. Intramuscular (into muscular layer of tissue)
a. Appropriate syringe with 1½ to 2½ inch long 22- or 20-gauge needle is used; never more than 3 ml is given into same area
b. Skin is cleansed with disinfectant
c. Injection is given at 60 to 90 degree angle to skin, depending on size of patient; aspirate before injecting medication
d. Injection is given mainly into deltoid muscle, gluteus maximus (buttock), and quadriceps femoris (large muscle of leg)
e. Area is massaged after injection
4. Tract method of intramuscular injection
a. Use 3 or 5 ml syringe with 2 to 4 inch long 20-gauge needle, depending on size of patient
b. Draw solution plus 0.5 cc of air into syringe
c. Change needle
d. Cleanse skin with disinfectant
e. Displace skin by pulling firmly in one direction
f. Insert needle at 90 degree angle, aspirate, and then inject medication and air slowly
g. Wait 10 seconds
h. Withdraw needle and release skin simultaneously
i. Massage area only if indicated

G. Intravenous administration (venoclysis) is infusion of large quantity of fluid into a vein
1. Purposes are to
a. Supply fluids to restore or maintain electrolyte balance
b. Supply drugs for immediate effect
c. Replace nutrients and vitamins
d. Replace blood loss
2. Only trained personnel should administer and regulate fluid administration
3. Amount of fluid to be given is ordered by physician; drip rate should be checked frequently by nurse
4. Venipuncture site care is performed daily or by institutional policies
5. Site is cleansed from venipuncture site outward
6. Limb used for venipuncture should be supported with arm board
7. When infusion is discontinued, site is checked frequently for bleeding

H. Hypodermoclysis is administration of large amounts of fluid into subcutaneous tissue
1. Purpose is to supply fluid and electrolytes when patient is unable to take them orally or by intravenous routes
2. Equipment used is same as for intravenous administration except that two 21-gauge needles are inserted at a 20 degree angle
3. Site is selected according to availability of subcutaneous tissue

I. Other routes are sometimes used
1. Purpose is to administer medication to a specific area
2. Method may be continuous drip, swabs, gargles, sprays, or direct injection
3. Sites may be throat or joints or others
4. Method is specifically ordered by physician
5. Medication is administered by trained personnel

Safety factors

A. Medicine cabinet is kept locked when not in use
B. Precautions are taken to protect patient when medication-induced limitations occur
C. Proper disposal of needles and syringes is important; break needles on disposable syringes to prevent reuse
D. Nondisposable needles are properly cleansed and sterilized
E. Nurse checks label three times to make sure it is correct medication and be cautious of spelling and trade and generic names
F. Nurse confirms patient's identity by asking name and checking ID bracelet with the name on medicine card
G. Nurse charts medications after they are given
H. Medication errors are reported *immediately*

WOUND CARE

Dressings

A. Dressing is any material placed on a wound or incision to protect, to absorb drainage, or to promote healing
B. Dressings are classified by method of application
1. Clean
2. Sterile

C. Types of material used are
   1. Gauze
   2. Petrolatum gauze
   3. Telfa
   4. Flannel
D. Nurse may be responsible for changing dressing or assisting physician in changing dressing

Bandages

A. Purposes—applied to give support, to immobilize a part, to apply pressure, or to hold dressings
B. Types of bandages
   1. Strips or rolls of gauze, cotton, flannel, or elastic materials
   2. Many widths, depending on purpose and part to be bandaged
C. Types of basic turns
   1. Circular
   2. Spiral
   3. Spiral reverse
   4. Recurrent
   5. Figure-of-eight
D. Direction—applied from distal to proximal

Binders

A. Binders are usually of heavy materials to support abdomen or chest or to hold large dressing in place
   1. Straight, such as abdomen or chest
   2. Tailed, such as T binder, four-tailed, or scultetus
B. Purposes are to
   1. Support
   2. Hold dressings in place
   3. Apply pressure

Wound irrigation

A. Irrigation is done to remove secretions or excessive discharge from surfaces or body cavities or to apply moist heat
B. It may be sterile or clean, depending on area to be irrigated
C. Equipment needed will depend on irrigation to be done
   1. Container to hold solution to be used
   2. Container for return flow of solution
   3. Means of measuring temperature of solution
   4. Irrigator
   5. Protection for patient and bedding
D. Charting of irrigation is always done

Application of heat and cold

A. Physiologic principles
   1. Cold applications (constrict blood vessels) prevent or reduce swelling, stop bleeding, and decrease suppuration
   2. Heat applications (dilate blood vessels) increase supply of oxygen and nutrients to body cells and increase amount of toxins and excess fluids carried away
B. Types of cold
   1. Dry—ice bag, ice cap, ice collar, and hypothermic device
   2. Moist—cold packs and compresses
C. Nursing observations
   1. White, mottled skin
   2. Frostbite
   3. Numbness
   4. Lowered body temperature
D. Precautions
   1. Caps and bags are two-thirds filled and air removed
   2. Containers are closed securely
   3. Caps and bags are always covered
   4. Application is removed every half hour for 1 hour
   5. Ice is replaced frequently
   6. These treatments are contraindicated in patients with poor circulation or impaired sensation
   7. Physician's order is always needed
E. Types of heat
   1. Dry—hot water bottle, sunlight, heating pad, and incandescent, ultraviolet, and infrared lights
   2. Moist—warm compresses, hot packs, and K-units
F. Nursing observations
   1. Burns
   2. Swelling
   3. Pain
   4. Changes in vital signs
   5. Loss of function of part
G. Precautions
   1. Always have a physician's order
   2. Observe carefully those body parts that are very sensitive and burn easily (eyes, neck, inner aspect of arm)
   3. Bottles and pads are always covered
   4. Never allow patient to lie on heating device
   5. Check for faulty electric wiring

6. Never use safety pins with electric devices
7. Check body temperature frequently
8. Check distance of heating bulbs from body area; should be at least 18 inches away
9. Wring out compresses well to prevent burn; if area is infected, use compress only once and discard

H. Baths
1. Hot or cold
2. Medicated

Application of counterirritants

A. Counterirritants produce a local effect improving circulation and relieve congestion caused by inflammatory process

B. They are classified according to effect or degree of irritation produced
1. Rubefacients
2. Vesicants
3. Pustulants
4. Keratolytics

C. Chemical counterirritants are used in same manner and with same effect as hot applications

Wound infections

A. Infections are systemic (general) or local; type depends on infecting organism

B. Signs of local infection result from increased circulation and accumulation of waste in area
1. Redness
2. Heat
3. Pain
4. Swelling
5. Loss of function
6. Changes in vital signs

C. Signs of general infection are
1. Increase in TPR
2. Nausea and vomiting
3. General malaise
4. Loss of appetite

D. Basic principles of treatment are
1. Physical and mental rest or rest of infected part
2. Elevation of part
3. Application of heat or cold

E. Specific treatment may include
1. Chemotherapy (sulfonamides, antibiotics)
2. Incision and drainage of area

F. Infections Control Committee investigates and follows up infections occurring in the institution

EYE, EAR, NOSE, AND THROAT PROCEDURES

Eye treatments

A. Drops
1. Equipment consists of medication, dropper, gauze pad, and tissue wipe; dropper may come with individual medicine
2. Instillation of correct strength, amount, and medication into correct eye is imperative
3. Nurse explains procedure to patient and washes hands
4. Medication is to be at room temperature, sterile, and checked for signs of deterioration (cloudiness, precipitation)
5. Nurse holds lower lid down, instructs patient to look upward, instills drops into conjunctival sac, releases lid slowly, and instructs patient to roll eye with lids closed unless contraindicated
6. Excess medication may be removed with tissue, wiping from inner to outer canthus

B. Ointments
1. Equipment consists of sterile gauze pad and tube of ointment
2. Nurse holds lower lid down and spreads ointment from inner to outer corners in conjunctival sac; after application nurse has patient roll eyeball with lid shut to help spread medicine

C. Hot compresses
1. Equipment consists of sterile basin of solution as ordered, gauze pad, heating device, and paper bag
2. Nurse explains procedure to patient and washes hands
3. Thin layer of petrolatum is applied over lid
4. Nurse wrings out gauze pad with hands if clean technique or with two pairs forceps if sterile technique and allows pad to stop steaming; nurse applies compresses slowly until patient is accustomed to heat or allows patient to apply compresses if able. (Nurse should try to keep compresses just on eyelid; if lid is inflamed, compresses may be placed on lid and cheek; if eyeball is inflamed, compresses may be placed on lid and brow)
5. Compresses are changed every 30 to 60 seconds for 15 to 20 minutes as ordered
6. If discharge is present, clean pad is used each time compress is applied
7. Two sets of equipment are used if both eyes are involved

8. Nurse applies petrolatum to eyelid following procedure
9. After procedure pads in paper bag are discarded; equipment is washed in hot, soapy water and disinfected or sterilized

D. Irrigation
1. Equipment consists of basin of sterile solution as ordered at 95° to 100°F, medicine dropper or ear syringe, basin for return flow, cotton balls to protect uninvolved eye and to dry treated eye, and face towel to protect bed; separate tip is needed for each eye
2. Nurse explains procedure to patient and washes hands
3. Flow of solution is directed into conjunctival sac from inner angle to outer angle of eye; nurse turns patient toward affected side
4. After procedure burnable material is discarded; remaining equipment is washed with hot, soapy water and sterilized

Ear treatments

A. Drops
1. Assemble equipment—medication, dropper, small cotton pledget
2. Explain procedure to patient and wash hands
3. Position patient's head flat with affected side up
4. Retract pinna to expose orifice of external canal, instill drops against internal wall of canal, and place cotton pledget at orifice if ordered
   a. Patient 3 years of age or older—retract pinna upward and posteriorly
   b. Patient younger than 3 years—retract pinna downward and posteriorly

B. Irrigations
1. Assemble equipment—sterile ear syringe, solution (105° to 108°F), basin for return flow, towel to protect bed
2. Explain procedure to patient and wash hands
3. Position patient—patient may lie, but sitting position is preferred, with head tilted slightly so affected ear is downward; patient may hold basin for return solution, if able
4. Retract pinna, according to age, to expose orifice of external canal; direct flow gently against side of canal and interrupt irrigation; if pain or dizziness occurs, notify physician

Nose treatments—administering drops

A. Assemble equipment—medication, dropper, tissue wipes
B. Explain procedure to patient; have patient breathe through mouth
C. Wash hands
D. Place prescribed number of drops in each nostril; tilt head back by placing pillow under shoulders or hanging head over side of bed
E. Instruct patient to retain position for 5 minutes and expectorate any medication that enters pharynx

Throat treatments

A. Throat swab
1. Assemble equipment—sterile applicators, tongue blade, medication as ordered, tissue wipes, flashlight, paper bag
2. Explain procedure to patient and wash hands
3. When swabbing throat, avoid stimulating gag reflex by touching uvula
4. Discard applicators, tongue blade, and tissues in paper bag to be burned

B. Nose and throat culture
1. Assemble equipment—sterile culture tube, applicator, tissue wipes
2. Explain procedure to patient and wash hands
3. After touching sides and back of throat with applicator, put in culture tube without contaminating inside of tube by breaking off top of applicator touched with fingers
4. Discard tissues in paper bag to be burned

C. Throat irrigation
1. Assemble equipment—irrigating container, solution at 110°F, tubing with rubber tip on end, tissue wipes, basin for return flow, bath towel to protect patient
2. Explain procedure to patient; have patient do treatment if able; instruct to tilt head forward over basin and breathe through nose; discourage deep breathing
3. Hold container slightly above patient's mouth; direct flow toward affected area
   a. Irrigation may be interrupted for patient's comfort
   b. Flow should not be directed toward uvula or base of tongue
4. Tilt patient's head to one side and then to other to facilitate results

D. Steam inhalations
   1. Inhalations supply warmth and moisture directly to mucous membranes of the respiratory tract
   2. Many types are made commercially
   3. Both hot and cold steam inhalers are available
   4. Continuous or intermittent inhalations may be ordered
   5. Nurse explains equipment and procedure
   6. Care is taken to protect patient from burns
   7. Steam is directed so that it surrounds patient's head
   8. Nurse prevents chilling of patient
   9. Linen is changed when damp
   10. Nurse encourages patient to expectorate

RESPIRATORY PROCEDURES

Administration of oxygen

A. Nasal catheter or nasal cannula (nasoinhaler)
   1. Explain procedure to patient
   2. Assemble equipment; and check for supply of oxygen and humidification
   3. Connect and lubricate nasal catheter; turn on oxygen to make sure tube is open; turn off oxygen
   4. For catheter, measure from tip of nose to ear for depth
   5. Insert nasal catheter as directed
   6. Turn on oxygen slowly; usual flow is 3 to 6 L per minute
   7. Tape catheter in place or adjust earpieces, and then adjust oxygen flow as ordered

B. Tent
   1. The major principle in administering oxygen by tent is that oxygen is heavier than air
   2. There are closed tents and open-top tents
   3. Oxygen is cooled by being run through ice and humidified by being run through water before it reaches tent
   4. Tent is tucked in around bottom of mattress; sheet is folded in half and doubled back over edge of tent
   5. Tent should be airtight with no holes; mattress should be rubber covered

C. Mask
   1. Explain carefully because covering face and mouth is frightening to the patient
   2. Fit mask over nose and mouth
   3. Turn on oxygen to liters per minute ordered
   4. Stay with the patient to help him adjust
   5. Remove mask and cleanse face every 2 hours; check skin and ears for irritation from mask and elastic band

D. Precautions—caution patients and visitors that no smoking is permitted wherever oxygen is in use

Chest physical therapy

A. Postural drainage is the use of various positions so that gravity can assist in removal of secretions
B. Percussion is a manual technique of striking the chest wall over the affected area with cupped hands in rhythmic motion
C. Vibration is a manual compression and tremorlike motion with hands or mechanical device against chest wall of affected area done during exhalation
D. Nurse positions patient so affected areas are vertical and gravity can assist in drainage
E. Position also depends on diagnosis and condition
F. Nurse provides emesis basin and tissues and gives oral hygiene after treatment
G. This therapy is contraindicated in patients with lung abscess or tumors, pneumothorax, and disease conditions of chest wall

Special respiratory treatments

A. Gases and drugs in vapor can be administered by way of the lungs for systemic effects
B. Drugs that act on the respiratory system can be classified as
   1. Stimulants or depressants
   2. Those that act on mucous membranes
   3. Those that change size of bronchioles
C. Common respiratory stimulants are CO_2 and atropine
D. Opiates depress respirations
E. Antiseptics, demulcents, and expectorants act on the mucous membranes; they are administered orally or as spray or vapor
F. Warm water vapor, nitrites, and adrenergic agents increase the size of bronchioles
G. Inhalant drugs must be added to vaporizer or nebulizing agent to be utilized
H. Steam (hot or cold) is chief treatment agent; it is very soothing
I. Water vapor therapy increases humidity of inspired air to secretions so they may be expectorated
J. Oxygen-helium therapy is used to reduce fatigue resulting from inhaling heavy gas (nitrogen) by substituting a lighter gas (helium); oxygen attached to

helium passes tracheal obstructions and constricted bronchioles

K. Intermittent positive pressure breathing machine administers oxygen and drugs under pressure to force them into lungs
   1. Pressure is applied during inspiration
   2. Pressure is ordered by physician
   3. Oral hygiene is necessary before and after treatment; if treatment is continuous, nurse gives mouth care every 2 hours

Thoracocentesis

A. Thoracocentesis is aspiration of pleural fluid to relieve pressure or obtain specimen for diagnostic purposes
B. Explain procedure to patient; obtain sterile thoracocentesis tray
C. Position patient leaning forward with head and arms supported on overbed table; expose side of chest as indicated
D. Assist the physician
E. Observe and record character and amount of fluid obtained
F. Observe and record patient's vital signs frequently after procedure
G. Care for equipment as directed

Suction

A. Purposes are to remove accumulated secretions of respiratory tract, to facilitate respiration, or to provide sputum specimen for diagnostic purposes; suction may be oral, nasal, or tracheal
B. Assemble equipment—suction machine, sterile whistle-tip suction catheter, sterile glove (may be disposable)
C. Explain procedure to patient
D. Take patient's pulse. Give patient oxygen by Ambu bag, or have patient take five deep breaths. Encourage patient to cough before suctioning
E. Turn on machine, put on glove, attach catheter to machine, insert catheter deep enough to remove secretions, apply suction using whistle-tip control, and gently rotate catheter while withdrawing
F. Suction intermittently no longer than 10 seconds at a time, to prevent long periods of hypoxia
G. Give patient oxygen following suction
H. Take pulse; do not suction again until pulse returns to normal (unless airway is obstructed by copious secretions)
I. Rotate patient's head from side to side to facilitate removal of bronchial secretions
J. Use sterile catheter and glove for *each* suctioning of tracheostomy
K. Observe and record amount and character of secretions, patient's color, and respiratory rate

GASTROINTESTINAL PROCEDURES

Enema

A. Cleansing enema—given to promote elimination of feces and flatus or to cleanse lower bowel
   1. Assemble equipment (may be disposable)
   2. Explain procedure to patient
   3. Position patient on left side, and ensure privacy
   4. Hold bag 18 inches above level of hips, lubricate rectal tube 2 to 3 inches, instruct patient to bear down, and insert tube 3 to 6 inches into rectum
   5. Give as much solution (105°F) as patient can tolerate (usually 500 to 1000 ml)
   6. Cramping and inability to retain solution may be relieved by temporarily interrupting flow of solution, lowering the container to reduce rate of flow, lowering container below level of patient to allow gases to escape, and encouraging slow, deep breathing through mouth
   7. Instruct patient to turn from left to right side when one half of solution is taken; this helps cleanse colon
   8. Assist patient to bathroom or with bedpan as indicated
   9. Observe and record character and amount of return and patient's tolerance of procedure
B. Retention enema—usually oily preparation given for lubricant action; it should be retained for short period of time; some are to be absorbed
   1. Assemble equipment (may be disposable)
   2. Explain procedure to patient
   3. Position patient on left side, and ensure privacy
   4. Regulate container height and depth of insertion according to type of enema ordered
   5. Give room temperature solution slowly in small amounts (about 150 ml) to aid patient in retaining solution
C. Other types of enemas
   1. Colonic irrigation (lavage)
   2. Proctoclysis
   3. Harris flush

Rectal tube

A. Rectal tube is used to assist in expelling flatus
B. Assemble equipment
C. Explain procedure to patient, and ensure privacy
D. Position patient on side; lubricate and insert tube as described for enemas. Tube is usually left in place 20 to 30 minutes; it may be necessary to tape tube to buttocks
E. Use flatus bag or vented drainage container (essential). "Bubbling" of water in vented container is indicative of effectiveness of procedure

Rectal suppository

A. Assemble equipment (may come prepacked with lubricant and finger cot)—suppository, lubricant, toilet tissue
B. Explain procedure to patient, and ensure privacy
C. Insert suppository; apply pressure over anus until defecation reflex has passed

Colostomy irrigation

A. Irrigation is done to regulate the discharge and drainage of fecal contents and flatus
B. Time of irrigation depends of physician's order and patient's established routine; when colostomy has become regulated, irrigation may only be every other day
C. Equipment consists of
   1. Irrigating applicance (types vary)
   2. Irrigating container
   3. Tubing and catheter (size is dependent on stoma size). (One may be used)
   4. Irrigating solution—usually 500 to 1000 ml tap water or physiologic saline at 100°F
   5. Lubricant
   6. Drainage bag or basin to direct or catch return flow
   7. Colostomy drainage bag and dressing or stoma pad
D. Nurse explains procedure to patient and ensures privacy
E. Irrigation is convenient if patient is seated on toilet. When patient is confined to bed, a side-lying position near the edge of the bed is desirable
F. Nurse holds irrigation container $1^1/_2$ to 2 feet above the stoma, clears catheter of air, lubricates catheter, introduces catheter through irrigating appliance, inserts into stoma, and advances 2 to 6 inches (unless irrigating cone is used). Nurse then allows solution to flow into stoma, removes catheter, and allows for return flow, which is usually completed within 45 to 60 minutes. When return is completed nurse removes appliance, washes and dries abdomen, and applies colostomy drainage bag, dressing, or stoma pad as indicated
G. Catheter is never forcibly advanced
H. Catheter may be advanced slightly to reduce excessive backflow
I. Ointments, lubricants, or medication may be ordered for stoma or skin surrounding stoma
J. Soiled equipment should be rinsed with cool water, then washed in hot soapy water or discarded if disposable
K. Nurse observes and records procedure (return of contents and patient's tolerance)

Gastric intubation

To administer liquid (pureed) feedings (gavage), to obtain specimens, to irrigate or cleanse (lavage), or for decompression

A. Tube insertion
   1. Nose to stomach—nasogastric
   2. Mouth to stomach—orogastric
   3. Artificial opening into stomach—gastrostomy
B. Technique of intubation
   1. Equipment needed is flashlight, tongue blade, stethoscope, cup of water, irrigating syringe (bulb), water-soluble lubricant, 12- to 18-gauge French tube
   2. If rubber tube is used, it should be chilled in ice
   3. Nurse explains procedure
   4. Patient should be in semi-Fowler's position
   5. Nurse protects patient's clothing with towel
   6. Approximate length of tube is from tip of nose to xiphoid process
   7. Nurse applies water-soluble lubricant to tip of tube; if intubation is for cytology study, then tube is lubricated with water or saline
   8. Tube is held 3 inches from tip, placed into nostril (or mouth), and advanced forward and downward
   9. Nurse has patient flex neck and take repeated shallow breaths when tube passes into pharynx (about 3 inches)
   10. As patient swallows, tube is advanced
C. Checking placement of tube
   1. Check back of throat with tongue blade and flashlight to see if coiling has occurred

2. Aspirate stomach contents; may need to advance tube if no contents obtained
3. While injecting 5 cc of air, use stethoscope to listen for air entering stomach
4. Place end of tube in water and observe for air bubbles or listen for air escaping from tube; either indicates tube is in lungs
5. Note patient's ability or inability to speak; patient will be unable to speak if tube is in trachea

D. Securing tube
1. Anchor with strip of tape, and secure to nose and cheek if nasogastric
2. Anchor with strip of tape, and secure to chin and cheek if orogastric

E. Removal of tube
1. Clamp tube
2. Remove anchoring tape
3. Draw tube through towel so it is wiped of secretion
4. Have patient inhale and then exhale slowly
5. Pull tube with one continuous, rapid motion
6. Wrap and discard tube if disposable

F. Tube feeding (gavage)—amount, frequency, and type ordered by physician
1. Feeding should be kept refrigerated and then warmed to room temperature before administration
2. Placement of tube should be checked
3. Patient should be in sitting position or on right side as condition indicates
4. Suction apparatus should be available if patient is unconscious
5. Feeding is poured into container and flow is regulated by adjusting clamp or height
6. Flow should be slow (30 to 45 minutes per 200 ml)
7. Feeding should be followed by ordered amount of water
8. Drugs may be administered, crushed, using feeding or water
9. Tube should be clamped to prevent air from entering stomach
10. If nausea, vomiting, or cramps occur, rate may be too fast or patient may be intolerant of feeding or volume
11. Tubes may be left in place between feedings or removed with each feeding as ordered by physician
12. Continuous tube feedings may also be ordered. Nurse must keep end of tubing in bottom of container and add water or feeding solution as solution gets low

G. Gastric lavage—as ordered by physician
1. Insert tube
2. If specimen is to be obtained, aspirate contents, label, and send to laboratory
3. If gastric washing is ordered, instill ordered solution and repeat until return is clear
4. Carefully measure solution instilled and solution returned

H. Charting
1. Size of tube inserted
2. Type and amount of tube feeding
3. Type, amount, and specimen disposition
4. Type and amount of return

Suction and irrigation

A. Nasogastric or GI tubes (Levin, Miller-Abbott, or Salem Sump) may be connected to mechanical suction apparatus

B. Irrigation is done to ensure patency of tube (solution is usually normal saline)

C. Irrigation technique follows
1. Check orders for frequency, solution type, amount, and method of aspiration (force or gravity)
2. Obtain equipment
3. Explain procedure and wash hands
4. Fill syringe and free of air
5. Instill solution into tube slowly and gently
6. If ordered, aspirate solution
7. Remove syringe and reconnect to suction if ordered

D. Patients with indwelling tubes should be given frequent mouth and nose care

E. Accurate measurement of intake and output is essential

Abdominal paracentesis

A. Puncture and withdrawal of accumulated fluid from peritoneal cavity

B. Explain procedure to patient

C. Gather equipment

D. Have patient void, take vital signs, and weigh patient

E. Place patient in semi-Fowler's position

F. Expose lower abdomen
G. Assist physician while observing patient
H. After procedure, make patient comfortable and observe and record vital signs
I. Record and label specimen if ordered

GENITOURINARY PROCEDURES

Catheterization

A. Assemble equipment—catheterization tray (sterile), containing catheter, basin, jar with lid, cotton balls, antiseptic solution, lubricant, sterile gloves, sheet for drape (disposable sets are available)
B. If the catheter is to be left in place, add
   1. Foley catheter
   2. Syringe
   3. Solution for inflating bulb (usually found is disposable catheter setups)
   4. Tape for securing in place
C. Explain procedure to patient, and ensure privacy
D. Place patient in dorsal recumbent position, and drape; set out equipment between legs
E. For female patient, cleanse vulva and meatus well, always going toward vagina; use applicator for one stroke only before discarding; cleanse meatus last; for male, cleanse glans then meatus, in circular motion
F. Insert catheter into meatus (3 to 4 inches in female and 6 inches in male) until urine flows; drain off urine into basin (no more than 750 ml at one time to prevent bladder collapse); pinch and remove catheter and discard
G. Make patient comfortable; clean and dispose of equipment as directed
H. Chart size of catheter used and amount of urine returned

Retention catheter irrigation

A. Open technique
   1. Assemble equipment—basin of sterile solution, 30 ml bulb syringe, basin for return flow
   2. Explain procedure to patient, and ensure privacy
   3. Disconnect catheter from drainage tube over empty basin; protect from contamination
   4. Allow solution to flow in by gravity or gentle pressure, drain, repeat until clear
   5. Connect catheter, and make patient comfortable
B. Closed techniques
   1. Y-connector and fluid reservoir—a sterile Y-connector is placed between the catheter and the drainage tubing. A large bottle or bag of sterile irrigating solution is hung on an IV pole with sterile tubing attached, same as three-way irrigation is set up. The cross-section of the catheter has three openings—drainage channel, channel to retention balloon, and irrigating channel. The fluid tubing is attached to the Y-connecter and other part of Y has a sterile bulb.
      a. Have clamp ready, and explain procedure to patient
      b. Clamp the draining tubing
      c. Open the fluid tubing from irrigation solution
      d. Allow the prescribed amount to flow in, usually 50 to 100 ml
      e. Close the fluid tubing
      f. The bulb is gently squeezed to circulate solution in bladder (often for transurethral resection surgery)
      g. Open the drainage tubing, and allow the fluid to flow into the drainage bag
      h. Observe fluid return for clots
      i. Record finding, and when totaling output subtract irrigation solution from total output
   2. Syringe-and-needle method
      a. Assemble equipment—20 to 30 ml syringe with needle, alcohol swabs, solution ordered, clamp
      b. Draw up the solution into syringe using sterile technique
      c. Use alcohol swab to clean resealable rubber entry port on the drainage tubing
      d. Insert needle into port
      e. Clamp tubing distal to needle entry area
      f. Inject fluid into catheter
      g. Remove needle
      h. Release clamp and allow fluid to drain into drainage bag
      i. Observe fluid return
      j. Repeat as necessary to use the amount of fluid ordered
      k. Chart observations, and when totaling output subtract amount of irrigant from total in irrigation bag

Bladder instillation

A. Explain procedure to patient, and ensure privacy
B. Do as for catheterization; while catheter is in place, instill medication ordered with 30 ml bulb syringe
C. Finish procedure as for catheterization

Urethral suppository

A. Explain procedure, and have patient empty bladder
B. Clean meatus and adjacent area
C. Lubricate tip of suppository with water or water-soluble lubricant
D. Insert into urethra (if patient is male, milk suppository down urethra until it is no longer palpable)
E. Apply firm pressure to meatus until suppository melts or spasm subsides
F. Instruct patient not to void for at least 30 minutes

VAGINAL PROCEDURES

Perineal care

A. Assemble equipment—container of prescribed solution, cotton balls for cleansing and drying, forceps, perineal pad, bedpan
B. Explain procedure to patient, and ensure privacy
C. Put patient on bedpan; pour solution over vulva, cleaning with cotton balls; dry vulva; make patient comfortable
D. Clean equipment
E. If using bottle method, fill bottle with warm water and squeeze solution over vulva; dry with tissue, wiping from urinary meatus to anus with one swipe; discard tissue

Vaginal irrigation (douche)

A. Assemble equipment—irrigating container with prescribed solution, rubber tubing, clamp, douche tip, cotton balls for drying, forceps, perineal pad, bed protection
B. Explain procedure to patient, have her void, and ensure privacy; if patient is able, she can administer irrigation to self in bathroom
C. Insert tip down and back
D. Give irrigation under low pressure; have solution flowing before inserting douche tip; rotate douche tip until prescribed amount is used
E. If patient on bedpan, raise head of bed slightly to allow fluid to drain into bedpan
F. After procedure make patient comfortable; dispose of equipment

Vaginal instillation

A. Assemble equipment—applicator and tube of medication, perineal pad
B. Explain procedure to patient, have her void, and ensure privacy
C. Insert syringe into vagina, and instill medication; put perineal pad in place
D. Discard equipment as directed

Vaginal suppositories

A. Explain procedure to patient, have her void, and ensure privacy
B. Insert suppository with rubber-gloved hand or applicator
C. Make patient comfortable; instruct patient to remain in bed for 15 to 20 minutes

PREOPERATIVE NURSING CARE

Psychosocial preparation

A. Nurse evaluates patient's knowledge and expected results of surgery
B. Anxiety may interfere with learning
C. Extremely frightened patients respond poorly to surgery
D. Planned, individualized, simple explanations will enhance patient cooperation
E. Nurse assesses and responds to patient's religious needs
F. Common preoperative fears are
   1. Fear of mutilation
   2. Fear of death
   3. Fear of change in family role
   4. Fear of pain
G. Family must understand measure taken to prepare patient
H. Family should participate in explanation and encouragement
I. Family presence usually will allay pateint's feeling of aloneness and display their concern and interest

Physical preparation

A. Explain preoperative tests (CBC, ECG, urinalysis, x-ray examinations), and give proper preparation
B. Explain, demonstrate, and have patient practice any special postoperative exercises he or she will do (turning, deep breathing, pumping feet)
C. Follow preoperative orders as prescribed by physician (enema, diet, medication)
D. Prepare skin (see hospital manual)
E. Care for valuables
F. Follow preoperative checklist
   1. Consent for surgery signed
   2. Nail polish, prothesis, jewelry, and make-up removed

3. Patient gown put on
4. Hygienic measures (bath with mouth care, void or catherize) performed
5. Vital signs checked
6. Identification bracelet placed on patient

G. Record observations and procedures on chart

POSTOPERATIVE NURSING CARE

Immediate care

A. Ensure patent airway
B. Maintain adequate circulation
C. Observe for complications at operative site and in general (hemorrhage, shock, swelling, severe pain)
D. Secure drainage and intravenous tubing
E. Position patient properly; keep patient warm
F. Assess mental status
G. Observe vital signs as ordered
H. Follow physician's orders
I. Report signs of restlessness, excessive drainage, or abnormal reactions
J. Support patient by answering questions briefly

Routine care

A. Follow physician's orders
B. Observe and record vital signs frequently during first 24 hours; report changes immediately
C. Check surgical site frequently
D. Give oral hygiene as needed
E. Have patient turn, cough, deep breathe (unless contraindicated), and exercise the legs every 2 hours
F. Observe and record accurate intake and output
G. Help patient with passive or active exercises unless contraindicated
H. Perform daily assessment
   1. Lungs—cough and breath sounds
   2. Circulation—pain in legs, chest, and intravenous site
   3. GI tract—nausea, vomiting, distention, bowel sounds
   4. Urine—color, odor, character, amount
   5. Mental status—depression, confusion, anxiety, restlessness
I. Offer pain medication

RADIATION PROCEDURES

Radiation

A. Radiate is to send out rays (light, heat, roentgen)
B. Radiation is used in diagnosis and therapeutic treatment of various conditions
C. Types of radiation are
   1. Alpha rays—harmless, do not travel far
   2. Beta rays—more penetrating, stop at patient's body
   3. Gamma rays—very penetrating

Types of therapy

A. Infrared lamp
B. Ultraviolet
C. Diathermy
D. Roentgen ray (x-ray—low voltage, external)
E. Betatron, cobalt, and cesium (high voltage, external)
F. Internal radiation
   1. Implants (skin surface, intratumor, intracavitary)
   2. Liquid forms of radioisotopes)
   3. Injection (intracavitary, systemic)

Radiation therapy and the nurse

A. General nursing care
   1. Explain procedure and precautions to patient and family
   2. If radiation sickness (nausea, vomiting) or skin irritation occurs, have physician discuss with patient
   3. Place linens in closed can
   4. Wear gown and rubber gloves while handling excreta and utensils
   5. Wash contaminated gloves with soap and water before removing
   6. Wash hands with soap and water
   7. If no means of disposing of excreta, dilute with large quantities of water and dispose of in normal manner
   8. Use precautions at all times
   9. Tell visitors to remain only for short periods of time
B. Nursing care and precautions for specific situations
   1. Therapy involving mouth
      a. Oral hygiene with brushing of teeth (or dentures) should be done three times a day
      b. Smoking should be discouraged
      c. Teeth should be examined for change in conditions; if changes are observed, physician should be notified
      d. Male patient should not shave if jaw is treated
   2. Uterine therapy
      a. Bed rest is maintained to prevent displacement of implant

b. Bedpan is inspected for loss of implant before contents are discarded
c. Foley catheter with continuous irrigation may be ordered to reduce bladder irritation
d. Vaginal irrigation may be ordered following removal of implant

3. Radioactive gold given intraperitoneally
    a. Leakage in dressings appears bright red and may be confused with blood
    b. Dressing should be wrapped in newspaper and disposed of in special container

C. General nursing care and precautions
1. Increase daily intake of fluids
2. Do not give milk of magnesia for therapy involving intestinal tract
3. Observe patient for symptoms of systemic radiation sickness
    a. Nausea, vomiting, anorexia, malaise
    b. Scarlet color of skin with shedding dermis
    c. Erythema of mucous membranes

PATIENT'S DEPARTURE

Transferring patient

A. Patient may be transferred from one service to another, from one floor to another, and from one hospital to another
B. Physician's order is necessary
C. Transfer patient ambulatory, by wheelchair, or on stretcher as ordered by physician; follow institution's procedure
D. Explain to patient, and be sure he or she has all personal effects
E. Do not transfer during mealtime or visiting hours to avoid confusion
F. Make proper charting notations

Discharging patient

A. Written order by physician is necessary
B. Nurse's responsibilities are to
1. Check to see that patient has clothes and personal effects and check them with him or her
2. Make certain patient has all instructions regarding diet, medications, treatments, and follow-up appointments
3. Notify relatives as necessary
4. Accompany patient to exit
5. Make proper charting notations

C. Discharge planning
1. Discharge planning begins following initial nursing assessment and planning for care
2. Nursing interventions are directed to eventual discharge of patient
3. Discharge planning consists of teaching patient and family
    a. Cause of illness
    b. Drugs, treatments, and diet
    c. Health care follow-up
    d. Functions within limitations

Caring for dying and dead

A. Signs of approaching death
1. Patient is pale with pinched expression of anxiety
2. Eyes are glazed and dull in appearance; pupils do not react to light
3. Mouth remains partially open unless patient attempts to speak; speech is mumbled and confused
4. Muscle tone becomes flaccid
5. Skin is cold and clammy and may be mottled; this is caused by slowed circulation; body temperature is usually elevated
6. Respirations are rapid and shallow, progressing to Cheyne-Stokes
7. Pulse becomes weak and thready
8. Patient may be diaphoretic, thirsty, and incontinent of urine and feces

B. Five stages in process of dying that nurse should recognize
1. Denial
2. Anger
3. Bargaining
4. Grief/depression
5. Acceptance

C. Nursing care of dying
1. Give symptomatic nursing care
2. Give good personal hygiene
3. Turn patient frequently
4. Give treatments and medication as long as possible or until discontinued
5. Carry out desires of patient and family as far as possible
6. Be available to provide emotional support and privacy to patient and family

D. Spiritual needs of patient
1. Fulfill needs as requested by patient or family
2. Adhere to patient's individual religious beliefs

E. Care of body after death
1. Lower headrest on bed

2. Leave one pillow under head to prevent congestion of blood in vessels of face
3. Close eyes
4. Be sure dentures are placed into mouth immediately; close mouth
5. Clean body; follow institution's procedure for packing and removal of drains, intravenous tubing, and endotracheal tubes
6. Straighten body and place in natural position
7. Allow viewing of body by relatives if they desire
8. Wrap in shroud and label with tag
9. Record observations, procedures, and time of death; complete records

EMERGENCY NURSING AND FIRST AID

Nursing assessment of victim

A. Examine for bleeding and apply pressure with dressing or fingers or, as last resort, tourniquet
B. Examine patient for breathing or lack of breathing; if there are no respirations, check patency of airway, remove any foreign bodies, and begin artificial respiration (mouth-to-nose or mouth-to-mouth methods)
C. Examine for indications that poison has been ingested; unless there are visible signs that mucous membrane is burned, give patient some emetic, allow him to vomit, and give more emetic
D. Always send to hospital with patient any empty bottles or containers found near patient when poisoning is suspected

General principles in giving emergency care

A. Maintain body temperature with external heat as necessary
B. Do not give oral liquids to unconscious patient
C. Keep crowds away from injured; loosen all tight clothing
D. Do not move patient unless there is immediate danger of another accident
E. Keep patient flat
F. Remain calm to reassure injured
G. Initiate first aid; have physician or ambulance called immediately, being sure to give exact location of accident
H. If it is necessary to move patient, do so cautiously, as if patient had broken neck or back

Basic life support

A. Definition—emergency measures (artificial circulation and artificial respiration) taken to sustain life until such time as the victim's heartbeat and respirations begin or resume (cardiopulmonary resuscitation [CPR])
B. General principles
   1. Clinical death—breathing and circulation have ceased
   2. Biologic death—brain has been without oxygen for 6 minutes or more
   3. Respiratory arrest—breathing has ceased; artificial respiration is necessary
   4. Cardiac arrest—breathing, pulse, and circulation have ceased; artificial respiration and circulation are necessary
   5. Steps in CPR—steps are airway, breathing, and circulation (ABC)
C. Artificial respiration—may be done mouth to mouth, mouth to nose, or mouth to stoma; basic necessity is for patent airway
   1. Mouth to mouth
      a. Open airway by tilting head backward as far as possible
      b. Put ear near mouth, listen, and look at victim's chest and feel to determine if victim is breathing
      c. If victim is not breathing, take a deep breath, make a tight seal with your mouth around the victim's and give four breaths into victim's mouth while nostrils are pinched
      d. Remove mouth and allow victim to exhale
      e. Check for pulse and breathing for 5 seconds
      f. Repeat every 5 seconds until respirations have been restored
      g. For infants and small children, do not hyperextend neck; cover the mouth and nose, and use small breaths with less volume (puffs)
D. CPR
   1. Need for CPR is recognized by pulselessness, deathlike appearance, and absent breathing
   2. Procedure should be done on hard surface
   3. Rescuer opens airway and gives four quick breaths
   4. Rescuer checks for carotid pulse
   5. Rescuer places heels of hands (one on top of other) two to three fingerbreadths above xiphoid process
   6. Rescuer rhythmically compresses $1\frac{1}{2}$ to 2 inches
   7. One rescuer should perform 15 compressions and 2 breaths 80 times per minute (15:2)

8. Two rescuers should perform 5 compressions and 1 breath 60 times per minute (5:1)
9. Infant cardiac massage is administered over the midsternum with the tips of two fingers at a rate of 100 compressions per minute (5:1)
10. Child cardiac massage is administered with the heel of one hand only, at the infant ratio

E. Basic guidelines
   1. Pupils should constrict if oxygen is reaching the brain
   2. Carotid pulse should be palpable during external cardiac massage
   3. If pupils remain dilated and patient shows no signs of response, efforts should be ceased
   4. Victim should be transported to the hospital as soon as possible

General emergency situations

A. Hemorrhage
   1. Signs and symptoms
      a. Weak, rapid pulse
      b. Pallor
      c. Cold, clammy skin
      d. Excessive thirst
   2. External (see first step—Nursing assessment of victim, p. 87)
      a. Direct pressure with clean dressing should be applied over bleeding vessel
      b. Digital pressure should be applied at one of six pressure points (temporal, facial, carotid, subclavian, brachial, femoral) to block blood from bleeding part
      c. Application of tourniquet implies decision to sacrifice limb rather than life and should be used only as last measure; tourniquet should be flat band at least 2 inches wide positioned just above wound; if wound is in area of joint, tourniquet should be placed just above joint; tourniquet should be tightened just enough to stop bleeding; note should be attached to victim's clothing indicating location of tourniquet and time applied; application of tourniquet demands immediate care by physician; tourniquet should not be released until victim is seen by physician
      d. Rope or wire should never be used
   3. Internal—keep victim flat, quiet, and warm

B. Shock
   1. Signs and symptoms
      a. Weak, rapid, thready pulse
      b. Pallor
      c. Cold, clammy skin
      d. Restlessness or unconsciousness
   2. Treatment—keep patient flat, quiet, and warm. Shock position is used unless contraindicated by type of injury

C. Asphyxiation
   1. Signs and symptoms
      a. Rapid, difficult breathing
      b. Cyanosis of mucous membranes and nail beds
      c. Congested face
      d. Dilated pupils
      e. Anxious expression
      f. Convulsions
      g. Coma
   2. Treatment
      a. Loosen clothing, cover patient, and turn patient on side; check to see that airway is clear
      b. Remove to fresh air
      c. Begin CPR if indicated

D. Wounds—classified as incised, lacerated, abraded, punctured, or contused
   1. Cover all wounds with clean dressing
   2. If cared for in home, clean well with soap, irrigate well with water, and apply clean dressing
   3. If wound was obtained outside home or from some soiled instrument, inquire concerning injection of tetanus antitoxin
   4. Always see physician unless wound is considered minor
   5. See physician if signs of infection occur

E. Fainting
   1. Lay victim flat with head lower than legs, and loosen clothing
   2. If patient is standing, help to floor to prevent injury
   3. Administer some form of smelling salts

Specific emergency situations

A. Extremes of temperature
   1. Heat stroke
      a. Symptoms consist of flushed, hot, dry skin; dizziness; nausea; dryness of mouth; rapid, full pulse; and high temperature
      b. Patient should be moved to shade with head and shoulders elevated; apply cold wet sheets or immerse in cold water, and loosen clothing; cold should be applied to head first and to rest of body as soon as possible

   c. Check rectal temperature every 15 minutes until a body temperature of 100°F is obtained
2. Heat exhaustion
   a. Symptoms consist of pale, cold, clammy skin; profuse perspiration; weak, thready pulse; shallow respirations; dizziness; and nausea and vomiting
   b. Patient should be moved to circulating air, kept flat and warm, and given 1/2 teaspoon salt in glass of water; when possible dose can be repeated every 15 minutes for 1 hour
   c. If victim vomits, no more fluids should be given
3. Frostbite
   a. Symptoms consist of grayish-white area of body and pain during early stages
   b. Area should be protected from further injury
   c. Frozen part should be covered until patient can be brought indoors; after prolonged exposure, patient should be placed in cool room and temperature gradually raised; patient should be given warm drink; frozen part should be thawed gradually; the part must not be rubbed
   d. Victim should not be allowed to smoke

B. Burns
1. If small area is burned, immerse in cold water and apply sterile gauze
2. If large area is burned, over with clean dry dressing (may use ironed linen); seek medical help
3. Do not bathe or break blisters
4. Never put grease on burns
5. Do not remove adhered clothing
6. Treat patient for shock if indicated

C. Fractures
1. Move part as little as possible
2. Apply splint that extends above and below joint of broken limb and break
3. Be sure splints are wide enough for support; pad well
4. Transport patient carefully; remember possibility of broken neck or back

D. Drowning
1. Remove victim from water, and loosen clothing
2. Check for open airway
3. Begin artificial respiration immediately

E. Injuries to eye, ear, nose, and throat
1. Foreign bodies
   a. Eye
      (1) Grasp eyelashes and turn eyelid back over small straight object (pencil, matchstick, cotton swab)
      (2) If object is seen, gently wipe off with sterile cotton swab or absorbent cotton
      (3) For chemical injuries only, flush eye with water
      (4) Bandage wounds of eye lightly; they should be treated by physician
   b. Ear
      (1) Do not irrigate ears to remove beans or peas since they swell and become more difficult to remove; you may instill few drops of alcohol to shrink dried vegetables
      (2) Kill insects by instilling heavy oil
      (3) Have physician remove object from ear
   c. Nose
      (1) Do not try to remove object if it cannot be seen
      (2) Blow nose slightly with both nostrils and mouth open
      (3) For nosebleed, have patient sit up with head tilted forward; apply cold compress over nose or pressure to bleeding side; if bleeding does not stop, call physician
   d. Throat—Heimlich maneuver (abdominal thrust)
      (1) Lean victim forward. With heel of hand, deliver sharp blow between victim's shoulder blades. If object is not dislodged, proceed with next steps
      (2) Stand behind victim. Wrap arms around victim's waist
      (3) Grasp your fist. Place thumb side of your fist against victim's abdomen (just above navel and below xiphoid process)
      (4) Press your fist in an upward, quick thrust
      (5) Repeat several times
2. Acid or alkali burn—flush with copious amounts of water immediately and cover with thick gauze

F. Bites
1. Animal
   a. Wash wound thoroughly; scrub with soap and water, and rinse with clear water
   b. Apply clean dressing

c. Take patient to physician
d. Determine whether animal has had rabies immunization

2. Snake
   a. Keep patient quiet and flat; immobilize extremities
   b. Tie constricting band above bite to stop flow of blood in veins
   c. Apply oral suction to site of bite unless there are sores in your mouth
   d. Move band up limb as swelling progresses
   e. Call ahead and transport patient to physician or hospital immediately
3. Insect
   a. Remove stinger if present
   b. Apply mixture of baking soda and cold cream or ammonia compresses to releive sting and itching; spider bites are nonpoisonous with the exception of those from black widow and brown recluse spiders, which may cause death in very young or very old persons
   c. Keep patient quiet and warm; call physician

G. Poisons
1. Immediate care is essential
2. Poisoning by mouth is treated by
   a. Diluting or neutralizing poison as quickly as possible (usually with water or milk)
   b. Inducing vomiting (except when corrosive poisons were taken or when convulsions or unconsciousness are present), usually with mustard water (1 teaspoon mustard to glass of tepid water until victim vomits) or 1 tablespoon syrup of ipecac and 2 glasses of water
   c. Maintaining respiration and vital functions
   d. Seeking medical help immediately
3. Inhaled poison gases are treated by
   a. Removing victim to source of fresh air
   b. Maintaining respiration; resuscitating if indicated
   c. Loosening tight clothing
   d. Seeking medical help immediately
4. Contact poisons are treated by
   a. Removing clothing; flushing affected area with water or other liquid
   b. Seeking medical help
   c. Washing area with soap and water for at least 5 minutes
   d. Maintaining airway; giving artificial respiration if indicated

Disaster

A. Definition—catastrophic occurrence causing suffering, helplessness, and disruption of daily patterns of life

B. Types
1. External—tornado, hurricane, acts of war, flood
2. Internal—fire in hospital, bomb threats, radiation accidents

C. Nurse's role in disaster
1. Adapts nursing skills in recognizing and meeting physical and emotional needs of victims and families with assistance of other trained professionals and volunteers
2. Attempts to get to hospital or emergency treatment center to assist as soon as possible
3. Applies principles of first aid in caring for victims
4. Assists with triage or sorting of patients based on the need to assign medical priorities

D. Government programs
1. Medical self-help training
   a. Training is developed through state health department or the civil defense office of individual locality
   b. More information is available from U.S. Department of Health and Human Services, Public Health Service, Washington, D.C.
2. Federal Disaster Relief Act
   a. Administered by the President of the United States
   b. Provides funds, military aid, and medical assistance to states that have exhausted their resouces as a result of disaster
3. Trauma centers—set up in various parts of United States for emergency treatment of trauma; following emergency situation, patient is transferred to a regular hospital

E. Red Cross programs

The American Red Cross does not make loans to families or individuals in need as a result of a disaster. Red Cross assistance is an outright gift from the American people with no obligation to repay
1. Emergency mass care assistance
   a. Food for disaster victims and emergency workers
   b. Temporary shelter for victims
   c. Medical and nursing aid of victims
   d. Clothing for victims
   e. Blood and blood products for sick and injured victims

2. Immediate assistance on individual family basis
   a. Welfare inquiry and information services
   b. Emergency assistance for food, clothing, rent, bedding, selected furnishings, transportation, medical needs, temporary home repairs and occupational supplies, other essentials
   c. Referral to government disaster programs
3. Aid for recovery to families for whom government programs are not available
   a. Casework services
   b. Food, clothing, and other maintenance until normal sources of support are restored
   c. Building and repair of owner-occupied homes
   d. Household furnishings
   e. Medical and nursing care
   f. Personal occupational supplies and equipment

F. Hospital disaster plans
   1. The Joint Commission on Accreditation of Hospitals requires that every hospital develop, maintain, and practice a disaster plan
   2. Disaster plans incorporate services of all hospital departments, with the Emergency Department being the center for mass casualty handling

FUNDAMENTALS OF NURSING REVIEW QUESTIONS

Read each question carefully and consider all possible answers. When you have decided which answer is **best,** blacken the corresponding space on the answer sheet. There is only **one** best answer for each question.

1 The nurse's primary objective in care of patients is to maintain the individual's state of health. The individual perceives health as
1. Having no bodily disturbances
2. Having the ability and capacity to function normally
3. Having had no illness that required hospitalization
4. Being different for each person, depending on where the person lives

2 How the individual determines the presence of illness depends on
1. The person's culture and the culture's expectations of the individual
2. Whether or not the person frequently seeks medical assistance
3. The individual's socioeconomic level
4. The normal functioning of the individual's body

3 In assessing the factors that affect one's health, the nurse would determine the patient's
(A) Perception of health
(B) Family structure and functions
(C) Socioeconomic and physical environment
(D) Religious, ethical, and moral values
1. A, B, and C
2. A, C, and D
3. B, C, and D
4. A, B, and D

4 The family should be included in planning patient care because
1. The patient and the family are concerned with how the illness will affect roles and responsibilities in the family
2. They are more familiar with the patient's habits and attitudes
3. The family will resent total care of patient by others
4. The family is more familiar with religious constraints on health care than the nurse

5 Communication is an important aspect in developing and delivering patient care. Good communication is based on
1. Listening to what another says and recording the information
2. Writing messages rather than verbal communication
3. Observing nonverbal communication rather than listening to spoken word
4. Listening, observing, interpreting, and reporting the communication

6 Therapeutic communication between the nurse and the patient provides communication that is
1. Easily understood and meets basic communication needs
2. Beneficial to the nursing staff in determining attitudes
3. Purposeful and directed toward goals that benefit the patient
4. Representative of the type of communication to which the patient is accustomed

7 To prevent the nurse from physical fatigue during the work day, the nurse must
1. Wear a girdle and not lift heavy objects

2. Maintain good posture and utilize good body mechanics
3. Use back muscles when moving or lifting patients
4. Make beds smoothly on one side at a time

8 The most effective means by which the nurse can protect other patients and self from infections is
1. Washing hands between patients, before and after performing care or procedures
2. Wearing a mask around patients with an upper respiratory infection
3. Discarding linen in hamper and not dropping it on the floor
4. Maintaining enteric isolation

Situation: Mr. Harris is admitted to the hospital for the first time in his life.

9 Environmental factors that will affect Mr. Harris's adjustment to the hospital are
(A) Lighting and decor of the room
(B) Previous contact with ill friends
(C) Noise and odors
(D) Personal privacy and safety
1. A and C
2. A, B, and C
3. B, C, and D
4. A, B, and D

10 Mr. Harris complains of the room being hot. You notice the air conditioner's thermostat is set on 74°F. You would
1. Open the door to his room to allow for ventilation
2. Open the window to allow a small draft of cool outside air
3. Increase the humidity in the room by obtaining a humidifier
4. Offer Mr. Harris a cold, wet washcloth to wipe his face

11 Daily care of Mr. Harris's room would consist of
1. Disinfecting and sterilizing items in his immediate area
2. Providing fresh water for his flowers
3. Scrubbing and waxing the floor
4. Damp dusting and straightening

12 Strict isolation is prescribed for Mr. Harris. After donning mask, gloves, and gown, you would be careful *not* to
1. Hold Mr. Harris's arm with gloved hand to take his pulse
2. Use a disposable stethoscope
3. Touch a wet item to the nurse's isolation gown
4. Get gloves wet with the soiled linen

13 Before leaving Mr. Harris's room, you would
1. Remove the dietary tray to the bedside table
2. Remove the gown, gloves, and mask
3. Remember to wash and sterilize the thermometer before taking the next patient's temperature
4. Reach into dirty linen hamper to push down the piled linen

14 While performing a sterile dressing change, you spill a glass of sterile normal saline on the sterile field. The area that becomes wet would
1. Be considered contaminated
2. Be a good place to put the sterile sponges for cleaning the wound later
3. Need to be removed or covered with a dry towel
4. Need to be dried before continuing the dressing change

15 Since bed rest is prescribed for Mr. Harris you would be especially careful to
1. Use a waterproof mattress and foam rubber padding on the bed
2. Keep his bed flat to prevent the bottom sheet from slipping
3. Keep bedrails down and the bed wheels locked
4. Make his bed wrinkle free and bathe him with long smooth strokes

16 You need to gather equipment besides bed linen to bathe Mr. Harris. This would include
1. Toothpaste, toothbrush, washcloth, and lotion
2. Lotion, washbasin, emesis basin, cloth, and water
3. Soap, water, and washcloth
4. Wash basin, soap, mouthwash, lotion, and washcloth

17 While bathing Mr. Harris's legs, you would be careful *not* to
1. Massage the lower legs
2. Heat bath water when changing
3. Wash the bottom of his feet since he is ticklish
4. Bend the knee while washing posterior aspect of leg

18 During the bath, observations of the skin include
1. Temperature, integrity, and condition
2. Color, warmth, and bruising
3. Markings made by wrinkles in the sheets or crumbs
4. Distribution and color of the hair

19 While cleaning Mr. Harris's dentures, you would be careful to
1. Hold dentures over basin of water
2. Soak in cold water before brushing dentures
3. Soak in very hot water before brushing dentures
4. Hold dentures with tissue paper under running water

20 You notice Mr. Harris to have a reddened skin discoloration over his coccyx area. He does not complain of it hurting. The probable cause of this problem is
1. Pressure over a bony prominence
2. Frequent moving up and down in the bed
3. Inadequate nutrients in his regular diet
4. Body lice that have embedded in the skin

21 To prevent further breakdown of the skin on Mr. Harris's coccyx, you would
1. Change the linen twice a day

2. Change his position at least every 2 hours
3. Place a waterproof pad under the area
4. Keep the area moist with warm water

22 In the evening, before Mr. Harris goes to sleep, you can help him to relax by
1. Reading him a story or the newspaper
2. Adjusting television so he can see the picture without straining
3. Rubbing his back, tightening the bed covers, and washing his face, hands, and back
4. Offering him oral hygiene, reading him the newspaper, and dimming the lights

23 Mr. Harris is embarrassed because he is incontinent of feces. To prevent further emotional stress and soiling of bed linen, you can
1. Place an absorbent diaper over his perineal area
2. Administer an antidiarrheic drug
3. Allow Mr. Harris to keep pan of water near his bed to keep himself clean
4. Offer Mr. Harris the bedpan at frequent intervals

24 Important documentation on Mr. Harris's chart concerning his incontinent feces is the
1. Frequency, color, and consistency of the stools
2. Emotional reaction of the patient before and after soiling of linen
3. Diet consumed by Mr. Harris at breakfast
4. Number of absorbent pads used during your shift

25 While charting on Mr. Harris's chart, you make an error. To correct the error, you would
1. Erase the mistake
2. Draw one line through and initial error
3. Scratch over the mistake and rewrite
4. Tear out and discard the page

26 Included as a part of charting is the recording of observations and assessment of the patient. Basic skills used by the nurse in assessment are
1. Subjective and objective observations
2. Communications of the patient
3. Laboratory data and patient's response to tests
4. Recording of all data in a legal manner

Situation: Dottie Allen is 24 years old. You are caring for her in the emergency room while the physician examines her for the cause of the abdominal pain.

27 The term used for the feeling of Dottie's abdomen is
1. Inspection
2. Palpation
3. Percussion
4. Auscultation

28 To prepare Dottie for a vaginal examination by the physician, you would assist Dottie into a
1. Knee-chest position
2. Sims's position
3. Prone position
4. Lithotomy position

29 While seeing about another patient, you leave Dottie alone. When you return to her room, she screams, "I'm too sick to be left just sitting here." The best response to make is
1. "I'm sorry to have kept you waiting. Let me help you into bed."
2. "We nurses understand, but we're very busy."
3. "Why don't you lie down, Mrs. Allen?"
4. "Don't worry, Mrs. Allen, I'll get to you when I can."

30 As you consider what Dottie said to you, your assessment would be that Dottie is
(A) Afraid
(B) Insecure in the new situation
(C) Anxious about the source of the pain
(D) Disrespectful to those trying to help her
1. A, B, and D
2. C
3. A, B, and C
4. B, C, and D

31 Dottie drank a glass of cold water before you were able to take her temperature. To obtain an accurate oral temperature, you must wait
1. 5 minutes
2. 10 minutes
3. 15 minutes
4. 30 minutes

32 Dottie's body temperature represents the balance between
1. Heat conversion and heat conduction
2. Heat produced and heat lost
3. Heat convection and heat conduction
4. Heat convection and heat conversion

33 A normal rectal temperature would be
1. 97.6°F
2. 98.6°F
3. 99.6°F
4. 100.6°F

34 You notice that Dottie's radial pulse is irregular. To obtain an accurate count of the pulse, you would
1. Seek assistance from another nurse to obtain apical-radial pulse rate
2. Press index and third fingers over radial aspect of forearm and count for 60 seconds
3. Press index finger over femoral artery and count for 15 seconds
4. Take apical pulse for 30 seconds

35 To count Dottie's respirations, you would be sure to
1. Count the respirations when she is not talking or aware of what you are doing
2. Count both the inspirations and expirations with Dottie in semi-Fowler's position

3. Count respiratory rate with Dottie in orthopneic position
4. Count periods of apnea as one respiration

36 The triage nurse tells you that Dottie's blood pressure was 120/80. This blood pressure would be considered
1. Hypertensive
2. Hypotensive
3. Normal for Dottie's age
4. A value with increased pulse pressure

37 Dottie is admitted to the hospital for further diagnostic tests to determine the cause of her abdominal pain. A routine urinalysis, clean-catch method, is ordered. To obtain the specimen, you would
1. Cleanse the urinary meatus and obtain urine in midstream of voiding
2. Catheterize the urinary meatus to obtain sterile urine
3. Save all of Dottie's urine for 24 hours
4. Obtain the first voided specimen in the morning

38 Chest x-ray films indicate that Dottie possibly has a lung lesion. To collect a sputum specimen, you
1. Collect emesis and send the specimen to the laboratory properly labeled
2. Request respiratory therapy to obtain specimen immediately
3. Obtain early morning sputum specimen and follow with oral hygiene
4. Have Dottie inhale and exhale several times to bring sputum out of lower lung lobe

39 To obtain a stool specimen from feces, you would
1. Run warm water over stool and collect water that runs off stool
2. Use a tongue blade to obtain small stool sample from bedpan
3. Use a sterile biopsy tray to obtain stool specimen
4. Give patient waterproof cup to collect stool

40 Dottie is scheduled for a lung biopsy in the morning. She is NPO after midnight. The best way to explain NPO is
1. "We do not want you to eat or drink anything after midnight."
2. "Dottie, you will be NPO after midnight."
3. "Having food or drink in your stomach when being anesthetized can cause you problems, so do not eat or drink anything after midnight. Do you have any questions?"
4. "Dottie, give me the cookies you are eating. You can't have any more food or water tonight. Do you have any questions?"

41 Dottie asks you what "biopsy" means. You would explain that a biopsy is
1. Obtaining a specimen of tissue
2. Obtaining cancer cells by cutting a piece of tissue away from an organ
3. An x-ray examination of an area to determine the depth of a lesion in the body
4. Recording of the amount of air exhaled by her lungs

42 At 9:00 PM the physician ordered Dottie Nembutal gr $\frac{\cdot\cdot}{\text{i ss}}$ PO for sleep. Before you administer the drug, you must know
(A) That the medication can be given to Dottie IM or PO
(B) The actions and side effects of drugs
(C) That Dottie is allergic or sensitive to certain drugs
(D) The dosage range for the drug
(E) How to explain contraindications of the drug to Dottie
1. A, B, and C
2. B, C, and D
3. A, B, C, and D
4. B, C, D, and E

The following information should be used to answer questions 43 through 51: Dottie returns to the unit following the lung biopsy procedure. The physician's report states that Dottie has lung cancer, probably secondary to uterine cancer that has metastasized. Dottie will be scheduled in a few days for a hysterectomy.

43 Antibiotic douches have been ordered for two days. To perform the douche, you would have Dottie lie in a dorsal recumbent position and insert the nozzle tip
1. Down and back into the vagina
2. Four inches into the vagina
3. One-fourth inch into vaginal orifice
4. Two inches into the vagina in an alternating in-and-out motion

44 Following the douche, you are to insert a vaginal suppository. You would instruct Dottie to
1. Push as if she needed to defecate
2. Remain in the bed for 15 or 20 minutes
3. Hold her legs together for 30 minutes
4. Void immediately after inserting the suppository

45 The morning of Dottie's surgery, the physician orders a cleansing enema in addition to the douche. Which procedure should be performed first?
1. Douche
2. Perineal care
3. Enema
4. Bed bath

46 What position would be best for Dottie to receive the enema?
1. Right lateral Sims's
2. Fowler's
3. Reverse Trendelenburg's
4. Left lateral Sims's

47 Immediately before Dottie leaves for surgery, you are ordered to catheterize her. Urinary catheterization is performed to
1. Decompress the bladder to prevent accidental injury during the hysterectomy

2. Prevent contamination of the sterile field by incontinent urine
3. Maintain accurate intake and output
4. Ensure Dottie's comfort during and after surgery

48 While catheterizing Dottie, you touch the catheter tip to her leg. You would
1. Cleanse the urinary meatus and insert the catheter
2. Change your sterile gloves to another pair
3. Discard the catheter and obtain another sterile catheter the same size
4. Dispose of the catheterization tray and begin again

49 You notice that 750 ml of urine has emptied and the urine continues to flow. You would
1. Empty the urine container and continue measuring output
2. Clamp the catheter, wait 15 minutes, and resume flow
3. Remove the catheter and report to physician the amount of urine obtained
4. Connect the catheter to the bedside drainage system

50 Following surgery, Dottie complains of a severe sore throat and nasal congestion. You obtain a sterile throat culture by
1. Touching a sterile applicator to both sides and back of throat
2. Having Dottie cough and collecting the product in a sterile container
3. Irrigating throat, directing flow toward affected area, and then sending return fluid to lab
4. Tilting Dottie's head back, having her inhale steam, and collecting a specimen

51 To relieve Dottie's nasal congestion, the physician has ordered Afrin nose drops. To instill nose drops, you have Dottie tilt her head back and
1. Breathe through her nose while you place drops in each nostril
2. Place specified number of drops in each nostril and hold that position for 5 minutes
3. Have Dottie blow her nose before instilling nose drops
4. Wait 5 minutes for gag reflex to subside before administering nose drops

---

Situation: Mr. Harlin is 60 years old and has chronic obstructive pulmonary disease.

52 Mr. Harlin is given oxygen by nasal catheter. To provide oxygen by this method you would
1. Insert catheter the length measured from patient's nose tip to ear
2. Have patient swallow ice chips as you insert nasal catheter
3. Turn on oxygen to 10 L per minute to remove any obstructions
4. Tape catheter to cheek to be sure catheter was not inserted too deeply

53 Any time oxygen is used in an area, safety precautions would consist of
(A) No smoking or igniting matches
(B) No use of friction-type toys or equipment
(C) Using gases that mix with oxygen to prevent explosions
(D) Making sure room is airtight
1. A, B, and C
2. A, B, C, and D
3. A and B
4. A and D

Situation: Mr. Collins is admitted for an excision of bilateral cataracts.

54 When giving Mr. Collin's intramuscular preoperative medications, the practical nurse must remember to inject into one site no more than
1. 1 ml
2. 2 ml
3. 3 ml
4. 4 ml

55 In giving an intramuscular injection, the needle is inserted at an angle of
1. 25 degrees
2. 45 degrees
3. 60 degrees
4. 90 degrees

56 Data that must be included on Mr. Collin's preoperative chart are
1. Hemoglobin, history and physical examination, record of last voiding, and lumbosacral spine films
2. Signed consent forms, vital signs, record of last voiding, hemoglobin, and hematocrit
3. Physicians' order sheet, nurses' notes, signed consent form, and radiology reports
4. Insurance forms, laboratory data, social and medical data, and signed consent form

57 In administering eye drops to Mr. Collins, the practical nurse
1. Holds the upper eyelid while instilling drops directly onto the cornea
2. Instructs the patient to look upward while instilling drops into the pupil
3. Instructs the patient to look upward while drops are instilled into the conjunctival sac
4. Instills the drops into the tear ducts and instructs the patient to squeeze eyes tightly

58 Mr. Collins develops a postoperative infection. The physician orders hot compresses applied to O.D. q.i.d. The nurse interprets this order as hot compresses to the
1. Left eye four times daily
2. Right eye four times daily
3. Left eye every 4 hours
4. Right eye every 4 hours

59 When applying hot compresses to Mr. Collins's eye, the practical nurse must
(A) Apply a thin layer of petrolatum over the affected eyelid
(B) Change compresses every 30 to 60 seconds for 15 to 20 minutes
(C) Use a single set of equipment for treating both eyes
(D) Apply compresses quickly to obtain the full effect of the intense heat
(E) Use a clean gauze with each application of the hot compresses
1. A, B, and C
2. B, D, and E
3. A, B, and D
4. A, B, and E

60 Signs of a local infection include
1. Redness, pain, swelling, and decreased temperature
2. Increased temperature, malaise, and decreased blood pressure
3. Redness, pain, heat, and swelling of the area
4. Increased temperature, pain, redness, and decreased urine output

---

Situation: Joey Anglin, aged 5, is admitted for evaluation of chronic otitis media.

61 Signs and symptoms often seen with systemic or general infections include
(A) Increased TPR
(B) Nausea and vomiting
(C) Elevated blood pressure
(D) General malaise
1. A, B, and D
2. B, C, and D
3. A, C, and D
4. A, B, C, and D

62 In administering ear drops to Joey, the nurse must retract the pinna of the ear
1. Upward and posteriorly to instill drops against the internal wall of the auditory canal
2. Downward and posteriorly to instill drops directly on the tympanic membrane
3. Upward and posteriorly to instill drops directly on the tympanic membrane
4. Downward and posteriorly to instill drops against the internal wall of the auditory canal

63 In preparing equipment for irrigation of the ear canal, the irrigating solution should be warmed to
1. 98° to 99°F
2. 105° to 108°F
3. 115° to 120°F
4. 120° to 125°F

Situation: Mrs. Ann Douglas, aged 40, is admitted for excision of her gallbladder.

64 Intravenous infusion of dextrose solution was ordered for Mrs. Douglas primarily to
1. Restore or maintain electrolyte balance
2. Restore platelets and hemoglobin
3. Replace proteins and fats
4. Increase urinary output

65 The nurse must check Mrs. Douglas's intravenous infusion frequently for
(A) Obstruction of the tubing
(B) Redness or swelling at the puncture site
(C) Maintenance of the prescribed drip rate
(D) Temperature of the solution
(E) Electrolyte concentration of the solution
1. A, B, and C
2. A, B, C, and D
3. B, C, D, and E
4. A, B, C, and E

66 Mrs. Douglas has poor circulation in her lower extremities. To which position should you adjust her bed to prevent impairment of circulation?
1. Reverse Trendelenburg's
2. Semi-Fowler's
3. Trendelenburg's
4. Low Fowler's

67 After supper you notice that Mrs. Douglas is lying on her side smoking a cigarette and flicking the ashes into the trash can. What should you explain to Mrs. Douglas about smoking in bed?
1. You tell Mrs. Douglas that she must be careful not to catch the bed on fire and you leave the room
2. You ask Mrs. Douglas to sit up in bed, give her an ashtray, and come into her room frequently until she has finished smoking
3. Pay no attention to what she is doing and check on her later
4. You tell the nurse in charge that Mrs. Douglas is causing a fire hazard and to please have the doctor talk with her

68 Mrs. Douglas tells you to get her medicine out of the suitcase because it's time to take her medicine. Your response should be
1. Nothing. The patient has the right to take her own medicine
2. "Mrs. Douglas, we will give you only the medication ordered by your doctor. I'll take these with me to the nurses' station."
3. "Mrs. Douglas, Dr. Sam will order the medications he wants you to have while you are in the hospital."
4. To hand the medications to her as she requested and notify the physician immediately

69 Mrs. Douglas is to receive a tub bath this morning. You should plan your work so that
1. The tub bath is given before breakfast
2. The tub bath is given at a time when you can stay with the patient or at least remain within calling distance
3. The tub bath can be taken by the patient while you are feeding a helpless patient
4. All other assignments are completed before starting this bath, since Mrs. Douglas will need your help

70 The physician writes the following order, "Obtain a sterile urine specimen for C & S." Which of the following is true concerning a *sterile* urine specimen?
1. May be obtained from the catheter bag if the patient has a Foley catheter
2. May be obtained using the "clean-catch" or "midstream" method as long as you use a sterile container
3. Must be obtained either by catheterizing the patient or from the catheter itself if the patient has a Foley catheter
4. May be obtained *only* by clamping off a Foley catheter for 15 minutes and then taking the specimen from the catheter tubing

71 You are ordered to obtain a 24-hour urine specimen from Mrs. Douglas. Which of the following best describes the proper method for this procedure?
1. Have patient void at 8:00 AM. Then have her void again at 8:00 AM the next day. Send both specimens to the laboratory
2. Have the patient empty her bladder at 8:00 AM; and discard this specimen. Then collect all urine voided for the next 24 hours. Ask patient to void at 8:00 AM the next day, and place this last specimen in the container. Send urine to the laboratory
3. Have patient empty the bladder at 8:00 AM and discard this specimen. Then collect all urine for 24 hours. At the end of the 24 hour period or 8:00 AM the next day, have patient empty bladder again, and discard urine. Send the collected urine to the laboratory
4. Have the patient void at 8:00 AM, and place urine in the container. Collect all urine for 24 hours. At 8:00 AM the next day, have her void, and add this specimen to the container. Send to the laboratory

72 To help Mrs. Douglas to void freely, which of the following nursing measures may you use?
(A) Insert a three-way Foley catheter
(B) Elevate the head of the bed and assist Mrs. Douglas to a natural position for voiding
(C) Provide privacy for Mrs. Douglas
(D) Pour warm water over the vulva while Mrs. Douglas is on the bedpan
(E) Increase her intake of fluids
1. A, B, and E
2. A, B, C, and D
3. A, C, and E
4. B, C, D, and E

73 Preoperative preparation for Mrs. Douglas before removal of her gallbladder will include
(A) Demonstration and practice of turning, coughing, and deep breathing
(B) Explanation of the complications associated with the surgery
(C) Simple explanations of the operative procedure and the postoperative equipment to be used
(D) Discouragement of family members from becoming involved in her surgical preparation
1. A and C
2. B, C, and D
3. B and D
4. A and B

74 When Mrs. Douglas returns from the recovery room to the floor, the *immediate* nursing action would be to
1. Take the blood pressure and pulse
2. Ensure a patent airway
3. Secure drainage and intravenous tubings
4. Observe the surgical dressing

75 Nursing observations that should be reported to the physician *immediately* include
1. Weak, thready pulse, hypotension, and decreased urinary output
2. Obstruction of the intravenous tubing and inflammation at the puncture site
3. Removal of the nasogastric tube by the patient
4. Three hundred fifty milliliters of yellow-green drainage from nasogastric tube during the 8-hour shift

76 In order to reinsert Mrs. Douglas's nasogastric tube, the nurse should
1. Place the patient in Trendelenburg's position to facilitate passage of the tube
2. Have Mrs. Douglas flex her neck and take repeated shallow breaths until the tube passes the pharynx
3. Measure from the tip of the nose to the umbilicus to determine length of insertion
4. Instruct Mrs. Douglas to hold her breath as the tube is passed to prevent gagging

77 Normal urine output per hour usually averages approximately:
1. 10 ml
2. 25 ml
3. 30 ml
4. 60 ml

78 The reason for Mrs. Douglas's nasogastric tube postoperatively is most likely
1. For diagnostic purposes
2. To aspirate gastric contents and decrease gastric distention
3. To feed her
4. To establish an adequate airway

79 To check the placement of nasogastric tube the nurse can
1. Order a chest x-ray examination after injecting 5 cc of air into the stomach
2. Ask the patient if the tube feels as if it is in the stomach
3. Ask the patient to take three deep breaths while pinching the nasogastric tube
4. Inject 5 cc of air into the nasogastric tube while listening with a stethoscope for air entering the stomach

80 Frequent oral hygiene for a patient with a nasogastric tube is necessary because
1. The patient breathes through his mouth
2. Patient will become hungry
3. Oral hygiene will prevent irritation from the tube
4. Food is regurgitated frequently

81 The best measure to prevent contamination of other patients following Mrs. Douglas's dressing change is
1. Hand washing
2. Sterilization
3. Isolation
4. Disinfection

Postoperatively, Mrs. Douglas develops "gas pains." The physician orders a Dulcolax suppository first and if no results, a rectal tube.

82 The correct procedure for administration of rectal suppositories includes
(A) Lubricating the suppository with water-soluble jelly before insertion
(B) Inserting the suppository 6 to 8 inches into the rectum
(C) Applying pressure over the anus until the defecation reflex has passed
(D) Applying several layers of sterile gauze over anus to prevent drainage of stool
1. A and B
2. B and C
3. A and D
4. A and C

83 A rectal tube used for postoperative distention achieves maximum results after
1. 30 minutes
2. 1 hour
3. 2 hours
4. 3 hours

84 Because of Mrs. Douglas's history of poor circulation, the physician orders heparin, 5000 units subcutaneously b.i.d. Subcutaneous injections are administered so that the medication is placed
1. Into the superficial muscle tissue
2. Into the superficial veins
3. Between the layers of skin
4. Under the first layer of skin

85 At what angle to the skin must a subcutaneous injection be inserted?
1. 15 degree angle to the skin
2. 45 degree angle to the skin
3. 60 degree angle to the skin
4. 90 degree angle to the skin

86 Correct procedure for the administration of heparin is to insert at
1. 45 degree angle, aspirate, massage briskly
2. 45 degree angle, do not aspirate, do not massage
3. 15 degree angle, aspirate, massage briskly
4. 15 degree angle, do not aspirate, do not massage

87 Three days postoperatively, the site of Mrs. Douglas's intravenous infusion becomes red and edematous. The physician orders continuous warm compresses to the site, which will have the effect of
1. Vasodilation
2. Vasoconstriction
3. Inhibition of microorganisms
4. Decreasing circulation to the area

88 Cold applications to the same site would have the effect of
(A) Vasodilation
(B) Vasoconstriction
(C) Increasing circulation
(D) Decreasing circulation
1. A and C
2. A and D
3. B and C
4. B and D

---

89 Mrs. Benjamin was admitted to the hospital in an unconscious condition after an auto accident. Her clothing must be removed quickly without too much movement. The nurse would
1. Cut them in any way necessary in order to remove quickly
2. Cut along seams so they could be mended
3. Leave her clothes on until she returns from the operating room

90 When mouth-to-mouth resuscitation is administered to an adult it is important that
1. There is an open airway
2. The nose is pinched
3. The jaw is jutted forward
4. All of the above

91 The external cardic massage ratio for one rescuer is
1. 5:1
2. 6:1
3. 15:2
4. 20:2

Situation: You and a friend are walking along a street when you see a car hit two children and speed away.

92 You would first examine the children for
1. Patent airway
2. Hemorrhage
3. Fractures
4. Possible head injury

93 You would use the following method of artificial respiration
1. Mouth-to-mouth
2. Prone-pressure
3. Back-pressure
4. Mouth-to-nose

94 In order to stop oozing bleeding you would first try
1. Pressure points
2. Direct pressure to the wound
3. Tourniquet
4. Ice packs

95 You notice one of the children has a severe burn on her arm and clothing is adhered to it; you would
1. Not remove the clothing
2. Apply petrolatum
3. Debride the wound
4. None of the above

96 In the meantime you send your friend to call a physician, instructing that the most important information to give the physician is the
1. Extent of injuries
2. Location of the accident
3. First aid already given
4. Time of the accident

---

97 The basic principle in unknown poisoning by mouth is to
1. Have patient vomit
2. Call physician
3. Give mustard and water
4. Dilute immediately with milk or water

98 Characteristic signs of heat exhaustion are
1. Profuse perspiration, normal body temperature, and fainting
2. Unconsciousness, incontinence, and bradycardia
3. Elevated body temperature, hot dry skin, and tachycardia
4. Flushed face, rigidity of body muscles, and excessive salivation

99 If a patient asks you to pray with him you should
1. Summon the hospital chaplain or minister of the patient's faith
2. Ask him about his faith because you may not agree with his religious beliefs
3. Comply with his request, asking him if he has any special prayer he would like to say
4. Ignore his request, realizing that illness often causes a patient concern about spiritual welfare

100 While putting Mr. Long's room in order you notice that he has a vase of wilted flowers on the dresser. He asks you not to disturb them; in this situation, it would be best if you
1. Tell him that dead flowers are depressing and he would feel better if they were removed
2. Ask him why on earth he wants to keep dead flowers in his room
3. Put fresh water in the vase and leave them as the patient requested
4. Ask his wife to discard the flowers when she comes for a visit

5 NURSING THE ADULT PATIENT

REFERENCES

Anderson, H.C.: Newton's geriatric nursing, ed. 5, St. Louis, 1971, The C.V. Mosby Co.

Brunner, L., Emerson, C.P., Ferguson, L.K., and Suddarth, D.S.: Textbook of medical-surgical nursing, ed. 3, Philadelphia, 1975, J.B. Lippincott Co.

Elhart, D., et al.: Scientific principles in nursing, ed. 8, St. Louis, 1978, The C.V. Mosby Co.

Freeman, R.: Community health nursing practice, Philadelphia, 1970, W.B. Saunders Co.

Garb, S., Crim, B.J., and Garf, T.: Pharmacology and patient care, ed. 3, New York, 1970, Springer Publishing Co., Inc.

Govoni, L.E., and Hayes, J.E.: Drugs and nursing implications, ed. 3, New York, 1978, Appleton-Century-Crofts.

Hahn, A.B., Barkin, R.S., and Oestreich, S.J.K.: Pharmacology in nursing, ed. 15, St. Louis, 1982, The C.V. Mosby Co.

Hasler, D., and Hasler, N.B.: Personal, home and community health, New York, 1967, Macmillan Publishing Co., Inc.

Hood, G.H., and Dincher, J.R.: Total patient care: foundations and practice, ed. 5, St. Louis, 1980, The C.V. Mosby Co.

Mason, M.A.: Basic medical surgical nursing, ed. 4, New York, 1978, Macmillan Publishing Co., Inc.

Phipps, W.J., Long, B.C., and Woods, N.F.: Shafer's medical-surgical nursing, ed. 7, St. Louis, 1980, The C.V. Mosby Co.

Shackelton, A.D.: Practical nurse nutrition education, ed. 3, Philadelphia, 1972, W.B. Saunders Co.

Shafer, K.N., et al.: Medical-surgical nursing, ed. 6, St. Louis, 1975, The C.V. Mosby Co.

Smith, D.W., and Germain, C.P.: Nursing of adults, Philadelphia, 1972, J.B. Lippincott Co.

Tucker, S.T., et al.: Patient care standards, ed. 2, St. Louis, 1980, The C.V. Mosby Co.

Before studying this unit it is important for the student to review Units 3 and 4. Principles and concepts reviewed in the earlier chapters are the foundations of nursing care presented in this unit. The nursing process is emphasized in establishing the plan of care that is based on problems identified. Examples of nursing care plans are provided but are by no means complete, and they are intended to serve only as examples.

CLASSIFICATION OF DISEASE

A. Congenital—condition present at birth
   1. Hereditary diseases that occur in families
   2. Acquired congenital diseases, such as those resulting from metabolic and nutritional problems during pregnancy
   3. Diseases that may be caused by chromosomal anomalies
B. Neoplastic—new growth, masses, or tumors
   1. Benign
   2. Malignant
C. External
   1. Trauma—mechanical injury to soft tissue or bone or both
   2. Physical—condition resulting from environmental agents, such as radiant energy, electricity, temperature, and atmospheric pressure
   3. Chemical—condition produced by caustic or corrosive agents, acids, metallic poisons, phosphorus, lead, and arsenic
   4. Oxygen deficit—condition caused by a lack of oxygen resulting from obstruction of oxgyen intake or oxygen utilization
   5. Allergic reaction—natural or acquired hypersensitivity to substances usually of a protein nature or to pollens, drugs, or foods
D. Metabolic—disease related to alterations in the anabolic and catabolic processes of the body caused by endocrine malfunction (such as hyperthyroidism and diabetes mellitus)

E. Organic—disease related to visible structural changes in tissues or organs
F. Functional—disease that affects bodily functions without any apparent organic changes
G. Further classification—onset and duration
   1. Acute—refers to the sudden onset, rapid course, and severe symptoms of a condition
   2. Chronic—long-term disease, such as arthritis

ESTABLISHMENT OF DIAGNOSIS

Introduction

A. Important function of practical nurse is to assist physician in establishing correct diagnosis
B. Properly collected and prepared specimens, accurately taken vital signs, and effectively communicated information assist in making diagnosis

History

Completed by physician or registered nurse

A. History of present illness
   1. Chief complaints
   2. Duration and severity of problems
   3. What patient believes causes illness
B. Medical history
   1. Question patient about medical history
   2. Note communicable diseases, surgery, and injuries
C. Systemic review
   1. Beginning at the head, review the various systems in detail
   2. Note patient's daily habits and routines
D. Family history
   1. Immediate family's health, beginning with grandparents
   2. Number of family members dead and cause of death
   3. Presence of allergies, tuberculosis, mental diseases, cancer, heart disease, or diabetes in family
E. Social history—socioeconomic, ethnic, religious, and educational background
F. Personal habits
   1. Factors influencing diagnosis and treatment are amount and frequency of
      a. Exercise
      b. Rest
      c. Sleep
      d. Drinking
      e. Smoking
      f. Diet
      g. Use of coffee, tea, and drugs
   2. Occupation and conditions of one's work also influence diagnosis and treatment

Physical examination

A. General appearance of patient and chief complaints are noted
B. Vital signs are observed
C. Beginning at the head, each system is examined thoroughly by
   1. Inspection
   2. Auscultation
   3. Palpation
   4. Percussion
D. Rectal and vaginal examinations are performed
E. Findings are summarized
F. Tentative diagnosis is made

Laboratory diagnosis (see Unit 4)

A. Preparation of patient
   1. Patient must be properly prepared and instructed for the test
   2. Proper preparation is responsibility of nurse and those designated to assist in that care
   3. Improper preparation of patients increases their hospital cost, lengthens their hospital stay, and increases time necessary to establish a diagnosis, thereby delaying treatment
B. Pathologic diagnosis—made on the basis of biopsy, Papanicolau's test (Pap smear), scrapings, specimens of body fluids or wastes, or any combination of the four
C. Roentgenographic diagnosis
   1. Fracture
   2. Foreign body
   3. Calcified lesion
   4. Organs—visualized with aid of iodine and barium solutions
D. Endoscopic diagnosis—made on basis of direct visualization
   1. Sigmoidoscopy
   2. Bronchoscopy
   3. Gastroscopy
   4. Arthroscopy

Autopsy

A. Autopsy gives most complete picture of disease
B. Nurse can assist medical team in securing autopsy permit

C. Autopsy may be beneficial to immediate family
D. Medical science advances on basis of knowledge the pathologist gains at autopsy

INFLAMMATION

Definition

Local reaction of the body to an irritant; it may be classified as serous, fibrinous, hemorrhagic, or purulent

Causes

A. Bacteriologic
B. Chemical
C. Physical
D. Traumatic

Pathophysiologic conditions

A. Congestion—characterized by initial transitory vasoconstriction, followed by vasodilation, followed by decreased blood flow
B. Exudation—characterized by diapedesis and leukocytosis and by local infiltration of tissues by serum and cells, causing edema; if irritant is bacteria, phagocytosis occurs
C. Resolution—when irritant is removed and debris of healing is removed through lymphatics; tissues return to normal

Symptoms

A. Rubor, or redness—hyperemia resulting from congestive phase
B. Calor, or heat—caused by vasodilation
C. Edema, or swelling—resulting from exudative phase
D. Dolor, or pain—produced by pressure of exudate on nerve ending
E. Loss of function—inability to use an inflamed part because of extent of the process
F. Changes in vital signs—temperature may be elevated and pulse rate increases with infection

Variations of the inflammatory process

A. Cellulitis—suppuration of subcutaneous tissue characterized by a rigid, swollen area
B. Abscess—localized collection of pus, which may rupture externally or internally
C. Ulcer—localized destruction of tissue on cutaneous or mucous surface
D. Boil, or furuncle—infected hair follicle
E. Carbuncle—multiple infected hair follicles
F. Sinus—tract leading from an abscess to the body surface
G. Fistula—connecting tract between two body surfaces or cavities

Repair

A. First intention—clean, incised wound that heals after suturing with a minimum of granulation and scar tissue
B. Second intention—healing from the bottom of the defect upward by granulation tissue; it results from loss of tissue or infection
C. Keloid (scarring)—large, shiny, irregular-shaped scar that continues to enlarge

Other types of changes produced by inflammation

A. Deteriorative changes
   1. Atrophy—reduction in size of cells and organs that were once normal in size
      a. Caused by inactivity or disuse
      b. Normal physiologic change, such as in postmenopausal reproductive organs
   2. Degeneration—alteration of cytoplasm, which may result in cellular death
   3. Necrosis—death of tissue within a circumscribed area, often called gangrene
      a. Necrotic area undergoes further changes and putrefaction from lack of venous circulation
      b. Necrotic area induced by loss of arterial blood supply
      c. Cells infected with toxigenic anaerobic clostridia and characterized by presence of gas in tissue. This type of gangrene spreads rapidly and can be fatal
B. Progressive changes
   1. Hypertrophy—increase in size of cell or organ
   2. Hyperplasia—increase in number of cells, such as in hyperthyroidism
   3. Regeneration—replacement of tissue that has been destroyed by tissue similar to that lost

NEOPLASMS (TUMORS)

In the treatment of tumors the main emphasis will be on cancer. Benign tumors are introduced as a comparison to malignant tumors

Classification

A. Benign
   1. Grow slowly

2. Do not usually cause death unless they interfere with a vital function
3. Are made of mature types of tissue
4. Are often encapsulated
5. Do not metastasize
6. Do not return once excised

B. Malignant
1. Grow rapidly
2. Extend into normal tissue
3. Are made of immature tissue
4. Interfere with normal life span if not treated early
5. Tend to metastasize by blood and lymph channels as well as by direct extension
6. Further classified as TNM system (primary tumor, regional nodes, and metastasis)

Causes

A. Cause is unknown
B. Causative factor theories are
1. Chemicals
2. Parasites
3. Hormones
4. Trauma
5. Inheritance
6. Viruses

Symptoms of cancer

A. Lump or thickening of breast
B. Sore that does not heal
C. Change in bowel or bladder habits
D. Persistent coughing or hoarseness
E. Difficulty in swallowing
F. Irregular bleeding or discharge from body orifices
G. Changes in wart or mole
H. Other symptoms—usually specific for area affected

Diagnostic tests

A. Complete physical examination
B. History narrative
C. Specific tests
1. Biopsy
2. Hormone levels
3. Phosphatase
a. Alkaline
b. Acid
4. Pap smear

D. Mammography—thermography and xerography
E. Endoscopic procedures

Treatment

A. Medical
1. Chemotherapy (antimetabolites, alkylating agents, antibiotics)
2. Radiation therapy (cobalt, radon seeds)
3. Immunotherapy—based on immunologic phenomena
4. Hormonal therapy (adrenocorticotropic hormone [ACTH], prednisone, androgens, estrogens) (sometimes included as chemotherapy)
5. Supportive therapy (analgesic, counseling)

B. Surgical
1. Radical
2. Palliative
3. Prophylactic

General nursing care principles

A. Perform preventive care by teaching early recognition of signs of cancer
B. Assist in preparation of patient for diagnostic tests and physical examination
C. Prepare patient physically and mentally for x-ray therapy or radioactive isotope therapy
1. Awareness of hazards involved in radiation therapy
2. Awareness of control of "hot" excreta
3. Awareness of local and systemic effects of radiation on body

D. Recognize role of various chemical agents, mode of administration, and anticipated responses and toxic reactions
E. Be aware of role of various treatments in cure, palliative therapy, and inhibition of cancer
F. Encourage confidence in physicians, hospital staff, and selected medical treatment
G. Reassure patient and family by acceptance and nonjudgmental attitude
H. Administer good general nursing care and specific care as the condition indicates
I. Assist patient to cope with increasing responsibility for own care if capable (patient with cystectomy or colostomy)
J. Accurately record observation and patient's condition and reactions
K. Be very supportive to patient and family

Agencies

Assist in detection, prevention, public education, research treatment, and rehabilitation

A. National Cancer Institute, Bethesda, Maryland
B. American Cancer Society and its major city and state chapters
C. Religious and international organizations
D. Hospice groups

Diseases of ear, nose, and throat

EAR

Introduction

A. Hearing impairment is deafness, or a loss of ability to hear, which may occur gradually or suddenly. Impairment is classified as
   1. Conductive—caused by disease or injury that interferes with sound wave conduction to inner ear
   2. Sensorineural—produced by disorder of inner ear, auditory nerve, or auditory center in brain
   3. Mixed—results from combination of the preceding
B. Impairment is diagnosed by audiometry, tuning fork tests (Weber, Rinne), and symptoms specific to condition
C. Treatment depends on cause and amount of impairment
   1. Surgical
      a. Fenestration, or creation of new windows for sound wave transmission (rarely done today)
      b. Stapedectomy, or removal of stapes and replacement by prostheses
   2. Supportive—hearing aid, lip reading
   3. Chemotherapeutic—vitamins, antibiotics

General nursing care principles

A. Educating and assisting patient (safety, community resources, appliances)
B. Understanding psychosocial aspects of hearing impairment
   1. May suffer depression and insecurity because of impairment of communication and loss of auditory background
   2. May refuse treatment or use of appliance as a result of attitudes conveyed by others or denial of disability
   3. May view appliances as a nuisance or annoyance
C. Providing postoperative care
   1. Patient should be cautioned to avoid blowing nose for at least 1 week
   2. Patient should maintain head position recommended by surgeon
   3. Nurse should change cotton in external ear canal as necessary
   4. Analgesics are given as patient indicates need
   5. Antibiotics are used prophylactically
   6. Safety measures are used since vertigo is common
   7. Strict aseptic technique is used (ear is close to brain)

Diseases of the ear

A. Otosclerosis
   1. Problems include
      a. Gradual hearing loss
      b. Tinnitus
      c. Safety
   2. Otosclerosis is a gradual loss of hearing resulting from fixation of ossicles of ear, which interferes with transmission, or conduction, of sound patterns. Heredity is a causative factor, but the underlying cause is unknown
   3. Diagnosis is based on examination by otologist, family history, and symptoms
   4. At present there is no cure. Hearing loss can be corrected by surgery (stapedectomy) and use of hearing aid
   5. Nursing care plan is same as general nursing care principles
B. Otitis media
   1. Problems include
      a. Decreased hearing
      b. Echoing of own voice
      c. Fever
      d. Malaise
      e. Pain and sensation of pressure in ear
      f. Drainage (foul smelling)
      g. Itching
   2. Otitis media, middle ear inflammation, may be classified as
      a. Serous—fluid forms in middle ear because of obstruction (infection, allergy, tumor, sudden change in altitude)
      b. Acute purulent—results from spread of microorganisms from eustachian tube (upper respiratory infections)

c. Chronic—preventable condition that results from not treating acute otitis media
3. Diagnosis is based on symptoms and otoscopic examination
4. Treatment of serous type is aspiration of fluid after paracentesis and treatment of the underlying cause. Treatment of acute purulent type is use of antibiotics and incision into eardrum (myringotomy). Complications may include mastoiditis, meningitis, and labyrinthitis
5. Nursing care plan is same as general nursing care principles

C. Ménière's disease
1. Problems include
   a. Vertigo
   b. Tinnitus
   c. Progressive hearing loss
2. Ménière's disease is a condition in which pathologic changes occur in the inner ear from unknown cause
3. Diagnosis is based on symptoms and otoscopic examination
4. Treatment is symptomatic or surgical (labyrinth destroyed) and includes
   a. Low sodium diet to lessen edema
   b. Sedatives to relieve apprehension
   c. Nicotinic acid for vasodilation
   d. Antiemetics (Dramamine, Antivert)
   e. Bed rest
5. Nursing care plan consists of preventing aggravation of symptoms
   a. Prevent jarring of bed
   b. Explain all movements to patient and carry out slowly
   c. Protect from falls caused by vertigo, and provide safety rails

NOSE

Diseases of the nose

A. Epistaxis
1. Problems include
   a. Hemorrhage
   b. Halitosis
   c. Preexisting condition
2. Epistaxis is defined as nosebleed. It may be caused by trauma, severe sneezing, coughing, lack of humidity, scurvy, lack of vitamin K, hypertension, or ulceration of vessels or tissue
3. Treatment consists of the following procedures
   a. Emergency—have patient sit with head tilted slightly forward. While patient breathes through mouth, pinch anterior nares until clotting occurs
   b. Medical
      (1) Posterior nasal packings
      (2) Cauterization
      (3) Application of vasoconstrictors
      (4) Daily check of hematocrit
      (5) Ascertainment of prothrombin times in males (check for hemophilia)
      (6) Thorough physical examination
4. Nursing care plan consists of instructing patient not to swallow blood, applying cold compresses to bridge of nose, monitoring vital signs, and assisting the physician

B. Sinusitis
1. Problems include
   a. Headache
   b. Pain and pressure over affected sinus
   c. Halitosis
   d. Nasal discharge, producing nausea at times
   e. Dizziness
2. Sinusitis is inflammatory reaction of paranasal sinuses, which can become chronic. It is one of the most commom upper respiratory problems in otolaryngology
3. Treatment is aimed at overcoming infection. Medical treatment consists of antibiotics, analgesics, antihistamines, decongestants, and increased fluid intake. Surgical treatment may be in the form of antral irrigation or Caldwell-Luc operation on maxillary sinuses
4. Nursing care plan (postoperative) involves
   a. Promoting wound healing
      (1) Have patient spit out drainage; note amount and character
      (2) Elevate head of bed 45 degrees
      (3) Observe nasopharynx for slipped nasal packing
      (4) Encourage fluids to 3000 ml in 24 hours
   b. Observing for complications
      (1) Hemorrhage
      (2) Airway obstruction

THROAT

Diseases of the throat

A. Laryngitis
  1. Problems include
    a. Hoarseness
    b. Loss of voice
    c. Pain in throat
  2. Laryngitis is inflammation and swelling of membranous lining of the larynx, which usually occurs with upper respiratory tract infection. It can be caused by excessive use of voice and irritation
  3. Treatment is complete voice rest, with antibiotics if infection is present. Laryngoscopic examination may be done if condition persists
  4. Nursing care plan involves
    a. Promoting healing
    b. Preventing infection

B. Laryngeal carcinoma
  1. Problems include
    a. Hoarseness
    b. Dysphagia
    c. Dyspnea
    d. Weight loss
    e. Weakness
    f. Anemia
  2. Cancer of the larynx is believed to be caused by chronic irritation (laryngitis, smoking, alcohol) and possibly heredity
  3. Diagnosis is confirmed by laryngoscopy, biopsy, and x-ray examination. Treatment is surgical removal of tumor and in many cases removal of larynx (laryngectomy). A permanent opening (tracheostomy) is necessary since trachea no longer connects to nasopharynx
  4. Nursing care plan involves
    a. Promoting patient preparation for surgery
      (1) Explain availability of appliances patient may use postoperatively (pad and pencil, magic slate) and permanently (electric larynx, esophageal speech)
      (2) Explain tracheostomy function and care to be expected postoperatively
      (3) Have member of Lost Chord Club or Nu Voice Club visit (with physician's approval)
    b. Promoting wound healing
      (1) Perform suction on and clean tracheostomy wound frequently
      (2) Position patient on side with head of bed elevated 45 degrees
      (3) Observe patency of airway, and humidify air breathed through tracheostomy
      (4) Observe patency of Hemovac and amount, color, and character of drainage
    c. Promoting self-care activities by patient
      (1) Instruct patient to care for self (feeding, tracheostomy care)
      (2) Instruct patient to avoid swimming, preventing water and debris from entering tracheal opening

EYE

Introduction

A. National Society for the Prevention of Blindness attempts to educate public about ways to prevent sight impairment
B. Early treatment may prevent serious problems
C. Ophthalmologist is physician qualified to diagnose and treat eye diseases and should not be confused with optician and optometrist, although these roles are expanding
D. Reduction or disturbance of vision is a common occurrence, affecting physical, social, and emotional aspects of an individual's life
E. Corrective lenses (glasses, contact lenses) may be employed to reduce certain disabilities
F. Standard for normal vision is expressed as a fraction (20/20). It indicates ability to read a certain line of Snellen chart from distance of 20 feet
G. Blindness is legally defined as central visual acuity of 20/200 or less in the better eye, even with corrective lenses
H. American Foundation for the Blind, state agencies, and the Library of Congress in Washington, D.C., provide information and assistance in securing Braille teachers, books, and additional aids for the visually handicapped

General nursing care principles

A. Speak before touching patient for any reason
B. Explain all treatments thoroughly
C. Adjust blinds and move bed as necessary to reduce glare; patient may be instructed to wear dark glasses when photophobia is a problem
D. Orient patient to room and ward, indicating placement of furniture, bathroom, personal items, and especially nurse call bell. Alert patient to any change in placement

E. Allow patient to do self-care with assistance as needed; encourage independence
F. At mealtime indicate position of utensils and placement of food items on dish using clock principle (meat is at 3 o'clock and vegetables are at 9 o'clock)
G. Preoperative preparation includes
   1. Observing elderly sedated patients closely; employing safety measures (siderails up)
   2. Doing hair and facial grooming since postoperative positioning of head may prohibit this being done by patient
   3. Reporting any detected respiratory condition or allergy causing sneezing or coughing since this may result in postoperative hemorrhage
H. Postoperative care involves
   1. Following physician's order for positioning of head and other restricted activities
   2. Encouraging family member to stay with patient if possible to provide support and reassurance
   3. Reorienting patient to room, showing position of call bell
   4. Keeping side rails up and in place
   5. Gently turning head to side if vomiting occurs. Do not raise head. Administer antiemetic as ordered
   6. Feeding patient with fixed head position or covered eyes
   7. Avoiding sudden movement of equipment or bed to prevent eye injury
   8. Performing frequent skin care (especially to bony prominences) since turning is not permitted. Keep linens smooth and clean without changing
   9. Instructing patient to avoid straining on defecation
   10. Instructing patient to avoid bending, stooping, or lifting heavy objects
   11. Instructing patient in performance of treatments to be done at home (eyedrops) (See Unit 4, Fundamentals of nursing, Eye procedures)

Common disorders

A. Refractive disorders—inability to refractive media (cornea, aqueous humor, lens, vitreous humor) to converge light rays to focus on retina
   1. Types
      a. Myopia (nearsightedness)—eyeball too long or lens too thick
      b. Hyperopia (farsightedness)—eyeball too short or lens too thin
      c. Astigmatism—defective curvature of cornea or lens
      d. Presbyopia—loss of elasticity of lens
   2. Symptoms—mainly associated with reduction in visual acuity
   3. Treatment—prescription lenses (glasses, contacts)
B. Eye infections
   1. Common types
      a. Uveitis
      b. Conjunctivitis (pinkeye)
      c. Keratitis
      d. Hordeolum (stye)
      e. Chalazion
   2. Some symptoms
      a. Edema of various eye parts
      b. Eye pain
      c. Increased or reduced tearing
      d. Purulent exudate
   3. Diagnosis—based on visual examination, symptoms, and culture and sensitivity
   4. Treatment—according to diagnosis. May include antibiotics, mydriatics, chemotherapeutic agents, applications of heat and cold, and sometimes surgical intervention

Diseases of the eye

A. Cataract
   1. Problems include
      a. Gradual vision loss
      b. Safety
   2. This condition is opacity of lens or lens capsule. Occurs most often in older persons during seventh, eighth, and ninth decades of life. May be congenital or caused by trauma
   3. Cataract is treated by surgical removal of lens or lens capsule, usually from one eye at a time, with consideration for patient's age and maturity of the cataract. Corrective lenses may be prescribed after patient is discharged
   4. For nursing care plan see general nursing care principles
B. Glaucoma
   1. Problems include
      a. Severe eye pain
      b. Blurred vision
      c. Headaches

d. Halos seen around lights (especially at night)
e. Reduced peripheral vision
f. Nausea and vomiting

2. Glaucoma is caused by increased intraocular pressure resulting from imbalance in absorption and production of aqueous humor. Glaucoma is classified as acute or chronic
3. Diagnosis is based on symptoms and tonometer reading indicating increased intraocular pressure (usually above 25 mm Hg)
4. Medical treatment includes miotic drugs (pilocarpine, timolol maleate [Timoptic]), carbonic anhydrase inhibitors (acetazolamide [Diamox]), and analgesics for pain. Surgical drainage operations are sometimes performed (iridectomy, sclerectomy)
5. For nursing care plan see general nursing care principles. Nurse should check eye drops carefully before administration to patient with glaucoma. An error in administration (mydriatic rather than miotic) may cause an acute attack resulting in blindness

Other eye conditions

A. Detached retina—sensory layer of the retina pulls away from the pigmented layer and vitreous humor leaks into the space, occupying the position the retina normally assumes; condition may occur following eye surgery (cataract removal)
   1. Characterized by loss of vision in affected area (may be complete loss). Moving spots and flashes of light may be seen. Patient may describe episode as a curtain dropping over visual field
   2. Diagnosed by retinal examination with ophthalmoscope and by symptoms
   3. Treated by bed rest and administration of mydriatics (atropine); scleral buckling is often performed

B. Corneal abrasions—interfere with vision and are treated by corneal transplant

C. Malignant eye tumors—are uncommon and are usually treated by enucleation of entire eyeball, including muscles. Prosthesis (glass eye) may be fitted following enucleation

Diseases of the skeletal system

MUSCULOSKELETAL

Introduction

Musculoskeletal problems may be caused by trauma, nutritional disorders, or degenerative phenomena. Proper nutrition and exercise are essential for maintenance of the musculoskeletal system

Assessment

A. Functional ability of affected and unaffected joints and limbs
B. Adaptations made because of disabilities
C. Pain evaluation (onset, cause, description)
D. Evaluation of skin integrity

SKELETAL

A. Fractures
   1. Problems include
      a. Pain, tenderness, and edema
      b. Immobility
      c. Shock of varying degrees
      d. Malalignment of bone
   2. Fracture is break in continuity of bone caused by trauma, bone weakness, or tumors and classified according to severity (simple or compound). Types of fractures are listed in Glossary. Symptoms are unnatural movement, crepitus, pain, tenderness, swelling and discoloration, and shortening of extremity
   3. Diagnosis is confirmed by x-ray examination. Main objectives of treatment are to regain correct alignment (reduce fracture), maintain alignment (skin or skeletal traction, casts, immobilizers), and regain function (physical therapy, exercises)
   4. Nursing care plan involves
      a. Maintaining proper bone alignment (cast, traction, immobilizer, internal fixation)
         (1) Support movable limbs at joints
         (2) Supply firm mattress
         (3) Check circulation of extremity distal to cast frequently; cast may inhibit circulation
         (4) Handle wet cast with flat part of hands; apply no pressure to wet cast
         (5) "Finish" edges of cast by petaling or with stockinette

(6) If cast covers wound, observe cast for drainage; smell cast for foul odor denoting infection
(7) After cast is removed, apply oil or lanolin to dry areas
(8) Check operative site for hemorrhage (swelling, discoloration)

b. Promoting comfort
(1) Assess onset and cause of discomfort and pain
(2) Administer analgesics
(3) Reposition patient if possible
(4) Administer frequent skin care

c. Preventing deformities
(1) Have patient turn, cough, and deep breathe at least every 2 hours
(2) Assess skin integrity every shift
(3) Assess range of motion of unaffected limbs
(4) Administer frequent skin care

B. Arthritis
1. Problems include
a. Sore, red, swollen joints
b. Muscle weakness
c. Fever
2. Arthritis is an inflammation of a joint caused by infection, trauma, endocrine abnormalities, or allergic reactions, or it may be of unknown cause
3. Diagnosis is established on the basis of symptoms
4. Treatment includes analgesics (aspirin), antiinflammatory drugs (prednisone, ibuprofen [Motrin]), and gold salts. Total joint replacements may be indicated
5. Nursing care plan involves
a. Reducing strain on joints
(1) Splints as ordered
(2) Heat as ordered
(3) Analgesics and antiinflammatory medications as ordered
(4) Rest periods and activity

b. Observing for postoperative complications (total joint replacement: total hip, for example)
(1) Hemorrhage—check dressing and vital signs frequently
(2) Fat embolus—report chest pain and tachycardia
(3) Dislocation of prosthesis—keep hip abducted postoperatively
(4) Wound infection—note drainage; keep dressing clean and dry

DISEASES OF THE INTEGUMENTARY SYSTEM OR SKIN

Introduction

The skin may be affected by external irritants or internal irritants. Proper nutrition, exercise, rest, and cleanliness are important in preventing skin problems and promoting healing. Large areas of skin loss may predispose patient to fluid and electrolyte imbalance

Assessment

A. Describe lesions in terms of size, shape, recent changes, and exudate
B. Observe skin integrity, especially over bony prominences
C. Evaluate for symptoms of fluid and electrolyte imbalance
1. Hypokalemia
2. Hyponatremia

Common dermatologic conditions

A. Acne vulgaris
1. Problems include
a. Altered body image because of facial disfigurement
b. Infection
2. Acne vulgaris is a disorder characterized by pustules, cysts, blackheads, and nodules, usually during adolescence. The increase in oil secretion stimulated by adolescent hormonal changes obstructs sebaceous glands, predisposing to cyst development. Secondary infections develop, leading to scarring
3. Diagnosis is made by symptoms and physical examination
4. Treatment is to prevent follicular obstruction (abrasive soap), reduce inflammation (steroids), alleviate predisposing factors (diet low in fats and carbohydrates), remove damaged skin (dermabrasion), and prevent infections (antibiotics)
5. Nursing care plan involves
a. Preventing infection and reducing inflammation
(1) Cleanse area as ordered
(2) Administer antibiotics as ordered

(3) Instruct patient to avoid touching lesions
b. Providing supportive environment
(1) Allow patient to ventilate feelings
(2) Encourage emphasis on attributes
c. Providing adequate nutrition
(1) Evaluate dietary habits
(2) Encourage proper diet
(3) Instruct patient to avoid excessive fats and carbohydrates

B. Furuncles (boils)
1. Problems include
a. Pain
b. Swelling with cellulitis
2. Furuncles are bacterial infection causing inflammation of one or more hair follicles
3. Treatment consists of hot wet compresses, topical antibiotic ointment and systemic antibiotics, and surgical incision and drainage
4. Nursing care plan involves
a. Instructing patient to avoid picking at lesions
b. Offering understanding

C. Athlete's foot
1. Problems include
a. Rash on feet
b. Pruritus
2. Athlete's foot is a superficial fungal infection that is usually found on the feet and is characterized by a chronic rash causing itching and burning
3. The organism may be cultured to confirm diagnosis
4. Treatment consists of foot soaks with potassium permanganate or Burow's solution, fungicidal creams, and systemic antibacterial agents if there is a superimposed infection
5. Nursing care plan involves
a. Preventing reinfection
(1) Keep feet clean and dry
(2) Have patient wear clean dry white socks
(3) Have patient wear clogs in community showers
b. Promoting comfort
(1) Encourage bed rest until acute phase resolved
(2) Elevate feet
(3) Administer foot soaks as ordered

D. Pediculosis capitis
1. Problems include
a. Itchy scalp
b. Excoriation of scalp
c. Live insects
d. Nits attached to strands of hair
2. Pediculosis capitis is the infestation of the hair of the head by lice, characterized by itching, excoriation, and crusting
3. Treatment consists of shampoos with gamma benzene hexachloride (Kwell) by patient and all family members or close contacts
4. Nursing care plan involves removing infestation
a. Shampoo with Kwell as directed
b. Comb hair after shampoo with a fine-toothed comb until all eggs are gone
c. Treat all family members

E. Herpes zoster (shingles)
1. Problems include
a. Fever
b. Pain
c. Vesicular eruptions
2. Herpes zoster is caused by a virus (varicella) that produces an inflammatory condition along the nerves from one or more posterior ganglia and is characterized by severely painful vesicular eruption and fever
3. Treatment consists of analgesics to control pain, barbiturates to control nervousness, antihistamines to control itching, steroids (systemically and locally) to promote healing, and cool wet compresses
4. Nursing care plan involves
a. Promoting comfort
(1) Administer analgesics, barbiturates, and antihistamines as ordered
(2) Apply cool wet dressing if ordered
(3) Ensure adequate fluid intake
b. Promoting healing
(1) Apply steroid locally and administer systemically
(2) Keep nails short
(3) Provide nutritional diet

F. Psoriasis
1. Problems include
a. Dry scaly skin
b. Pruritus
2. Psoriasis is a chronic, noninfectious, inflammatory condition of unknown cause, which is characterized by small, scaly papules that develop into deep red, scaling lesions covered by silvery scales

3. Treatment is palliative; there is no known cure. Treatment consists of wet dressings, steroid preparations, anthralin preparations, coal tar preparations, and methotrexate to relieve symptoms
4. Nursing care plan involves
   a. Reducing scaling
      (1) Provide daily tub bath
      (2) Remove scales with soft brush
      (3) Apply ointments as ordered
   b. Reducing discomfort
      (1) Keep patient's nails short
      (2) Encourage moderate exposure to sun

G. Cancer of the skin
1. Problems include
   a. Lesion that may ulcerate
   b. Emotional impact of diagnosis
2. The most common lesion is basal cell carcinoma, which is usually caused by prolonged exposure to skin irritants and is characterized by small nodules with pearly translucent borders that crust and ulcerate
3. Diagnosis is confirmed by biopsy
4. Treatment depends on location, cell type, cosmetic desires of patient, and invasiveness of lesion. Radiation and surgical removal may be indicated
5. Nursing care plan involves
   a. Protecting irradiated skin areas
      (1) Apply lanolin to irradiated area
      (2) Keep skin clean and dry; avoid abrasive soaps
      (3) Keep radiation markings intact
   b. Educating patient
      (1) To wear protective clothing or lotions while exposed to sun
      (2) To report any unusual skin changes, especially changes in moles

Allergic skin diseases

A. Problems include
1. Pruritus
2. Swelling

B. Allergic skin diseases are defined as conditions in which there is an allergic response of the skin caused by substances coming in contact with the skin (contact dermatitis) or by substances taken internally (foods or medication) and characterized by dilation of blood vessels causing redness and swelling

C. Diagnosis is confirmed by patch testing

D. Treatment consists of desensitization and removal of the cause

E. Nursing care plan involves controlling initiating event
1. Identify initiating event (contact, emotional upset)
2. Desensitize protocol

Burns

A. Problems
1. Fluid and electrolyte imbalance
2. Loss of skin protection
3. Pain
4. Shock

B. Definition—wounds caused by excessive exposure to heat (fire, steam, radiation, electricity, chemicals). Classification depends on depth of burn: first degree (erythema), second degree (blisters containing water and electrolytes), and third degree (massive edema, necrosis because entire dermis is destroyed). "Rule of nines" is used to calculate percent of body burned and fluid replacement

C. Treatment
1. Shock phase (first 48 hours)
   a. Respiratory evaluation; tracheostomy may be done
   b. Replacement of fluids and electrolytes
   c. Wound care
      (1) Debridement followed by topical antiinfectives (silver sulfadiazine [Silvadene], mafenide [Sulfamylon])
      (2) Open dressing method
      (3) Occlusive dressing method
      (4) Reverse isolation method
   d. Treatment of shock
   e. Administration of drugs
      (1) Narcotics to relieve pain
      (2) Systemic antibiotics
      (3) Tetanus toxoid given prophylactically
2. Turning point (2 to 5 days)
   a. Restricted fluid intake; diuresis is occurring
   b. Wound care
   c. Pain relief
3. Recovery phase
   a. High-protein, high-carbohydrate diet
   b. Wound care; skin grafts may be done
   c. Systemic antibiotics
   d. Physical therapy
   e. Occupational therapy

D. Nursing care plan
  1. Shock phase
    a. Maintain adequate oxygen to body cells
      (1) Monitor vital signs
      (2) Observe for restlessness
      (3) Administer oxygen as ordered
      (4) Monitor arterial blood gases (ABG)
      (5) Assess level of consciousness
    b. Replace fluid loss
      (1) Maintain intravenous fluid
      (2) Monitor fluid administration
      (3) Monitor hemoglobin, hematocrit, and electrolytes
    c. Monitor kidney function
      (1) Insert Foley catheter
      (2) Provide care necessary with catheter
      (3) Monitor output every hour
      (4) Measure specific gravity
      (5) Monitor blood urea nitrogen (BUN) and creatine clearance
    d. Control pain
      (1) Administer narcotics
      (2) Administer oxygen
    e. Prevent infections
      (1) Assist physician with debridement and dressing application
      (2) Position patient for comfort in anatomically correct manner
      (3) Reverse isolation
  2. Turning point
    a. Monitor respiratory status
      (1) Observe for restlessness
      (2) Note rate and depth of respirations
      (3) Auscultate chest every shift
      (4) Monitor blood gases
    b. Promote hydration and kidney function
      (1) Maintain accurate intake and output
      (2) Maintain intravenous fluid
      (3) Monitor urine specific gravity
      (4) Report symptoms of fluid overload
      (5) Weigh daily
    c. Promote wound healing
      (1) Establish reverse isolation
      (2) Change dressing as ordered
      (3) Provide adequate nutrition
      (4) Position patient to prevent deformity
    d. Control pain
      (1) Administer analgesic before dressing change
      (2) Reposition frequently
    e. Provide emotional support for patient and family
      (1) Be sympathetic—allow patient and family to verbalize feelings
      (2) Encourage patient to see daily accomplishments and improvements
  3. Recovery phase
    a. Promote wound healing
      (1) Encourage diet high in carbohydrates and proteins
      (2) Change dressing as ordered
      (3) Observe for symptoms of infection
    b. Prevent contractures
      (1) Encourage movement of unaffected areas
      (2) Position affected areas in anatomically correct manner
    c. Observe for complications
      (1) Curling's ulcer—stress ulcer in stomach mucosa
      (2) Anemia—caused by blood loss
      (3) Renal failure—complication resulting from shock
    d. Provide emotional support and diversional activities

DISEASES OF THE URINARY TRACT

Introduction

Urinary tract disorders involve disturbances in function and structure and abnormal conditions of the urinary tract. Patients with disorders suffer from physical discomfort, embarrassment, and anxiety. The urinary tract functions as one of the body's waste disposal systems for by-products of metabolism and regulates balance of body fluids and electrolytes. Frequently gastrointestinal symptoms will be related to urologic conditions because of anatomic proximity, renointestinal reflexes, and peritoneal irritation (nausea, vomiting, diarrhea, abdominal discomfort)

Assessment

A. Obtain information about patient's voiding patterns
B. Observe character, color, and amount of urine
C. Observe appearance of genitalia
D. Note weight, any signs of edema, and skin condition

Infections

A. Cystitis
  1. Problems include
    a. Urgency
    b. Hematuria

c. Frequency
d. Perineal and suprapubic pain
2. Cystitis is inflammation of the urinary bladder. The condition may be caused by obstruction, infection *(Escherichia coli),* or upper urinary tract infection
3. Diagnosis is based on patient history, physical examination, urinalysis, and culture and sensitivity
4. Treatment is directed to evaluating cause (organism, structural problem, obstruction) and correcting causative factors. It may consist of
a. Use of antibiotic or chemotherapeutic drugs
b. Use of analgesics (phenazopyridine [Pyridium]), antispasmodics, and heat to perineum to relieve spasm, pain, and urgency
c. Maintenance of acid urine (pH 5.5); organisms are unable to live in acid urine
5. Nursing care plan is based on encouraging rest, maintaining accurate intake and output, and instructing patient in ordered treatments

B. Pyelonephritis
1. Problems include
a. Headache
b. Fatigue
c. Anorexia
d. Weight loss
2. Pyelonephritis is inflammation of renal pelvis and lining of collecting system. The condition may be caused by renal disease, trauma, pregnancy, or obstruction or may result from ureterovesical reflux. During acute and chronic stages, the urine contains pus, bacteria, and albumin
3. Diagnosis is made on the same basis as in cystitis
4. Treatment is based on combating the organism that causes infection
5. Nursing care plan is based on encouraging rest, maintaining accurate intake and output, and instructing patient in ordered treatments

C. Acute glomerulonephritis
1. Problems include
a. Generalized edema
b. Fatigue
c. Anorexia
d. Mild hypertension
e. Anemia
f. Oliguria
2. This is an inflammatory process involving both kidneys. It is commonly seen following an upper respiratory tract infection (beta-hemolytic streptococci), impetigo, or a pneumococcal or staphylococcal infection
3. Diagnosis is based on symptoms, patient history, urinalysis, blood chemistry (elevated BUN and serum creatinine and rise of C-reactive protein), and needle biopsy
4. There is no specific treatment. Management is directed to controlling symptoms and pathologic conditions. Diet is restricted in sodium and protein according to degree of edema and renal damage. Antibiotics, antihypertensives, and antiinflammatory agents (prednisone) are given
5. Nursing care plan involves preventing progression of renal damage
a. Maintain bed rest
b. Monitor intake and output and daily weights
c. Observe for signs of renal failure, cardiac failure, pulmonary edema, and increasing hypertension

Obstructions

A. Renal calculi
1. Problems include
a. Flank pain as stone moves
b. Hematuria
c. Infection
2. Calculi are found frequently in the urinary tract. Etiologic factors are stasis of urine, infections, vitamin deficiencies, and hyperparathyroidism
3. Diagnosis is based on symptoms, physical examination, cystoscopic examination, and intravenous pyelogram. Stones smaller than 1 cm are expected to pass on their own or with increased fluids; sometimes glycerin introduced by way of ureteral catheter and cystoscope will dilate ureter and assist passage of stone
4. Some bladder stones, if too large for cystoscopic removal, may be crushed and removed by way of litholapaxy. Larger stones are removed through abdominal surgery. Analgesics and antibiotics are administered for pain and to combat or prevent infection
5. Nursing care plan involves facilitating passages of stone
a. Force fluids to 3000 ml in 24 hours
b. Strain all urine to note passage of stone
c. Administer antibiotics and analgesics as ordered

Neoplasms

A. Renal tumors
  1. Problems include
    a. Hematuria
    b. Pain
    c. Weight loss
    d. Malaise
    e. Fever
  2. Hypernephroma (renal adenocarcinoma) is the most common malignancy of the kidney in adults
  3. Diagnosis is based on physical examination, biopsy, and x-ray examination
  4. Treatment is surgical removal as early as possible. Chemotherapy and radiation therapy may may also be used
  5. Nursing care plan (postoperative care) involves
    a. Promoting wound healing
    b. Observing for complications
      (1) Pneumonia
      (2) Renal failure

Renal failure

A. Problems include
  1. Edema
  2. Oliguria
  3. Nausea and vomiting
  4. Hypertension
  5. Confusion and irritability
  6. Reduced level of consciousness
  7. Convulsions
B. Renal failure is malfunctioning of the kidneys. Waste products are not excreted and remain in bloodstream (uremia). It may be classified as acute or chronic. Failure may be caused by obstruction, hypertension, and poisoning. Elevated BUN, creatinine, uric acid, potassium, and phosphorus are found in renal failure
C. Diagnosis is based on history and evaluation
D. Treatment consists of the attempt to reverse or remove cause; a dietary regimen directed toward reduction of sodium, fluids, and proteins; mild sedation for restlessness; antimicrobial therapy to prevent infection; and peritoneal dialysis or renal dialysis by way of artificial kidney machine to rest kidneys
E. Nursing care plan is directed to close observation of patient and adherence to physician's regimen
  1. Prevent further renal failure
    a. Observe for signs of complete renal shutdown
    b. Observe and protect patient who has behavioral changes (irritability, complaints of headache, reduced level of consciousness)
    c. Teach patient importance of strict adherence to diet
    d. Restrict activity
  2. Promote comfort
    a. Give oral hygiene and meticulous skin care for uremic frost
    b. Provide emotional support to family and patient
    c. Assist patient to adapt ordered treatment to daily living patterns

DISORDERS OF THE FEMALE REPRODUCTIVE SYSTEM (GYNECOLOGIC DISORDERS)

Introduction

Disorders of the female reproductive tract other than those caused by pregnancy may interfere with health status and/or childbearing capacity. Regardless of pathologic conditions, early diagnosis and prompt medical attention are important. Many persons are reluctant to discuss matters concerning their reproductive system and sexual functioning, and consideration of these feelings is a must for health team members

Assessment

A. Note pattern of menstrual cycle
  1. History of menstrual pattern
  2. Character, amount, and length of menstrual flow
B. Observe appearance of vulva, perineum, and anus
C. Observe for presence and character of vaginal discharge
D. Obtain information about patient's voiding patterns and bowel habits
E. Observe appearance of breasts
  1. Size, symmetry, contour
  2. Condition of skin, nipples

Infections

A. Nonvenereal
  1. Problems include
    a. Abnormal vaginal discharge
    b. Pruritus and edema of perineal area
    c. Fever
    d. Dysuria

2. Most common are caused by *Trichomonas vaginalis* (protozoan) or *Candida albicans* (fungus). The presence of the infectious organism initiates a localized inflammatory response resulting in the previously mentioned problems
3. Diagnosis is made by microscopic examination of vaginal secretions
4. Treatment is according to causative organism and may be in the form of douche, vaginal suppository or cream, or oral medication. *Candida* is treated primarily with nystatin or miconazole. *Trichomonas* is treated primarily with metronidazole (Flagyl)
5. Nursing care plan involves
   a. Reducing perineal discomfort
      (1) Administer medications as ordered
      (2) Administer perineal care every 3 to 4 hours (sitz bath may be included)
      (3) Encourage fluid intake to 3000 ml unless contraindicated
   b. Promoting healing
      (1) Administer medications as ordered
      (2) Use careful hand-washing technique to prevent spread and recurrence
      (3) Instruct patient on principles of hygiene

B. Venereal
1. Gonorrhea
   a. Problems include
      (1) Abnormal vaginal discharge
      (2) Dysuria
      (3) Pruritus and pain in vulvar region
   b. *Neisseria gonorrhea* is contracted by sexual intercourse with a person infected with gonorrhea. The primary site of infection is the genital tract. Infection may spread to other body parts. Symptoms occur 3 days to 2 weeks after intercourse with an infected person. Occasionally infections are asymptomatic for long periods of time. Abscesses of Skene's or Bartholin's glands may develop
   c. Diagnosis is based on stained smear of urethral discharge and cultures using special medium
   d. The infection is treated with antibiotics (penicillin), sitz baths, douches, and surgery as needed to drain abscesses
   e. Nursing care plan involves
      (1) Reducing perineal discomfort
         (a) Administer medications as ordered
         (b) Administer perineal care every 3 to 4 hours (sitz bath may be included)
         (c) Encourage fluid intake to 3000 ml unless contraindicated
      (2) Promoting healing
         (a) Administer antibiotics as ordered
         (b) Use careful hand-washing technique to prevent spread and recurrence
         (c) Instruct patient regarding communicability (avoid direct contact with the wet discharge)
2. Syphilis
   Additional assessment consists of observing, recording, and reporting chancre of genitalia, nipple, or mouth; skin rashes; condylomas; alopecia; and lymph node changes
   a. Problems include
      (1) Pain in vulvar region
      (2) Other symptoms present according to severity of infection
   b. Syphilis *(Treponema pallidum)* is contracted by sexual intercourse or other types of intimate contact with an infected person (it may be congenital); syphilis is classified by stages (primary, secondary, tertiary) according to progression of disease. In the primary stage, symptoms include chancre of the genitalia, nipple, or mouth. Secondary stage symptoms include skin rash, condylomas, alopecia, and lymph node changes. The tertiary stage, seen less frequently since the advent of antibiotics, includes serious complications commonly affecting the aorta, the eye, and the central nervous system
   c. Diagnosis is based on Venereal Disease Research Laboratories (VDRL), Rapid Plasma Reagin (RPR), and Fluorescent Treponemal Antibody Absorption (FTA-ABS) tests. In early stages treatment is with antibiotics (penicillin). In later stages antibiotics are used, but treatment is also directed at damaged structures according to pathologic conditions and symptoms
   d. Nursing care plan involves reducing perineal discomfort
      (1) Administer medications as ordered
      (2) Administer perineal care every 3 to 4 hours (sitz bath may be included)
      (3) Encourage fluid intake to 3000 ml unless contraindicated

Tumors of lower reproductive structures

In making additional assessment, keep in mind that tumors may be asymptomatic. Note disturbances in normal menstrual pattern. Changes in amount and character of vaginal discharge should be noted as well as any changes in overall feeling of well-being (fatigability, depression)

A. Problems include
   1. Dysmenorrhea
   2. Fatigability
   3. Lower abdominal pain
   4. Constipation

B. Uterine fibroids are the most common benign tumors of the uterus. They are believed to be hormonal in origin, resulting in dysmenorrhea, anemia caused by excessive flow, and fatigability. Benign ovarian cysts are fairly common tumors of the female reproductive system. Because of hormonal influence they are often associated with acute and/or chronic lower abdominal pain and fertility problems. Malignant tumors may involve any reproductive structure. Cervical cancer is usually asymptomatic, while uterine cancer is rare before the onset of menses. Problems and symptoms for the patient are a result of the presence of the malignancy and may vary

C. Diagnosis is based on pelvic examination, Pap smear, biopsy, Schiller's test, dilation and curettage (D&C), and various radiologic examinations. Hormonal therapy is sometimes used in treatment of benign tumors, as well as hysterectomy, myomectomy, and oophorectomy

D. Treatment of malignancies will vary according to tumor classification, childbearing status, and pathologic condition of tumor itself. Modes of treatment include surgery, chemotherapy, radium inserts, radioactive cobalt, and x-ray therapy (see Unit 4, Radiation procedures, and Unit 5, Neoplasms)

E. Nursing care plan in patient having total abdominal hysterectomy is as follows
   1. Preoperative
      a. Reduce anxiety concerning surgery
         (1) Explain purpose and administration of preoperative treatments
         (2) Administer preoperative treatments as ordered (may include vaginal suppository, douche, enema, or urinary catheterization)
         (3) Instruct patient regarding turning, coughing, deep breathing, requesting pain medication postoperatively, and commonly expected postoperative treatments
   2. Postoperative
      a. Promote wound healing
         (1) Monitor vital signs every 4 hours
         (2) Observe for signs of hemorrhage, infection, and urinary retention
         (3) Administer ordered medications (antibiotics, antipyretics)
         (4) Change dressing as ordered and perineal pad as needed
      b. Reduce pain
         (1) Assess character, duration, and intensity of pain
         (2) Administer ordered analgesics and narcotics
         (3) Perform comfort measures to enhance pain relief
      c. Prevent complications
         (1) Turn, cough, and deep breathe every 2 hours
         (2) Encourage fluids
         (3) Have patient ambulate as ordered
         (4) Instruct in ordered self-care treatments before discharge
         (5) Administer nursing measures associated with radiation therapy if appropriate (see Unit 4, Radiation procedures)

Functional disorders

A. Ectopic pregnancy

   In making additional assessment, observe for usual signs of pregnancy, vaginal bleeding or concealed internal bleeding, abdominal tenderness, or severe abdominal pain
   1. Problems include
      a. Hemorrhage
      b. Abdominal pain
   2. Ectopic pregnancy refers to pregnancy occurring in areas other than the uterus. Tubal pregnancy is most common. This condition is considered an acute abdominal emergency and requires surgical intervention
   3. Diagnosis is based on symptoms and positive cul-de-sac puncture (culdocentesis)

4. Treatment includes surgical removal of products of conception and accumulated blood, as well as treatment for shock
5. Nursing care plan is same as for hysterectomy, including nursing implications for treatment of shock

B. Endometriosis
In making additional assessment, observe for progressively severe pain and pelvic discomfort (dragging) during menstruation. Sterility is often associated with endometriosis
1. Problems include
   a. Severe dysmenorrhea
   b. Depression
   c. Menorrhagia
2. This is a condition in which tissue resembling endometrium is found outside of the uterus on the ovaries, in the pelvic cavity, and sometimes in the abdominal cavity. Symptoms are a result of hormonal influence on the seeded endometrium and may result in anemia and sterility
3. Treatment includes synthetic oral hormones to prevent ovulation and breakthrough bleeding. Menopause may naturally relieve the condition, but surgical or radiologic intervention may be necessary
4. Nursing care plan includes general principles for care of the gynecologic patient preoperatively and postoperatively

Structural disorders

A. Uterine displacement
1. Problems include
   a. Vaginal discharge
   b. Fatigability
   c. Dyspareunia
   d. Constipation
   e. Pelvic dragging sensation
2. This is an abnormal position of the uterus (usually congenital). It is classified as retrocession, retroversion, or retroflexion. It may be caused by irregular bowel routine, poor posture or body mechanics, and trauma.
3. Diagnosis is by pelvic examination, history, and symptomatology
4. Treatment may include manual manipulation with a pessary inserted vaginally to maintain correction or surgical correction if untoward symptoms develop
5. Nursing care plan includes general principles for care of the gynecologic patient, with instruction in correct posture and ordered exercises

B. Relaxation of pelvic muscles
1. Problems include
   a. Fatigability
   b. Backache or pelvic pain
   c. Stress incontinence
   d. Protrusion of tissue below vaginal orifice
2. Poor muscular support in the pelvic area causes displacement or sagging of one or more structures. This condition may be classified as
   a. Cystocele—protrusion of bladder into the vagina
   b. Rectocele—bulging of rectum into the vagina
   c. Prolapse—descent of uterus into the vaginal vault
3. Treatment may be by surgical correction, or when the condition is found in older women with complications, a pessary may be used
4. Nursing care plan following surgical intervention involves
   a. Promoting healing
      (1) Observation for signs of bleeding and infection
      (2) Administration of ordered antibiotics and stool softeners
      (3) Administration of ordered treatments (perineal care, sitz baths, Foley catheter care)
      (4) Positioning as ordered to reduce pressure to operative area
   b. Relieving discomfort
      (1) Administer comfort measures as indicated
      (2) Administer analgesics as ordered
      (3) Instruct patient to avoid straining on defecation

C. Vesicovaginal and rectovaginal fistulas
In making additional assessment, observe for passage of urine or stool from vagina or urine from rectum and signs of infection
1. Problems include
   a. Edema, inflammation of perineum
   b. Abnormal vaginal or rectal discharge
2. These fistulas are openings between vaginal tract, either anteriorly with the bladder or posteriorly with the rectum. They are characterized by loss of flatus, fecal material, and urine by way of the respective fistula

3. These conditions are diagnosed by pelvic examination, symptomatology, and x-ray examination. They require surgical repair
4. Nursing care plan is same as for patient having surgery for relaxation of pelvic muscles

D. Sexual dysfunction
1. Problems include
    a. Dyspareunia
    b. Frigidity
    c. Infertility
2. Sexual dysfunction is a physical and/or emotional disorder affecting normal sexual function or reproductive capacity. It may be caused by gonorrhea, immature organs, endometriosis, pelvic inflammatory disease, congenital anomalies, uterine tumor or displacement, trauma, endocrine dysfunction, and mental or emotional disturbances
3. Diagnosis is based on physical examination, which may include endocrine and fertility studies as well as psychologic evaluation when indicated
4. Treatment includes correction of physical disorder when possible and additional counseling or psychotherapy when indicated
5. Nursing care plan is specific according to cause, with particular accent on accepting, nonjudgmental attitude toward the patient

Breast diseases

A. Cystic disease (chronic cystic mastitis)

In making additional assessment, observe for appearance of lump in axilla or breast tissue, change in firmness, and pain or tenderness in breast
1. Problems include
    a. Pain and breast tenderness
    b. Anxiety
2. Cystic disease is an abnormal proliferation of breast tissue forming fibrotic masses throughout the breasts. These masses block the ducts and cause cyst formation. The disease may be asymptomatic other than palpable lumps or tenderness and pain premenstrually. Lumps are usually movable on palpation but may cause the patient anxiety because of fear of breast cancer
3. Diagnosis is based on breast examination and symptoms. Mammography, thermography, xerography, or biopsy may be done to rule out the possibility of malignancy
4. Treatment may include supportive brassiere to reduce discomfort, or simple mastectomy with insertion of implants may be done for chronic or multiple cystic disease
5. See nursing care plan for patient with breast surgery

B. Tumors

In making additional assessment, observe for appearance of lump in axilla or breast tissue, pain or tenderness in breast, redness, chapping or orange peel appearance of skin, and nipple discharge (bloody, brown, or clear fluid is especially significant)
1. Problems include
    a. Pain or tenderness in breast
    b. Anxiety
2. Tumors of the breast may be benign or malignant, but all are considered potentially malignant until diagnosis is confirmed by biopsy. Breasts are the most common site of cancer in American women
3. Diagnosis is based on symptoms, breast examination, mammography, thermography, xerography, and biopsy
4. Treatment may include surgical excision of benign tumor, simple mastectomy, modified radical mastectomy, or radical mastectomy. Hormonal therapy, radiotherapy, and chemotherapy may be instituted for adjunctive therapy or metastatic disease
5. Nursing care plan for patient having breast surgery includes the following
    a. Preoperatively
        (1) Reduce anxiety
            (a) Be available to patient to allow venting of feelings and provide emotional support
            (b) Know what the physician has told the patient, and exhibit a positive attitude toward necessity of surgery
        (2) Explain and perform ordered treatments (skin preparation, medications); instruct patient regarding turning, coughing, deep breathing, requesting pain medication postoperatively, and commonly ordered postoperative treatments
    b. Postoperatively (radical mastectomy)
        (1) Promote wound healing
            (a) Monitor vital signs every 4 hours

(b) Observe dressing and any drains (Hemovac) for amount, color, consistency, and odor of drainage
(c) Check beneath the patient since drainage may not be obvious on front of bandage
(d) Upper arm of affected side should be restricted from motion (especially abduction) whether bandaged or not
(e) Observe hand on affected side for signs of impaired circulation
(f) Arm on affected side should be elevated above breast level with pillow for at least 24 hours
(g) Avoid injections, vaccinations, venipuncture, or taking blood pressure in arm on affected side
(h) An elastic sleeve or bandage may be ordered to control arm edema
(i) For about 2 weeks, support arm in sling when patient is walking
(j) Exercises ordered by physician should be explained before patient is discharged

(2) Relieve pain
(a) Assess character, duration, and intensity of pain
(b) Administer analgesics and narcotics as ordered

(3) Promote adjustment to altered body image
(a) Be with patient at time of discovery of loss of breast
(b) Offer emotional support and answer questions
(c) Assist patient to look at incision before discharge, but do not insist that she do so
(d) With physician's order, make arrangements with the American Cancer Society's "Reach to Recovery" program
(e) Make an improvised prosthesis, using patient's brassiere, for wear on dismissal and at home until physician tells patient she may be fitted for permanent prosthesis
(f) Improvised prosthesis should not exert pressure on the incision or shoulder
(g) With physician approval provide information for fitting and purchase of prosthesis

(4) Prevent complications
(a) Observe for signs of infection
(b) Assist patient to cough and deep breathe as chest may be restricted by dressing
(c) Instruct patient before discharge to observe hand and arm on affected side for signs of infection or edema
(d) Instruct patient to protect affected arm against scratching, insect bites, trauma, and injections
(e) Individuals with metastatic disease require extensive follow-up care, and instruction specific to treatment may be ordered

DISORDERS OF THE MALE REPRODUCTIVE SYSTEM

Introduction

Close association of the reproductive system with the lower urinary system in the male frequently causes both systems to be affected by a disorder. Patient may be hesitant to discuss his condition because of fear of embarrassment and impotence

Assessment

A. Obtain relevant information from health history
B. Observe appearance of penis, scrotum, perineum, and anus
C. Obtain information about patient's voiding patterns and bowel habits

Infections

A. Venereal—see Infections, Venereal, under Disorders of the female reproductive system
B. Epididmyo-orchitis
   1. Problems include
      a. Chills and fever
      b. Scrotal tenderness and pain
      c. Erythema and edema of scrotum
   2. This is a simultaneous infection and inflammation of the epididymis and testis, which may be caused by prostatitis and occasionally untreated gonorrhea. Mumps may cause orchitis without epididymitis
   3. Diagnosis is based on symptoms and physical examination

4. Treatment may include antibiotics, scrotal elevation (Bellevue Bridge) with application of ice bags to reduce pain, and bed rest. Chronic bilateral epididymitis may be treated by vasectomy. Sterility results when bilateral vasectomy is performed
5. Nursing care plan is specific to treatments ordered

Structural disorders—torsion

A. Problems include
   1. Sharp pain in testicle
   2. Edema of testicle
   3. Chills, fever, and nausea and vomiting associated with severe pain

B. Torsion is a condition in which the spermatic cord becomes twisted. It may result from strenuous exercise; however, simple movement may also be the cause

C. Diagnosis is based on symptoms and physical examination

D. Immediate surgery is necessary to preserve fertility and prevent spermatic cord atrophy

E. Nursing care plan (postoperative) involves
   1. Promoting wound healing
      a. Observe wound for signs of bleeding and infection
      b. Monitor vital signs every 4 hours
      c. Administer antibiotics as ordered
      d. Apply scrotal elevation as ordered
      e. Apply heat or cold as ordered
   2. Relieving pain
      a. Assess location, character, and intensity of pain
      b. Administer analgesics and narcotics as ordered
      c. Elevate scrotum as ordered

Functional disorders—hydrocele

A. Problems include pain in scrotum and scrotal edema. However the condition may be asymptomatic

B. This is an abnormal accumulation of fluid between testis and tunica vaginalis (membrane surrounding testis) or along the spermatic cord. It may be caused by infection or trauma, or the cause may be unknown. A change in both testicular size and weight occurs with increased pain and swelling when condition is acute

C. Diagnosis is based on symptoms and physical examination

D. Conservative treatment includes wearing of scrotal support. Surgical excision or needle aspiration of fluid may be performed. Scrotal support is worn for several weeks postoperatively

E. See nursing care plan under Structural disorders, Torsion

Tumors of the prostate—benign prostatic hypertrophy

A. Problems include
   1. Dysuria
   2. Nocturia
   3. Hesitancy
   4. Urinary retention
   5. Urinary infection

B. This condition is an enlargement of periurethral glands from an overgrowth of glandular and muscle tissue. It is one of the most common manifestations of obstruction. It usually occurs in men during the fourth or fifth decade of life. Symptoms are primarily associated with impingement of glands on the urethra and bladder

C. Diagnosis is made by digital rectal examination, cystoscopic examination (observe enlargement), excretory urogram (note back pressure of urine), and catheterization after voiding (residual urine)

D. Treatment is based on severity, cause, and condition of the patient. Conservative treatment includes prostatic massage and antiseptics. Prostatectomy may be required

E. Nursing care plan for prostatectomy involves
   1. Promoting wound healing
      a. Report frank bleeding (although some hematuria is expected)
      b. Check catheters for patency since clots may cause spasm, pain, and bleeding
         (1) Check tubing for kinks
         (2) "Milk" catheter tubing
         (3) Follow physician's orders for intermittent or continuous irrigation
      c. Observe and record output from each catheter separately
      d. Observe bladder for distention
      e. Change dressings frequently to keep patient clean and dry, being careful to avoid displacement of any drains

2. Reducing pain
   a. Check patency of all catheters
   b. Assess character, location, duration, and intensity of pain
   c. For bladder spasm not caused by catheter obstruction, antispasmodic drugs (propantheline [Pro-Banthine], opium and belladonna suppositories) should be administered as ordered
   d. Administer analgesics and narcotics as ordered
3. Preventing complications
   a. Encourage fluid intake to 3000 ml in 24 hours unless contraindicated
   b. Turn, cough, and deep breathe every 2 hours
   c. Avoid use of rectal tubes, rectal thermometers, and enemas unless ordered otherwise
   d. Instruct patient to avoid straining
   e. Administer stool softeners as ordered
   f. Instruct patient in perineal exercises as ordered

DISEASES OF THE RESPIRATORY SYSTEM

Introduction

Respiratory diseases are the most common cause of illness in humans. Prompt treatment is necessary to prevent acute problems from becoming chronic illness, causing disability and requiring early retirement. Many times respiratory and cardiac problems are closely related. Respiratory therapist, nurse, and physician must work closely for optimal effect of treatment

Assessment

A. History, including that of present illness and past history of respiratory problems
B. Rate and rhythm of respiratory pattern
C. Position assumed by patient
D. Cough (productive, nonproductive)
E. Sputum (characteristics)
F. Pain (initiating factors, association with inspiration and expiration)
G. Systemic effects of lung function (clubbing of fingers, polycythemia)
H. Anatomic appearance of external chest (barrel, retractions, abnormal configurations)

Traumatic chest injuries

A. Chest injuries caused by trauma are life-threatening because they compromise the body's oxygen supply (see Glossary for types of chest injuries)
B. Problems include dyspnea, chest pain, shock, and cyanosis
C. Diagnosis is confirmed by chest x-ray examination, ABG, and history
D. Treatment centers around restoration of respiratory function, controlling pain, and treating shock. Some conditions may require thoracotomy tube insertion, while others may require open-chest surgery
E. Nursing care plan involves the following procedures
   1. Preoperative
      a. Assess respiratory function
         (1) Monitor laboratory values (ABG, hemoglobin)
         (2) Observe level of consciousness; report increasing restlessness (a sign of hypoxia)
         (3) Record rate, depth, and character of respiration
      b. Increase oxygen to body cells
         (1) Maintain oxygen per ordered method (endotracheal tube, mask)
         (2) Provide calm, reassuring atmosphere
         (3) Maintain patent airway
      c. Reduce emotional stress
         (1) If possible, explain and demonstrate postoperative procedures (coughing, deep breathing)
         (2) Provide calm, reassuring atmosphere
   2. Postoperative
      a. Maintain oxygen to all body cells
         (1) Keep airway patent (suctioning, repositioning)
         (2) Monitor vital signs every 15 minutes
         (3) Elevate head of bed
         (4) Administer oxygen as ordered
      b. Promote drainage of chest cavity
         (1) Keep drainage bottles below level of chest
         (2) Reposition frequently
         (3) Provide adequate hydration to liquify secretions
         (4) Encourage deep breathing and coughing
         (5) Milk tubes, in direction of drainage bottle, hourly
         (6) Observe chest tubes for fluctuation, which indicates proper functioning
         (7) Chart amount and character of drainage
         (8) Observe for leaks as indicated by bubbling

(9) If bottles are damaged, tubes may need to be clamped, unless tension pneumothorax is suspected
(10) If tubes become dislodged from chest, cover incision with petroleum gauze and notify physician immediately

c. Provide comfort
   (1) Administer analgesics as ordered
   (2) Reposition as ordered
   (3) Provide back care
   (4) Teach range of motion exercises

Allergic respiratory diseases—asthma

A. Problems include
   1. Shortness of breath (expiratory wheeze)
   2. Tachycardia
   3. Cyanosis and hypoxia
   4. Anxiety
   5. Productive cough

B. Asthma is an allergic response caused by the antigen-antibody reaction. Infections and environmental irritants are factors. An increase in the concentration of allergens leads to accumulation of mucus. Histamine is released, causing constriction of the bronchioles

C. Treatment consists of
   1. Attempting to determine source of allergy by eliminating possible allergens (substances that produce allergic reactions and may be introduced into body by inhalation, ingestion, injection, and direct contact)
   2. Desensitizing patient by parenteral injection of minute doses of a specific allergen in successively larger doses over a period of time
   3. Providing symptomatic relief
      a. Adrenalin (epinephrine), 1:1000, injected subcutaneously in nonhypertensive patients is usually effective
      b. Aminophylline, 0.5 g, is administered intravenously for mild episodes
      c. Aminophylline rectal suppositories and theophylline compound containing ephedrine and phenobarbital (Tedral) are used
      d. Antibiotics are used to treat infections
      e. Potassium iodide and ammonium chloride afford patient an opportunity to expectorate (characteristic tenacious, mucoid, eosinophil-laden sputum)
      f. Prednisone or beclomethasone dipropionate (Vanceril) is effective orally or parenterally (nurse should observe patient carefully for signs of edema and steroid toxicity)
      g. Bronchodilators such as isoproterenol (Isuprel) may be used as aerosols
      h. Oxygen may be given, but intermittent positive pressure breathing (IPPB) with the usual face mask does not afford relief for the expiratory phase
      i. Apprehension is best treated by calm, efficient personnel, moving quickly to relieve patient
      j. Patient should be taught prophylactic measures
         (1) Avoid situations that will aggravate an episode
         (2) Avoid cold and high humidity
         (3) Avoid outdoor exertion in damp conditions
         (4) Spend winters in warm, dry climates, which are beneficial in avoiding respiratory diseases
         (5) Avoid emotional and physical stress
         (6) Live with a positive, wholesome attitude toward condition. This is important for person with asthma

D. Nursing care plan involves
   1. Relieving shortness of breath and hypoxia
      a. Administer medication as ordered
      b. Administer oxygen as ordered
      c. Provide calm, reassuring atmosphere
   2. Preventing future attacks
      a. Teach patient to control or avoid factors initiating attack
      b. Help patient to recognize limitations and deal with them
   3. Providing emotional support
      a. Remain calm
      b. Perform procedures with expertise
      c. Remain with patient while he is anxious
   4. Maintaining patent airway
      a. Help patient into high Fowler's position
      b. Provide padded, over-bed table for orthopneic position
      c. Administer oxygen by catheter if ordered
      d. Suction p.r.n.
      e. Monitor vital signs every 4 hours; observe skin color and level of consciousness

Infectious lung diseases

A. Pneumonia
 1. Problems include
  a. Elevated temperature and chills
  b. Productive cough
  c. Chest pain
 2. Pneumonia is an inflammation of the lungs caused by infectious agents such as bacterial, viral, or perhaps aspirated materials. Debilitated patients or those with chronic respiratory diseases are most at risk. The invading organism initiates the inflammatory response causing chest pain, cough, and elevated temperature
 3. Diagnosis is confirmed by sputum culture
 4. Treatment is based on culture and sensitivity report for appropriate antibiotic therapy. Oxygen, fluid therapy, and codeine for pain are used to treat symptoms
 5. Nursing care plan involves
  a. Controlling chest pain
   (1) Administer codeine as ordered
   (2) Splint chest during coughing
   (3) Elevate head of bed
   (4) Encourage fluids
  b. Promoting comfort
   (1) Give sponge bath frequently (avoid chilling)
   (2) Provide frequent mouth care

B. Tuberculosis
 1. For problems, see Glossary, Table 6
 2. Diagnosis is established by
  a. Roentgenologic examinations of chest
   (1) Planigraphy
   (2) Bronchography
   (3) Photofluorography
   (4) Fluoroscopy
  b. Physical examination for correlative signs and symptoms
  c. History
   (1) Exposure
   (2) Family contacts
   (3) Home conditions
   (4) Alcoholism
  d. Gastric lavage
  e. Skin tests
   (1) There are two preparations of tuberculin—old tuberculin (OT) and purified protein derivative (PPD)
   (2) Administration techniques are Mantoux (intradermal), jet injection, and multiple-puncture (tine)
   (3) Test is usually read 48 to 72 hours after injection; erythema without induration is not important in reading reaction
   (4) Reactions are as follows
    (a) In the Mantoux test and jet injection, a 10 mm area or more of induration is positive; an area up to 4 mm is negative
    (b) In multiple-puncture test, largest single reaction is measured; 5 mm of induration is positive; less than 2 mm is negative
    (c) Positive skin test indicates presence of, but not activation of, tuberculosis
   (5) Tuberculin converter is one who has history of negative skin test and change to positive in 12-month period; no evidence of disease is found on bacteriologic or x-ray examination
  f. Surgical diagnostic procedures
   (1) Bronchoscopy
   (2) Pleural biopsy
   (3) Scalene and mediastinal node biopsy
   (4) Lung biopsy
 3. Medical treatment consists of
  a. Isolation or medical asepsis to prevent spread of tuberculosis (proper sputum disposal and proper hand washing)
  b. Diet modified in regard to caloric requirements (protein, calcium, and vitamins A, C, and B_6 requirements are increased)
  c. Medications
   (1) Streptomycin, 1 g daily
   (2) Ethambutol, a tuberculostatic, given in dose of 15.25 mg per kg daily
   (3) Isoniazid (INH)
    (a) Inhibits growth of tubercle bacilli
    (b) May be given orally or parenterally
    (c) Has low toxicity
    (d) Is given in daily dose of 300 mg with pyridoxine (to prevent peripheral neuritis)
   (4) *p*-Aminosalicylic acid, 12 to 15 g per day, in three doses after meals
   (5) Other tuberculostatic drugs are pyrazinamide, viomycin sulfate, cycloserine, ethionamide, and rifampin
   (6) Combined therapeutic regimens are usual

4. Nursing care plan involves
   a. Emotional support
      (1) Actively listen and support patient and family
      (2) Assist patient and family in accepting diagnosis
      (3) Encourage diversional activities
   b. Prevention of spread of infection
      (1) Teach patient how to cough and not spread droplets and how to wash hands
      (2) Maintain isolation
   c. Enhancement of patient resistance to debilitating disease
      (1) Provide frequent mouth care
      (2) Provide diet as ordered, in small feedings
      (3) Alternate rest and activity
      (4) Encourage fresh air and sunshine

Chronic diseases—pulmonary emphysema

A. Problems include
   1. Dyspnea caused by exertion, cold air, and nonproduction of sputum in respiratory infections
   2. Coughing (in paroxysms on awakening or exposure to cold air)
   3. "Barrel chest" deformity resulting from inspiratory position characteristic of chronic emphysema
   4. Less active respiratory center; center is not as active in controlling respirations because of chronic carbon dioxide tension of arterial blood

B. Pulmonary emphysema is a chronic respiratory disease characterized by overdistention of the alveoli, preventing adequate oxygenation of blood

C. Diagnosis is confirmed by history, symptoms, and chest x-ray and pulmonary function examinations

D. Treatment consists of teaching rest, energy conservation, breathing exercises, and relaxing breathing; discouraging smoking to reduce irritants; and providing bronchodilator drugs (intravenous, oral, or inhalation). Oxygen therapy should be administered with great caution because of carbon dioxide narcosis. Tracheostomy may be required if bronchial obstruction is associated problem

E. Nursing care plan involves
   1. Maintaining patent airway
      a. Administer medications as ordered
      b. Encourage fluids to liquefy secretions
      c. Position patient to promote postural drainage
      d. Assist patient to expectorate mucus
      e. Assess frequently for adequate oxygenation (observe color and level of consciousness and auscultate chest)
   2. Maintaining nutrition
      a. Provide high-protein diet, in small feedings
      b. Force fluids
      c. Provide frequent mouth care

VASCULAR CONDITIONS

Introduction

Peripheral vascular diseases include all conditions that affect the circulatory system excluding those affecting the heart. Vessel changes (arteriosclerosis, atherosclerosis) are the usual causative factors of arterial insufficiency. These changes are the subject of much research nationwide. Prompt medical treatment is necessary to prevent further disability such as amputations. General assessment of the peripheral vascular system should include the following

A. Assess peripheral pulses (femoral, popliteal, radial, pedal, brachial, carotid)
   1. Quality of force
   2. Presences
   3. Comparison of one side of body to the other

B. Observe integrity of skin
   1. Temperature
   2. Color
   3. Edema
   4. Taut, shiny skin

C. Assess pain
   1. Tenderness along vein
   2. Cramping
   3. Positive Homan's sign (calf pain during dorsiflexion of the foot)

D. Assess status of sensation (dimension may indicate diminished blood supply)

E. Observe characteristics of any discolored or ulcerated areas

F. Assess presence of risk factors
   1. Cigarette smoking
   2. Obesity

3. Hypertension
4. Elevated serum cholesterol level
5. Sedentary existence
6. Diabetes
7. Family history

Diseases of the arteries

A. Arteriosclerosis
  1. Problems include
    a. Cramplike pain in affected extremities
    b. Numbness and tingling
    c. Poor circulation to area which may cause ulcers
    d. Trophic skin changes
  2. Arteriosclerosis is hardening and thickening of arterial wall, ultimately restricting blood supply. Certain disease states (diabetes) may be predisposing factors
  3. Diagnosis is confirmed by arteriography to visualize major arterial circulatory channels
  4. Treatment objectives are to limit intake of saturated fats, lower cholesterol levels (colestipol), control risk factors, and increase blood flow to area (vasodilators and anticoagulants). Amputation may be necessary
  5. Nursing care plan involves
    a. Protecting affected extremity
      (1) Use bed cradle
      (2) Provide heel guards and elbow pads
      (3) Reposition frequently
      (4) Assess integrity of skin
      (5) Encourage daily hygiene
      (6) Keep skin dry
      (7) Assist out of bed
      (8) Provide uncluttered environment
    b. Increasing blood flow to area
      (1) Administer anticoagulants and vasodilators as ordered
      (2) Observe for side effects of medications
    c. Educating patient for care at home
    d. Preventing complications postoperatively (amputation)
      (1) Hemorrhage
        (a) Check vital signs
        (b) Keep tourniquet at bedside
        (c) Elevate stump
      (2) Flexion contracture—keep stump flat after 24 hours
      (3) Dependence—promote mobility
      (4) Stump necrosis—condition stump as ordered
      (5) Phantom pain
        (a) Administer medication
        (b) Listen to and support patient

B. Hypertensive vascular disease
  Additional assessment factors include changes in level of consciousness, in vision, in sensation, and in blood pressure
  1. Problems include
    a. Headache
    b. Blurred vision
    c. Nausea
    d. Fatigue
    e. Irritability
    f. Edema
  2. Hypertension affects primarily small vessels, increasing the peripheral resistance, and therefore affects blood pressure. Ultimately, heart, brain, kidney, and eyes are adversely affected. The condition is characterized by persistent levels of blood pressure in which systolic pressure is above 150 mm Hg and diastolic pressure is above 90 mm Hg
    a. Primary hypertension (essential) is a condition in which there is no apparent cause (may be benign or malignant)
    b. Secondary hypertension is blood pressure elevation associated with another condition such as toxemia, renal disease, coarctation of aorta, and pheochromocytoma
  3. The actual cause of hypertension is unknown, but control of risk factors is proved to be of help. Diagnosis is confirmed by history and physical examination
  4. Main treatment objectives include measures to lower blood pressure, such as antihypertensive drugs, weight control, restriction of sodium and cholesterol intake, and elimination of vasoconstrictors (nicotine)
  5. Nursing care plan involves
    a. Controlling blood pressure
      (1) Administer antihypertensives, diuretics, and sedatives as ordered
      (2) Weigh daily
      (3) Provide diet low in sodium and cholesterol as ordered
      (4) Administer stool softeners

b. Maintaining safe environment
   (1) Observe for orthostatic hypotension
   (2) Keep room uncluttered
   (3) Negotiate care plan to include rest periods
c. Observing for complications
   (1) Renal
      (a) Check intake and output and specific gravity
      (b) Record characteristics of urine
   (2) Visual—report blurring
   (3) Cerebral—report changes in level of consciousness, increase in irritability, and seizures
d. Educating patient
   (1) Explain medications and side effects
   (2) Explain risk factors and how to control them

Diseases of the veins

A. Phlebitis
1. Problems include
   a. Pain along path of vein and positive Homan's sign
   b. Edema and localized redness
   c. Elevated temperature
2. Phlebitis is inflammation of walls of veins usually following conditions that promote venous stasis (bed rest, pregnancy, trauma). Thrombophlebitis (clot formation caused by inflammation) may lead to pulmonary embolism, myocardial infarction, or cerebrovascular accident
3. Diagnosis is confirmed by history and physical examination
4. Treatment is aimed at promoting venous return, thereby decreasing clot formation. Medical treatment includes bed rest, elevation of affected limb, warm moist compresses, anticoagulant drugs, and elastic stockings. Surgical treatment may include ligation above and below thrombosed area to prevent movement of clot to major vessels and other areas
5. Nursing care plan involves
   a. Promoting venous return
      (1) Apply warm moist compresses
      (2) Reposition frequently
      (3) Do not use knee gatch
      (4) Elevate lower extremities if ordered
      (5) Administer anticoagulants as ordered
      (6) Maintain elastic stockings; remove daily to assess skin integrity and reapply
      (7) Promote passive or active exercises and early ambulation; do not dangle legs; have patient sit with legs elevated
      (8) Do not massage legs
   b. Educating patient
      (1) Avoid crossing legs and wearing garters and girdles
      (2) Avoid extremes in heat and cold
      (3) Avoid hard soaps
      (4) Explain medication administration, side effects, and purposes

B. Varicose veins
1. Problems include
   a. Large tortuous leg veins leading to disfigurement
   b. Leg fatigue
   c. Leg cramps and pain
   d. Predisposition to leg ulcers resulting from venous stasis
2. Varicose veins are dilated, tortuous veins. They result from incomplete closure of venous valves leading to blood backflow, which further congests and distends the veins. Predisposing factors include heredity, pregnancy, obesity, and aging process with loss of tissue elasticity
3. Diagnosis is made using Trendelenburg's test for valvular competence, venography, and physical examination
4. Medical treatment includes weight reduction and restriction of activities and devices that cause venous stasis. Surgical treatment includes vein ligation and stripping
5. Nursing care plan involves
   a. Promoting venous return
      (1) Elevate foot of bed
      (2) Maintain elastic bandages
      (3) Encourage and assist with walking
      (4) Have patient avoid sitting
   b. Promoting comfort and safety
      (1) Administer analgesics as circumstances may require
      (2) Assist when out of bed
      (3) Observe, record, and report increase in bleeding

CARDIAC CONDITIONS

Introduction

A. Cardiovascular deaths account for approximately 51% of all deaths in the United States. To diminish mortality, the two major aims are to (1) control the disease progression and (2) reduce the risk factors predisposing to cardiovascular conditions. Nursing plays a significant role in both aims by encouraging prompt evaluation and treatment for chronic throat infections, encouraging proper prenatal care, and identifying high-risk patients and encouraging them to seek medical assistance for proper treatment
B. General assessment of the cardiovascular system should include the following (see also assessment of peripheral vascular system under Vascular conditions)
   1. Heart rate and rhythm
   2. Character of respiration
   3. Blood pressure evaluation
   4. Presence of dyspnea, pain, productive cough, syncope, fatigue, neck vein distention, and edema
   5. Complete blood count (CBC), ABG, electrocardiogram (ECG), and serum enzymes

Angina pectoris

A. Problems include
   1. Radiating chest pain
   2. Anxiety
   3. Shortness of breath
   4. Tachycardia
B. Angina is chest pain caused by increased demand for oxygen when supply is diminished. Angina is usually preceded by physical or emotional exertion. Atherosclerosis of the coronary arteries is most common cause of insufficient blood supply to heart muscle. The already diminished supply of blood (oxygen) is further compromised by exertion, thus causing pain
C. Diagnosis is established by ECG during the acute episode, patient history and physical, and coronary angiograms
D. Treatment consists of relief of chest pain (nitroglycerin), sedatives, analgesics, and increased blood supply to myocardium (long-acting nitrates such as isosorbide dinitrate [Isordil], nitroglycerin ointment [Nitrol], and propranolol [Inderal])
E. Nursing care plan involves
   1. Relieving pain
      a. Administer nitroglycerin, sedatives, and analgesics as ordered
      b. Encourage bed rest
      c. Administer oxygen
      d. Monitor vital signs
   2. Controlling recurrence
      a. Explain drug therapy and how to comply
      b. Investigate precipitating factors
      c. Avoid constipation
      d. Increase activity as tolerated
      e. Help patient stop smoking
      f. Report to physician if pain persists longer than 20 minutes after taking nitroglycerin

Myocardial infarction (MI)

A. Problems include
   1. Chest pain
   2. Shortness of breath
   3. Shock
   4. Anxiety and restlessness
   5. Tachycardia
   6. Elevated temperature (48 hours)
B. Myocardial infarction is the total obstruction of a coronary artery that results in the death of the tissue supplied by the coronary artery. The obstruction may be caused by atherosclerosis, thrombus, or embolus
C. ECG changes usually confirm the diagnosis. Supplemental diagnostic procedures include elevated sedentary rate, white blood count (WBC), creatinine phosphokinase (CPK), lactic dehydrogenase (LDH), and alum-precipitated toxoid (APT)
D. Treatment includes control of pain, prevention of complications, and promotion of healing and scar formation
E. Nursing care plan involves
   1. Controlling chest pain and anxiety
      a. Administer analgesics as ordered (morphine, meperdine [Demerol])
      b. Administer oxygen
      c. Maintain intravenous tubing for administration of medications
   2. Observing for complications
      a. Shock
         (1) Vital signs
         (2) Intake and output
         (3) Cool moist skin
         (4) Restlessness

b. Arrhythmias
(1) Abnormal heart rate rhythm
(2) Chest pain
c. Embolitic phenomenon
(1) Positive Homan's sign
(2) Sudden chest pain
(3) Shortness of breath
3. Reducing workload of heart
a. Bed rest
b. Oxygen
c. Sedatives as ordered
4. Providing emotional support
a. Provide calm supportive atmosphere
b. Help patient to recognize limitations and accept them
c. Identify fears and discuss them
d. Educate patient and family concerning illness

Nursing care plan for complications of cardiac disease

A. Congestive heart failure (failure of heart to pump adequate amounts of blood to meet body's needs)
1. Reduce workload of heart
a. Administer digitalis preparations
b. Monitor intake and output
c. Administer diuretics
d. Provide low-sodium diet
2. Prevent recurrence by observing
a. Right ventricular failure—preceded by dependent edema, neck vein engorgement, and ascites
b. Left ventricular failure—preceded by dyspnea, orthopnea, cough, and hemoptysis
B. Acute pulmonary edema (sudden excessive fluid in lungs that has leaked through the capillary walls into the air pathways)
1. Decrease workload of heart
a. Apply rotating tourniquets
b. Administer digitalis preparations and diuretics
c. Administer morphine to allay apprehension and decrease respiratory rate
d. Place patient in semi-Fowler's position
2. Increase oxygen to all cells
a. Administer oxygen
b. Administer bronchodilators as ordered (aminophylline)
C. Arrhythmias (disturbances in heart rhythm or rate)—maintain adequate cardiac output
1. Administer antiarrhythmic drugs as ordered
2. Monitor vital signs (assess pulse frequently)

HEMATOLOGIC AND LYMPHATIC CONDITIONS

Introduction

Diseases of the blood and lymph can be caused by poor nutrition, genetic disorders, toxic exposure, or tumor invasion. Public education, especially during formative years, helps to establish proper nutritious dietary patterns. Public awareness of the dangers of toxic chemicals and radiation exposure will serve to promote prevention

General assessment of the blood and lymphatic system

A. Review of cardiovascular and peripheral vascular systems (tachycardia, chest pain, murmurs)
B. Detailed family history
C. Environment (exposure to chemicals)
D. Drugs presently used (prescribed or over-the-counter)
E. Pain
F. Fever pattern
G. Skin (bruises, texture changes)
H. Eye, ear, nose, and throat (eyes for jaundice, gums for bleeding and ulcerations)
I. Abdomen (increase in size of liver or spleen)
J. Musculoskeletal system (pain, deformity)
K. Nervous system (changes in behavior or motor function)
L. Lymph nodes (report complaints of pain, tenderness, and enlargement)

Anemias

A. Iron deficiency anemia
1. Problems include
a. Weakness and fatigue
b. Vertigo
c. Anorexia
d. Tachycardia
e. Chest pain
f. Dyspnea on exertion
2. Iron deficiency anemia is caused by inadequate dietary intake of iron, impaired absorption, increased requirements, or blood loss. Lack of iron necessary for hemoglobin formation leads to hypoxemia or insufficient oxygen to body tissues

3. Diagnosis is made based on physical examination, decrease in red blood cells, hemoglobin, hematocrit, and iron stores
4. Treatment focuses on iron replacement (ferrous sulfate, iron dextran [Imferon]) and correcting the cause (dietary education, blood transfusions)
5. Nursing care plan involves
   a. Maintaining safe, quiet environment
      (1) Have patient ambulate with assistance
      (2) Maintain clutter-free room
      (3) Encourage rest periods
   b. Maintaining comfort
      (1) Administer antiemetics and analgesics as ordered
      (2) Provide frequent, meticulous skin care
      (3) Administer stool softeners as necessary
   c. Replacing iron stores
      (1) Six small, attractive, nutritious feedings
      (2) Frequent oral hygiene
      (3) Dietary education
      (4) Iron preparations as ordered—intramuscular (use Z-track methods) or orally (explain that stool color will be black)

B. Pernicious anemia
1. Problems include
   a. Dyspnea
   b. Soreness of tongue and mouth
   c. Visual disturbances
   d. Paresthesia of extremities
   e. Behavioral changes
2. Perncicious anemia is a condition in which the body produces inadequate red blood cells and hemoglobin because of lack of the intrinsic factor in the stomach. Lack of the intrinsic factor prevents the absorption of vitamin B_{12} (extrinsic factor). Vitamin B_{12} is necessary for the maturation of red blood cells
3. Diagnosis is confirmed by gastric analysis (lack of free hydrochloric acid), Schilling test, bone marrow examination, gastroscopy, and blood smear
4. Treatment includes parenteral supply of missing Vitamin B_{12}
5. For nursing care plan, see Iron deficiency anemia

C. Polycythemia vera
Additional assessment factors include inspection of hands, feet, and face for reddish-purple discoloration and investigation of bleeding from skin and mucous membranes
1. Problems include
   a. Headache
   b. Weakness
   c. Dyspnea
   d. Pruritus
   e. Complications such as peptic ulcer, congestive heart failure, leukemia, and cardiovascular accident
2. Polycythemia vera is a condition in which there is an increase in the production of red blood cells, white blood cells, and platelets. This increase in blood cells increases the viscosity of the circulating blood and leads to engorgement of organs
3. Diagnosis is confirmed by elevation of red blood cell, white blood cell, and platelet counts and bone marrow examination
4. Treatment objectives are aimed at lowering red cell mass by phlebotomy or chemotherapy to suppress bone marrow function (chlorambucil [Leukeran], melphalan [Alkeran]) and restriction of iron-containing foods and drugs
5. Nursing care plan involves the following (see also Iron deficiency anemia, excluding diet)
   a. Maintain comfort
      (1) Ensure meticulous, frequent skin care
      (2) Encourage active and passive range of motion
      (3) Assist patient to get up
      (4) Assess skin for bleeding
      (5) Give soothing baths and keep nails short for pruritus
   b. Reduce red cell mass and viscosity of blood
      (1) Administer medications as ordered
      (2) Assist with phlebotomy
      (3) Encourage fluid intake up to 3000 ml per day
      (4) Provide diet as ordered
   c. Observe for complications
      (1) Monitor vitals signs four times a day
      (2) Observe, report, and record stools and urine
      (3) Auscultate chest every shift
      (4) Check extremities for signs of phlebitis
      (5) Assess neurologic status every day
   d. Provide emotional support to patient, family, and significant others

D. Leukemias
  1. Problems include
    a. Anemia (fatigue, weakness, tachycardia, dyspnea on exertion)
    b. Decreased resistance to infection
    c. Excessive bleeding from gums, nose, and wounds
    d. Elevated temperature
    e. Anorexia, nausea, and vomiting
    f. Pain (from infarctions)
  2. Leukemias are diseases of the blood-forming tissue characterized by excessive production of both mature and immature white blood cells. They are classified according to type of white blood cell involved (granulocyte, monocyte, lymphocyte) and according to maturity of cells involved (acute for immature, chronic for mature). The leukemia process leads to a depression in the production of red blood cells and platelets, predisposing the patient to infections, hemorrhage, and anemia
  3. Diagnosis of leukemia is confirmed by evaluation of blood studies, bone marrow examination, and lymph node biospy
  4. Treatment is aimed at inducing remission via chemotherapy. Antimetabolites (methotrexate) to inhibit cell growth, alkylating agents (cyclophosphamide [Cytoxan]) to interfere with chemical processes in the cell, antibiotics (doxorubicin [Adriamycin]) to interfere with cell proteins, plant alkaloids (vincristine) to inhibit cell division, and hormones (prednisone) to diminish growth of lymphocytes. Radiation therapy may also be used on localized lymph nodes (testes, brain). Blood transfusions may also be given
  5. Nursing care plan involves
    a. Maintaining patient comfort and safety
      (1) Reverse isolation
      (2) Observe for complications from chemotherapy (monitor CBC)
      (3) Provide frequent mouth care with swabs
      (4) Encourage soft nutritious diet
      (5) Administer comfort measures such as back care, frequent repositioning, soothing baths, and analgesics as ordered
      (6) Assist patient to get up
      (7) Administer oxygen as needed
      (8) Use small-gauge needles; watch for excessive bleeding
    b. Provide emotional support for patient and family
      (1) Listen and allow patient to verbalize feelings
      (2) Explain procedures
      (3) Allow family to participate in care giving

E. Hodgkin's disease
  1. Problems include
    a. Pruritus
    b. Pyrexia
    c. Dysphagia
    d. Anemia (weakness, fatigue)
    e. Dyspnea
  2. Hodgkin's disease is a malignancy of unknown cause of the lymphoid tissue. Lymph nodes enlarge, causing pain and pressure in specific areas (cervical, axillary, inguinal, and mediastinal areas)
  3. Diagnosis is confirmed by lymph node biopsy (presence of Sternberg-Reed cells), CBC, and liver and spleen scans. Exploratory laparotomy with splenectomy may also be done to determine prognosis and treatment
  4. Treatment measures are to reduce tumor size (radiation, cyclophosphamide, vincristine)
  5. For nursing care plan see Leukemias

F. Bleeding disorders
  1. Problems include
    a. Excessive bleeding from wounds, gums, and nose or internally from all body systems
    b. Shock
    c. Pain (especially if bleeding occurs into internal organs)
  2. Bleeding disorders result from decrease in components necessary for proper blood clotting (platelets or other clotting factors). The causes of platelet disorders can be acquired (thrombocytopenia), or they may be unknown (idiopathic thrombocytopenic purpura). Most coagulation disorders are either acquired (hepatic diseases, decreased vitamin K levels) or congenital (hemophilia)
  3. Diagnosis is confirmed by blood analysis revealing absence or diminution of specific clotting component
  4. Major treatment aims are to replace deficient factor (fresh frozen plasma, platelet infusion, cryoprecipitate) and to treat the patient symptomatically during acute episodes (prednisone, vi-

tamin K). Splenectomy may be performed when platelet decrease is cause of hemorrhage. Splenectomy is performed to remove the site of platelet destruction. Genetic counseling is recommended for those conditions that are congenital

5. Nursing care plan involves
   a. Maintaining patient comfort and safety (see Leukemias)
   b. Observing for shock
      (1) Make careful observation of urine and stool
      (2) Assess vital signs
      (3) Observe for restlessness
      (4) Investigate complaints of pain (may be bleeding into joints or internal organs)
   c. Reducing pain
      (1) Ensure meticulous skin care
      (2) Support extremities and joints
      (3) Change positions frequently

DISEASES OF THE GASTROINTESTINAL TRACT

Introduction

Disorders of the gastrointestinal tract involve disturbances in ingesting, digesting, absorbing nutrients, and eliminating waste products. Throughout life, eating is a means of establishing and maintaining social and cultural ties. This often complicates adjustment of patients to ordered therapeutic regimens. Frustration and repressed anger are known to cause an increase in secretions and motility of the gastrointestinal system

Assessment

A. Relevant information from health history
B. Nutritional habits (dietary intake, diet therapy)
C. Bowel elimination pattern (including use of laxatives and enemas)
D. Incidence of indigestion, flatulence, vomiting, pain associated with ingestion of food
E. Psychosocial adjustment to stress (coping patterns)

Stomatitis

Additional assessment includes observation of mucosa of mouth and tongue for ulcers, bleeding, and halitosis

A. Problems include
   1. Ulcers
   2. Pain and burning sensation
   3. Bleeding gums
   4. Halitosis
B. Stomatitis is an inflammation of mouth and tongue. Its cause may be primary (herpes, Vincent's angina), systemic (avitaminosis, pernicious anemia), or drug induced (steroids, cancer chemotherapeutic agents)
C. Diagnosis is based on oral and general physical examination
D. Treatment depends on identified cause
E. Nursing care plan consists primarily of frequent oral hygiene, administration of ordered medications, and treatment of identified causal condition

Parotitis

A. Problems include
   1. Swelling of gland
   2. Pain in ear
   3. Dysphagia
B. This inflammation of the parotid gland is usually caused by staphlococci
C. Diagnosis is based on oral and general physical examination
D. The condition is usually treated with sulfonamides or penicillin
E. Nursing care plan consists primarily of administering ordered medications and applying ice bags to swollen area as ordered

Hiatal hernia

A. Problems include
   1. Heartburn
   2. Eructation
   3. Feeling of fullness after meals
   4. Substernal pain
B. In this condition part of the upper stomach herniates into the lower thorax through an enlargement of the opening in the diaphragm. It may be caused by trauma or it may be congenital. Symptoms are primarily related to reflux of stomach contents, distension, and spasms in stomach
C. Diagnosis is made by physical examination, barium swallow, and upper gastrointestinal (GI) series.
D. Medical management consists of antacids, weight reduction, small frequent bland meals (four to six per day), and avoiding a recumbent position after eating. Elevating the head of the bed and using two to three pillows may help to prevent pain at night. If medical treatment is unsuccessful or complications occur, surgery may be done to correct the structural problem
E. Postoperative nursing care plan is same as for laparotomy or thoracotomy

Peptic ulcer

A. Problems include
   1. Gnawing sensation 1 to 3 hours past meals
   2. Eructation
   3. Nausea
   4. Vomiting
   5. Hematemesis
   6. Melena
   7. Anxiety

B. This is an erosion of the mucosa in areas of the GI tract that come in contact with hydrochloric acid and other gastric juices. Ulceration may occur in the lower part of the esophagus, in the stomach, or in the duodenum. It occurs more frequently near the pylorus, and symptoms become more severe in relationship to the extensiveness and invasiveness of the ulcer. Stress, heredity, and certain drugs and foods may contribute to ulcer formation

C. Diagnosis is made by upper GI series, gastric analysis, gastroscopic examination, and patient history

D. Medical treatment consists of use of sedatives and tranquilizers to provide physical and mental rest and anticholinergic drugs, antacids, and histamine antagonists (cimetidine) to decrease and/or control gastric acidity. Also a bland diet usually is prescribed. Surgical treatment consists of gastric resection

E. Nursing care plan for postoperative gastric resection involves
   1. Promoting wound healing
      a. Maintain nasogastric suction; note and record character and amount of drainage
      b. Observe wound for drainage, signs of bleeding, and infection
      c. Administer antibiotics
   2. Reducing pain
      a. Assess location, duration, and intensity of pain
      b. Administer analgesics and narcotics as ordered
   3. Maintaining fluid balance
      a. Monitor intravenous fluids
      b. Administer ordered electrolyte replacements
      c. Begin oral fluids as ordered when bowel sounds are audible
   4. Preventing complications
      a. Hemorrhage—monitor vital signs every 4 hours, and report any bleeding immediately
      b. Acute gastric dilation—observe for tachycardia, hypotension, and epigastric pain, and maintain patency of nasogastric tube
      c. Dumping syndrome (a rapid emptying of gastric contents into jejunum)—observe for weakness, vertigo, palpitations, and diaphoresis after meals; have patient eat small frequent meals low in sugar and salt, avoid drinking fluids with meals, and lie down after meals
      d. Malabsorption—observe for weight loss, weakness, and fatigue postoperatively

Ulcerative colitis

A. Problems include
   1. Fever
   2. Bloody diarrhea
   3. Anorexia
   4. Weight loss
   5. Dehydration
   6. Anxiety

B. This is an inflammatory process involving submucosa and mucosa of the intestines and rectum. It is seen more often in the young adult (20 to 40 years)

C. Diagnosis is made by sigmoidoscopy, barium enema, symptoms, and physical examination

D. Medical treatment consists of replacement of blood volume; bed rest in acute phases; control of stools by narcotic agents (diphenoxylate [Lomotil], paregoric); relief of cramps by belladonna alkaloids or anticholinergic drugs; reduction of anxiety with tranquilizers and sedatives; antibiotic therapy (penicillin, streptomycin, kanamycin [Kantrex], cephalothin [Keflin]); slowly absorbed sulfonamides with azo dyes (sulfasalazine [Azulfidine]); steroid therapy; low-residue diet; and in some cases psychotherapy. Surgical treatment (colectomy with ileostomy) is necessary when massive hemorrhage or perforation occurs

E. Nursing care plan for postoperative colectomy with ileostomy involves
   1. Promoting wound healing
      a. Maintain integrity of ileostomy appliance; drainage is constant and liquid
      b. Note character, amount, and consistency of drainage
      c. Observe wound for bleeding and signs of infection

d. Administer stoma skin care as drainage is constant and irritating
e. Administer ordered antibiotics
2. Relieving pain
a. Assess location, duration, and intensity of pain
b. Administer ordered analgesics and narcotics
3. Maintaining fluid balance
a. Monitor intravenous fluids
b. Monitor patient for signs of electrolyte imbalance
c. Administer ordered electrolyte replacements
4. Promoting adjustment to altered body image
a. Display supportive, nonjudgmental attitude
b. Encourage patient participation in self-care, including ileostomy care
c. With physician's approval, refer patient to United Ostomy Association, 1111 Wilshire Blvd., Los Angeles, Calif. 90017, for further educational materials

Appendicitis

A. Problems include
1. Acute abdominal pain in lower right quadrant that radiates
2. Fever
B. This is an inflammation of the vermiform appendix caused by infection, obstruction, or interrupted blood supply
C. Diagnosis is based on symptoms, physical examination, and an elevated WBC
D. Treatment is surgical removal of appendix and administration of systemic antibiotics
E. Nursing care plan consists of general nursing care to promote wound healing, reduction of pain postoperatively, and prevention of complications. With peritonitis avoid laxatives before surgery, and observe patient for fever, increased pain, and changes in vital signs

Intestinal obstruction

A. Problems include
1. Vomiting fecallike material
2. Constipation
3. Wavelike abdominal pain
B. Intestinal obstruction is inability of intestinal contents to flow normally along intestinal tract. It is classified as either organic (tumor) or mechanical (paralytic ileus)
C. Diagnosis is confirmed by physical examination and x-ray examination of small bowel
D. Medical treatment consists of relieving distention (Miller-Abbott tube, NPO), correcting fluid and electrolyte imbalance, and administering systemic antibiotics. Surgical intervention may include resecting obstructive lesion and necrotic tissue or performing a colostomy
E. Nursing care plan is same as for ileostomy, with the exception that stoma drainage will be formed fecal material that may be regulated according to the individual patient

Hemorrhoids

A. Problems include
1. Rectal pain
2. Rectal itching
3. Bleeding during defecation
B. Hemorrhoids are varicose veins found in the anal canal; they may be internal or external and are caused by pregnancy, chronic constipation, or heredity
C. Diagnosis is made by visual examination and proctoscopy
D. Medical treatment consists of stool softeners, witch hazel compresses, and sitz baths. Surgical treatment is removal (hemorrhoidectomy)
E. Nursing care plan consists primarily of carrying out ordered treatments and promoting wound healing

DISEASES OF THE ACCESSORY ORGANS

Pancreatitis

A. Problems include
1. Pain
2. Nausea
3. Vomiting
4. Shock
B. Inflammation of pancreas is caused by digestive actions of enzymes secreted by pancreas. The condition is usually associated with bacterial infections, excessive intake of alcohol, or obstructions in biliary tract from gallstones
C. Diagnosis is made by physical examination, symptoms, elevated WBC, and elevated serum lipase and amylase
D. Treatment consists of controlling pain with meperidine (Demerol); treating shock with blood replacement and plasma; gastric decompression to assist in

resting pancreas from secreting enzymes for digestion; administering anticholinergic drugs; and replacing electrolytes

E. Nursing care plan consists primarily of performing ordered treatment and providing emotional support

Cirrhosis of the liver (Laennec's)

A. Problems include
   1. Indigestion
   2. Flatulence
   3. Nausea
   4. Vomiting
   5. Weight loss
   6. Jaundice
   7. Ascites
   8. Esophageal varices
   9. Hepatic coma

B. This is fibrosis of liver parenchyma resulting from prolonged malnourishment (vitamin D deficiency or chronic alcoholism), causing fatty degeneration and tissue necrosis; hobnail or atrophic appearance follows scarring process

C. Diagnosis is based on physical examination and liver biopsy

D. Treatment consists of parenteral therapy to help maintain fluid and electrolyte balance (imbalances are caused by renal complications, ascites, hydrothorax, and hemorrhage from varices) and periodic relief of ascites by paracentesis. Treatment of esophageal hemorrhage is by insertion of the Sengstaken-Blakemore triple-lumen tube, which is anchored in cardiac end of stomach and inflated in esophagus to apply hemostasis and decompress stomach. Elimination of alcohol intake is essential to reverse or arrest early cirrhotic changes. Provide rest by sedation inasmuch as there is some renal and liver damage that may interfere with metabolism and with excretion of drugs. Diet should be high in carbohydrates and proteins; proteins are restricted during hepatic coma. Vitamin supplements, iron, and folic acid are needed to correct anemias that develop

E. Nursing care plan involves
   1. Preventing progression of cirrhosis
      a. Evaluate neurologic status, ascites, jaundice, and weakness
      b. Monitor weight, intake and output, vital signs, color, and number and consistency of bowel movements
   2. Promoting comfort
      a. Provide meticulous skin care
      b. Provide frequent oral hygiene
      c. Offer emotional support to patient and family

Viral hepatitis

A. Problems include the following
   1. Preicteric phase—fever, rash, anorexia, nausea, vomiting, weakness, pain on palpation of liver
   2. Icteric phase—jaundice, dark urine, hepatomegaly, nausea, epigastric distress

B. This is a contagious and infectious disease caused by a virus, resulting in inflammation of the liver. Classification is
   1. Infectious (Type A)—transmitted by contaminated food, stools, or water or by close contact with carriers. Incubation period is 2 to 7 weeks
   2. Serum (Type B)—transmitted parenterally (blood transfusion, contaminated needles) and by skin puncture (contaminated instrument). Incubation period is 2 to 5 months
   3. Noninfectious—caused by exposure to toxic or chemical substances

C. Condition is diagnosed by clinical evaluation (enzyme studies, presence of Australia antigen, counterelectrophoresis)

D. There is no known successful medical therapy. Treatment is based on supportive regimen
   1. Diet high in proteins and carbohydrates, with vitamin supplements (especially vitamin B complex)
   2. Bed rest and relaxation
   3. Isolation precautions according to type of hepatitis

E. Nursing care plan is based on ensuring proper rest, encouraging dietary intake, observing for signs of hepatic coma (minor to complete mental disorientation and motor disturbances), and supporting during diagnostic procedures and convalescence

Cholecystitis (inflammation) and cholelithiasis (stones) of the gallbladder

A. Problems include
   1. Colicky pain (mild to severe)
   2. Dyspepsia on ingestion of fatty foods
   3. Pruritus
   4. Nausea and vomiting

B. Chronic cholecystitis is rare without presence of stones. Cause of cholelithiasis is not definitely known, but it is believed that bile stasis, infection, and hypercholesterolemia are predisposing factors
C. Diagnosis is based on
   1. Cholecystography—visualization of shape and position of gallbladder by administration of iodide-containing dye (ipodate calcium/sodium [Oragrafin], iopanoic acid [Telepaque]) or intravenously (iodipamide meglumine [Cholografin])
   2. Cholangiography—direct injection of dye into biliary tree
D. Medical treatment consists of diet control with elimination of fried, high-fat, spicy, and rich foods (essential); relief of biliary colic and pain (atropine and meperdine [Demerol]); bile salts in addition to dietary restriction to allay gastric distress; antispasmodics and anticholinergics to allay muscle spasms; and antibiotics for infection (ampicillin). Surgical treatment consists of surgical removal of gallbladder with stones, with exploration of common bile duct (cholecystectomy). Following surgery, T tube is left in bile duct to drain bile until normal flow is established. Sometimes patient will experience postcholecystectomy syndrome, which mimics symptoms that occurred before removal of gallbladder
E. Nursing care plan for cholecystectomy involves promoting wound healing
   1. Proper positioning for comfort and promotion of drainage from T tube; unless there are orders to irrigate tube, nurse simply records character and amount of drainage
   2. Observation of changes in color of skin, sclerae, and stool to determine return of proper drainage of bile into duodenum
   3. Protection of skin around incision from irritation by bile
   4. Instruction in low-fat diet

DISORDERS OF THE ENDOCRINE SYSTEM

Introduction

Hormones secreted by endocrine system assist in regulation of many vital functions such as reproduction, growth and development, fluid and electrolyte balance, and metabolism for energy production. Overproduction or underproduction of hormones interferes with normal physiologic function and therefore disables the patient. Symptomatology may appear in the form of observable abnormalities that may cause the patient embarrassment. Nurse should be aware of the interrelationship of all the endocrine glands. Malfunction of one gland may produce alterations in activity of other glands. Nurse should encourage the symptomatic individual to seek immediate medical care

Assessment

Assessment of the endocrine system should include
A. Skin color and texture
B. Hair texture
C. Abnormalities in menstruation
D. Abnormalities in hair distribution
E. Excessive urine output and thirst
F. Fatigue or excessive energy (energy level)
G. Disproportion in bone structure or overall growth
H. Absence of secondary sex characteristics at appropriate age

Disorders of the pituitary gland

A. Hyperpituitarism
   1. Problems include
      a. Excessive oiliness and diaphoresis
      b. Overgrowth of bones
      c. Emotional problems caused by irreversible physical changes
      d. Joint and back pain
   2. Giantism (increase in length and width of bones in children) and acromegaly (increase in bone transversely, cartilage, and soft tissue in adults) can be caused by a pituitary tumor or increase in size and function of the gland
   3. Diagnosis is established by physical examination and presence of increased growth hormone
   4. Acromegaly may be treated by radiation of the gland or hypophysectomy
   5. Nursing care plan involves
      a. Assisting patient to accept altered body image
         (1) Listen and allow patient to verbalize feelings
         (2) Anticipate needs; avoid awkward situations
      b. Ensuring patient comfort
         (1) Maintain alignment
         (2) Support painful joints
         (3) Encourage active and passive range of motion exercise
         (4) Reposition frequently
         (5) Assist patient to get up
         (6) Control pain as ordered

B. Diabetes insipidus
  1. Problems include
    a. Polyuria
    b. Polydipsia
    c. Anorexia and weakness
    d. Dehydration
  2. Diabetes insipidus is caused by lack of antidiuretic hormone (ADH), which is secreted by posterior lobe of pituitary. Causes of the failure may result from tumors, hypophysectomy, or irradiation of the pituitary. Lack of ADH causes excessive water excretion from the body
  3. Diagnosis is confirmed by history and by measuring urine specific gravity
  4. Treatment consists of hormone replacement intramuscularly (pitressen tannate) or by nasal spray (lypressin). Lifelong therapy is necessary
  5. Nursing care plan involves
    a. Monitoring fluid and electrolyte status
      (1) Weigh daily at same time and with same clothing
      (2) Measure urine specific gravity
      (3) Provide sufficient fluids (may be up to 18 L daily)
      (4) Monitor intake and output
      (5) Observe for symptoms of electrolyte imbalance
    b. Preparing for surgery if hypophysectomy indicated

Disorders of the thyroid gland

A. Hyperthyroidism (toxic goiter, Graves' disease)
  1. Problems include
    a. Excessive irritability
    b. Tachycardia
    c. Heat intolerance and perspiration
    d. Increased appetite
    e. Muscle weakness, fatigue, and tremor
  2. Hyperthyroidism results when there is an overproduction of thyroid hormones. This excess speeds up all metabolic processes, and therefore more oxygen is used and energy expended. Death may occur from heart failure
  3. Diagnosis is confirmed with elevation of laboratory values such as T_3, T_4, ^{131}I uptake, and BUN
  4. Medical treatment consists of antithyroid drugs to reduce thyroid production (propylthiouracil) and drugs to control systemic effects of hormone, such as Inderal to reduce tachycardia, tremors, and nervousness. Surgical intervention (subtotal thyroidectomy) may be indicated
  5. Nursing care plan involves
    a. Promoting calm, safe environment
      (1) Provide quiet, well-ventilated, cool room
      (2) Plan care to prevent overstimulation
      (3) Provide diversional activities
      (4) Keep linen dry
      (5) Provide measures to promote sleep (medications, back care, warm drinks)
    b. Maintaining adequate nutrition
      (1) Provide high-caloric, high-protein diet
      (2) Provide between-meal snacks
      (3) Avoid beverages with caffeine
      (4) Force fluids—3000 to 4000 ml daily
    c. Observing for complications of medications
    d. Preparing for surgery (if indicated)
    e. Observing for postoperative complications
      (1) Laryngeal edema—check quality of voice every hour
      (2) Hemorrhage—check dressing at side and behind neck
      (3) Tetany—check reflexes every 2 hours; calcium replacement may be indicated
      (4) Thyroid storm—check for increase in temperature and pulse, confusion, and widening pulse pressure

B. Hypothyroidism
  1. Problems include
    a. Subnormal temperature and intolerance to cold
    b. Mental dullness and lethargy
    c. Anorexia and constipation
    d. Dyspnea on exertion
  2. Hypothyroidism results from lack of thyroid hormone secretion by thyroid gland. Primary inhibition may be a result of thyroid inability or secondarily from lack of pituitary stimulation. Cretinism is caused by thyroid deficiency at birth. The lack of thyroid hormone reduces rate of all metabolic activity
  3. Diagnosis is confirmed by same laboratory test as for hyperthyroidism
  4. Treatment is aimed at restoration of normal metabolic rate by replacing thyroid hormone (thyroglobin [Proloid], levothyroxine [Synthroid])
  5. Nursing care plan involves
    1. Providing adequat rest
      (1) Plan care to allow rest periods
      (2) Provide six small feedings

b. Ensuring safety
   (1) Provide uncluttered environment
   (2) Administer sedatives and hypnotics carefully—may be unusually sensitive
   (3) Assist patient to get up
c. Observing for side effects of medications
d. Observing for complications
   (1) Myxedema coma—coma, hypotension, convulsions
   (2) Myocardial infarction
   (3) Congestive heart failure

Disorders of the parathyroid gland

A. Hyperparathyroidism
   1. Problems include
      a. Muscle weakness and fatigue
      b. Arrhythmias
      c. Kidney stone formation
      d. Bone pain, deformities, and pathologic fractures
   2. Hyperparathyroidism is characterized by overproduction of parathormone, causing decalcification of the bones, increasing serum calcium, and decreasing serum phosphorus levels. Elevated serum calcium levels depress neuromuscular control and can lead to fatigue, clumsiness, and cardiac standstill
   3. Laboratory values show increase in calcium levels and decreased phosphorus levels; x-ray examination reveals skeletal changes
   4. Treatment may include surgical removal of gland
   5. Nursing care plan involves
      a. Preventing and observing for complications caused by excessive parathormone
         (1) Pathologic fractures—position carefully
         (2) Kidney stones—monitor intake and output; force fluids
         (3) Gastrointestinal ulceration—observe stools and vomitus; check vital signs
         (4) Arrhythmias—observe for confusion; check vital signs four times a day
      b. Preparing for parathyroidectomy
      c. Observing for postoperative complications (see postoperative procedures under Diseases of the thyroid gland, Hyperthyroidism)

B. Hypoparathyroidism
   1. Problems include
      a. Irritability
      b. Hypersensitive reflexes and seizures
      c. Anxiety and apprehension
   2. Hypoparathyroidism results from diminished secretion of parathormone. Calcium levels fall, and phosphorus levels are increased, causing muscular hyperirritability
   3. Diagnosis is confirmed by serum calcium levels and physical examinations (Chvostek's sign—spasm of facial muscles when facial nerve tapped—and Trousseau's sign—carpopedal spasm of hands and fingers)
   4. Treatment includes calcium replacement
   5. Nursing care plan involves
      a. Replacing calcium
         (1) Administer calcium as ordered
         (2) Monitor intravenous drip with calcium
         (3) Increase dietary intake of vitamin D to increase calcium absorption
         (4) Observe for vomiting—first symptom of hypercalcemia
      b. Allaying apprehension
         (1) Provide calm reassuring atmosphere
         (2) Respond when tetany symptoms reported

Disorders of the adrenal glands

A. Adrenal cortex hypofunction (Addison's disease)
   1. Problems include
      a. Muscle weakness and hypoglycemia
      b. Sodium and water depletion—dehydration
      c. Gastrointestinal disturbances—anorexia, nausea, vomiting
   2. This is a deficiency of adrenocortical hormones caused by destruction of the cortex or atrophy of the cortex because of prolonged steroid therapy or pituitary dysfunction. Symptoms result from disturbances in sodium and potassium metabolism
   3. Diagnosis is based on changes in blood chemistry, urine studies, and injection of adrencocorticotropic hormone (ACTH) to assess response
   4. Treatment consists of replacing missing hormone (hydrocortisone) and restoring of electrolyte balance (high-sodium, low-potassium diet and fluids)
   5. Nursing care plan involves
      a. Restoring electrolyte balance
         (1) Administer medications as ordered
         (2) Observe for toxicity of medications (edema, headache)
         (3) Administer fluids as ordered

b. Observing for complications
(1) Dehydration
(2) Hypoglycemia
(3) Addisonian crisis

B. Adrenal cortex hyperfunction (Cushing's syndrome)
1. Problems include
a. Emotional problems resulting from altered body image (hirsutism, breast atrophy, clitoral enlargement, deepend voice)
b. Thin fragile skin
c. Osteoporosis
d. Increased susceptibility to infection
e. Hypertension
2. Cushing's syndrome results from hypersecretion of cortisol from the adrenal cortex. Causes of oversecretion may be tumors or overstimulation by ACTH
3. Diagnosis is made on the basis of symptoms, urine studies, and blood chemistry (hyperglycemia, elevated cortisol, decreased potassium, and reduced number of eosinophils)
4. Treatment is aimed at removal of cause and hormonal replacement following surgical removal of adrenal cortex (cortisol, fludrocorticortisone acetate [Florinef], sodium chloride)
5. Nursing care plan involves
a. Assisting patient to accept altered body image
b. Maintaining skin integrity
(1) Provide careful skin care
(2) Reposition frequently
(3) Prevent skin drying
c. Ensuring safety
(1) Maintain alignment
(2) Screen visitors for upper respiratory infections
(3) Assist patient to get up
d. Providing hormonal replacement following adrenalectomy—administer medications as ordered
e. Providing therapeutic diet
(1) Encourage diet high in potassium and low in sodium
(2) Explain necessity of compliance

Disorder of the pancreas—diabetes mellitus

A. Problems include
1. Polydipsia
2. Polyuria
3. Polyphagia
4. Weight loss
5. Strength loss
6. Drowsiness
7. Slow-healing wounds
8. Glycosuria
9. Elevated blood glucose level (hyperglycemia)

B. Diabetes mellitus a metabolic disease related to body's inability to oxidize carbohydrates. Disturbances usually are caused by faulty pancreatic activity and interference with production of insulin. Condition is believed to be inherited as mendelian recessive trait

C. Diagnosis is made by evaluation of symptoms and results of glucose tolerance test, postprandial blood glucose test, Dextrostix, Tes-Tape, and Clinitest

D. Treatment consists of the following
1. Continuous medical supervision, urine and blood testing, and insulin (used by approximately half of diabetic patients) are indicated; insulin is prepared in units per milliliter (U100)
a. Isophane (NPH) and Lente insulin are intermediate-acting insulins
b. Regular and Semilente insulin are short-acting insulins
c. Ultralente and protamine zinc (PZI) insulin have prolonged duration of activity
2. Oral hypoglycemic agents (tolbutamide [Orinase], chloropropamide [Diabinese]) are used by newly diagnosed adult diabetic patients who have mild nonketotic diabetes and whose condition cannot be controlled by diet alone but who do not require insulin. These agents stimulate pancreas to produce insulin
3. Diet is an important aspect of treatment and is calculated by age, sex, height, and weight. Diet may be instituted without insulin, or insulin may be a vital part of regimen. Carbohydrates are essential and necessary for energy, but sugar, potatoes, spaghetti, and macaroni are limited. Proteins are essential for tissue building; they are found in eggs, milk, and meat. Fats must be watched in complications involving liver, where fats are oxidized

E. Nursing care plan involves the following
1. Educate patient education
a. Hygiene
b. Administration of insulin—rotate sites; use sterile equipment

c. Action of oral hypoglycemic drugs
d. Dietary restrictions
e. Foot care—inspect routinely (corns, blisters, abrasions), bathe daily in warm water, massage feet, wear noncompressive shoes and clean socks, do foot exercises, and avoid injury (see physician if injury occurs)

2. Observe for complications—signs of acidosis (ketoacidosis, coma)
a. Increased weakness
b. Dull headache
c. Malaise
d. Insatiable thirst
e. Nausea and vomiting
f. Hot, dry, flushed appearance
g. Kussmaul's respirations
h. Sweet odor to breath
i. Hypotension

3. Observe for complications—signs of shock (hypoglycemia). Complications can be diminished by patient compliance to treatment regimen (keeping blood glucose within normal range)
a. Weakness and faintness
b. Dizziness and double vision
c. Restlessness and confusion
d. Profuse perspiration
e. Pallor
f. Rapid pulse

4. Eye problems—retinitis, cataracts, glaucoma
5. Circulatory problems—atherosclerosis, arteriosclerosis

CONDITIONS OF NERVOUS SYSTEM

Introduction

The nervous system helps to regulate and coordinate body functions and enables the body to function as a whole

Assessment

A. Assess level of consciousness
B. Assess motor, sensory, and reflex function
C. Assess pupil reaction
D. Obtain information regarding previous mental and motor function

Intracranial lesions

A. Problems include
1. Headache
2. Decreased level of consciousness
3. Visual disturbances
4. Pupil changes
5. Projectile vomiting
6. Altered vital signs (decreased pulse and respirations)
7. Changes in motor, sensory, or reflex activity

B. Any type of lesion that takes up space in the cranial cavity usually produces an increase in intracranial pressure. All tumors of the brain are considered malignant. Head injuries produce conditions similar to intracranial tumors in that they encroach on vital centers in a closed compartment. Head injuries may vary from a slight bruising of brain tissue to vascular rupture causing hemorrhage or hematoma

C. Diagnosis is complex and may include neurologic examination, lumbar puncture, brain scan, electroencephalogram (EEG), pneumoencephalogram, and cerebral arteriography

D. Treatment is aimed at removing the lesion, evacuating the hematoma, or alleviating the symptoms by decreasing intracranial pressure. Medical treatment includes radiation therapy (may be done for palliation, preoperatively to reduce a tumor and also postoperatively); diuretics and steroid drug therapy (used to reduce intracranial pressure); and sedatives and narcotics (seldom used because they mask symptoms and depress level of consciousness). Surgical treatment may include craniotomy to remove a portion of cranium and get to the lesion site; decompression to remove part of the bony skull to relieve intracranial pressure; and evacuation of hematoma

E. Nursing care plan involves
1. Maintaining quiet environment and promoting rest
2. Observing for signs of increased intracranial pressure
3. Arousing patient frequently to check level of consciousness
4. Elevating head of bed to facilitate drainage of cerebrospinal fluid
5. Changing position frequently and helping patient with range of motion exercises
6. Performing frequent mouth care
7. Positioning patient off operative side

Cerebrovascular accident

A. Problems include
1. Headache
2. Dizziness
3. Coma

4. Convulsions
5. Elevated blood pressure
6. Labored respirations
7. Aphasia
8. Dysphagia and hemiplegia

B. This condition is rupture of cerebral blood vessel or embolism or thrombosis of cerebral blood vessel; contributing causes include hypertension, atherosclerosis, aneurysm, trauma, systemic disease, acute infections, and noxious agents

C. Diagnosis is confirmed through history and physical examination plus cerebral arteriography

D. Treatment is aimed at maintaining physiologic function and preventing complications

E. Nursing care plan for cerebrovascular accident involves the following
   1. Acute phase
      a. Protect from further injury
         (1) Loosen tight clothing
         (2) Use soft object to protect tongue and keep airway clear during convulsions
         (3) Monitor vital signs
      b. Maintain patent airway
         (1) Turn head to side
         (2) Remove any food particles in mouth
         (3) Use suction, if facilities are available
   2. Convalescent phase—restore and maintain optimal functioning
      a. Align patient in bed, and utilize equipment (sandbags) to prevent inward shoulder rotation and outward hip rotation
      b. Support affected side with pillows if hemiplegia is present
      c. Turn patient every 2 hours to prevent skin breakdown
      d. Avoid foot drop by use of foot board
      e. Perform oral hygiene frequently to prevent aspiration of food not swallowed as a result of dysphagia
      f. Perform skin care—necessary because of incontinence
      g. Use indwelling catheter to facilitate accurate measurement of intake and output, as well as nursing care
      h. Encourage patient, who is often discouraged if nurse does not understand garbled speech
      i. Treat hemiplegia as health team; physician and physical therapist decide approach; nurse should be aware of role in rehabilitation
      j. Use nasogastric feedings for comatose patients
      k. Encourage ambulation, which is encouraging to patient and family
      l. Keep family involved in care and rehabilitation of patient

Spinal cord lesions—tumors

A. Problems include
   1. Pain
   2. Numbness
   3. Tingling
   4. Weakness or paralysis

B. This is an abnormal growth of cells that may occur outside or inside the spinal cord. It may be benign or malignant. However, any growth compressing or interfering with nerve function is considered serious

C. Diagnosis is made by history, neurologic examination, and myelogram

D. Treatment is primarily centered on surgical removal of such growth when possible. Chemotherapy and radiation may be used in certain situations

E. Nursing care plan involves
   1. Relieving pain
   2. Maintaining joint motion
   3. Maintaining proper alignment and support of spine at all times
   4. Maintaining constant assessment of motor, sensory, and reflex function

Spinal cord injuries

A. Problems include
   1. Same as for spinal tumors
   2. Respiratory distress (see Diseases of the respiratory system)
   3. Injuries at C4 and above

B. Spinal cord may be completely or partially severed or destroyed. Complete severance of spinal cord results in permanent paralysis of body parts below the site of injury. Spinal shock may cause temporary paralysis and is caused by edema in the partially damaged cord

C. Diagnosis is based on physical examination and symptoms

D. Treatment is aimed at preventing further damage and restoring the natural contour of the spinal cord. Emergency treatment consists of keeping patient flat, log rolling for transfer, and supporting head and neck so that there is no movement. Hospital treatment consists of administration of steroids (dexamethasone [Decadron]) and application of traction, Crutchfield tongs, body cast, or back brace

E. Nursing care plan involves
   1. Maintaining strict alignment of spine as set with traction
   2. Maintaining respiratory function (suction, oxygen, respiratory assistance)
   3. Maintaining skin integrity (turning frames, skin care)
   4. Maintaining fluid balance and nutrition
   5. Maintaining urinary and fecal elimination
   6. Maintaining medical regimen (avoid injections below the level of lesion)
   7. Promoting acceptance of altered body image

Herniated intervertebral disk

A. Problems include
   1. Pain in the affected area radiating to the extremity
   2. Weakness and loss of sensation in body part supplied by affected nerves

B. This is a rupture or herniation of the membranous covering that surrounds the intervertebral disk. The herniated tissue pushes outward and compresses the nerve roots as they exit the spinal column. Symptoms will be localized to the area innervated by the affected nerve root

C. Diagnosis is confirmed by history, physical examination, and myelogram

D. Medical treatment consists of bed rest, bed boards with firm mattress, cervical or pelvic traction, moist heat, and analgesics and muscle relaxants. Surgical intervention may be employed when conservative treatment is unsuccessful (laminectomy or spinal fusion)

E. Nursing care plan is same as for spinal cord tumor. (See Rehabilitation nursing for long-term care)

Parkinson's disease

A. Problems include
   1. Muscle tremors
   2. Slow speech
   3. Shuffling gait
   4. Drooling
   5. Masklike expression
   6. Pill-rolling hand action

B. This is a progressive degenerative disease of the nervous system. The cause is unknown

C. Treatment is aimed at relieving the symptoms. Medical treatment consists of antispasmodics (trihexyphenidyl [Artane], benztropine mesylate [Cogentin]); muscle relaxants; antiviral agents (amantadine [Symmetrel]); and levodopa (L-dopa) and levodopa with carbidopa (Sinemet). Surgical interventions have varying degrees of success and may consist of chemopallidectomy, chemothalamectomy, or cryogenic surgery

D. Nursing care plan is aimed at maintaining continuation of independent living activities as long as possible. Postoperative nursing care is similar to that of postcraniotomy (see Rehabilitation nursing for long-term care)

Multiple sclerosis

A. Problems include
   1. Disturbance in motion
   2. Spasticity
   3. Visual disturbances
   4. Speech difficulties

B. Multiple sclerosis is degeneration and scarring of the myelin sheath that surrounds individual nerve pathways; degenerative changes interfere with conduction of motor nerve impulses

C. Treatment is aimed at helping patient to live as effectively as possible and remain independent as long as possible. This is done with physical therapy, vasodilator drugs (nicotinic acid), and muscle relaxants (dantrolene [Dantrium], baclofen [Lioresal])

D. Nursing care plan involves the following (see Rehabilitation nursing for long-term care)
   1. Maintaining adequate rest
   2. Maintaining optimal nutrition
   3. Maintaining skin integrity
   4. Maintaining independent activities as long as possible

GERIATRIC NURSING

Introduction

There are 20 million persons in the United States over 64 years of age; there are estimates that number will reach 30 million by year 2000. Average life expectancy is 77 years for women and 72 years for men. Less than 5% of persons over 65 years of age live in institutions. Factors increasing life expectancy are heredity, advances in medical science, daily living improvements, and attitude

Physiologic aspects of aging

A. Aging is a normal, gradual slowing of body functions, beginning with conception and proceeding at a different rate in each individual
B. Factors contributing to aging process are
   1. Degenerative diseases
   2. Poor health habits
   3. Excesses of tobacco, food, and alcohol
   4. Inactivity
C. Changes that may occur are
   1. Calcium stored in bone shifts to tissues and blood vessels
   2. Teeth are lost
   3. Progressive hearing loss is experienced
   4. Circulation, especially to lower extremities, lessens
   5. Sensory and motor impulses and reactions are slowed
   6. Bowel becomes sluggish
   7. Urinary stress incontinence may develop
   8. Changes in the shape of the lens may cause visual disturbances
   9. Glandular secretions, circulatory impairment, and loss of fatty tissue contribute to skin breakdown
   10. Hair becomes gray and dry
   11. Lessened activity lessens need for sleep
   12. Taste buds atrophy
D. Three fourths of individuals over 65 years of age have a chronic disease, such as
   1. Heart disease
   2. Chronic respiratory disease
   3. Arthritis

Psychosocial aspects of aging

A. Persons should prepare in advance for retirement financially and psychologically
B. Healthy attitude and zest for living help in making adjustment
C. Person may need to adjust to loss of spouse and friends
D. Income is usually fixed
E. Persons should establish social contacts with persons of his or her own age

General nursing care of older persons

A. Nurse should accept patient as he or she is and not criticize
B. Nurse should be patient and allow aged patient to perform self-care as much as possible
C. Safety is vital; bones are more brittle, reflexes are slowed, and vision is impaired
D. Nurse should serve simple, well-balanced meals
E. Nurse should speak clearly, facing patient
F. Daily use of laxatives should be discouraged
G. Patient should be protected from temperature extremes; skin is very sensitive to heat and cold
H. Nurse should not bathe patient daily with soap; it contributes to drying skin
I. Nurse should allow for intervals of rest but encourage activity
J. Care should be taken to prevent odors and keep patient clean
K. Nurse should treat patient with respect
L. Visits from family and friends should be encouraged
M. Nurse should be aware of any chronic disease patient has and make daily assessments accordingly

Rehabilitation of the older patient

A. Patient should be encouraged to accept limitations and function within them
B. Compulsory retirement may be demoralizing
C. Alternative activities should be explored
D. Nurse should accentuate abilities, not disabilities
E. Older persons are valuable contributors to community

Community plans and programs

A. Social Security—while person is employed, part of salary is put into fund; monthly income from this source depends on time person was enrolled and amount contributed
B. Medicare—this is health insurance for persons over age 65, covering hospitalization and physicians' services
C. Retirement plans—business and industry provide plans to be utilized after retirement
D. Clubs—many Golden Age Clubs provide recreation for older persons; hobbies are cultivated
E. Churches and civic organizations—these organizations realize how much older persons have to offer
F. Housing—federally funded apartment complexes are available to older persons on fixed incomes
G. Nursing homes—these are available for older persons with chronic illnesses, who cannot care for themselves

COMMUNITY HEALTH NURSING

Introduction

A. Community health is an organized effort in the prevention of disease, prolongation of life, and education of public
B. Public health nursing is professional practice of nursing skills (technical, interpersonal), which are applied to health problems that affect a community
C. Emphasis is placed on the community as a whole, with care directed toward individual health care problems
D. The nurse must constantly assess the health situation in regard to welfare and development of family and community
E. William Rathborne is considered to be the father of public health nursing (PHN)

Organizational structure

A. Federal level
 1. Department of Health and Human Services (HHS) is branch of federal government in which all health agencies are grouped
 2. Public Health Service (PHS) is responsible for the advancement and protection of health for the United States
 3. Food and Drug Administration (FDA) is a scientific institution and law-enforcement agency that is responsible for safeguarding the public's health and finance in regard to drugs, foods, and cosmetics
B. State level
 1. Each state's public (tax-supported) and voluntary (not tax-supported) health agencies are organized to meet the needs of the citizens of the state and to coordinate financial aid from federal branch. They are directly accountable to governor
 2. Responsibilities of state health department are to
  a. Assist and advise local departments
  b. Provide direct services to counties without local agency
  c. Coordinate activities of all agencies and personnel within health departments
  d. Promote legislation by providing information on health problems
  e. Enforce health laws and regulations and publicize these facts
C. Local level
 1. Local agencies function as the direct contact with the people
 2. They play major role in providing services and fulfilling goals
 3. Examples of duties are
  a. Management and internal affairs
  b. Vital statistics
  c. Mental health
  d. Environmental health

Role of nurse in community health

A. Provider of personal care to the sick in their home
B. Advocate for the individuals in the community. He or she works with the physician, family, health services, and schools
C. Advisor to those whom he or she serves (teacher, counselor, collaborator)
D. Sensitive observer who reports to the physician and follows his or her orders
E. Person who can influence decisions made by individual, family, and community in the direction of health care
F. Organizer and manager
G. Participant in community planning and action

Home health care

A. Basic nursing principles
 1. Use same principles in home as in hospital
 2. Adapt procedure to patient and equipment available
 3. Have necessary supplies and equipment; nurse and family may improvise most equipment needed
 4. Rent equipment, such as hospital bed and wheelchair, from hospital supply company if needed; investigate loan possibilities
 5. Keep patient's record and observations of reactions and condition as physician orders. Include the following in record: date, medicines, treatments, intake and output, nurse's notes, and physician's order sheet
 6. Keep physician's and ambulance's telephone numbers easily available
 7. Review Units 3, 4, 5, and 6
B. Consider patient and position in family
 1. The child (restrictions and limitations caused by illness and family's adjustment)
 2. The adolescent (treat as young adult, assist in self-help activities)

3. The homemaker (gradual resumption of household activities)
4. The wage earner (assist in ascertaining information about available resources)

Communicable disease nursing*

A. Communicable diseases—those diseases passed from one person to another either by direct or indirect contact or by insects as intermediate hosts; they may affect individuals at any age; many more commonly occur in children
   1. Direct contact means close contact with patient having communicable disease or with carrier (carrier may be human or intermediate host)
   2. Indirect contact includes infection from contact with dust, excretions from patient, and contaminated food, water, or milk
   3. Practical nurse may care for communicable disease patients in their homes as well as in hospital
   4. Some communicable diseases are more common in children, but when large reservoir of susceptible adults exists, severe epidemics may occur
   5. Communicable diseases common in adults may be transmitted to children
B. Causes of most common communicable diseases
   1. Bacteria, such as streptococci, staphylococci, and bacilli (tuberculosis, diphtheria, typhoid fever)
   2. Viruses, large and small, that are nonbacterial (atypical pneumonia, common cold)
   3. Rickettsiae (Rocky Mountain spotted fever)
   4. Spirochetes (syphilis)
   5. Parasites (pinworms, *Trichinella*)
C. Sources of infection
   1. Human beings
   2. Animals
   3. Insects
   4. Food
   5. Water
D. Portals of entry
   1. Respiratory tract
   2. Gastrointestinal tract
   3. Genitourinary tract
   4. Skin

*For specific diseases see Appendix, Table 6, Communicable disease chart.

E. Portals of exit
   1. Discharges from any body system (sputum, urine, feces)
   2. Discharges and drainage from wounds
F. Important words to know (see Glossary for definitions)
   1. Disinfection
   2. Immunity
   3. Toxin
   4. Incubation period
   5. Isolation
   6. Quarantine
   7. Inoculation
   8. Vaccine
   9. Serum
   10. Booster dose
G. Community protection against communicable diseases
   1. Certain diseases should be reported to city, county, or state health departments; nurse should know regulations and reportable diseases in community
   2. Federal government's responsibilities are
      a. Establishment of quarantine stations at ports; quarantine regulations are under jurisdiction of PHS
      b. Medical examination of all immigrants for communicable disease
      c. Maintenance of officers in foreign ports to examine immigrants before embarkation
      d. Inspection of all ships and airplanes coming from foreign ports
      e. Spraying interiors of airplanes coming from tropical countries with insecticide
      f. Establishment of regulations concerning immunization of persons traveling outside United States
      g. Assistance of state and local health departments with investigation and control of specific epidemics
      h. Maintenance of Centers for Disease Control in Atlanta, Georgia
   3. Education in treatment and prevention of communicable diseases is now carried out in every community by both government and private agencies through
      a. Newspapers
      b. Magazines

c. Radio
d. Television
e. Schools
(1) Courses in health
(2) Parent-teacher associations

H. Protection of nurse, patient, and family
1. Responsibilities of nurse
a. Should be informed about basic facts in communicable disease control and treatment
b. Should be experienced in carrying out isolation technique
c. Should know about organisms causing disease
(1) Virulence
(2) How they enter and leave body
(3) Period of incubation
(4) How long patient, belongings, and family need to be isolated
(5) Vaccines, antitoxins, serums, or other measures available for protection of patient, family, and community
2. Special nursing precautions
a. Wash hands after any contact with contaminated area or articles
b. Use gown, mask, and rubber gloves as indicated by infection control and knowledge about how disease spreads
c. Disinfect bed linen, dishes, and clothing as indicated
d. Teach patient and family
(1) Precautions necessary
(2) Regulations for institutional and home care
3. General nursing
a. Assist with tests and special treatments
b. Give specific medicines as ordered
c. Perform nursing care during fever
d. Protect patient during convalescence
e. Know about complications and report first symptom
f. Perform accurate charting at all times

REHABILITATION NURSING

Introduction

Basic philosophy of rehabilitation should include assisting all physically or mentally handicapped persons to achieve greatest degree of total independence and self-realization possible within limits of their handicaps

A. Basic principles
1. Emphasize individual's assets rather than handicap
2. Consider total patient (mind, body, emotions, education, training, age)
3. Emphasize self-help; it is important factor in all diseases but is especially important in chronic illness, paralysis, and loss of limb or vital functions, such as sight or hearing
4. Teach patient to use resources

B. Result of modern medical advances
1. Early diagnosis, adequate treatment, and prevention of diseases, such as poliomyelities, reduce aftereffects
2. Methods, such as splinting and light casting, help to prevent deformity in arthritis
3. Surgical and orthopedic techniques help in repairing diseased and injured tissues
4. Early ambulation helps keep muscles in good tone
5. Application of rehabilitation techniques early in disease helps to prevent or reduce deformity

C. Result of community health actions
1. Rehabilitation of physically handicapped is accepted and supported economically
2. Financial support to institutions and agencies in this field comes from
a. Private funds through agencies such as the National Foundation–March of Dimes (formerly the National Foundation for Infantile Paralysis)
b. Public funds through state rehabilitation programs; they provide medical care and retraining and educational programs (Vocational Rehabilitation Act of 1954); programs are being expanded to include some kinds of disabilities
c. Social Security Act, which provides benefits to disabled eligible persons under 62 years of age
3. Many agencies make provision for all phases of rehabilitation
a. Voluntary agencies
(1) These are supported by private donations and United Fund
(2) Arthritis Foundation is one example
b. Agencies supported by local, state, or federal taxes

(1) Federal aid is given to states to carry out programs of vocational education and rehabilitation
(2) State aid is available for medical care, hospitalization, nursing care, and prosthetic appliances

4. Employment of handicapped persons is increased by
   a. President's Committee on Employment of Physically Handicapped, which spurred state employment services, voluntary groups, and private business to increase employment of handicapped workers
   b. Special workshops where severely disabled persons unable to return to employment because of handicaps can find employment (Abilities, Inc.; Paraplegics Manufacturing Company; Unlimited Skills, Inc.; Goodwill Industries)
5. Prevention depends on
   a. Development of safeguards in industry
   b. Better traffic laws and enforcement
   c. Safety education for individuals
   d. Early diagnosis and treatment of diseases
   e. Training in water and work safety
   f. Government control of certain drugs that may contribute to birth defects and accidents

D. Phases of rehabilitation
1. Acute illness
   a. Goal and first consideration is to provide good medical and nursing care
   b. Classification of disability is made concerning extent and probable duration
   c. Emotional support to patient's family is important
2. Recovery and restorative care
   a. Motivate patient to achieve independence and self-realization
   b. Teach activities of daily living
   c. Utilize facilities for physical therapy, occupational therapy, and speech therapy
   d. Provide continuity in all teaching
   e. Allow patient to express feelings and frustrations; provide acceptance, understanding, and encouragement
3. Economic and vocational guidance
   a. Patient may have fears that he or she will become dependent on family and community
   b. Importance of retraining and reeducating handicapped person should be stressed
   c. Vocational rehabilitation is now carried out with state and local funds
      (1) Primary objective is to make patient employable
      (2) Rehabilitation depends on evaluation, retraining, and continued education of patient
      (3) Rehabilitation plan assists in finding employment
4. Nurse and physically handicapped patient
   a. Often patient is cared for in own home or institution for chronic diseases
   b. Nurse should be familiar with program for individual patient in order to cooperate with treatment
   c. Nurse should provide encouragement and optimism; results may be slow

E. Teamwork
1. Nurse—valuable member of team (physician, therapists, and social worker)
2. Physical therapist
   a. Trained in use of physical agents (exercises, hydrotherapy, electrotherapy, light therapy, and others)
   b. Capable of interpreting patient's condition and restoring function of muscles and nerves
3. Occupational therapist
   a. Activities are designed to interest patient; they may lead to training for vocation
   b. Programs are designed for patient during long convalescence of limited activity, for patients who will always be confined to bed, and for patients with limited motion of hands and arms; group therapy is utilized and is valuable experience for patient
4. Social worker
   a. Studies home and total environment to help patient make adjustments
   b. Interprets patient's condition and activities to teachers, employers, and members of family
   c. Knows agencies and facilities in community through which patient may obtain job training and placement and special appliances and prostheses
5. Rehabilitation centers—offer specialized assistance to handicapped. There are special centers for blind, deaf, and mentally retarded persons

6. Family, school, and employing agency—cooperation is important
7. Community agencies
8. Team—basic purposes are to help patient
   a. Carry on activities of daily living (ADL)
   b. Train in balance and ambulation
   c. Train for gainful employment if no longer able to do accustomed work because of handicap
   d. Find recreational outlets
   e. Adjust emotionally to handicap
   f. Find status and satisfactory role in family, work, and community groups

F. Classification of physically handicapped patient
   1. Cause of handicap
      a. Disease
      b. Accident—traffic or industrial
   2. Examples of handicaps and assisting agencies
      a. Visual (the blind)—American Foundation for the Blind and National Society for the Prevention of Blindness
      b. Audible (the deaf)—American Society for Hard of Hearing, with local chapters
      c. Vocal—The Lost Cord Club

General nursing care

A. Acute stage
   1. It is important that all nurses inspire confidence and hope for future in patient
   2. Patient should be restored to optimal physical health as quickly as possible
   3. Most important nursing function is to prevent conditions, such as contractures and decubiti, that would increase patient's limitations

B. Chronic stage
   1. Convalescence may be long, depending on defect
   2. Nurse must help patient develop independence as quickly as possible within limitation and condition; patient should be encouraged to
      a. Be responsible for personal hygiene
      b. Be responsible for feeding and dressing self
      c. Develop independence in ambulation (wheelchair, artificial limbs, crutches, braces)
      d. Develop recreational interests within limits of handicap; these often can be part of muscle retraining
   3. Cooperation of family is important if patient is to develop self-reliance

C. Specific nursing techniques
   1. Help to maintain safe, sanitary, and congenial environment for all patients
   2. Use mechanical aids to prevent deformities and preserve good body alignment (sandbags, foot boards, bed boards, pillows)
   3. Work with therapist in carrying out therapeutic exercises as indicated (passive, active, active-assistive, resistive, stretching)
   4. Help patient to use mechanical devices (wheelchairs, braces, prostheses, crutches, canes)
   5. Teach techniques applicable to elimination of body wastes (training in bladder and bowel control)
   6. Prevent and care for ulcers
      a. Examine skin daily (look for reddened areas), and keep skin dry at all times
      b. Examine any part of body where rubbing against brace or cast may occur
      c. Bathe all paralyzed parts daily
      d. Use foam pillow and other devices to prevent pressure on any reddened part
      e. Help patient to change position frequently and to sit up in chair if allowed; encourage ambulation
      f. Serve high-protein diet unless otherwise ordered
      g. Cooperate with team members in teaching patient and family so that patient becomes self-sufficient

D. Use of crutches, braces, wheelchairs, appliances, and prostheses
   1. Crutches
      a. All crutches should be fitted individually and provided with rubber tips to protect against slipping
      b. Bed patients are prepared by exercises and sitting in chair before attempting to walk with crutches (strengthens weak muscles after inactivity)
      c. Patient will usually have practiced with parallel bars in the physical therapy department or with a "walker"
      d. Technique of crutch walking is
         (1) Crutches should be measured for each patient and should have rubber tips
         (2) Patient should wear strong, well-fitting shoes

(3) Type of crutch walking depends on patient's disability
(4) Four-point gait is right foot and then left crutch, then left foot and right crutch, moving alternately
(5) Two-point gait is rapid type of four-point gait; patient is able to move right foot and left crutch together then left foot and right crutch
(6) Three-point gait is used when patient is unable to bear weight of body on one leg; both crutches and weak or artificial leg move together, then good leg moves ahead
(7) Nurse should be sure physician's instructions are understood before attempting to teach and supervise patient in crutch walking

2. Braces
   a. Braces are ordered by physician for support and to prevent or correct deformities and are fitted to patient
   b. Leg braces include acceptable shoe into which brace fits or is attached; it is important that shoes be kept in good condition and give good support
   c. If patient is child, nurse should watch for signs that he or she is outgrowing brace
3. Wheelchairs
   a. Type of wheelchair is prescribed by physician to meet needs of individual patient
   b. Brakes should be kept in good working condition
4. Appliances
   a. These are used mainly for maximum use of hands and upper extremities
   b. They are devised to help with use of telephone, eating, writing, use of typewriter, and many other activities
5. Prostheses
   a. A prosthesis is any artificial part of body
   b. Type is chosen and fitted by physician and prosthetist
   c. Stump is dressed, cleaned, and massaged according to physician's instructions
   d. Unused muscles weaken; therefore, patient should use prosthesis as soon as possible

E. Care of aids
1. Manufacturer's instructions for care should be followed
2. Patient or family should keep instructions for future reference

NURSING THE ADULT PATIENT REVIEW QUESTIONS

Read each question carefully and consider all possible answers. When you have decided which answer is **best,** blacken the corresponding space on the answer sheet. There is only **one** best answer for each question.

Situation: Mrs. Moore, a 65-year-old widow, is admitted to the hospital for a diagnostic workup. She has never been hospitalized.

1 The practical nurse recognized Mrs. Moore's complaints of pain, tingling, and numbness as a group of symptoms described as
1. Functional
2. Objective
3. Personal
4. Subjective

2 Mrs. Moore has been treated for arthritis as an outpatient. Her arthritis is best classified as
1. Acute
2. Chronic
3. Subacute
4. Semichronic

3 Inflammatory reactions in arthritis include which of the following symptoms?
1. Loss of function, resolution
2. Pain, infection
3. Pain, swelling
4. Resolution, swelling

4 Mrs. Moore falls out of bed and sustains a 3-in. scalp laceration. If it is quickly sutured, it will heal by
1. First intention
2. Secondary intention
3. Keloids
4. Scar formation

5 Mrs. Moore complains of dizziness after falling and is placed on bedrest for several weeks. Her thigh muscles may undergo a change known as
1. Atrophy
2. Hyperplasia
3. Hypertrophy
4. Regeneration

6 During Mrs. Moore's physical examination, the methods utilized in examining the joints are
1. Auscultation, palpation
2. Inspection, palpation
3. Inspection, endoscopy
4. Percussion, auscultation

7 The practical nurse's primary role during Mrs. Moore's hospitalization is that of
1. Anticipation, teaching
2. Friendliness, comfort
3. Reassurance, emotional support
4. Sympathy, cheerfulness

Situation: Mr. Merlin Jenkins, a 70-year-old man, is admitted with a diagnosis of congestive heart failure. His presenting symptoms are dyspnea; frothy, blood-tinged sputum; and anxiety. Pedal edema and cyanosis are also present.

8 Congestive heart failure is best described as
1. Collection of fluid in the tissues
2. Inability of the heart to meet the body's demands
3. Reduced body needs as opposed to increased heart activity
4. Venous-return retardation by a compensatory heart

9 Dyspnea, experienced by Mr. Jenkins, is best relieved by placing him in a position called
1. Trendelenburg's
2. Orthopnic
3. Sims's
4. Supine

10 Mr. Jenkins' symptoms that indicate left-sided heart failure are
1. Cyanosis and pedal edema
2. Frothy sputum and dyspnea
3. Pedal edema and anxiety
4. Sputum and ascites

11 In the diagnostic workup, electrocardiography was performed to ascertain
(A) Causes of heart failure
(B) Complications of heart failure
(C) Presence of congestive heart failure
(D) Presence of heart block
1. A, B, and D
2. B, C, and D
3. A, C, and D
4. A, B, and C

12 Rotation of tourniquets was instituted to
1. Decrease blood loss
2. Decrease workload of heart
3. Reduce blood flow
4. Test various pressures

13 The nurse should discontinue Mr. Jenkins' tourniquets as ordered. The usual order is to remove
1. One tourniquet every 15 to 20 minutes
2. One tourniquet every hour
3. All tourniquets at the same time
4. All tourniquets after 1 hour of rotating

14 Digitalis is effective in Mr. Jenkins' therapy because it has
(A) Contractile effects on the heart
(B) Diuretic properties
(C) Mild vasoconstrictive properties
(D) Slowing effect on heart rate
1. A, B, and C
2. B, C, and D
3. A, C, and D
4. A, B, and D

15 An early symptom of digitalis intoxication is
1. Anorexia
2. Constipation
3. Tachycardia
4. Photophobia

16 A parenteral diuretic drug effective in right-sided heart failure is
1. Chlorpromazine
2. Diamox
3. Donnatal
4. Furosemide

17 Mr. Jenkins is placed on a 500 mg sodium diet. He should avoid
1. Pork and beans with franks
2. Fresh fruit, broiled chicken
3. Pickles, pork chops
4. Fish, pot roast

18 The nurse's major role in administering care to Mr. Jenkins is that of
1. Assessing his level of endurance
2. Conserving his energy and lessening the demands on his heart
3. Teaching him the low-sodium foods
4. Working quickly and quietly

19 An accurate picture of the effectiveness of diuretic therapy is best ascertained through
1. Daily weight measurement
2. Intake-output records every 8 hours
3. Testing for pedal edema daily
4. Type of diuretic administered

20 The electrolyte usually lost during diuretic and digitalis therapy is
1. Calcium
2. Chloride
3. Potassium
4. Sodium

21 Foods necessary for replacement of the electrolyte lost during diuretic therapy might include increased amounts of
1. Meat, dairy products, and eggs
2. Orange juice, bananas, and canteloupe
3. Apples, pears, and plums
4. Farina, rice, and tapioca

22 Cyanosis develops in heart failure as a direct result of
1. Arterial hypoxemia
2. Fluid in the pleura
3. Gas exchange impairment
4. Pulmonary edema

Situation: Mr. Allen, a 50-year-old advertising executive, experiences an acute myocardial infarction. He is unmarried and lives with and supports his mother and sister.

23 Precordial pain that promptly responds to nitroglycerin is diagnosed as
1. Angina pectoris
2. Coronary insufficiency
3. Coronary occlusion
4. Myocardial infarction

24 Serum enzyme elevations that are suggestive of myocardial infarction include
(A) APT
(B) PTT
(C) CPK
(D) LDH
1. B, C, and D
2. A, C, and D
3. A, B, and D
4. A, B, and C

25 The basic emotional reaction experienced by Mr. Allen is most likely to be
1. Anxiety
2. Depression
3. Fear
4. Hostility

26 The nurse should pay careful attention during the first 24 hours for increase in Mr. Allen's
1. Blood pressure
2. Pulse
3. Respirations
4. Temperature

27 During the first week of Mr. Allen's illness, the nurse should enforce bed rest to
1. Prevent arrhythmias
2. Arrest congestive heart failure
3. Prevent heart rupture
4. Promote healing of scar

28 Shock may occur during the early stages of infarction because of
1. Cardiac failure
2. Hypovolemia
3. Psychic trauma
4. Peripheral vasodilation

29 The most effective position for cardiogenic shock is
1. Fowler's
2. Orthopnea
3. Supine
4. Trendelenburg's

30 Perhaps the most potent of the vasopressors utilized in raising blood pressure is
1. Aramine
2. Ephedrine
3. Levophed
4. Wyamine

31 Rapid digitalization may be effected in Mr. Allen by the use of intravenous
1. Cedilanid
2. Digitoxin
3. Digoxin
4. Isuprel

32 Mr. Allen's anxiety might be allayed by
(A) Analgesia
(B) Psychotherapy
(C) Reassurance
(D) Sedation
1. A, B, and C
2. B, C, and D
3. A, C, and D
4. A, B, and D

33 To prevent thromboembolic phenomenon after infarction, the physician prescribes a long-term anticoagulant known as
1. Warfarin
2. Heparin
3. Protamine
4. Vitamin K

34 In heparin administration the nurse must avoid
1. Administration of steroids
2. Cleansing of injection site
3. Pinching and rubbing of the skin
4. Rapid administration of drug

35 Mr. Allen's mother should be told that for best recovery her son needs
1. Limited visitation
2. Frank discussion of problem
3. Freedom from worry
4. Restful environment

36 When Mr. Allen refused to use the bedpan, the physician ordered which of the following
1. Bathroom privileges
2. Bedside commode
3. Bedpan on toilet seat
4. Twice-daily, toilet privileges

37 Mr. Allen is experiencing nausea and vomiting. Appropriate action would be to
1. Order digitoxin level
2. Notify the physician
3. Place him on a bland diet
4. Notify the dietian

38 Miss Allen asked how long her brother would be hospitalized. The nurse replied
1. "As long as necessary for his heart to heal"
2. "It varies with the patient, it's hard to say"
3. "What has his doctor told you?"
4. "Until his ECG is normal"

39 Arrhythmias that develop suddenly in acute infarctions may result in
1. Death
2. Scarring
3. Shock
4. Tamponade

Situation: Mr. Paul Stein, a 45-year-old bachelor alcoholic, develops a cold that "hangs on" for weeks. The bed is usually wet from "night sweats," and a productive cough has been present for a few weeks. A Tuberculosis Society mobile unit x-ray examination was suggestive.

40 Tuberculosis is
1. Congenital
2. Infectious
3. Hereditary
4. Neoplastic

41 Dr. Mixon performed an intradermal test with PPD. A positive result is read in reference to
1. Areas of erythema
2. Areas of induration
3. Both erythema and induration
4. Number of red puncture marks

42 A positive tuberculin test indicates
1. Lung cancer
2. Cavitation
3. Nonactive disease
4. Presence of disease

43 Isolation precautions for the tuberculosis patient consist of
1. Confinement to sanitarium
2. Daily terminal disinfection
3. Mask, cap, gown, and shoe covering
4. Proper sputum disposal and handwashing

44 Mr. Stein's diet should consist of
(A) Milk
(B) Fruits
(C) Candies
(D) Meat, fish, and poultry
1. B, C, and D
2. A, C, and D
3. A, B, and D
4. A, B, C, and D

45 If chest tubes become dislodged the nurse's immediate action should be to
1. Cover incision with petroleum gauze
2. Cover incision with gauze pad
3. Cover incision with Telfa dressing
4. Cover incision with tape

46 The postoperative patient who exhibits pyrexia, purulent drainage, and congestion around the incision may be said to have
1. Exudation
2. Resolution
3. Postoperative infection
4. Rubor

47 The most widely used antituberculosis agents are
1. Cycloserine, Viomycin, INH
2. Isoniazid, PAS, and streptomycin
3. *p*-Aminosalicylic acid, INH, ASA
4. Streptomycin, PAS, and Mantoux

Situation: Mr. Bond had been experiencing dyspnea on exertion, cough, and cyanosis for several months. He developed signs of cor pulmonale and died 2 days later.

48 Pulmonary emphysema is a disease of the
1. Alveolar sacs
2. Bronchi
3. Pleural sac
4. Subcutaneous tissue

49 Observation of the pulmonary emphysematous patient for cor pulmonale reveals
1. Dyspnea, cyanosis
2. Lethary, bradycardia
3. Nystagmus, convulsion
4. Suppression, coughing

50 The respiratory center of the emphysematous patient is
1. Controlled by rate of respirations
2. Controlled by oxygen content of blood
3. Not as active in controlled respirations
4. Not functioning at all

51 Autopsies are beneficial because they
(A) Contribute to medical science
(B) Establish cause of death
(C) Promote the study of pathologic conditions
(D) Promote medical personnel's knowledge of physiology
1. A, B, and C
2. B, C, and D
3. A, C, and D
4. A, B, and D

Situation: Miss Pepin, 35 years old, has recently become the secretary of an industrial firm's president. She visits her physician complaining of burning stomach pain that is relieved by intake of food. She also has hunger pains at night that are relieved by food intake. She is tense and anxious over her new position. She is hospitalized on the weekend for "tests"; she fears cancer.

52 An ulcer is a(n)
1. Circumscribed lesion with loss of mucosal cover
2. Inflammatory tract leading from a suppurating cavity
3. Tract connecting two body cavities
4. Tumorlike mass on the mucosa

53 In caring for Miss Pepin the nurse would expect her to be
1. Courteous and friendly
2. Anxious and demanding
3. Quiet and depressed
4. Excessively cheerful

54 Most peptic ulcers are located in the
1. Pylorus
2. Greater curvature
3. Esophagus
4. Septum

55 Tests most likely to give a positive diagnosis in Miss Pepin's case are
1. Barium enema, upper GI series
2. Gastroscopy, barium enema
3. Graham-Cole test, barium swallow
4. Upper GI series, gastroscopy

56 Medications that allay production of gastric juices are
1. Cholinergics
2. Androgenics
3. Anticholinergics
4. Steroids

57 The purposes of the treatment of gastric ulcers are
(A) Allay anxiety
(B) Prevent complications
(C) Prevent recurrence
(D) Promote healing
1. A, B, and C
2. B, C, and D
3. A, C, and D
4. A, B, C, and D

58 After partaking of cocktails, Miss Pepin would experience
1. Dyspepsia
2. Cirrhosis of the liver
3. Gastritis
4. Pancreatitis

59 In the medical treatment of gastric ulcers, it is necessary to avoid
1. Lean meats
2. Potatoes
3. Fried chicken
4. Dairy products

60 Gastric resection is performed on ulcer patients who have
1. Pernicious anemia
2. Dumping syndrome
3. Perforation
4. Psychotic behavior

61 Gastric resections may result in the following sequelae
1. Diabetes insipidus
2. Dumping syndrome
3. Esophageal varices
4. Thrombocytopenia

Situation: Mrs. Strong, a 55-year-old woman with hypertension, is admitted with a diagnosis of cerebrovascular accident. Mr. Strong is a brewery worker; they have no children. She is comatose.

62 The comatose patient must be protected from which of the following?
1. Aspiration, myocardial infarction
2. Deformities, contractures
3. Atelectasis, decubti
4. Injury, convulsions

63 Mrs. Strong's eyes should be closed to prevent
1. Astigmatism
2. Corneal scarring
3. Conjunctivitis
4. Choroiditis

64 Gastric intubation may be for all of the following purposes
(A) Gastric decompression
(B) Gavaging foods
(C) Maintaining electrolytes
(D) Promoting oral hygiene
1. B, C, and D
2. A, C, and D
3. A, B, and D
4. A, B, and C

65 Suctioning should be done frequently on Mrs. Strong because
1. Aspiration of secretions may cause pneumonia
2. Food lodging in buccal cavity causes tooth decay
3. She may snore
4. Suctioning prevents stomatitis

66 An oxygen catheter should be changed at least every 8 hours and an alternate nostril used to prevent
1. Allergic reaction
2. Mucosal irritation
3. Deviated septum
4. Rhinophyma

67 Objects coming in contact with Mrs. Strong should be checked carefully for temperature extremes because of
1. Paralysis
2. Decreased superficial reflexes

3. Decreased deep reflexes
4. Loss of cutaneous sensations

68 Aphasia is a problem Mrs. Strong will have because of disturbances in the
1. Circle of Willis
2. Medulla
3. Speech areas
4. Cerebellum

69 The nurse should encourage Mr. Strong to
1. Do range of motion exercises for his wife
2. Limit her intake and output
3. Communicate with his wife using sign language
4. Visit only at visiting hours so he does not tire Mrs. Strong

70 The agency to assist in Mrs. Strong's rehabilitation at a nominal cost is the
1. NAA (Nurses Aide Association)
2. NLN (National League for Nurses)
3. VA (Veterans Administration)
4. VNA (Visiting Nurses Association)

71 A hot-water bottle burns Mrs. Strong on the ankle, causing a blister. The burn is of the
1. First degree
2. Second degree
3. Third degree
4. Fourth degree

72 Legally, Mrs. Strong might sue the nurse for
1. Damages
2. Expenses
3. Malpractice
4. Neglect

73 Laboratory reports indicate a blood glucose level of 240. The nurse recognizes this is
1. Normal
2. Decreased
3. Significantly elevated
4. Significantly decreased

74 The type of insulin administered in parenteral fluids for the acidotic patient is
1. Globin
2. NPH
3. Protamine zinc
4. Regular

75 Mrs. Strong should do the following daily while convalescing at home
(A) Ambulate
(B) Take automobile rides
(C) Remain confined to her wheelchair
(D) Perform exercises
1. A, B, and C
2. A, C, and D
3. A, B, and D
4. A and C

76 Patients diagnosed as having hearing impairment may refuse to wear hearing aids. The nurse should understand that
1. Hearing aids are too expensive to wear
2. Society will shun them for their disability
3. Patients may believe that wearing the aid would be admission of the disability
4. Application of the hearing aid demands manual dexterity

77 Symptoms associated with Meniere's disease will necessitate which of the following nursing actions?
1. Side rails, uncluttered environment
2. Strict aseptic technique while changing dressings
3. Caution to avoid nose blowing for at least 1 week
4. Changing nose packing frequently

78 The nurse should check carefully to make certain the eye drops administered to the glaucoma patient are
1. Mydriatics
2. Sterile
3. Miotics
4. Warmed before administration

79 Which of the following symptoms demonstrated by the throat surgery patient postoperatively would warrant an immediate call to the surgeon?
1. Frequent swallowing, hypotension
2. Hoarseness, thirst
3. Hematemesis of dark blood, drowsiness
4. Pain, hypertension

80 For the patient with otitis media, nursing care is centered on reducing the severity or alleviating the following problems
1. Dizziness and decreased hearing
2. Fever and tinnitus
3. Pain and pressure in the ear
4. Nausa and vomiting

81 Emergency treatment for epistaxis includes the following actions
(A) Have the patient sit with head tilted forward
(B) Perform antral irrigation with iced saline
(C) Pinch anterior nares until clotting occurs
(D) Instruct patient to breathe through mouth
1. A and C
2. A and D
3. A, C, and D
4. A, B, and D

82 When a patient describes a loss of vision in a specific area of the visual field (moving spots) and says he remembers seeing a "curtain fall" over his field of vision, you might expect this to be characteristic of
1. Glaucoma
2. Cataracts
3. Corneal abrasions
4. Detached retina

Situation: Mrs. Ford, 50 years of age, was seen in the gynecologic clinic. Cancer of the cervix was suspected.

83 The test most often used to aid in detecting cervical cancer is
1. Huhner test
2. Papanicolaou's test
3. Rubin's test
4. Schiller's test

84 The screening cancer detection test for the most common cancer in women is
1. Biopsy of cervical tissue
2. Dilation and curettage
3. Positive Kahn's test
4. Breast self-examination

85 The early symptoms that Mrs. Ford complained of probably were
1. Leukorrhea and/or vaginal bleeding
2. Sacral backache and lower abdominal pain
3. Dysuria and swelling of the labia
4. Enlargement of the abdomen

86 The test result was returned as "Suspicious of cancer." A test to confirm the diagnosis of cervical cancer is
1. Biopsy of the area
2. Smear or culture of the area or both
3. Schiller's test
4. Papanicolaou's stain

87 Mrs. Ford is now admitted for a radium implant procedure. The physician's written orders include which of the following?
(A) Cleansing enema
(B) Betadine vaginal irrigation
(C) Indwelling catheter
(D) Surgical abdominal preparation
1. B, C, and D
2. A, C, and D
3. A, B, and D
4. A, B, and C

88 Preoperatively Mrs. Ford should receive information in relation to her postoperative course to include which of the following?
(A) She will have a three-way Foley with a genitourinary irrigant
(B) She should breathe deeply to help prevent pneumonia
(C) She can have bathroom privileges with assistance
(D) She should tell her family to limit their visiting as long as the radium is in place
(E) The nurse should monitor her exposure in terms of time, distance, and shielding while the radium is in place
1. A, D, and C
2. A, B, and C
3. B and D
4. A, B, D, and E

89 A purulent discharge is an early symptom of gonorrhea. The causative organism is
1. *Neisseria* gonococcus
2. Welch's bacillus
3. *Treponema pallidum*
4. Ducrey's bacillus

90 The lesion seen on the patient with syphilis in the infectious stage is
1. Chancre
2. Chancroid
3. Condyloma
4. Gumma

91 The causative organism of syphilis is
1. Ducrey's bacillus
2. *Neisseria* gonococcus
3. *Treponema pallidum*
4. Welch's bacillus

92 The chief mode of transmission of the causative organism of syphilis is
1. Contaminated articles
2. Direct contact
3. Droplet infection
4. Fomites

93 Mrs. Ford has persistent blood pressure of 160/110. This blood pressure is considered to be
1. Hypotensive
2. Hypertensive
3. Normotensive
4. Antihypertensive

94 Nursing assessment of a patient with a blood pressure such as Mrs. Ford's would include
1. No special assessment since this is a normal blood pressure
2. Pulse evaluation, urine specific gravity, and work history
3. Level of consciousness, vision changes, and changes in sensation
4. Urine culture and sensitivity, presence of dysuria, and complaints of dizziness

Situation: Mrs. Andrews was admitted to the hospital for a complete urologic workup.

95 The excretory function of the kidneys can be determined by
(A) Urine culture
(B) Creatinine clearance
(C) Intravenous pyelogram
(D) KUB film
1. A and B
2. B and C
3. A and C
4. B and D

96 A cytoscopic examination was done on Mrs. Andrews on admission. When a cystoscopic examination is done, it is understood that
1. A roentgenogram is made of the abdomen so that the kidneys, ureters, and bladder are shown
2. The bladder is inspected by means of an electric-optic instrument
3. A dye is injected intravenously, and a study made of the function of the kidneys
4. A dye is injected through ureteral catheters, and a roentgenogram is made of the kidney pelves

97 The patient is scheduled for an intravenous pyelogram tomorrow morning. The instructions to be followed before the procedure is done include
(A) Eat anything but exclude fluids
(B) Drink large amounts of water
(C) Restrict food and water from midnight until after the procedure
(D) Give cleansing enemas until clear the night before
1. A and D
2. A and B
3. C and D
4. B and D

98 To prevent progression of kidney damage from acute glomerulonephritis the nurse should
(A) Maintain bed rest
(B) Monitor intake and output
(C) Weigh daily
(D) Force fluids to promote sodium absorption
1. A and C
2. B, C, and D
3. A, B, and C
4. A, B, and D

99 A common blood test is that is used in a urologic workup is the blood urea nitrogen (BUN) test. The normal level for this test is
1. 10 to 20 mg/100 ml of whole blood
2. 25 to 40 mg/100 ml of whole blood
3. 50 to 80 mg/100 ml of whole blood
4. 70 to 120 mg/100 ml of whole blood

Situation: Mr. Tate, 60 years of age, was admitted to the hospital. On completing the physical examination, the physician found that Mr. Tate has a markedly enlarged prostate gland. A tentative diagnosis of benign hypertrophy of the prostate was made.

100 Anatomically, the prostate
1. Lies in front of the bladder and behind the pubis
2. Surrounds the urethra as it emerges from the bladder
3. Lies in back of the bladder and in front of the rectum
4. Is bean shaped and composed of glandular tissue

101 The symptoms indicative of benign prostatic hypertrophy are
1. Frequency, hesitancy, straining, and hematuria
2. Nocturia, hesitancy, straining, and anuria
3. Frequency, pyuria, straining, and hematuria
4. Hesitancy, straining, suppression, and urgency

102 Cystitis is often a complication occurring with benign prostatic hypertrophy. Treatment of cystitis consists of
(A) Antibiotics
(B) Analgesics (Pyridium)
(C) Maintenance of acid urine
(D) Avoiding use of bubble bath and bath oils
(E) Restricting fluids
1. A, B, and D
2. B, C, and E
3. A, C, and E
4. A, B, C, and D

103 Diagnosis of prostatic hypertrophy is made by
(A) Digital rectal examination
(B) Kidney, ureter, and bladder x-ray (KUB) examination
(C) Cystoscopic examination
(D) Excretory urogram
(E) Catheterization for residual urine
1. A, B, and C
2. A, C, D, and E
3. A, C, D, and E
4. B, C, and E

104 Following a prostatectomy the nurse may help to promote wound healing by
(A) Reporting all bleeding to the physician
(B) Checking catheters for patency
(C) Milking catheter tubing to keep it patent
(D) Recording observations and amount of output from each catheter
1. A, B, C, and D
2. B, C, and D
3. B and D
4. A and D

105 The nurse may best help to reduce pain following a prostatectomy by
1. Assessing pain and administering antispasmodics for bladder spasms and analgesics for incisional pain
2. Assessing for bleeding, signs of infection, and hemorrhage and administering antibiotics as ordered
3. Reporting frank bleeding and following physician's orders for bladder irrigations
4. Assessing pain and administering narcotics as ordered

106 The most common complication occuring soon after a prostatectomy is
1. Bladder spasms
2. Hemorrhage
3. Dribbling of urine
4. Sterility

107 Complications following a prostatectomy may be prevented by
(A) Turning, coughing, and deep breathing every 2 hours
(B) Instructing patient in perineal exercises as ordered
(C) Administering stool softeners as ordered
(D) Taking temperatures rectally to facilitate mouth breathing
(E) Instructing patient to take oil retention enemas only to soften stools
1. A, C, and E
2. A, B, D, and E
3. A, B, C, and E
4. A, B, and C

108 Mr. Tate's discharge instructions from the nurse should include
(A) Refrain from straining and heavy lifting for at least 3 weeks
(B) Do not become constipated; use a mild laxative
(C) Drink at least 10 to 12 glasses of water (liquids) each day
(D) Watch for bleeding
1. A, B, and D
2. B, C, and D
3. A, C, and D
4. A, B, C, and D

109 Mr. Tate is to have a suprapubic prostatectomy. In this procedure the gland is approached through the
1. Bladder
2. Perineum
3. Urethra
4. Ureters

110 Nursing measures to prevent the formation of thrombophlebitis following surgery would include
1. Active and passive range of motion exercises for lower extremities and early ambulation
2. Massage of the gastrocnemius muscles at least every shift and early ambulation
3. Administering anticoagulants and encouraging sitting and dangling
4. Trendelenburg's position and Homan's sign

111 When checking the drainage from the urethral catheter, the nurse noticed that the drainage was bright red. The initial nursing action is to
1. Exert traction on the urethral catheter
2. Notify the surgeon immediately
3. Milk the drainage tube
4. Irrigate the catheter immediately with normal saline solution

---

Situation: William Carr awakened with a sharp pain in his loin. It was not like any other pain he had ever felt. The pain was not constant but seemed to radiate around the flank of the groin and into the testes. The remainder of the day William noticed that the pain would come and go, leaving a dull, aching pain on the opposite side. When he went to the bathroom, he noticed that his urine was slightly bloody. That evening William called the physician who sent him to the hospital. After a physical examination, the physician made a diagnosis of renal calculi.

112 Calculi of the renal system can be caused by
(A) Stasis of urine for a long period of time
(B) Excessive fluid in the kidneys
(C) Excessive intake of vitamin D
(D) Hyperparathyroidism
(E) Debilitating disease with decalcification of the bones (gout)
1. A, B, C, and D
2. B, C, D, and E
3. A, C, D, and E
4. A, B, C, and E

113 Two small calculi were found in the ureter, and the physician removed them. Mr. Carr had no further trouble and was allowed to go home shortly after the stones were removed and it was certain that he had no infection. Dismissal instructions would include
(A) Restricting fluids
(B) Encouraging him to take an increased amount of fluids
(C) Telling him to return to the physician for a follow-up visit
(D) Diet restrictions if necessary
1. A, C, and D
2. A, B, and E
3. B, C, and D
4. A, B, and C

114 Dietary treatment of renal calculi depends on the chemical composition of the stone. If the stone is the result of uric acid, a low-purine diet is given. The patient should avoid
1. Eggs
2. Greens
3. Liver
4. Milk

Situation: Mr. Robert Jacobs, 66 years of age, came to the hospital for treatment for malignant bladder tumor.

115 The most important single symptom of bladder tumor is
1. Urinary frequency with dysuria
2. Painless hematuria
3. Cystitis
4. Enlargement of the abdomen because of the size of the tumor

116 The usual treatment for a malignant renal tumor includes
(A) Surgical removal
(B) Radiation therapy
(C) Chemotherapy

(D) Administering Pyridium
(E) Straining all urine
1. A, B, and C
2. A, C, D, and E
3. A, C, and E
4. A, B, and E

117 Problems often seen with renal tumors include
(A) Pain
(B) Hematuria
(C) Polyuria
(D) Weight loss
(E) Polydipsia
1. A, B, and D
2. B, C, and D
3. B and D
4. B, C, D, and E

---

118 Renal failure is malfunctioning of the kidneys. Waste products not excreted include
1. Phosphorus, albumin, and sodium
2. Creatinine, urea, and potassium
3. Calcium, creatinine, and sodium
4. Potassium, albumin, and bilirubin

119 Problems often seen in the patient with renal failure include
1. Edema, hyperactivity, and hematuria
2. Convulsions, polyuria, and irritability
3. Edema, hypotension, and anemia
4. Hypertension, oliguria, and confusion

120 Treatment for renal failure includes
(A) Diet restrictions on sodium and protein
(B) Peritoneal dialysis
(C) Force fluids to 3000 ml daily NO
(D) Strong sedation to prevent convulsions
(E) Antimicrobials to prevent infection
1. A, B, and C
2. B, C, and D
3. A, B, C, and E wrong
4. A, B, and E

121 The patient with renal failure who is beginning hemodialysis will most likely
1. Be very cooperative and extremely grateful for this treatment
2. Be dependent on his or her family for all decision making
3. Express anger as his or her independence is lost
4. Reject any offers for emotional support at this time

122 A substance used for its analgesic and physiologic effects in patients who have cystitis is
1. Gantrisin
2. Mandelic acid
3. Pyridium
4. Urea

123 Pyridium changes the color of the urine. You would anticipate the color of the urine to be
1. Purple
2. Black
3. Red-orange
4. Robin's-egg blue

124 When caring for a patient with a Foley catheter, the nurse *should*
(A) Check for patency
(B) Check for kinks in tubing
(C) Collect a specimen of urine for culture from the end of the drainage tube
(D) Change the drainage bottle when necessary
1. A, B, and C
2. B, C, and D
3. A, B, and D
4. C and D

125 The diet for a patient with a fractured bone should be
1. High in carbohydrates and protein
2. High in protein and calcium
3. Low in protein and high in potassium
4. High in fats and minerals

126 The nurse should remember that the fractured part will be immobilized for a time, which can result in loss of muscle tone. Complications of loss of muscle tone are
(A) Muscle hypertrophy
(B) Atrophic muscles
(C) Hypoelastic muscles
(D) Contracted muscles
1. B, C, and D
2. A, B, and C
3. A, B, and D
4. A, C, and D

127 If the part was placed in traction, the nurse should know that the purposes of traction are to
(A) Relieve muscle spasm
(B) Alleviate pain
(C) Promote good body alignment
(D) Prevent rotation
1. B, C, and D
2. A, C, and D
3. A, B, and D
4. A, B, C, and D

128 Skin traction may be applied by
1. Insertion of a Steinmann pin
2. Tape, moleskin, and foam boots with strap attachments
3. Insertion of a Kirschner wire through the end of the bone
4. Crutchfield tongs

129 After a cast has been applied, the nurse should suspect circulatory impairment if the patient complains of
1. Stiffness of the digits
2. Itching of the part
3. Numbness or tingling of the digits or both
4. Excessive sweating under the cast

130 When a patient complains of intense pain while in a cast, the nurse should
1. Explain that this will gradually leave
2. Report it to the physician at once
3. Support the extremity on a pillow
4. Apply an ice bag

131 Signs of arterial impairment are
1. Cold, pallor, numbness, and swelling
2. Blotchiness, petechiae, and tingling
3. Swelling, pain, and tiny water blisters under the cast

132 Following an amputation, which of the following should be at the bedside?
1. Tourniquet
2. Mayo stand
3. Kirschner wire
4. Stockinette

133 Heat therapy can
1. Lessen the possibility of contractures
2. Increase circulation of the affected part
3. Prevent the recurrence of such conditions as arthritis
4. Increase the muscle tone of the part

134 Diagnosis of a fracture is confirmed by
1. X-ray examination
2. Endoscopic examination
3. Serum calcium
4. Schilling test

135 Daily assessment of a fracture patient should include
(A) Smelling the cast
(B) Petaling
(C) Blanching
(D) Temperature
1. B, C, and D
2. A, B, and C
3. A, C, and D
4. A, B, C, and D

136 Exercises to prepare for crutch walking should include
(A) Sit-ups
(B) Push-ups
(C) Straight leg raises
(D) Quadriceps setting
1. A and C
2. B, C, and D
3. A, B, and C
4. A, B, C, and D

Situation: Mrs. Dent, 72 years of age, was admitted with a left intratrochanteric fracture.

137 The symptoms associated with this type of fracture would probably be
1. Shock, pain, and adduction with hip and knee flexion
2. Pain, external rotation, and lengthening of the extremity
3. Pain, external rotation, and shortening of the extremity
4. Shock, internal rotation, and shortening of the extremity

138 Mrs. Dent was put in Buck's traction as a temporary, conservative treatment. The principles of traction include
(A) Must be secure
(B) Must be continuous
(C) Should be applied by a physician
(D) May be released carefully for the patient to have x-ray examination
(E) Must be applied in a straight line
1. B and C
2. A, B, and E
3. A, B, and C
4. A, B, C, and D

139 After a few days Mrs. Dent was taken to surgery, where an internal fixation was done. The advantages of this type of reduction are that it
(A) Permits early ambulation
(B) Lessens danger of nonunion
(C) Decreases danger of hemorrhage
(D) Prevents flexion or contracture of the hip
1. A and B
2. B, C, and D
3. A, B, and D
4. A, B, C, and D

140 The postoperative total hip replacement must maintain abduction of the joint. This is accomplished by
1. Logrolling to the affected side
2. Pillow to keep legs separated
3. Keeping the head of the bed at a 45-degree angle
4. Ambulating the patient the first postoperative day

141 Aseptic necrosis is a complication, especially when the fracture site is in or near the end of the bone. Aseptic necrosis is caused by
1. Wound infection
2. Loss of blood supply to the head of the bone
3. Weight bearing or using of the part before the fracture is properly healed
4. Improper reduction of the bone

---

142 Information necessary for a complete pain assessment would include
1. Precipitating event, description, and location
2. Medication preference and location
3. Emotional state of patient and nutritional needs
4. Time since last injection and physician's order

143 Streptomycin is used in the treatment of infections. The nurse should be observant for
1. Agranulocytosis
2. Edema, especially of the face
3. Impairment of hearing and equilibrium
4. Oliguria

144 Acetylsalicylic acid is frequently used on the orthopedic service. Some of its purposes are
(A) To keep the patient from going into alkalosis
(B) To relieve mild to moderate pain
(C) The treatment of arthritis
(D) Antipyretic action
1. A and C
2. B and C
3. B, C, and D
4. A, B, C, and D

145 Some of the signs of acetylsalicylic acid poisoning may be
(A) Nausea and vomiting
(B) Edema
(C) Tinnitus
(D) Severe headache
1. A and C
2. B and C
3. A, C, and D
4. A, B, C, and D

Situation: Mrs. Brown complains of loss of hearing. Her physician used a device to determine her hearing acuity.

146 This device is called a(n)
1. Audiograph
2. Audiometer
3. Tuning fork
4. Audioscreen

147 If Mrs. Brown's deafness is sensorineural, it is probably true that
1. Her voice is very loud and she hears poorly over the phone; she would benefit from a hearing aid, but surgery offers little hope
2. Her voice is soft and she hears well over the phone; she would not benefit from a hearing aid, but surgery offers hope
3. She hears poorly over the phone and her voice is very loud; she would benefit very little from a hearing aid, and surgery offers little hope
4. She hears well over the phone and her voice is soft; she could benefit from a hearing aid, and surgery offers hope for better hearing

148 If Mrs. Brown's deafness is of the conduction type, then
1. Her voice is very loud and she hears poorly over the phone; she would benefit from a hearing aid, and surgery offers her little hope for better hearing.
2. Her voice is soft and she hears well over the phone; she would not benefit by a hearing aid, but surgery offers hope
3. She hears poorly over the phone and her voice is very loud; she would benefit very little from a hearing aid, and surgery offers little hope
4. She hears well over the phone and her voice is soft; she would benefit from a hearing aid, and surgery offers hope

Situation: Mr. Burch, 65 years of age, came to the clinic complaining of persistent hoarseness but no particular discomfort. He was told to rest his voice for a week and return for a laryngoscopic examination.

149 The function of the larynx is to
(A) Help produce speech
(B) Protect the lower respiratory tract from food and foreign bodies
(C) Help propel food into the esophagus
(D) Aid in the cough reflex
(E) Aid in respiration
1. A, and D
2. A, D, and E
3. A, C, D, and E
4. A, B, C, D, and E

150 After the examination and biopsy of the larynx, the physician made the diagnosis of cancer and recommended total laryngectomy. This procedure will consist of
1. Splitting the larynx and removing the vocal cords
2. Removing the laryngeal cartilages and inserting a tube into the trachea
3. Removing the vocal cords and inserting a tube into the larynx
4. Removing the laryngeal cartilages and making a connection with the trachea and pharynx

151 In preparing Mr. Burch psychologically for postoperative adjustment, the nurse would inform him that he will
1. Have to rest his voice as much as possible and will be fed through a tube instead of eating
2. Have to learn to suction the mucus from his throat with a rubber tube when he needs to cough
3. Be on a liquid diet and must use some other means of communication until he recovers his voice
4. Breathe through a metal tube at the base of his neck instead of through his nose and mouth

152 Following surgery, to keep Mr. Burch's airway patent, it is necessary to suction the trachea
1. Every hour for the first 2 days, and then every 4 hours
2. Whenever there is drainage in the tube or trachea
3. Before each meal, midmorning, and afternoon
4. Whenever he complains of difficulty in breathing

153 Humidified oxygen is administered via tracheostomy after a laryngectomy because
1. Humidified oxygen contains more water
2. The upper airway is no longer connected to the lower airway
3. The lower airway heals more quickly if humidity is utilized
4. Humidified oxygen administration facilitates suctioning

154 Initial symptoms of hypoxia are
1. Tachycardia and restlessness
2. Bradycardia and hypertension
3. Irritability and hyperactivity
4. Hypotension and edema

155 The purpose of steam inhalation is to
1. Produce thicker secretions, which may be expectorated more easily
2. Increase the oxygen content coming in contact with the mucous membranes
3. Increase the evaporation of water from the mucous membranes
4. Prevent drying of the trachea or tracheitis

156 Mr. Burch's tube-feeding solution is kept on the ward in the refrigerator. Before giving the feeding, the nurse should
1. Add half as much water as the quantity of feeding
2. Bring the feeding to a boil in order to eliminate any contamination
3. Heat the feeding to room temperature in order to make it more digestible
4. Serve the mixture as it comes from the refrigerator in order to make it more palatable

157 Demerol instead of morphine was given to Mr. Burch postoperatively because morphine
1. Would make him relax and forget that suctioning is necessary
2. Depresses the action of the ciliated epithelium
3. Dulls the cough reflex
4. Reduces the respiratory rate

158 The chief methods by which one can learn to speak after a laryngectomy are
(A) Laryngeal whisper
(B) Esophageal speech
(C) Electric larynx
(D) Artificial respiration
1. A and B
2. B and C
3. A, C, and D
4. A, B, C, and D

Situation: Mrs. Bens, a 49-year-old homemaker who is a known diabetic, was referred to the eye specialist by her family physician for evaluation. For about a month she had been having pain in her eyes and blurred vision, and she had been seeing colored rings when she looked at lights. The ophthalmologist's diagnosis was acute primary glaucoma.

159 The symptoms of acute glaucoma may include all of the following *except*
1. Blurred vision
2. Early loss of central vision
3. Inability to see well at night
4. Pain in the eyes

160 An eye medication definitely contraindicated in glaucoma is
1. Epinephrine
2. Eserine
3. Homatropine
4. Pontocaine

161 If glaucoma is untreated, the end result is
1. Aphakia
2. Astigmatism
3. Blindness
4. Uveitis

162 The normal intraocular pressure is
1. Approximately 20 mm of mercury
2. Approximately 25 mm of water
3. Approximately 35 mm of mercury
4. Approximately 35 mm of water

163 Intraocular pressure is measured with an instrument called a(n)
1. Oculometer
2. Perimeter
3. Tonometer
4. Tontamone

164 To relieve Mrs. Bens's increased intraocular pressure, the physician ordered pilocarpine eye instillations. Pilocarpine is classified as a(n)
1. Analgesic
2. Cyclopegic
3. Miotic
4. Mydriatic

165 Pilocarpine is valuable in the treatment of glaucoma because it
1. Constricts the pupil and draws the iris away from the cornea
2. Dilates the pupil and draws the iris away from the cornea
3. Constricts the pupil and allows the iris to adhere to the cornea
4. Dilates the pupil and allows the iris to adhere to the cornea

166 Treatment of acute glaucoma may include all of the following *except*
1. Correcting glasses
2. Cyclodialysis
3. Iridectomy, if performed early
4. Miotics locally

167 Absolute glaucoma is the condition that results in
1. Detachment of the retina
2. Hypertrophy of the conjunctiva
3. Severe pain and loss of vision
4. Temporary loss of vision

168 The most frequent operative procedure for glaucoma is
1. Cyclodialysis
2. Enucleation
3. Iridectomy
4. Trephining

Situation: Mrs. Palmer was admitted to the neurology department with a diagnosis of possible brain tumor.

169 In the early stages a tumor in the frontal cerebral area may cause which of the following symptoms?
1. Blurred vision, headache, and paralysis
2. Headache and paralysis
3. Blurred vision and headache
4. Personality changes and paralysis

170 Mrs. Palmer is scheduled for pneumoencephalography. This procedure, done in the x-ray department, consists of an injection of
1. Air directly into the ventricles
2. A dye into the lumbar subarachnoid space
3. A radioactive substance intravenously
4. Air into the lumbar subarachnoid space

171 After this procedure, Mrs. Palmer may be expected to
(A) Experience a headache
(B) Be unconscious
(C) Need the bed slightly elevated
(D) Require an analgesic
(E) Have to lie flat
1. B and C
2. A, C, and E
3. A, D, and E
4. C and D

172 Mrs. Palmer developed a constant headache, widening of pulse pressure, and projectile vomiting without nausea. This is a sign of
1. Brain tumor
2. Cerebrovascular accident
3. Increased hemorrhage
4. Increased intracranial pressure

173 A craniotomy is to be performed on Mrs. Palmer. It will be done under hypothermia because it minimizes
1. Bleeding
2. Blood pressure
3. Body temperature
4. Headache

174 Postoperatively, Mrs. Palmer's position in bed will be
1. Elevated 45 degrees, head turned toward operative site
2. Elevated 30 degrees, head turned away from operative site
3. Flat, head turned toward operative site
4. Flat, head turned away from operative site

175 Drugs used postoperatively to reduce cerebral edema are
1. Dilatin and phenobarbital
2. Decadron and Osmitrol
3. Dilaudid and 50% dextrose
4. Atropine and urea

176 In observing Mrs. Palmer for hemorrhage, the practical nurse should watch especially for
1. Dyspnea
2. High blood pressure
3. Restlessness
4. Slowed pulse

177 A description of normal pupil activity might include
(A) Equal
(B) Dilated
(C) Fixed
(D) Reactive to light
1. A and D
2. A, B, and D
3. A, B, and C
4. A, C, and D

178 If Mrs. Palmer develops a brain abscess, *early* symptoms may include
(A) Anorexia
(B) Fever
(C) Malaise
(D) Opisthotonos
1. A, B, and D
2. A, B, and C
3. B, C, and D
4. None of these

Questions 179 through 191 are concerned with drugs that affect the nervous system and the anatomy and physiology of the nervous system.

179 A drug that mimics the action of the parasympathetic nervous system is
1. Adrenergic
2. Anticholinergic
3. Cholinergic
4. Cholinergic-blocking

180 An example of a central nervous system stimulant is
1. Atabrine
2. Coramine
3. Dilaudid
4. Pentobarbital

181 A drug used to combat drowsiness and apathy that may accompany barbiturate therapy is
1. Decadron
2. Coriden
3. Ritalin
4. Valium

182 An example of a synthetic narcotic includes all the following *except*
1. Dilaudid
2. Leritine
3. Morphone
4. Talwin

183 The toxic dose of morphine for an adult is
1. gr 1/4
2. gr 1/6
3. 30 mg
4. 60 mg

184 A drug order states, "Morphine sulfate, gr 1/4 IM stat," and the label reads, 15 mg/ml (cc). The nurse therefore gives
1. 1 ml (cc)
2. 1.5 ml (cc)
3. 2 ml (cc)
4. 4 ml (cc)

185 A drug order states "Nembutal, gr 3 h.s.," and the nurse has on hand 100 mg capsules. The nurse gives
1. 1/2 capsule
2. 1 capsule
3. 2 capsules
4. 3 capsules

186 The brain receives its blood supply by way of the
(A) Carotids
(B) Vertebrals
(C) Jugulars
(D) Subclavians
(E) Superior vena cava
1. B and D
2. A and B
3. D and E
4. A and C

187 The sympathetic nerves are concerned with the
1. Cranial nerves
2. Craniosacral nerves
3. Cerebellar nerves
4. Thoracolumbar areas

188 The chief function of the cerebellum is
1. Equilibrium
2. Conscious thought
3. Hearing
4. Sight

189 The large space below the medulla in which cerebrospinal fluid circulates is the
1. Cisterna magna
2. Foramen magnum
3. Foramen ovale
4. Submedulla

190 Cerebrospinal fluid has its origin in the
1. Aqueduct of Sylvius
2. Lateral ventricles
3. Choroid plexus of the third ventricle
4. Choroid plexuses of all the ventricles

191 Sedatives and strong narcotics are not frequently administered to patients with increased intracranial pressure because they
(A) Decrease level of consciousness
(B) Depress respiration
(C) Stimulate the sympathetic nervous system
(D) Mask neurologic signs and symptoms
1. C and D
2. A, B, and C
3. A, B, and D
4. A and B

---

192 The chief characteristic of herpes zoster is
1. Erythema along a nerve root
2. Painful vesicles along a nerve root
3. Paresthesia along sciatic nerve
4. Vesicles along a nerve root with no pain

193 Guillain-Barré syndrome is an infectious type of polyneuritis that primarily affects
1. Cranial or peripheral nerve roots or both
2. The cerebral meninges
3. The spinal cord
4. Peripheral nerves only

194 The nursing care plan for a patient with a diagnosis of Guillain-Barré syndrome will be similar to that used for
(A) Alcoholic in delirium tremens
(B) Serious head injury
(C) Paraplegics
(D) Cervical fractures
(E) Comatose patients
1. A
2. B, D, and E
3. E
4. C and D

195 It is suspected that a patient has meningococcal meningitis and should therefore be isolated
1. For his entire hospitalization
2. For the first 48 hours
3. Until his cultures are negative
4. For 24 hours after initiating antibiotic therapy

196 If a cerebrospinal fluid specimen is obtained from a meningitis patient it will characteristically appear
1. Bloody
2. Clear
3. Milky
4. Yellow

Situation: Mr. Drake displays the following symptoms: tremors; slow, monotonous speech; dysphagia; drooling; emotional lability; masklike face; and shuffling gait with trunk forward.

197 The symptoms Mr. Drake displays indicate
1. Multiple sclerosis
2. Myasthenia gravis
3. Parkinson's disease
4. Sydenham's chorea

198 The drugs used to alleviate Mr. Drake's symptoms are
1. ACTH and papaverine
2. Artane and Cogentin
3. Librium and Norflex
4. Prostigmin and Tensilon

199 Early symptoms of multiple sclerosis include
(A) Paralysis and excessive crying
(B) Blurred vision
(C) Paresthesia
(D) Transient muscle weakness
1. A and B
2. A, B, and C
3. C and D
4. B, C, and D

200 A lumbar puncture is done in order to obtain cerebrospinal fluid to
(A) Culture
(B) Obtain protein and white blood cell count
(C) Perform the Kahan test
(D) View under darkfield illumination
1. A
2. C and D
3. A and B
4. A, B, and D

201 The type of neurosyphilis that affects chiefly the cerebral cortex is
1. General paresis
2. Primary lues
3. Tabes dorsalis
4. Tertiary lues

202 When an individual is allergic to penicillin, the drug of choice used to reat syphilis is
1. Tetracycline
2. Atabrine
3. Streptomycin
4. Sulfadiazine

203 Emergency nursing care of the patient suspected of a spinal cord injury will be to
(A) Place in semi-Fowler's position to stabilize the vertebral column
(B) Keep flat with head and neck stabilized
(C) Logroll onto a stretcher for transport
(D) Place in orthopneic position to facilitate respiration
1. A and C
2. B and C
3. B and D
4. C and D

Situation: Mr. Green received third-degree burns in an attempt to rescue his father from their burning home. Mr. Green has burns covering the left arm, anterior chest, and face.

204 A third-degree burn means that
1. The skin and deeper tissues have been destroyed
2. The deepest third of the dermal tissues have been destroyed
3. The burn is less severe than a first-degree burn
4. The first layer has been destroyed

205 The use of any type of grease or oil on a third-degree burn is
1. Desirable because it prevents air from contacting tissues
2. Undesirable because it has to be removed later when the wound is cleaned
3. Questionable because some cases are helped while others are not
4. Desirable because it is a first-aid treatment

206 The best emergency measure in a third-degree burn is
1. To leave clothing in place and cover with a warm, wet, blanket
2. To leave clothing in place and cover burned area with a clean cloth
3. To strip charred clothing and flush with water
4. Keep it dry and open to air

207 Because Mr. Green was unable to save his father, he did not care whether he lived or died. Such an attitude
1. Cannot be changed and should be accepted
2. Will not affect the regeneration of tissues or his recovery
3. Will definitely hinder his recovery
4. Will aid the tissues in healing as anxiety is no longer a problem

208 If Mr. Green is conscious, the best kind of fluid to give him as an emergency treatment, and thereafter, is
1. Hot tea or coffee
2. Lactated Ringer's solution
3. Salt and soda-bicarbonate solution
4. Milk or high-protein milk

209 Closed dressings are applied to burned areas because they
1. Can absorb large quantities of fluids
2. Are the most comfortable
3. Help prevent fluid loss
4. Will immobilize the part

210 The skin for grafting was taken from Mr. Green's thigh. This is known as a(n)
1. Autograft
2. Heterograft
3. Homograft
4. Isograft

211 To promote postburn hydration and kidney function, the nurse should
1. Keep accurate intake and output, weight daily, and maintain IV fluids
2. Reverse isolation and measure urine specific gravity
3. Reposition frequently and administer analgesics
4. Note depth of respirations and measure intake and output accurately

212 The quantity of fluid needed by Mr. Green to replace his loss or expected loss should be given
1. Within 12 hours
2. Within 24 hours
3. Within 36 hours
4. Within 48 hours

213 Mr. Green's urinary output is measured hourly and should stay
1. Between 10 to 20 ml per hour
2. Between 30 to 50 ml per hour
3. Between 50 to 60 ml per hour
4. Between 60 to 100 ml per hour

---

214 Mrs. Post, who is admitted for treatment of breast cancer, knows that all of the following are true *except*
1. Incidence is highest after menopause
2. It seems to run in families
3. Injury to the breast leads to malignancy
4. It is more frequent in women whose mothers had it

215 Conclusive diagnosis is made in malignancy of the breast by
1. Feeling of lumps on physical examination
2. Biopsy and microscopic examination
3. X-ray examination, primarily mammography
4. Discharge from nipples and thermography

216 Important points to remember to stress in instructing a radical mastectomy patient before discharge are
1. Frequent changing of dressings and good nutrition
2. Promotion of rest
3. Prevention of infection and phlebitis
4. Teaching of good posture and prescribed exercise

217 Mrs. Post developed considerable edema of the left arm. The treatment that will give her relief is
1. Elevation of affected hand and arm and elastic sleeve
2. Use of a hot-water bottle and elevation
3. Massage of hand and arm with cocoa butter
4. Use of an ice bag and elastic sleeve

218 Self-examination of the breast should be done
(A) Monthly, following menstruation
(B) Monthly, preceding menstruation
(C) In all women
(D) Only at the time of medical examination
1. A and C
2. C and D
3. B and C
4. A, C, and D

219 Which of the following is not relevant to Mrs. Post's exercises?
1. The exercises should not be accompanied by a lot of pain
2. Exercises are done daily, with household and personal activities in mind
3. They are done only 2 weeks after surgery
4. They are done to protect muscle tone and prevent contractures

220 The hormone believed necessary for the growth of malignant cells of the breast is
1. Adrenalin
2. Estrogen
3. Testosterone
4. Thyroxine

221 The hormone for palliative therapy in terminal carcinoma of the breast in premenopausal women is
1. Adrenalin
2. Estrogen
3. Testosterone
4. Thyroxine

---

222 Diabetes mellitus is an endocrine disease characterized by which of these?
(A) The body's inability to metabolize carbohydrates normally
(B) Failure of the islands of Langerhans of the pancreas to produce adequate insulin
(C) Improper utilization of protein and fats
(D) Reduction of secretion of antidiuretic hormone by the pituitary
1. A
2. B and C
3. A, C, and D
4. A, B, and C

223 Diabetes is inherited as a mendelian recessive characteristic. The disease does not necessarily manifest itself early in life. Which of the following are correct?
(A) If both parents have diabetes, all the children may have diabetes if they live long enough
(B) If one parent has diabetes and the other is a carrier of the gene, the chance of their children developing diabetes is 50%
(C) If both parents are carriers, the chance of their children developing diabetes is 25%
(D) If both parents are carriers, their children have a less than 5% chance of developing diabetes
1. A, C, and D
2. A and B
3. A, B, and D
4. A, B, and C

224 Diabetes mellitus is increasing in incidence. This is often attributed to
(A) Exposure to harmful chemicals
(B) Changes in family unit
(C) Better diagnostic means
(D) Changes in cultural patterns
(E) Longer life-span
1. A and B
2. C and D
3. B and E
4. C and E

225 The most difficult age group in which to control diabetes is
1. Children 4 to 9 years of age
2. Young adults
3. Adolescents
4. Adults over 70 years of age

226 Diabetic coma may be caused by
1. Overdose of insulin
2. Increase of sugar in urine
3. Omission of prescribed insulin dose
4. Increase in physical activity

227 Symptoms that may be experienced by patients in diabetic coma are
1. Sweating, hunger, and trembling
2. Pallor, headache, and weakness
3. Slow pulse and difficulty in breathing
4. Hot dry skin, nausea, vomiting, and drowsiness

228 The treatment of diabetic coma by the physician may be to
1. Administer insulin and intravenous fluids (normal saline)
2. Order a high-protein diet and replace lost sugar
3. Place the patient in an oxygen tent, and administer D_5W intravenously
4. Administer dextrose and force fluids

229 Sugar and acetone (S & A) or clinitest and acetone urine specimens are collected to determine the
1. Amount of albumin in the urine
2. Time of day the retention of sugar is heaviest
3. Amount of insulin in the body
4. Time of day the excretion of sugar is heaviest

230 When interpreting the results of the Tes-Tape on urine, orange indicates
1. 1+ sugar
2. 2+ sugar
3. 3+ sugar
4. 4+ sugar

231 When using Clinitest to test for urine sugar, the nurse will use a
1. Capsule
2. Piece of tape
3. Piece of paper
4. Tablet

232 NPH insulin is best administered
1. Before dinner
2. Whenever the patient needs it
3. Before breakfast
4. After breakfast

233 Tolbutamide, commonly referred to by the trade name Orinase, is a sulfonamide derivative that is most often used to treat
1. Severe juvenile diabetes
2. Diabetic coma
3. Middle-aged and older persons whose blood glucose fluctuates widely
4. Older persons who have failing islands of Langerhans

234 Diabetes is a chronic disease; the patient needs careful instruction before leaving the hospital. The most important is
1. Take insulin as prescribed
2. Instruction in removing hangnails and corns
3. Carrying an identification card stating that he or she has diabetes
4. Special care of the feet

235 The carbohydrate in a diet for a diabetic patient is distributed primarily on the basis of
1. Height, weight, age, sex, and activity of the patient
2. Severity of the disease
3. Kind of insulin given and nutritional needs
4. Weight and prognosis

236 A diabetic patient may have ice cream if he knows how to work it into his diet plan. One-half cup of ice cream is equal to
1. One bread exchange
2. One milk exchange
3. One bread exchange plus two fat exchanges
4. One milk exchange plus two fat exchanges

237 The thyroid hormone affects all of the following *except*
1. Water and electrolyte metabolism
2. Proper growth
3. Reproduction
4. Visual acuity

238 A protein-bound iodine test is ordered to determine the
1. Degree of activity of the thyroid gland
2. Amount of iodine in the thyroid gland
3. Concentration of thyroxin in the bloodstream
4. Amount of cholesterol in the bloodstream

239 An overactive thyroid is the result of
1. An inability to cope with difficult problems and face reality
2. An inadequate intake of iodine
3. An excessive amount of thyroxin
4. A diet deficient in vitamins

240 Lugol's solution is used to
1. Prevent the decrease of basal metabolism and induce weight control
2. Reduce exophthalmos and decrease overactivity
3. Decrease glandular hyperplasia and basal metabolism
4. Cause an increase in clotting time

241 Lugol's solution is administered in fruit juice or milk and taken through a straw to
(A) Disguise its taste
(B) Provide additional nourishment
(C) Prevent infiltration of the gastric mucosa
(D) Prevent the reaction of iodine on teeth
1. A and D
2. A, B, and C
3. B, C, and D
4. A

242 Aphonia would lead one to suspect
1. Hemorrhage
2. Hysteria
3. Injury to the esophagus
4. Injury to the recurrent laryngeal nerve endings

243 Tetany, postoperatively, may be caused by
1. Invasion by the bacillus tetani
2. An increase in the amount of calcium in the blood
3. A decrease of phosphorus in the blood
4. A decrease in the amount of calcium in the bloodstream

244 Neomycin is used in preparation for intestinal surgery because
1. It is readily absorbed by the gastrointestinal tract
2. It is poorly absorbed by the gastrointestinal tract
3. It does not destroy beneficial bacteria in the gastrointestinal tract
4. It is nontoxic to most persons

245 Peptic ulcer patients are treated with antacid therapy. Which of the following are complications of such therapy?
1. Constipation with fecal impaction and acidosis
2. Acidosis and anemia
3. Alkalosis and kidney stones
4. Ureteral calculi and diarrhea

246 Diagnostic tests for carcinoma of the stomach include
(A) Gastrointestinal series
(B) Gastroscopic examination
(C) Cytologic examination
(D) Gastric vagotomy
1. A, B, and D
2. B and D
3. B
4. A, B, and C

247 Mechanical obstructions of the intestines are caused by
(A) Strangulated hernias
(B) Volvulus
(C) Intussusception
(D) Paralytic ileus
1. A
2. C
3. A, B, and C
4. B, C, and D

248 Neurogenic obstructions of the intestines are caused by
(A) Manipulation of the bowels during surgery
(B) Spinal anesthesia
(C) Spinal cord lesions
(D) Volvulus
1. A, B, and D
2. B and C
3. A, C, and D
4. A, B, and C

249 Decompression of the small intestines is accomplished by continuous aspiration of contents by a tube. The tube most often used is the
1. Miller-Abbott
2. Levin
3. Rehfuss'
4. Sengstaken-Blakemore

250 Mr. Thom has been receiving anticoagulant therapy. He has just had an emergency appendectomy. Postoperatively the nurse would use which of the following special precautions?
1. Soft bristle toothbrush, electric razor, and small-gauge needles
2. Antiemetic, narcotics for pain, and early ambulation
3. Uncluttered environment and antiembolism stockings
4. Oral medications only and Hematest on urine daily

251 In ruptured acute appendicitis the chief complication is
1. Intestinal obstruction
2. Ileitis
3. Colitis
4. Peritonitis

252 An early symptom of carcinoma of the sigmoid colon is
1. Change in bowel habits
2. Rectal bleeding
3. Abdominal distention
4. Fecal vomiting

253 The patient with ulcerative colitis is sometimes described as an individual who is
1. Euphoric
2. Independent
3. "High strung"
4. Placid

254 Nursing care of patients with ulcerative colitis includes which of the following?
(A) Supportive care, both mental and physical
(B) Keeping the skin surface around ileostomy clean and dry

(C) As patients improve, giving them restful recreation and mental diversion
(D) Keeping patients in quiet area alone so that they work out their problems
1. A and C
2. B and D
3. C and D
4. A, B, and C

255 One of the early symptoms of carcinoma of the rectum is
1. Tarry stools
2. Bright red blood in stools
3. Vomiting
4. Pain

256 Hemorrhoids are caused by which of the following?
1. Straining at stool and heavy lifting
2. Occupations requiring prolonged upright positions and rectal trauma
3. Pregnancy and infections
4. Straining at stool and pregnancy

257 The operation of choice for patients with cancer of the rectum is most often
1. Permanent colostomy
2. Gastroenterostomy
3. Abdominoperineal resection
4. Perineal colostomy

258 A patient with peritonitis is placed in low Fowler's position because it
1. Localizes the pain in the lower abdomen
2. Helps localize the infection
3. Facilitates breathing postoperatively
4. Eases the strain on the suture line

259 Nursing care of a colostomy includes which of the following?
(A) Daily cleansing routine
(B) Encouragement of patient to care for own colostomy
(C) Limitation of the intake of fluids
(D) Irrigation of the colostomy at the same time daily if ordered
1. B and D
2. A, B, and C
3. A and D
4. A, B, and D

260 If a patient complains of pain during a colostomy irrigation, the nurse should
1. Lower the irrigating can
2. Discontinue the irrigation
3. Clamp the catheter for a few minutes
4. Insert the catheter about 1 inch more

261 One of the accepted factors associated with peptic ulcers is the
1. Age of the patient
2. Eating habits of the patient
3. Emotional makeup of the patient
4. Cultural background of the patient

262 The most important aspect of the dietary treatment for peptic ulcer is giving
1. Many protein foods in order to buffer the acids in the stomach
2. Plenty of fats to slow down the secretion of the acids into the stomach
3. Frequent feedings so that there is always something in the stomach
4. Only soft-cooked foods so that the foods do not irritate the stomach

263 After a cholecystectomy, bile drainage from the T tube is most often
1. Measured and discarded
2. Mixed with food and administered to the patient
3. Administered to the patient through a stomach tube
4. Sent to the laboratory for analysis

264 A common discomfort in patients with jaundice is
1. Dermatitis
2. Excessive thirst
3. Pruritus
4. Petechiae

265 Cirrhosis of the liver is commonly associated with
1. Excessive drinking of alcohol
2. Faulty utilization of bile salts
3. Infection and jaundice
4. Malnutrition and alcoholism

266 The patient with cirrhosis of the liver is given a diet high in calories and protein. The principal purpose of the protein foods in this case is to
1. Provide calories in the diet in a very well-tolerated form
2. Provide an excellent source of vitamins and minerals, especially vitamins A and D, which are necessary for repair of the liver tissue
3. Provide the elements for the repair of the hepatic cells and the formation of bile salts
4. Provide a more concentrated source of calories, since these patients often have no desire to eat

267 When there is danger of hepatic coma, the protein content of the patient's diet is drastically reduced to no protein from 30 g of protein. This step is taken because
1. The liver is so damaged that it cannot digest protein, and thus any amount of protein taken will just be wasted
2. The liver is so damaged that it can no longer handle the products of deaminization of proteins, and thus ammonia enters the bloodstream and affects the central nervous system
3. The liver can no longer convert the proteins to body proteins to be used for growth and repair
4. The liver can no longer take care of the end products of protein metabolism, and thus the bile salts enter the bloodstream, a state of acidosis occurs, and the symptoms of hepatic coma begin to appear

268 Homologous serum hepatitis (hepatitis B) is contracted by
1. Exposure to infection
2. Parenteral inoculation
3. Physical damage to the liver
4. Improper utilization of bile salts

269 Dangerous complications of cirrhosis of the liver are
1. Ascites and esophageal varices
2. Hemorrhage and weight loss
3. Infection and hemorrhage
4. Weight gain and fluid loss

270 The patient with bleeding esophageal varices can be treated with a Sengstaken-Blakemore tube. In caring for the patient with this type of tube, the nurse should be most alert for
1. Loss of balloon pressure
2. Irritation of nares
3. Airway obstruction
4. Atelectasis

271 The patient with cirrhosis of the liver has many problems. Some of these are
(A) Indigestion
(B) Ascites
(C) Jaundice
(D) Vomiting
1. A and B
2. B and C
3. C and D
4. A, B, C, and D

272 The surgical treatment of cirrhosis of the liver with bleeding esophageal varices is
1. Portacaval shunt
2. Lobectomy
3. Gastroesophagectomy
4. Gastroenterostomy

6 MATERNAL AND CHILD HEALTH

REFERENCES

Broadribb, V.: Foundations of pediatric nursing, ed. 2, Philadelphia, 1973, J.B. Lippincott Co.

Broadribb, V., and Dorliss, D.: Maternal-child nursing, Philadelphia, 1973, J.B. Lippincott Co.

Chance, P.: Learning through play, New York, 1979, Gardner Press, Inc.

Chinn, P.L., and Leitch, C.J.: Child health maintenance: a guide to clinical assessment, ed. 2, St. Louis, 1979, The C.V. Mosby Co.

Clausen, J.P., et al.: Maternity nursing today, ed. 2, New York, 1977, McGraw-Hill Book Co.

Evans, M., and Hansen, B.: Guide to pediatric nursing: a clinical reference, New York, 1980, Appleton-Century-Crofts.

Goerzen, J.L., and Chinn, P.L.: Review of maternal and child nursing, St. Louis, 1975, The C.V. Mosby Co.

Hamilton, P.M.: Basic pediatric nursing, ed. 4, St. Louis, 1982, The C.V. Mosby Co.

Hunt, S., Groff, J., and Holbrook, J.: Nutrition: principles and clinical practice, New York, 1980, John Wiley & Sons.

Ingalls, A.J., and Salerno, M.C.: Maternal and child health nursing, ed. 4, St. Louis, 1979, The C.V. Mosby Co.

Iorio, J.: Childbirth: family-centered nursing, ed. 3, St. Louis, 1975, The C.V. Mosby Co.

Klaus, M., Leger, T., and Trause, M.A.: Maternal attachment and mothering disorders: a round table, 1975, Johnson & Johnson Baby Products Co.

Latham, H.C., Heckel, R.V., Hebert, L.J., and Bennett, E.: Pediatric nursing, ed. 3, St. Louis, 1977, The C.V. Mosby Co.

Marlow, D.R.: Textbook of pediatric nursing, ed. 5, Philadelphia, 1977, W.B. Saunders Co.

Petrillo, M., and Sanger, S.: Emotional care of hospitalized children, ed. 2, Philadelphia, 1980, J.B. Lippincott Co.

Reinhardt, A.M., and Quinn, M.D., editors: Family-centered community nursing: a sociocultural framework, St. Louis, 1980, The C.V. Mosby Co.

Scanlon, J.W., et al.: A system of newborn physical examination, Baltimore, 1979, University Park Press.

Trotter, S., and Thoman, E.: Social responsiveness of infants: pediatric round table–2, 1978, Johnson & Johnson Baby Products Co.

Waechter, E.H., Blake, F.G., and Lipp, J.P.: Nursing care of children, ed. 9, Philadelphia, 1976, J.B. Lippincott Co.

Whaley, L.F., and Wong, D.L.: Nursing care of infants and children, St. Louis, 1979, The C.V. Mosby Co.

INTRODUCTION

Important information to be reviewed

A. Normal physiologic changes of maturity
B. Physical changes—include beginning of menstruation and ovulation
C. Emotional changes during pregnancy
D. Community resources for mothers, infants, and children
E. Nursing techniques during pregnancy, during labor and postpartum
F. Principles of child health and disease
G. Growth and development of normal child

History of maternal and child health

A. Pregnancy in primitive cultures was a mysterious and superstitious subject
B. Children were not valued, and mortality was high, especially for female children and the weak
C. At first women delivered their own infants
D. Eventually husbands helped wives
E. Next, assistance was given by priests, wise women, medicine men, and most recently physicians
F. Instruments were used and cesarean sections were performed on dead mothers as far back as 3000 BC
G. Importance of children was recognized by Egyptians

H. Orientals had modern knowledge of menstruation and gestation as early as 600 BC
I. Hebrews recognized importance of nutrition for children; they had religious ceremony of circumcision
J. Greeks believed in body beautiful
K. Christianity promoted new theories of child care and charity
L. Middle Ages emphasized family life
M. Printing press made possible first books on obstetrics and pediatrics
N. Industrial Revolution had definite effect on maternal and child health; cities, slums, child labor, epidemics, and various social problems developed
O. Morton and Lister made possible use of anesthesia
P. Semmelweis advocated idea of cleanliness among patients
Q. Landsteiner made blood transfusions possible
R. Fleming made antibiotics possible through discovery of penicillin

Recent trends

A. Improved quality and availability of prenatal care
B. Rooming-in for mother and newborn (birthing rooms)
C. Prepared childbirth
D. Father present at labor and delivery
E. Total care of the family
F. Increased use of internal and external fetal monitoring devices
G. Increased availability of services for high-risk mothers and infants
H. Classes in parenting
I. Emphasis on strengthening maternal-infant bonding

Agencies

See Units 2 and 5

ANATOMY AND PHYSIOLOGY OF MALE AND FEMALE REPRODUCTIVE SYSTEMS

Review Unit 3

ANTEPARTAL GROWTH AND DEVELOPMENT OF INFANT

Embryo

From implantation to end of first 2 months
A. This is period of rapid growth
B. Muscle and bone formation begin
C. Nervous system develops
D. Head forms and is large in comparison to body
E. Organs form; heart begins to beat
F. Short arms and legs develop
G. Embryo resembles an infant at end of the second month

Fetus

From 2 months to term
A. Third month—fetus resembles human form and becomes active; sex can be determined visually
B. Fourth month—muscles are developed; movements may be felt by mother (quickening)
C. Fifth month—fetus is fully developed; fetal heart rate is heard by examiner
D. Sixth month—fat deposits are apparent; baby rarely viable outside uterus
E. Seventh month—weight gain continues
F. Eighth and ninth months—maturation continues with storage of proteins until birth

PREGNANCY

Introduction

A. Signs and symptoms
  1. Presumptive
    a. Amenorrhea
    b. Nausea and vomiting (morning sickness)
    c. Breast changes (enlargement, tingling, increased pigmentation)
    d. Quickening
    e. Urinary frequency
    f. Fatigue
  2. Probable
    a. Changes in uterine size and shape
    b. Braxton Hicks' contractions
    c. Chadwick's sign
    d. Pregnancy tests
      (1) Biologic—necessitates animal colony
      (2) Immunologic—is used more frequently; is faster and eliminates need for animal colonies; is 90% accurate (Gravindex)
  3. Positive
    a. Fetal movement felt by examiner
    b. Fetal heart tones heard by examiner
    c. Fetal skeleton seen by x-ray examination, including ultrasound
    d. Fetal electrocardiogram (ECG)
B. Duration
  1. Pregnancy is normally 9 calendar months, 10 lunar months, or 270 to 290 days from first day of last menstruation

2. Pregnancy is divided into first, second, and third trimesters
3. Delivery date, or estimated date of confinement (EDC), is computed by Nägele's rule—count back 3 months from the first day of last menstrual period (LMP) and add 7 days

Oct 10	First day LMP
− 3 months	
July 10	
+ 7 days	
July 17	EDC

Prenatal care

A. Initial prenatal visit
  1. Should be scheduled as soon as possible when pregnancy is suspected
  2. Includes complete medical history
     a. General health, diseases, and operations
     b. Allergies
     c. Previous blood transfusions
     d. Gynecologic history
     e. Obstetric history
     f. Family's medical history (diabetes, heart disease)
  3. Includes thorough physical examination by physician
     a. Routine examination of head, chest, extremities, and teeth
     b. Pelvic examination and measurements
     c. Abdominal examination
     d. Observation of vital signs, blood pressure, and weight
  4. Includes laboratory tests
     a. Maternal blood type and Rh factor
     b. Hemoglobin and hematocrit
     c. VDRL for syphilis
     d. Urinalysis (special attention to albumin and sugar)
     e. Other tests as indicated by patient's condition

B. General nursing care plan—includes patient instruction concerning continuous health supervision and routine return examinations
  1. Examinations are usually scheduled monthly until twenty-eighth week, then every 2 weeks until thirty-sixth week, then weekly to term
  2. They include
     a. Weight measurement
     b. Blood pressure reading
     c. Abdominal examination for fetal growth (fundal height)
     d. Auscultation of fetal heart
     e. Urinalysis for sugar, acetone, and albumin
     f. Continued patient instruction during pregnancy

C. General hygiene
  1. Dental examination and good dental hygiene are encouraged
  2. Clothing should be comfortable and nonrestrictive
     a. Well-fitting brassiere will provide comfort and support for breasts
     b. Shoes should be comfortable and promote good balance (low heels)
     c. Flattering apparrel and good posture help reduce anxiety over change in appearance
  3. Daily baths provide cleanliness and comfort, although showers are usually suggested in last 2 months because of danger of slipping in tub
  4. Occasional mild exercise is encouraged (often depends on previous habits)
  5. Rest periods are essential when indicated by fatigue
  6. Douching should be done only with physician's approval
  7. Sexual intercourse is not usually contraindicated during pregnancy; however, abstinence in last month may be advised to prevent onset of premature labor

D. Nutrition
  1. Fetus is dependent on mother for dietary needs
  2. Maximum weight gain of 20 to 25 pounds is recommended for entire pregnancy, with the pattern of weight gain being more significant than the total
  3. Sometimes salt restrictions may be ordered by physician during last trimester
  4. Diet should include Basic Four foods and 1 quart of milk daily
  5. More calories should be added (approximately 200 per day) during later half of pregnancy

E. Common discomforts
  1. Nausea and vomiting often occur after first trimester; they are controlled by high-carbohydrate diet and rest and relaxation
  2. Constipation is controlled by exercise, bulk in diet, plenty of fluids, and mild laxatives

3. Varicose veins are avoided by regular bowel habits, rest with elevation of legs and hips, and elimination of garters and constricting clothes
4. Pruritus is controlled by frequent bathing and medications as ordered
5. Leukorrhea should be reported if excessive; frequent bathing is helpful for its control
6. Backache is relieved by a well-fitting girdle and low-heeled, well-fitting shoes

F. Danger signals that should be reported to physician at once
1. Persistent headache
2. Persistent nausea and vomiting
3. Dizziness and visual disturbances
4. Edema
5. Diminution of urinary output
6. Constipation
7. Vaginal bleeding
8. Severe pain in lower abdomen
9. Shortness of breath
10. Apprehension and nervousness
11. Failure to feel fetal movements
12. Pain in lumbar regions in early months
13. Any illness or infection

G. Home delivery
1. At present, only a small percentage of patients, mostly in rural areas, have home deliveries. Recent trends show an increase in interest in home delivery as an alternative to hospital delivery
2. Nurse may work directly with physician
3. Nurse must know what equipment should be available
4. Nurse must know responsibility in preparing home for delivery
5. Patient and family must be instructed regarding symptoms of approaching labor and what to do when labor begins

Complications of pregnancy

A. Hyperemesis gravidarum
1. Problems include
   a. Nausea
   b. Excessive vomiting
   c. Dehydration
   d. Anxiety
2. This condition is characterized by excessive nausea and vomiting during pregnancy. The cause is unknown
3. Treatment is primarily supportive and includes bed rest, administration of intravenous fluids, and occasionally administration of sedatives
4. Nursing care plan involves
   a. Maintaining adequate hydration
      (1) Monitor vital signs and fetal heart tones (if of adequate gestational age) every 4 hours
      (2) Monitor intake and output, and note amount and characteristics of emesis every 8 hours
      (3) Provide frequent oral hygiene
      (4) Administer ordered intravenous fluids and medications
      (5) Administer diet as ordered, usually small frequent feedings
   b. Reducing anxiety
      (1) Allow time for patient to express feelings
      (2) Provide reassurance and information regarding ordered treatment

B. Abortion*
1. Problems include
   a. Vaginal bleeding
   b. Cramplike pain in lower abdomen
   c. Anxiety or grief
2. Abortion is the termination of pregnancy before the fetus is viable (before the fetus has developed enough to survive). Abortions are classified and treated in the following manner
   a. Induced
      (1) Therapeutic—performed legally by physician for medical reasons or at patient's discretion for unwanted pregnancy
      (2) Criminal—abortion is induced by patient, lay person, or professional medical personnel (physician, nurse) in an illegal manner. There is high incidence of infection with criminal abortions
   b. Spontaneous
      (1) Causes
         (a) Hormonal deficiencies
         (b) Endometrial problems
         (c) Incompetent cervix
         (d) Premature cervical dilation (may be prevented by suturing with plastic sutures)

*The U.S. Supreme Court has ruled that abortions performed by authorized medical personnel during the first 3 months of pregnancy are legal. The individual states are to decide the legality of abortions performed after the third month.

(2) Types
(a) Threatened—usually treated with bed rest
(b) Inevitable—characterized by cervical dilation and cramps; treated as stages dictate
(c) Incomplete—all products of conception are not expelled. Treatment may consist of dilation and curettage, blood volume replacement, and oxytocics (prescribed for stimulating uterine contractions)
(d) Complete—all products of conception are expelled
(e) Missed—retention of dead fetus despite apparent signs of abortion

3. Nursing care plan involves
   a. Preventing hemorrhage
      (1) Monitor vital signs and temperature every 2 to 4 hours as ordered
      (2) Observe and record amount and characteristics of vaginal bleeding (count perineal pads)
      (3) Administer ordered intravenous fluids and medications
      (4) Notify physician immediately of signs of shock or excessive bleeding
   b. Promoting comfort
      (1) Observe and record character, duration, and intensity of pain
      (2) Administer analgesics as ordered
      (3) Position patient for comfort as ordered. Oxytocics may stimulate uterine contractions and increase discomfort
   c. Reducing anxiety
      (1) Allow time for patient to express feelings
      (2) Remain with patient, as grief and sense of loss may cause feelings of guilt
      (3) Instruct patient regarding all ordered treatment

C. Placenta previa
1. Problems include
   a. Painless bleeding—vaginal or hidden
   b. Shock
   c. Fetal distress
   d. Asymptomatic until labor begins
2. Placenta previa occurs when the placenta is attached to the lower part of the uterus. It may be classified as complete or partial. Bleeding usually occurs in the last trimester
3. It is diagnosed by symptoms and x-ray examination
4. Treatment is ordered according to severity of condition and may include bed rest, fluid replacement, and/or cesarean section
5. Nursing care is primarily supportive (see Cesarean section)

D. Abruptio placentae
1. Problems include
   a. Bleeding—vaginal or hidden
   b. Shock
   c. Fetal distress
   d. Sudden severe pain and boardlike rigidity over abdomen
2. Abruptio placentae consists of premature separation of placenta. It usually occurs in last trimester
3. Diagnosis is based on symptoms and x-ray examination (as time permits)
4. Treatment is ordered according to severity of condition and fetal distress. It may include bed rest, fluid replacement, and/or cesarean section
5. Nursing care plan is primarily supportive (see Cesarean section)

E. Pregnancy-induced hypertension (PIH)
1. Problems include
   a. Elevated blood pressure
   b. Generalized edema
   c. Visual disturbances
   d. Headache
   e. Nausea
   f. Convulsions, unconsciousness, and coma
   g. Fetal distress
   h. Proteinuria and oliguria
2. Pregnancy-induced hypertension (sometimes referred to as toxemia) is a disorder of pregnancy characterized by hypertension, edema, and proteinuria. The cause is unknown. It is classified in the following manner
   a. Chronic hypertension—onset precedes pregnancy
   b. Preeclampsia—usually occurs in last trimester; additional symptoms include visual disturbances, headache, and nausea
   c. Eclampsia—convulsive stage following preeclampsia, characterized by convulsions, unconsciousness, coma, and oliguria

3. It is treated according to classification and severity. Medical treatment may include bed rest and reduction of environmental stimuli; low-sodium, high-protein, low-fat diet; administration of sedatives (phenobarbital or diazepam [Valium]), diuretics (chlorothiazide [Diuril]), and antihypertensives (magnesium sulfate, hydralazine, or methyldopa [Aldomet])
4. Nursing care plan involves
   a. Reducing blood pressure and preventing seizures
      (1) Monitor vital signs and fetal heart tones every 2 to 4 hours as ordered
      (2) Maintain seizure precautions (for hospitalized patient), and observe for signs of seizure activity
      (3) Reduce environmental stimuli (lights, noise; limit visitors)
      (4) Administer medications as ordered (sedatives, antihypertensives)
      (5) Observe for onset of labor
   b. Maintaining adequate nutrition and hydration
      (1) Monitor intake and output every 1 to 8 hours as ordered
      (2) Weigh daily
      (3) Observe site, degree, and extent of edema
      (4) Administer intravenous fluids and diet as ordered (usually low-sodium, high-protein, low-fat diet)

LABOR AND DELIVERY

Introduction

A. Signs of impending labor may include
   1. Lightening (further settling of fetal head into pelvis)
   2. Braxton Hicks' contractions of increased force
   3. Pinkish vaginal discharge referred to as "show"
   4. Spontaneous rupture of amniotic membrane
B. Patient's labor and delivery experience will be influenced by
   1. Antepartal care
   2. Structure of mother's pelvis and size and position of fetus' head
   3. Educational level and preparation (childbirth classes)
   4. Family support or participation or both
   5. Acceptance, skill, and assistance of nurse
   6. Method of analgesia and anesthesia selected
   7. Progression and course of the labor
C. Nurse should understand the following terms used to describe and evaluate labor
   1. Lie
   2. Presentation
   3. Position
   4. Station
   5. Cervical dilation
   6. Cervical effacement
   7. Uterine contraction
      a. Duration
      b. Frequency
      c. Intensity
D. Exact cause of the onset of labor is unknown; it is probably action of hormones
E. True labor is characterized by
   1. Regular, forceful contractions
   2. Dilation and effacement of cervix
   3. Descent of presenting part into pelvis

Anesthesia and analgesia in childbirth

A. Introduction
   1. Many kinds of anesthesia and analgesia are used, depending on patient's and physician's choice and approval
   2. Some obstetricians now advocate natural childbirth methods (Dick-Reed, Lamaze)
      a. These methods are based on belief that childbirth is a natural process
      b. They include preparation for labor and birth by educating prospective parents regarding
         (1) Physiology of birth process
         (2) Preparation and strengthening of muscles involved in birth process
         (3) Performance of proper breathing and relaxation techniques during birth process
      c. Some methods (Lamaze) include assistant or coach (usually the father) as an active participant in the birth process
   3. Medication (scopolamine) may be used to produce a form of amnesia. Use of this drug with morphine to produce twilight sleep is no longer recommended
   4. Hypnosis and relaxation therapy may be used
B. Types of anesthetics
   1. General anesthesia (nitrous oxide)

2. Regional anesthesia
   a. Paracervical block
   b. Pudendal block
   c. Caudal block
   d. Saddle block
3. Local anesthesia

First stage of labor

A. Basic needs of the mother are
   1. Acceptance, support, and reassurance
   2. Pain management and relief
   3. Safe delivery of healthy infant
B. First stage begins with onset of labor and ends with complete dilation of cervix (10 cm). It is divided into two phases
   1. Latent—weak, often irregular, contractions
   2. Active—increased frequency, duration, and intensity of contractions
C. Duration is approximately 14 hours for first baby; it may be shorter for subsequent pregnancies
D. Nursing care plan focuses on meeting basic needs of mother and includes the following nursing measures
   1. Perform routinely ordered procedures (enema, perineal shave)
   2. Observe and record
      a. Contractions
      b. Maternal vital signs
      c. Fluid intake and output
      d. Fetal heart tones (normal 120 to 160 beats per minute)
      e. Vaginal discharge (amniotic fluid, bleeding)
   3. Provide comfort measures as indicated (mouth care, back rub)
   4. Give explanations to mother concerning procedures to be performed and her progress in labor
   5. Assist mother in performing any learned exercises or breathing techniques
   6. Notify family of mother's progress
   7. Carefully observe and report abnormal symptoms
      a. Excessive vaginal bleeding
      b. Presence of meconium in vaginal discharge
      c. Prolapsed cord or extremity
      d. Sudden change or abnormality of fetal heart tones
      e. Sudden change or abnormality of maternal vital signs
      f. Sudden and severe abdominal pain
      g. Respiratory difficulty

Second stage of labor

A. Basic needs of the mother are same as in first stage but often increase in frequency and intensity as delivery approaches
B. Second stage begins with complete dilation of cervix and ends with delivery of infant
C. Duration is usually 1 hour for first pregnancy and shorter for subsequent pregnancies
D. Nursing care plan is the same as for the first stage with the addition of the following nursing measures
   1. Prepare delivery room and equipment
   2. Frequently observe maternal vital signs and fetal heart tones
   3. Support patient (and partner) in performance of breathing techniques and positioning, according to chosen childbirth method
   4. Place legs in stirrups, and apply wrist restraints
   5. Instruct patient to bear down during contractions as if having a bowel movement

Third stage of labor

A. Basic needs of mother are
   1. Safe delivery of healthy infant
   2. Normal involution of uterus
   3. Hygienic care of perineum
   4. Reassurance and support
B. Third stage begins with delivery of infant and ends with expulsion of placenta
C. Duration is short, usually lasting a few minutes
D. Vaginal bleeding is controlled by contraction of the uterus
   1. Use fundal massage
   2. Administer drugs (ergonovine maleate [Methergine], oxytocin [Pitocin]) as ordered
E. Nursing care plan focuses on meeting immediate basic needs of mother and includes the following nursing measures
   1. Frequently observe maternal vital signs and vaginal bleeding
   2. Check fundal contraction and massaging as indicated
   3. Administer ordered medications
   4. Remove legs from stirrups
   5. Cleanse perineum and apply perineal pad
   6. Clean and care for equipment used in delivery process

Complications of labor and delivery

A. Introduction
   1. Several preventive measures may be employed by the physician when patient's antepartal history or labor process indicates the need
      a. Application of internal or external fetal monitor or both to observe for signs of fetal distress
      b. Induction of labor by artificial rupture of membranes or administration of medication (Pitocin) or both to stimulate and regulate uterine activity
      c. Episiotomy, or incision of the perineum, to prevent tearing during delivery
      d. Application of forceps to fetal head to facilitate safe delivery
      e. Cesarean section, or removal of infant through abdominal incision, when vaginal delivery is contraindicated
   2. Dystocia (abnormal labor) may be caused by
      a. Malposition or presentation (breech, transverse lie)
      b. Cephalopelvic disproportion
      c. Uterine inertia or uterine tetany

B. Prolapsed cord—condition in which umbilical cord falls into vagina before the presenting part, causing cord compression between presenting part and pelvis

POSTPARTUM PERIOD (PUERPERIUM)

A. Postpartum period is time period beginning with birth and ending 6 weeks after delivery

B. Basic needs of mother include
   1. Normal involution of uterus
   2. Relief from discomfort and fatigue
   3. Healing of episiotomy and/or abdominal incision (if applicable)
   4. Onset of lactation, if breast feeding, or suppression of lactation if not nursing
   5. Hygienic care of perineum and breasts
   6. Return of normal elimination patterns
   7. Successful adjustment to new role

C. In caring for mother in the postpartum period it is important to assess the following physical changes that generally occur
   1. Uterus involutes to near normal size
   2. External genitals return to near normal
   3. Abdominal muscles regain tone
   4. Lochia (vaginal discharge) consists of blood, mucus, and lining of uterus
      a. Lochia rubra occurs in first few days; it is bright red and may be small clots
      b. Lochia serosa occurs from about fifth to tenth day postpartum; it is pink to brown
      c. Lochia alba occurs after about tenth day postpartum and is straw colored
      d. Abnormal amount, color, or foul odor of lochia should be reported at once
   5. Breasts of nursing mother are characterized by
      a. Colostrum (yellowish fluid), which is expressed in the first few days
      b. Engorgement as milk increases
   6. Afterpains, caused by contractions of the uterus, are more usual with second and later deliveries and usually begin after first 2 days postpartum
   7. Discomforts and fatigue from birth process combined with drop in hormone levels may cause depression (postpartum blues)

D. Nursing care plan for mother in postpartum period is centered on meeting basic needs and includes the following nursing measures and considerations
   1. Lochia—check daily (character, amount, odor)
   2. Breasts—examine after each nursing for cracked nipples and other problems
      a. Breast is cleansed daily with clear water
      b. Breast binder is used only as ordered by physician
   3. Uterus
      a. Check fundal height daily
      b. When instructed to, massage uterus; it helps in involution and slows down or stops uterine hemorrhage
   4. Perineum
      a. Apply double sterile pad after delivery, and hold in place with T binder
      b. Always remove and apply pad front to back to prevent contamination from rectum
      c. After each voiding or bowel movement, pour warm water (or antiseptic solution as ordered) over perineum without separating labia
      d. Use clean tissues in gentle, downward motion to dry perineum
      e. Give sitz baths only as ordered
      f. Use perineal light; it is soothing and beneficial (40 watt bulb placed 2 feet away)

g. Use medication such as Dermoplast or Tucks on stitches as ordered
h. Instruct mother in performance of own perineal care in most instances
5. Urination
a. Encourage patient to void 8 hours after delivery or when bladder appears distended
b. Watch for distended bladder (it will displace uterus)
c. Keep record of intake and output
6. Defecation—patient may be constipated
a. Encourage adequate diet and early ambulation
b. Give enemas and cathartics only as physician orders (usually before going home)
7. Temperature, pulse, respiration (TPR)—twice a day or as ordered
8. Diet
a. Unless otherwise ordered by physician, good, normal diet is given
b. Diet should be high in minerals and vitamins and consist of Basic Four foods
c. Lactation requires same diet as is required during latter half of pregnancy with additional $^1/_2$ quart of milk (and additional 1000 calories per day)
9. Early ambulation and exercise as ordered by physician
a. Is believed to help muscles return to normal quickly; simple exercises may be started on second day postpartum
b. Helps bladder and bowels return to normal
c. Helps in involution of uterus
10. Health instructions for mother
a. Personal hygiene instructions regarding bath, douches, coitus, and bowels according to physician's routine
b. Care of breasts; cleanliness and use of a well-fitting brassiere are important
c. Diet and fluid intake and output; mother should continue similar diet as was used before delivery
d. Planning work and increasing resumption gradually; she should avoid unnecessary lifting and heavy housework
e. Rest and sleep; she should get at least 8 hours' sleep at night and 2 hours' rest during day; she should plan rest periods for times when infant is sleeping
f. Fresh air, sunshine, and walking outdoors as soon as permitted
g. Postpartum examination as ordered by physician (usually in 6 weeks)
11. Rooming-in
a. This is plan whereby mother may have infant at bedside to care for as she is able and wishes to do
b. Some hospitals plan for rooming-in for normal mothers and infants
c. If conditions in home are normal, rooming-in should be encouraged
d. Father is included in the plan
e. Some institutions provide birthing rooms in which the entire labor, delivery, and postpartal care may be given with father and/or other family members present
12. Birth registration
a. Registration should be prompt and accurate
b. It is responsibility of hospital or physician
c. Proof of birth is very important for everyone

E. Complications of the puerperium include the following
1. Postpartum hemorrhage
a. This may be caused by
(1) Uterine atony
(2) Retained placental parts
(3) Cervical and vaginal lacerations
(4) Other causes (prolonged induction of labor, rapid delivery)
b. Problems include
(1) Vaginal bleeding
(2) Boggy consistency of uterus felt on palpation
(3) Symptoms of shock
c. Treatment may include
(1) Intravenous fluids
(2) Blood transfusion
(3) Administration of medications (Pitocin, Methergine)
(4) Specific treatment according to cause
d. Nursing care plan includes meeting basic needs of mother as well as nursing measures used in caring for the patient in shock
2. Puerperal infection
a. This is infection of birth canal occurring during puerperium; most common organisms responsible are streptococcus and staphylococcus

b. Problems include
   (1) Temperature above 100.4°F
   (2) Tenderness and purulent exudate from episiotomy incision (if involved)
   (3) Abnormal uterine involution with abdominal tenderness
   (4) Abnormal color or odor of lochia
c. Treatment may include
   (1) Administration of antibiotics
   (2) Warm sitz baths
   (3) Bed rest
   (4) Forced fluids
   (5) Isolation precautions
d. Strict aseptic technique by labor and delivery personnel is best prevention of puerperal infection
e. Nursing care plan includes meeting basic needs of mother within restrictions set by isolation procedures. Nursing measures associated with care of patient with an infection are listed above in treatment plan

3. Mastitis
   a. Mastitis is breast infection of nursing mother resulting from bacteria entering one or both breasts through fissured or cracked nipples. Most common organisms responsible are streptococci and staphylococci
   b. Condition is characterized on assessment by
      (1) Pain in nipple and breast affected
      (2) Swelling and heat in affected area
      (3) Temperature elevation
   c. Treatment may include
      (1) Administration of antibiotics and analgesics
      (2) Bed rest
      (3) Application of ice packs (to prevent abscess)
      (4) Cessation of nursing
      (5) Incision and drainage of formed abscesses
   d. Adequate prenatal preparation of breasts for nursing and careful observation for cracks or fissures of nipples are best methods of prevention
   e. Nursing care plan includes supportive nursing measures and performance of ordered treatments
4. Other complications may include
   a. Urinary tract infections
   b. Thromboembolic disease
   c. Inability of mother to bond with newborn

NORMAL NEWBORN

Assessment

Assessment of the normal newborn includes observation of

A. Vital signs
   1. Temperature is 97° to 99°F
   2. Pulse rate is 90 to 180 per minute, depending on activity
   3. Respirations may be irregular, from 32 to 48 per minute
   4. Blood pressure varies and is not usually measured
B. Weight
   1. Average is 7 pounds for girls and 7½ pounds for boys (6½ to 7½ pounds is average range)
   2. Some weight loss is normal; it should not exceed 9% of body weight
C. Length—ranges from 18 to 22 inches
D. Skin
   1. Skin is reddish, changing to pink
   2. It may have mottled appearance
   3. Initially extremities may be bluish (acrocyanosis)
   4. Common variations may include
      a. Milia neonatorum
      b. Mongolian spots
      c. Icterus neonatorum
E. Head
   1. Head is large in proportion to body
   2. It may be elongated with scalp edema (molding) resulting from head conforming to birth canal
   3. Anterior and posterior fontanelles (soft spots) allow for future brain growth
F. Activity
   1. Normal newborn has many reflexes at birth
      a. Moro or startle reflex—flexion of extremities in response to sudden noise or movement
      b. Tonic neck reflex—fencing position; it cannot be elicited
      c. Blinking of eyelids
      d. Grasp reflex—flexion of fingers around object
      e. Rooting—turning head in direction of stroked cheek
      f. Sucking
      g. Swallowing and gag reflexes
      h. Breathing
      i. Sneezing and coughing—used to clear air passages
   2. Normal newborn has lusty cry

3. Normal newborn freely moves arms and legs; listlessness should be reported

G. Gastrointestinal tract
   1. Stomach capacity is usually 1 to 2 ounces
   2. Newborn may swallow air with feeding; if he or she is not "bubbled" or burped during and after feeding, swallowed air may cause regurgitation
   3. Stools should be observed
      a. First stool contains meconium and is blackish green and tarry
      b. Stools gradually become soft and yellowish
      c. Absence of passage of stool in first 24 hours may be indicative of congenital defect (imperforate anus)

Immediate care

Usually done in delivery room

A. Airway is suctioned of mucus and fluid, usually by physician or midwife using rubber bulb syringe
B. Umbilical cord is clamped and cut
   1. Cord blood may be obtained to test for syphilis and Rh antibodies
   2. Cord is observed for presence of three vessels and bleeding
C. Identification procedure is done (usually ID bracelets for mother and newborn and footprinting)
D. Evaluation of newborn's condition is done by Apgar scoring consisting of five observations
   1. Heart rate
   2. Respiratory effort
   3. Muscle tone
   4. Reflex irritability
   5. Color
E. Eyedrops of 1% silver nitrate solution are instilled to prevent ophthalmia neonatorum (legal requirement in the United States)
F. Skin is dried, and newborn is placed in preheated crib or wrapped in warm blanket or both for warmth

General nursing care plan

A. First 24 hours are most important in observation of newborn; constant supervision is given for first 4 hours
B. Clothing should be lightweight and warm
C. Newborn is usually bathed daily or as physician orders
D. Feeding schedules vary according to institution, physician, and method (breast, bottle)
   1. Newborn is usually given nothing by mouth for first 12 hours of life, with sterile or glucose water given for first feeding
   2. Newborn is usually fed every 4 hours during hospital stay
   3. Demand feeding is popular; newborn is fed at time and amount he or she wishes
   4. Mother should be instructed in selected method of feeding and assume responsibility for newborn as soon as possible (see Formula preparation, p. 181)

HIGH-RISK NEWBORN

Introduction

A. Prematurity is indicated as follows
   1. Low birth weight newborn is 2500 g (5.5 pounds) or less at birth
   2. Gestational age of premature newborn is 37 weeks or less
   3. Newborn is classified according to gestational age and birth weight
      a. Small for gestational age (SGA)
      b. Large for gestational age (LGA)
B. Postmaturity indicates a newborn is of more than 43 weeks' gestational age
C. Nurses working with premature newborns should be specially trained and skilled in their nursing care
D. Physician relies on nurse for accurate report of newborn's condition
E. Complications associated with prematurity are
   1. Infection
   2. Hyaline membrane disease or respiratory distress syndrome (RDS)
   3. Hemorrhage
   4. Nutritional deficiencies
   5. Congenital anomalies
F. Immaturity of body systems of the premature newborn produces inefficient function, which often requires artificial assistance
   1. Incubator (Isolette)
   2. Temperature and humidity controls
   3. Oxygen therapy
   4. Special feeding methods (gavage) and schedules
   5. Strict aseptic technique to prevent infection
G. Assessment of the premature newborn includes observation of
   1. Thin, transparent skin with little subcutaneous fat
   2. Lanugo (fine downy hair) covering body, especially forehead and shoulders
   3. Limp, flaccid movements with poor muscle tone
   4. Shallow, irregular respirations

DISORDERS OF THE NEWBORN

Introduction

A. Symptoms to be reported as one assesses the newborn are
   1. Fever
   2. Lethargy or hyperirritability
   3. Vomiting
   4. Skin rash
   5. Blood or mucus in stool
   6. Persistent watery or frequent greenish stools
   7. Difficult grunting respirations
   8. Jaundice
   9. Cyanosis
   10. Anuria
   11. Abdominal distention

B. Parents of newborns with disorders should be included as much as possible in their care

C. Parents should receive instruction in care of newborn and plan for home care well in advance of dismissal

Specific disorders

A. Hemolytic disease of the newborn (erythroblastosis fetalis)
   1. Introduction—of all newborns, 1% have erythroblastosis fetalis; 95% of these have a chance of survival with prompt treatment by exchange transfusion. The condition is caused by antibody-antigen reaction resulting from Rh and ABO incompatibilities. Diagnosis can be made in utero. An essential factor is early detection and reporting of condition
   2. Assessment factors
      a. Appearance of jaundice at birth or soon after birth (most important sign)
      b. Yellow-tinged cord
      c. Yellow-tinged vernix caseosa
      d. Enlarged liver and spleen
      e. Petechial hemorrhages into skin
      f. Severe edema
   3. Exchange transfusions
      a. Rh negative blood is used
      b. Twice as much donor blood is given than is estimated blood volume of newborn
      c. Transfusion should replace about 85% of newborn's blood
      d. Transfusion may have to be repeated if bilirubin level remains elevated
   4. Nursing care plan—is primarily supportive and includes performance of specifically ordered treatments

B. Respiratory distress syndrome (RDS) or hyaline membrane disease
   1. Condition results from deficiency of enzyme (surfactant) in alveolar spaces causing atelectasis or complete collapse. This condition causes 67% of all neonatal deaths and is characterized by onset of respiratory distress within few minutes or hours after birth
   2. Treatment may include
      a. Transfer to neonatal intensive care unit when possible
      b. Administration of oxygen therapy (positive end-expiratory pressure [PEEP], continuous positive airway pressure [CPAP]) to maintain respiratory function
      c. Administration of intravenous fluids and antibiotics
   3. Nursing care plan includes maintenance of environment (Isolette), constant observation of the newborn, and performance of specifically ordered treatments

---

Infant

INTRODUCTION

A. Infancy begins at 4 weeks of age and continues until walking begins (approximately 1 year of age)

B. Infant learns to trust mother first, then other adults through contact and having basic needs met quickly and consistently

C. Basic needs are
   1. Food
   2. Pleasure of sucking
   3. Warmth and comfort
   4. Feeling of love and security
   5. Stimulation of senses by environment

D. Infant expresses sociability by smiling, making of sounds, and imitating (da-da) and then saying one or two words

E. Play provides a means of practicing motor skills, coordination, and specific eye-hand movements
   1. Play materials should be stimulating (bright in color), safe, and durable

2. Toy selection depends on
   a. Motor skills of infant
   b. Function of toy

F. Physical growth and development vary with each infant but proceed in an orderly sequence
   1. Motor development precedes cephalocaudal (head to feet)
   2. Muscular development precedes proximodistal (grasp rattler, pick up button with fingers)

G. Dentition varies with age. Lower two central incisors usually erupt first, followed by top two central incisors
   1. Deciduous teeth (20) are completely in by $2^1/_2$ years of age
   2. They are replaced by permanent teeth (32) by 6 or 7 years of age
   3. To prevent tooth decay, children need
      a. Good daily dental hygiene
         (1) For infants, teeth should be cleaned with gauze and water
         (2) After 2 years of age, small brush with soft bristles should be used
         (3) Yearly examination by dentist is necessary by 3 years of age
         (4) Elimination of too many sweets from diet is important
      b. Fluoridation of water supply—protects against dental caries

H. Medical supervision includes
   1. Routine examination by physician
   2. Immunization and tuberculin skin testing (see Appendix, Table 6, for immunization schedule)

NUTRITION

A. Psychologic considerations include
   1. Making infant comfortable while feeding
   2. Making all contacts with food happy and satisfactory to foster infant's development of trust
   3. Never using force or threats

B. Techniques of feeding are
   1. Demand—offer feeding when infant appears to be hungry
   2. Scheduled—offer feeding at routine time intervals

C. Introduction of foods and new tastes should be done gradually, and child should be observed for allergies to foods by introducing one at a time
   1. First month of life—formula or breast milk or both
   2. Second month—cereals and pureed fruits
   3. Third month—pureed vegetables and meats
   4. When able to chew—junior foods
   5. From 3 to 4 months of age—begin to use cup and spoon

D. Formula preparation consists of
   1. Terminal sterilization—method in which everything used is clean; bottles and formula are sterilized together in one operation
   2. Aseptic sterilization—method in which equipment, bottles, and formula are sterilized separately and assembled under aseptic conditions
   3. Tap water method—used with an inspected water supply; bottles and equipment are sterilized and stored in refrigerator; each bottle is then made up separately from canned milk and tap water immediately before feeding
   4. Prepared formulas—available with directions on cans
   5. Principles in preparation
      a. Cleanliness of all equipment
      b. Washing of hands thoroughly before making formula
      c. Sterilization of bottles, nipples, and containers
      d. Refrigeration of prepared formula for not more than 24 hours

E. Calories, vitamins, and minerals are increased according to activity and individual needs

F. Weaning usually occurs in the last half of the first year; infant will begin to handle bottle as an object rather than as source of food
   1. Begin weaning by eliminating one bottle- or breast-feeding during the day, preferably the midday feeding when cup can be offered with meal
   2. Progress with weaning by gradually decreasing number of times bottle or breast are offered during the day
   3. Night bottle- or breast-feeding should be last to be stopped

ASSESSMENT

Assessment of the normal infant includes observation of

A. Physical characteristics
   1. Weight—doubles by 6 months and triples by 12 months of age
   2. Height—increases 1 inch per month for first 6 months and $^1/_2$ inch for next 6 months

3. Head and chest circumferences—head circumference larger at birth than chest circumference; circumferences equal by 12 months of age
4. Fontanelles—posterior fontanelle closes by 2 months and anterior fontanelle closes by 18 months of age
5. Reflexes—primitive reflexes (Moro, tonic neck, sucking) gradually disappear by 4 months and completely lost by 8 months
6. Motor development
   a. Gross motor movements progress as follows: lifts head (birth), sits alone (8 months), crawls (9 months), creeps (11 months), cruises (12 months), and walks (13 months)
   b. Fine motor movements progress as follows: shows grasp reflex (birth), holds objects (3 months), reaches and grasps objects voluntarily (5 months), plays with objects (6 months), transfers objects from one hand to other (7 months), shows pincer grasp with thumb and index fingers (8 months), makes marks on paper with crayon (11 months), sequential play—fills container with objects by placing one at a time (12 months), and attempts to build two block tower (13 months)

B. Social characteristics
1. Vocalization—smiles (2 months), coos and laughs aloud (4 months), speaks one or two words (12 months), and speaks two more words other than "mama" and "daddy" (13 months)
2. Socialization—stares intently at faces (1 month), enjoys people interaction (4 months), plays peekaboo (7 months), fears strangers (9 months), repeats actions for attention (10 months), and demonstrates jealousy, affection, anger, and fear (13 months)

C. Sense of trust—personality develops from basic passivity to active interaction with parents and familiar others

HOSPITALIZATION
Introduction

A. Adjustment of the infant depends on nurse's ability to apply knowledge of normal growth and development, emotional and physical needs of infant, and familiarity with family background and routines

B. Common treatments and procedures specific to care of infants include
1. Restraints—used to ensure safety and applied only if absolutely necessary
   a. Mummy—infant is wrapped in such a manner as to temporarily immobilize extremities
   b. Elbow restraint—commercially available or made by covering tongue depressor with gauze and placed to prevent flexion of elbow
   c. Clove hitch—strips of gauze made into figure eight and placed as wadding to restrain wrists or ankles
2. Vital signs
   a. Blood pressure is difficult to obtain, and proper equipment must be used
      (1) Blood pressure cuff the width of two thirds of the upper arm
      (2) Sphygmomanometer or electronic devices for measurement
   b. Pulse is taken apically
   c. Temperature is taken rectally or axillary with either glass or electronic device. Rectal method is done last as it may influence pulse and respiration
3. Specimens
   a. Urine is collected in a plastic bag applied to perineum (urine strap)
   b. Blood is obtained from external jugular or femoral veins. Nurse is responsible for restraining infant
4. Medications (see Unit 4 for administration procedure)—accurate administration is essential
   a. Oral medications
      (1) Infant is held or raised to a sitting position
      (2) Liquid form or crushed tablet is mixed in honey or water and given slowly
      (3) Syringe (no needle), medicine dropper, nipple, or teaspoon is used for administration
   b. Intramuscular injections
      (1) This route is used when drug cannot be given orally or intravenously
      (2) Preferred sites for injection are midanterior and midlateral thigh
      (3) To reduce pain from injection, nurse should allow alcohol to dry, use sharp needle, insert needle quickly, inject drug slowly, and remove needle quickly
   c. Intravenous therapy (see Units 3 and 4)
      (1) Amount infused, rate, and site are checked hourly
      (2) Infant is weighed daily
      (3) Intake and output are monitored closely

5. Enema (see Unit 4)
   a. Assemble equipment—no. 10 to 12 French catheter, physiologic saline solution (no more than 300 ml), bedpan, diaper, and pillow
   b. Position buttocks on bedpan with pillow behind back and shoulders
   c. Wrap diapers around legs to restrain in position
   d. Insert catheter 2 to 4 inches into anus
   e. Hold enema can no higher than 18 inches above infant's hips
   f. Carefully record amount instilled and amount returned (minimal or no return may occur)

General nursing care plan

A. Encourage mother or principal care giver to be with infant during hospitalization
   1. Explain procedures to allay parents' anxiety
   2. Provide contact by cuddling, rocking, and stroking
   3. Allow family to participate in care (baths, feeding)
B. Provide opportunity for infant to experience pleasant stimuli
   1. Speak softly, cuddle, and soothe (especially after painful or uncomfortable procedures or treatments)
   2. Plan nursing care to allow for long periods of rest
   3. Provide environment that stimulates social, motor, and personality development (see Physical characteristics, pp. 181-182)
   4. Provide opportunity for sucking, displaying of emotions, and playing
C. Allow infant to regress in behaviors
   1. Infant may not desire to continue learned skills in hospital environment (refuses to drink from cup and wants bottle)
   2. Do not attempt to force infant into learning new behaviors (feeding self, walking, weaning)
   3. Recognize normal mood swings (laughing to crying); may be more frequent in hospital
D. Provide comfort and love when significant person cannot be with infant (see following section, Maternal-child separation)
   1. Swaddle young infant in blanket
   2. Provide familiar objects in immediate environment
   3. Plan nursing care to allow not only time to meet basic needs but also cuddling and play activities

MATERNAL-CHILD SEPARATION

A. "Maternally deprived"—term used to describe an infant who has not received a loving relationship from significant persons
   1. Degrees of deprivation are noted by infant's behavior
      a. Partial deprivation—infant displays acute anxiety and demonstrates need for love and affection
      b. Total deprivation—behavior denotes inability to form normal relationships
   2. Deprivation was first noted in institutions in which infants had all physical needs met but lacked individual "loving care"
B. Behavior of deprivation occurring in first 6 months of life
   1. Infant cries monotonously and uses rocking movement to comfort self
   2. Infant fails to gain weight and has slow motor development
   3. Sleep pattern is altered and a placid, then completely passive, facial expression develops
   4. Infant is very susceptible to infections
   5. Mortality is high if deprivation continues
C. Deprivation occurring in second 6 months of life
   1. Infant has had a warm and loving relationship
   2. He or she appears sad, cries, and is withdrawn
   3. Infant may refuse to eat and may lose weight
   4. Infant clings to a doll or other familiar object
   5. In deprivation lasting longer than 3 months, recovery from autoerotic behavior may be difficult
D. Stages of separation identified following 6 to 9 months of age
   1. Protest—constant crying
   2. Despair—behavior is passive and depressed
   3. Denial—inability to show a complete relationship with an adult

Toddler

INTRODUCTION

A. This stage is from time in which walking first occurs to 3 years of age
B. Child has sense of autonomy and increasing ability to help self
C. Child displays anger and hate when denied wants
D. In developing, child will have a degree of self-control or else a sense of shyness and shame

E. Child develops close relationship with total family
F. Basic needs are same as for infant with the addition of needing gradual independence and exploration
G. Child learns to understand others and to communicate through language
H. Characteristics of behavior are
   1. Negativism—is unable to handle frustration and behaves opposite of what is desired of him or her ("no-no")
   2. Ritualism—desires to have everything orderly and routine. This provides child with a feeling of security
   3. Slowness in meeting requests—is able to differentiate right and wrong and cannot decide which to choose
   4. Temper tantrums—reaction to frustration
I. Play is parallel (plays beside and not with)
   1. Play provides physical and social development
   2. Play provides a release of energy and means of sublimating desire in an approved manner
   3. Toys should be selected to
      a. Meet likes and dislikes of child
      b. Encourage motor skills and imagination
J. Medical and dental supervision should be provided
   1. Routine visits to physician and dentist by $2^1/_2$ to 3 years of age
   2. Immunizations (see Appendix)
K. Toilet training occurs in this stage
   1. Child must be developed enough physically and emotionally to be ready for training (approximately at $2^1/_2$ years of age)
   2. Tension should be avoided in all toilet training
   3. Interest and approval bring better results than punishment

NUTRITION

A. Diet should be balanced in essential nutrients for body function and increased exertion of energy
B. Physiologic anorexia occurs as result of decreased need for food (utilizes stored nutrients from infancy), personality characteristics (independence), and preferences for certain foods
C. Child should not be forced to eat but should be encouraged to eat essential food substances. Let child feed self when he or she shows desire to do so
D. Daily food requirements for children past infancy are
   1. Milk, 2 to 4 cups
   2. Egg, one
   3. Meat, poultry, fish, or cottage cheese or bland cheeses, one serving
   4. Liver, once a week
   5. Vegetable (green or yellow), two or more servings
   6. Raw vegetables, one serving
   7. Raw or cooked citrus fruit, two or more
   8. Cereals and bread, one to three servings
   9. Butter or fortified margarine

ASSESSMENT

Assessment of normal toddler includes observation of
A. Physical characteristics
   1. Height and weight increases are slow until age of 3 years
   2. Physiologic anorexia occurs as a result of slow growth
   3. Sphincter control develops (daytime control of bowel and bladder at $2^1/_2$ years)
   4. Gross motor movements develop—walks alone and creeps upstairs (15 months), jumps in place with both feet and throws ball overhand (18 months), aligns two or more objects and turns doorknobs and jar lids (24 months), and builds tower of eight blocks and holds crayons with fingers to draw a cross (30 months)
B. Social characteristics
   1. Vocalization—says "no" even when in agreement (18 months), has vocabulary of approximately 300 words (24 months), and can give first and last name (30 months)
   2. Socialization—can be separated from mother for short time and has temper tantrums (18 months), demonstrates "domestic mimicry" and awareness of ownership ("my . . .") (24 months), and demonstrates parallel play and notices sex differences (30 months)
C. Sense of autonomy—personality demonstrates feeling of self-importance, desire for control, and recognition

HOSPITALIZATION

Introduction

A. Maternal separation is major fear of toddler, and hospitalization, compounded with separation, evokes acute anxiety in toddler. Preparation of toddler in elective admissions is preferred to provide the child some familiarity with people and physical environment
B. For common treatments and procedures, see Infant, Hospitalization

C. Child's and mother's adjustment to hospitalization depend on cause of hospitalization, care and support received from personnel, and child's personality. Factors influencing anxiety resulting from hospitalization and separation are
   1. Mother and child relationship
   2. Psychosocial developmental level of child
   3. Previous experiences in separation from mother
   4. Preparation for hospitalization and/or previous hospitalizations
D. Responses to hospitalization include
   1. General responses—fear of the unknown and of punishment and fear of being separated from mother
   2. Specific responses—toddler may have frequent and violent temper tantrums, regress in toilet training, and become fearful of people; insomnia, overactivity, and possible aggressive behavior toward others are other responses (also see responses if separated from mother under Infant, Maternal-child separation)

General nursing care plan

A. Encourage mother or principal care giver to be with toddler during hospitalization
   1. If able, prepare toddler and parents for hospitalization by play-acting procedures and explanation
   2. Encourage mother (or other) to tell child when leaving immediate area
   3. Provide parents and child time to interact alone and child opportunity to play (activity appropriate for age and imposed restrictions)
   4. Allow parents to express feelings (concerns about hospitalization, child's change in behavior, discipline problems)
   5. Utilize mother-child relationship to foster trust of child in hospital personnel (allay mother's anxiety, allow mother to explain procedures to child, provide support to mother)
B. Plan nursing care to prevent situations that aggravate normal toddler behaviors (negativism, temper tantrums)
   1. Establish a trusting relationship with toddler
   2. Express desired behaviors directly ("Tommy, this medicine is for you to drink") and not by asking toddler a question
   3. Expect regression in normal behaviors, and do not attempt to enforce learned behaviors (a child who is daytime toilet trained begins to soil clothing after hospitalization). Do not attempt to toilet train while in hospital
   4. Arrange staffing of nurses to limit number of strangers toddler must contact during hospitalization
C. Provide familiar objects from home in toddler's immediate environment (security blanket, stuffed animal)
D. Understand family's and child's background and rituals to minimize conflicts and length of adjustment period

Preschool child

INTRODUCTION

A. This is stage of development between 3 and 6 years of age
B. Child has sense of initiative and desire to learn about the world and people around him or her
C. Child has a conscience and values
D. Child imitates adult of same sex and has elaborate imagination
E. Parent of opposite sex becomes love object (oedipal)
F. Sibling rivalry occurs with birth of a sibling
   1. Expression of jealousy may be direct (hitting) or indirect (clumsiness in holding infant)
   2. Parents should encourage preschooler to aid in caring for new sibling; also can give preschooler a new doll so child can imitate parents' actions
G. Child needs security (love, understanding) and independence (responsibilities, decision making)
H. Child learns moral values (religion) and sex information (where babies come from) during this stage
I. Feelings and ideas are expressed through language
J. Special problems of preschooler are
   1. Anxiety—caused by separation and fears (pain, darkness)
   2. Thumbsucking—possibly caused by inadequate sucking pleasure in infancy or unhappiness
   3. Enuresis—caused by poor toilet training (too early, too severe, overtraining), inability to cope with problems, environment (dark halls, cold), or physical problem (irritable bladder)
   4. Bad language—caused by learning improper word

5. Masturbation (excessive)—may be caused by child turning to self for pleasure that he or she is unable to receive elsewhere
6. Destructiveness (intentional)—caused by unhappiness and inability to control feelings (anger, jealousy)

K. Play is cooperative (exchange with other children)
   1. Play provides opportunity for child to deal with reality, develop personality, and control feelings
   2. Child displays imagination and imitation of adult world
   3. Play is means of expressing creativity
   4. Toys are selected to meet needs for creativity, imagination, and motor development

L. Medical and dental supervision is necessary at least every 6 months

NUTRITION

A. Nutrition should include Basic Four foods (see Toddler, Introduction and Nutrition)
   1. Child shows little interest in eating but enjoys social aspects of family meals
   2. Food should be served attractively and imaginatively but should be plainly cooked

B. Preschooler's food preferences are determined by the child's tastes, fads, and imitating preferences of others

ASSESSMENT

Assessment of normal preschooler includes observation of

A. Physical characteristics
   1. Vital signs
      a. At 3 years—pulse, 95 per minute, blood pressure, 100/67, respirations, 24 per minute
      b. At 5 years—pulse and respirations are decreased slightly in rate
   2. Weight and height—increase of 4 to 6 pounds and 2 to $2^1/_2$ inches in height since age of 2 years; remains constant through age of 5 years (birth length doubles at age 4)
   3. Nighttime control of bowel and bladder
   4. Motor development
      a. Gross motor movements—rides tricycle (3 years), skips and hops on one foot (4 years), and throws and catches ball and jumps rope (5 years)
      b. Fine motor movements—copies geometric samples (3 years), uses scissors (4 years), and ties shoelaces and can draw stick people with 7 to 9 parts (5 years)

B. Social characteristics
   1. Vocalization—has language ability in short complete sentences and frequently asks questions (3 years), tells exaggerated stories to make them more interesting and can repeat simple songs and rhymes (4 years), and names four or more colors and knows names of days of week (5 years)
   2. Socialization—imitates adult social interactions in play and with adults; shares personal objects; enjoys boasting, tattling, and entertaining; and begins cooperative play by 5 years of age

C. Sense of initiative—guided by a sense of conscience, preschooler demonstrates ability to have graded independence and desire to complete tasks; exhibits sexual curiosity

HOSPITALIZATION

Introduction

A. Because of preschooler's understanding of language, preparation for hospitalization and medical interventions is easier. Preschooler's major fear is bodily harm, and child should be approached honestly by hospital personnel and parents

B. For common treatments and procedures, see Infant, Hospitalization

C. Play therapy is useful. Utilizing play as the medium, the child can learn about illness, procedures (surgery), and hospital personnel. Since preschoolers use toys to learn functions of the adult world, toys can be used as a tool through which child expresses feelings in a manner suitable to child's developmental level

General nursing care plan

A. Prepare preschooler for hospitalization and procedures
   1. Decrease parents' anxiety by educating them in hospital routines, prescribed procedures, and treatments
   2. Allow parents to play through expected procedures with child. Hospital personnel need to work with parents and child to provide education and support (needle play)

3. As soon as condition allows, child is to be provided time to play (diversional activity, play therapy)
4. Preschooler's questions should be listened to carefully and answered in simple terms to avoid the child's imaginative thoughts from creating unrealistic assumptions

B. Encourage parents and others to express periods of separation from child in logical time frames ("I will be back before you eat supper")
C. Avoid creating feelings of guilt and inadequacy in the preschool child by allowing the child to express self
   1. Encourage child to cry when in pain rather than reinforcing cultural expectations ("Big boys don't cry")
   2. Explain to child in concrete terms ("The needle hurts your arm, but the hurting stops very quickly")

School-aged child

INTRODUCTION

A. This is stage of development between 6 and 12 years of age
B. Child has a sense of industry, enjoys people and doing things for people, and enjoys engaging in purposeful activities and tasks
C. Child hero-worships someone of same sex
D. Child is loyal to friends of own age, sex, and group (clubs)
E. Child plays fairly, following rules in a game, and is competitive
F. Rewards and recognition of achievement are motivations
G. Through school, family, and friends, child develops attitudes and social role
H. Child adjusts to school and community experiences
   1. Tensions may develop
   2. Child may rebel against rigid routines
   3. Child may be more interested in activities outside home
   4. Child learns how to get along with friends
I. Child demonstrates physical and mental ability through school and recreational activities
J. Child develops interest in group in contrast to individual activities of earlier age
K. Child becomes aware of how individuals react to one another
L. Play has less physical activity, and child has longer attention span
   1. Child is interested in hobbies and games
   2. Play is more sophisticated as age progresses to 12 years
M. Medical checkup should be done at least once a year
N. Dental examination should be done two to three times a year

NUTRITION

A. Nutrition should include foods from Basic Four food groups (see Toddler, Nutrition)
   1. School-aged child develops sense of industry by participating in meal preparation and selecting foods
   2. Caloric requirements decrease; obesity becomes a problem if overeating occurs
B. Mealtime should be enjoyable with no stress
   1. School-aged child becomes interested in table manners between ages of 10 and 12 years
   2. Most conflicts about meals occur because of time of meal (interference with child's preferred activities), not because of food fads or decreased desire of food, as occurred during preschool years

ASSESSMENT

Assessment of normal schoolchild includes observation of

A. Physical characteristics
   1. Vital signs—temperature, 98.6°F; pulse, 85 to 100 per minute; respirations, 18 to 20 per minute; and blood pressure, 95 to 108/62 to 67; close to adult ranges
   2. Height—slow growth in height until pubescence
   3. Weight—rapid gain
   4. Eruption of permanent teeth—occurs between ages of 6 and 21 years; 28 permanent teeth by age of 13 years
   5. Motor development—gross motor movements are refined from clumsiness (6 years) to equal those of an adult (12 years). Fine motor movements demonstrate ability to construct simple structures (6 years) to complex manipulations of small parts (12 years)

B. Social characteristics
   1. Vocalization—language ability is formed and child uses various types of sentence structures by age of 6 years
   2. Socialization—increasingly independent and interested in school activities, clubs, and organizations involving children of the same sex. Peer relationships and significant adults (schoolteacher, scout leader) are very important to the schoolchild. Adult role models provide child someone from whom to gain social acceptance and emotional support and with whom to identify

C. Sense of industry—enjoys accomplishing tasks, purposeful activity, and games; plays and interacts cooperatively with others; enjoys success and finds pride in schoolwork and building of toy models or sewing

HOSPITALIZATION

Introduction

A. Major fear in hospitalized schoolchild is loss of self-control. Schoolchild can understand explanations and pictorial demonstrations of what to expect. Child's previous experiences with illness, hospitalization, and developmental level will influence adjustment

B. For common treatments and procedures, see Infant, Hospitalization. Schoolchild is physically developed to permit medications and procedures to be administered in the same manner as to adults

C. With long-term hospitalization of schoolchild, provision of schoolwork and recreational and play activities are to be scheduled in day activities as permitted by physical condition

General nursing care plan

A. Provide guidance to schoolchild whose behavior vacillates from conforming to hospitalization to rebelling against adult authority
   1. Allow child to make some choice about care (bath time, site for injection, food)
   2. Allow child to assist in specified projects (helping to make bed, collecting medicine cups, drawing pictures for room)
   3. Affirm limitations on activities and behaviors while child is in hospital
   4. Encourage child to express feelings (fear of mutilation, death, and punishment)
   5. Identify coping mechanisms, and support child by gaining child's trust and providing explanations to questions from child

B. Utilize child's interest in learning and preference of nonfamily adult role models to teach child health and physical care

C. Respect older schoolchild's desire for privacy by being careful not to expose various body areas while giving care or performing treatments

Adolescent

INTRODUCTION

A. Stage of development begins when secondary sex characteristics appear and ends when psychologic maturity and somatic growth are completed (approximately 13 to 18 years of age)

B. Adolescent conflicts with any authority
   1. Parents
   2. School
   3. Church

C. Immature wish for independence and dependence at same time causes tensions and conflicts

D. Group recognition, fads (food, clothes, behavior), and later heterosexual relationships are important

E. Adolescent explores feelings about politics, religion, and philosophies

F. Recreation of girls and boys includes
   1. Social functions
   2. Movies and books
   3. Shopping and making self attractive
   4. Competitive sports
   5. Exercise and physical activities

G. There is increased interest in personal appearance and opposite sex

H. Normal desires of adolescent include
   1. Understanding of physical and emotional changes
   2. Acceptance of sexual changes
   3. Recognition as individual by family and friends
   4. Help in making decisions about school and work

I. Adolescent develops sense of identity and intimacy

J. Adolescent should assume responsibility for regular dental and medical checkups

NUTRITION

A. Appetite increases because of high energy need during period of rapid physical growth

B. Food faddism can result in inadequate intake of proper nutrients
C. Adolescent demonstrates a sense of identity by accepting or rejecting foods or meal preferences of parents
D. Nutritional requirements are same as for adult, except during growth spurts when the following nutrients need to be increased
   1. Calories—girls, 2400 calories per day; boys, 2800 to 3000 calories per day
   2. Protein
   3. Vitamins
   4. Minerals (especially iron)

ASSESSMENT

Assessment of normal adolescent includes observation of
A. Physical characteristics
   1. Physical changes in height and body proportions
      a. Male—rapid linear growth, widening of shoulders, increased muscle development, lean appearance
      b. Female—early cessation of linear growth as compared to boys', widening of pelvis, fatty deposits contour body more like adult female
   2. Hormonal changes
      a. Male—physical increase in size of testes and penis; growth of pubic, axillary, and facial hairs; voice change; production of mature spermatozoa (approximately 15 years of age), increase in sebaceous glands secretion
      b. Female—budding of nipples and breast formation, growth of pubic and axillary hairs, pigmentation of nipples, onset of menarche, deepening of voice tone
B. Socialization—adolescent prefers to be in groups of both sexes; spends countless hours talking to "dear friends"; responds to peer pressure and morals to interact in social activities
C. Sense of identity—adolescent desires to separate self from parents in various physical and emotional degrees and to be like "the group"; decides on vocation for adult years
D. Sense of intimacy—transition from childhood to adulthood is marked by determination of identity ("Who am I?") to responding with concern, care, and feeling for someone other than self

HOSPITALIZATION

Introduction

A. Hospitalization will be difficult if adolescent is placed on unit with small children. Adolescent has difficulty coping with illness, especially long-term, because of many problems already associated with normal growth and development. Adolescent has a sense of immortality and may have difficulty adjusting to concept of "being different from peer group." All efforts by hospital personnel should be directed to providing for privacy, the expression of feelings, and the opportunity to make some decisions in care
B. Health information should be provided for adolescent
   1. Teach health maintenance (nutrition, normal growth and development)
   2. Identify and correct misconceptions or old wives' tales (menses, limitations in activities during menses, reproductive process)
   3. Counsel adolescents in need of sexual information (birth control, menstrual cycle)
   4. Assist parents and adolescents to recognize normal psychologic and physiologic reactions during adolescence
C. Adolescent should be approached as an individual
   1. Differentiate normal behaviors in adolescents from behaviors that indicate a need for further evaluation and care
   2. Establish realistic limitations and expectations of the adolescent based on developmental level (hour of sleep, bath time, visitors)
   3. Interact with adolescent as health care provider and not authority figure
   4. Foster expressions of interests, goals, and worries from adolescent (lapse in school and social activities, guilt if responsible for hospitalization, burden on others)

Special psychosocial problems in children

Following are common psychosocial problems seen in children (preschooler to adolescent). The problems generally can be categorized as
A. Neurotic symptoms (finger sucking, nail biting, fears, school phobia)

B. Behavior problems (truancy, drug use)
C. Language problems (functional—stuttering; anomaly—cleft palate; cerebral lesions—cerebral palsy)
D. Psychosomatic illnesses (overeating, constipation, enuresis, abdominal pain)

GENERAL NURSING CARE PLAN (see also Unit 7)

A. Accurately observe and record behavior
B. Develop an interdisciplinary plan of care (therapist, physician, nurse, psychiatrist, social worker)
C. Establish regularly scheduled team conferences to discuss causes of problems, recent observations, and assessments based on established interventions

SPECIFIC PSYCHOSOCIAL PROBLEMS, CAUSE, AND CARE

Pathologic temper tantrums

A. Child has not learned to control feelings and frustrations
B. Child's behavior is directed toward environment or self
C. Child needs professional care to learn control and behavior appropriate to age

Childhood schizophrenia

A. Child has abnormal personality for age and developmental level
B. Child needs professional care to evaluate and treat underlying causes

Phobias

A. Child has irrational, unnatural fears of surroundings or objects (dark, dogs, water)
B. Child is slowly helped to cope with objects or situations initiating fear

Juvenile delinquency

A. Child does not behave in society in an acceptable manner
B. Cause is usually a combination of factors
   1. Poor family relationships
   2. Peer group pressures
   3. Decreased ability to make judgments
   4. Mental retardation
   5. Neurosis or personality disorders

Drug and alcohol abuse

A. Peer influence, modeling of parents, and ready access to substances are contributing causes for abuse
B. Recognition of problem, identification of causes, legal controls, and education of public and children to dangers and warning signs of addiction will curtail use of substances by children and adolescents

Sense of immortality

A. The child, and most particularly the adolescent, lacks maturity to be cautious and takes risks that can jeopardize life and health (speeding of automobiles, swimming alone in unprotected areas)
B. Education, without instilling fear in the child, is necessary to protect the child and others from harm

Health problems of infancy and childhood

The following section reviews common illnesses observed specifically in infants and children. See Unit 5 for review of conditions that occur in adults and children (otitis media, fractures, acne vulgaris, burns, pyelonephritis, acute glomerulonephritis, asthma, tuberculosis, pneumonia, anemias, leukemia, appendicitis, and diabetes insipidus and mellitus)

COMMON CONDITIONS CAUSING FLUID AND ELECTROLYTE IMBALANCE

Introduction

Disturbances in fluid and electrolytes are common in infancy and early childhood. Acute disturbances can occur rapidly and be life threatening (see Unit 5, Fluid and electrolytes)

Assessment

A. Observe child's appearance and behavior
   1. Dull appearance to eyes
   2. Anorexia
   3. Decreased activity and irritability
   4. Lethargy
B. Assess vital signs. Variations can occur rapidly and indicate possible cause of imbalance
   1. Temperature
      a. Elevation—indicates decreased fluid volume and excess sodium
      b. Subnormal—could indicate shock
   2. Pulse—assess quality and rate
   3. Respirations—assess rate and sounds
      a. Moist rales—could indicate fluid overload

b. Rapid, deep respirations—could indicate metabolic acidosis and respiratory alkalosis
4. Blood pressure
a. High blood pressure—could indicate fluid excess
b. Low blood pressure—could indicate fluid deficit
C. Observe skin texture and color
1. Skin turgor—poor skin turgor (dehydration), puffiness around eyes, edema (fluid retention)
2. Skin color—paleness could indicate deficiency in protein, fluid, or fluid shift; flushed skin could indicate fever and/or sodium excess
D. Observe changes in body weight (sudden increase or decrease)

General nursing care plan

A. Accurate measurement of intake and output
1. Fluid intake
a. Intravenous fluids—type, amount, and rate to be monitored hourly
b. Food and fluids—frequently child is allowed nothing by mouth (NPO) except for intravenous fluids. If child is allowed fluids by mouth, these should be measured
2. Fluid output
a. Urine output—amount, specific gravity, and character of urine are to be monitored hourly
b. Stool output—monitor amount and texture, and if diarrhea, stool needs to be weighed to determine fluid content
B. Frequent assessment of vital signs (temperature, pulse, respirations, and blood pressure)
C. Accurate history (medical, social) and physical examination to establish data base for future assessments and interventions
D. Frequent evaluation of child and condition to determine effectiveness of medical treatment and nursing care
E. Observation of intravenous fluid site for infiltration, phlebitis, and disconnection of tubing or needle from site
1. Restrain child only if necessary to protect intravenous therapy (see treatments and procedures under Infant, Hospitalization)
2. Immobilize extremity (arm, leg) to protect therapy and child from harm

Conditions producing fluid and electrolyte imbalance

A. Diarrhea
1. Problems include
a. Dehydration
b. Excoriation of skin around anus
c. Metabolic acidosis
d. Communicability (bacteriologic, viral)
e. Abdominal discomfort
2. Diarrhea is the major symptom of disorders involving digestion, absorption, and secretion of the alimentary tract. Various etiologic factors can cause diarrhea in infants and small children. Sudden change in frequency and consistency of stools is usually caused by an infectious process; other etiologic factors are malabsorption of water-soluble nutrients, congenital short bowel, poisons, and dietary indiscretions
3. Diagnosis is made on history, stool culture, and stool analysis (pH, leukocytes, fat, blood)
4. Treatment of diarrhea depends on severity
a. Mild—usually treated at home. Child's activity is decreased; child is NPO except for clear liquids (Gatorade), grated apples (or Kaopectate), and for older children, Lomotil (diphenoxylate with atropine)
b. Severe—treatment is directed toward associated physiologic disturbances (fluid loss and replacement) and meeting child's energy requirements (calories)
5. Nursing care plan involves
a. Maintaining adequate hydration
(1) Record admission weight and daily morning weights
(2) Monitor strictly intake and output (measure or weigh urine and feces)
(3) Administer prescribed intravenous fluids, and monitor hourly rate and intake
(4) Observe and record skin turgor, infant's fontanelles (sunken, bulging), and condition of periocular area (sunken, edematous)
b. Providing data to support determination of cause
(1) Monitor frequency, color, consistency, and amount of stools
(2) Report factors associated with feeding (method of feeding, complaints, types of food)
(3) Collect stool specimens for laboratory examination

c. Providing safe environment to staff and others
   (1) Isolate child (private room)
   (2) Maintain enteric precautions
   (3) Wash hands carefully before and after providing care to child and others
d. Providing emotional support to child and parents (see Hospitalization for specific age of child)
   (1) Explain diagnostic procedures and limitations
   (2) Encourage use of pacifier for infants to provide sucking while NPO, anxious, and isolated
   (3) Explain reason for restricted and gradual progression of diet
e. Preventing skin irritation and breakdown
   (1) Keep area dry and clean (frequent changing of diapers)
   (2) Use mild soap to cleanse area
   (3) Apply water-resistant ointment (Vaseline)
   (4) If area is excoriated, leave open to air and apply warm heat (heat lamp)

B. Vomiting
1. Problems include
   a. Dehydration
   b. Metabolic alkalosis
   c. Malnutrition
   d. Determination of cause
   e. Possibility of aspiration
2. Vomiting is common occurrence in infancy and is usually minor and temporary. Acute, persistent vomiting is usually a result of an infection or psychologic factors
3. Diagnosis is made on the determination of whether or not vomiting is a manifestation of another condition or the dominant clinical condition
4. Treatment is directed at determining cause, preventing complications (fluid and electrolyte imbalance, aspiration), drug therapy
5. Nursing care plan involves
   a. Observing to identify type of vomiting
      (1) Spitting up—liquid feeding returns after fast feeding or burp
      (2) Rumination (self-induced)—stomach contents vomited and reswallowed, usually a result of poor mother-infant relationship
      (3) "Wet burp"—liquid feeding returns with burp and shows no evidence of having been in contact with gastric juices (not curdled)
      (4) Projectile vomiting—intense forceful ejection of vomitus. May be caused by pyloric stenosis, increased intracranial pressure, and gastrointestinal obstruction (vomitus may contain bile and/or feces)
   b. Providing data to support determination of cause—observe character of vomitus (appearance and contents), frequency and persistence, amount, force of vomiting, relationship to feeding (formula or breast milk), feeding technique, mother-infant relationship, and history (vomiting associated with diarrhea, motion sickness, anxiety)
   c. Maintaining adequate hydration (see Diarrhea, Nursing care plan)
   d. Providing emotional support to child and family (see Diarrhea, Nursing care plan)

C. Hypertrophic pyloric stenosis
1. Problems include
   a. Vomiting
   b. Failure to gain weight
   c. Dehydration
   d. Decreased stools
2. Diagnosis is made based on history of clinical manifestations (sudden projectile vomiting, hunger evidenced by infant's willingness to refeed after vomiting) and radiologic diagnosis (upper GI series)
3. Surgical intervention is preferred treatment (Fredet-Ramstedt procedure)
4. Preoperative nursing care plan involves
   a. Maintaining adequate hydration (see Diarrhea, Nursing care plan)
   b. Maintaining nutritional status
      (1) Feed slowly thickened or unthickened feedings, in a semiupright position
      (2) Feed small amount, with burping before and after feedings
      (3) Handle infant minimally (especially after feedings)
   c. Preventing complications of gastric lavage (aspiration, fluid, and electrolyte imbalance)
      (1) Observe placement of gastric tube
      (2) Check for patency of all tubing
      (3) Monitor intake and output

5. Postoperative nursing care plan involves
   a. Maintaining infant in proper position (right side)
   b. Maintaining adequate hydration (see Diarrhea, Nursing care plan)
   c. Maintaining nutritional status
      (1) Following postoperative vomiting (initial 24 to 48 hours), observe tolerance to feeding
      (2) Offer feedings slowly; observe amount; observe maternal feeding technique
   d. Promoting healing at operative site
      (1) Observe incision site for drainage, signs of infection, and stages of healing
      (2) Provide care to incision as prescribed by physician (aseptic bandage changes)
   e. Providing emotional support to child and educate family
      (1) Provide explanation in aspects of hospital and home care
      (2) Allow maternal and infant care to foster trusting relationship and decrease anxiety in infant and parents

D. Burn—see Unit 5, Diseases of the integumentary system or skin

E. Nephrotic syndrome (for other renal conditions, see Unit 5, Diseases of the urinary tract)
1. Problems include
   a. Ascites
   b. Proteinuria
   c. Hypoproteinemia (results in malnutrition)
   d. Anorexia
   e. Irritability
2. Nephrosis is a complex group of symptoms that may or may not be an extension of another condition (glomerulonephritis). The syndrome can occur separately from an unknown cause
3. Diagnosis is based on history (weight gain, puffiness, anorexia), skin pallor and signs of malnutrition, and laboratory tests (proteinuria, hypoproteinemia, renal biopsy)
4. Treatment is aimed at correcting proteinuria, preventing infection, and establishing nutritional balance
5. Nursing care plan involves
   a. Monitoring and observing effect of treatment on reduction of edema
      (1) Monitor strictly intake and output (urine specific gravity)
      (2) Record daily morning weight
      (3) Observe daily for resolution or increase in edema
      (4) Test urine for albumin level
      (5) Observe color and texture of skin
   b. Preventing secondary infections
      (1) Provide daily hygienic measures with special skin care (apply lanolin); keep skin dry and clean
      (2) Isolate from contact with upper respiratory infections, keep turned and warm, and monitor for signs of infection
   c. Promoting optimal nutritional state
      (1) Interdisciplinary team approach to combat child's anorexia
      (2) High-protein diet to counteract negative nitrogen balance
      (3) Fluid and sodium restriction during period of massive edema
   d. Providing for emotional support of child and family
      (1) Deter persons from commenting on child's atypical appearance
      (2) Provide diversional activity and play therapy while bed rest is prescribed and afterwards
      (3) Instruct parents and child on hospital and home care

COMMON INFECTIOUS CONDITIONS IN CHILDREN

Introduction

Infectious conditions cover a wide spectrum of diseases and conditions that are transferable from one source to another. Infectious conditions can be classified as to type of infecting organism (bacterial, viral, parasitic, fungal). (See also Unit 5, Communicable diseases, and Appendix, Table 6)

Assessment

A. Obtain relevant history from parents (medicosocial)
B. Determine type of infectious process
C. Observe infected area (skin, products of gastrointestinal tract/stool)
D. Assess general condition (fever, nutritional state, lesions, and symptoms of cardiovascular, respiratory, and gastrointestinal diseases)

General nursing care plan

A. Prevent transfer of infection to others
   1. Isolate child and other infected persons (see Unit 4, Isolation)
   2. Identify organism and mode of transmission
   3. Ensure proper drug treatment as prescribed by physician

B. Institute general hygienic measures
   1. Identify external sources of infection and treat underlying cause
   2. Maintain body hygiene (daily medicated baths)
   3. Clean and/or disinfect environment

C. Provide comfort measures
   1. Provide diversional activity and play therapy
   2. Medicate (systemically, topically) any irritated areas as prescribed by physician

D. Frequently evaluate child and condition to determine effectiveness of medical treatment and nursing care

E. Provide environment conducive to fostering normal growth and development (review growth and development for specific age group)

F. Institute measures to reduce fever (if applicable)
   1. Administer antipyretic (aspirin, acetaminophen) as ordered by physician
   2. Dress child in light clothing
   3. Provide tepid sponge bath
   4. Frequently monitor rectal temperature
   5. Provide alcohol sponge bath (only if prescribed by physician)
   6. Observe for signs of change in levels of consciousness and febrile seizures

Bacterial infections

A. Impetigo
   1. In making additional assessment, observe vesicles on skin (rapidly spreading circinate erythematous lesions). Note type of drainage (purulent) and any crustation
   2. Problems include
      a. Mildly infectious organisms (staphylococcal or streptococcal)
      b. Susceptible to secondary infections (acute glomerulonephritis, rheumatic fever)
      c. Altered body image
   3. Impetigo is a superficial skin infection usually from secondary infections of insect bites
   4. Diagnosis is made on identification of organism (may be group A beta-hemolytic *Streptococcus* or *Staphylococcus aureus)*
   5. Treatment is systemic antibiotics (penicillin) and topical bacteriocidal ointments (gentamycin [Garamycin], polymyxin B [Neosporin])
   6. Nursing care plan involves the following (see also General nursing care plan on this page)
      a. Carefully remove crusts and debris with 1:20 Burrow's solution compresses (as prescribed by physician)
      b. Prevent transmission to others during period of communicability (until lesions are healed). Incubation period is 2 to 5 days. Transmitted by direct contact

B. Streptococcal pharyngitis
   1. In making additional assessment, observe throat for redness, edema of uvula, and exudate. Enlarged and tender anterocervical lymph nodes are palpable
   2. Problems include
      a. High fever
      b. Malaise and irritability
      c. Headache
      d. Anorexia
      e. Sore throat and painful swallowing
   3. Streptococcal pharyngitis is acute infection of upper respiratory tract usually occurring during winter and early spring months
   4. Diagnosis is determined by identification of group A beta-hemolytic streptococci from throat exudate
   5. Treatment is systemic antibiotic therapy (penicillin)
   6. Nursing care plan involves
      a. Obtaining sterile throat cultures
      b. Preventing poor nutrition and dehydration
         (1) Offer diet of warm liquids and soft, nonspicy foods
         (2) Administer throat analgesics (lozenges, gargles) as prescribed by physician to decrease pain of swallowing
      c. Preventing transmission to others during period of communicability (greatest during acute phase). Incubation period is 2 to 5 days. Transmitted by direct contact and large droplets

Viral infections

See Appendix, Table 6, for common childhood communicable diseases (chickenpox, measles, smallpox, mumps)

A. Warts (verrucae)
   1. Problems include
      a. Susceptible to secondary infections (staphylococcal) when skin integrity is lost
      b. Altered body image
   2. Warts are a common viral infection of the skin. They are flesh-colored papules
   3. Diagnosis is made by appearance of skin lesions
   4. Treatment may consist of surgical removal or medication (topical application of 40% salicylic acid) to cause atrophy of warts
   5. Nursing care plan involves
      a. Educating parents and child not to irritate or try to remove warts (picking)
      b. Observing for presence of secondary infection

B. Infectious mononucleosis (glandular fever)
   1. In making additional assessment, palpate for enlarged cervical lymph nodes and spleen. Tonsils are painful, erythematous, and enlarged with exudate
   2. Problems include
      a. High fever
      b. Abdominal pain
      c. Lymphocytosis (over 20% are atypical)
      d. Malaise
      e. Skin rash (occasionally observed)
   3. Infectious mononucleosis is self-limiting, acute, Epstein-Barr viral infection. Onset of symptoms may be acute or insidious, and symptoms may appear from 10 days to 6 weeks after exposure (direct or indirect contact)
   4. Diagnosis is made by confirming clinical manifestations with laboratory diagnosis (positive Monospot and heterophil antibody test)
   5. Treatment is supportive of symptoms (self-limiting disease) and includes prevention of complications (spleen rupture)
   6. Nursing care plan involves
      a. Relieving discomfort from symptoms
         (1) Administer aspirin for fever, malaise, and headache (as prescribed by physician)
         (2) Alternate periods of rest with limited activity
         (3) Lessen sore throat with gargles, warm drinks, and analgesics (as prescribed)
      b. Observing for signs of complications—hepatitis, ruptured spleen, pneumonitis (rarely occur). Precautions and care would include
         (1) Never attempt to palpate spleen
         (2) Place hand carefully when turning child (place on hip)
         (3) Provide secure environment to prevent possibility of trauma to abdomen
      c. Providing emotional support to child and family
         (1) Infectious mononucleosis usually occurs in teenagers who have very active lives. Explanation and education are essential to gain cooperation (see Adolescent, Hospitalization)
         (2) Promote understanding of parents in dealing with child's irritability and malaise

Parasitic infections

See also Unit 5, Diseases of the integumentary system or skin

A. Scabies
   1. In making additional assessment, observe for burrows into the skin (black, approximately 1/2 inch in length)
   2. Problems include
      a. Severe itching
      b. Secondary infections
   3. Scabies is skin infection by female mite *(Sarcoptes scabiei)*
   4. Diagnosis is made by symptoms and visualization of black burrows on thin, moist areas of skin (axilla, groin, between fingers and toes)
   5. Skin is treated with gamma benzene hexachloride (Kwell) lotion washings
   6. See General nursing care plan, p. 194

B. Helminthic infections
   1. In making additional assessment, determine infecting helminth and mode of transmission and reproduction, and observe for secondary complications (upper respiratory obstruction, anemia)
   2. Problems include
      a. Intestinal obstruction
      b. Circulatory impairment
      c. Respiratory obstruction
      d. Anemia, malnutrition, and abdominal pain and distention (in cases of severe infections)

3. Helminthic infections are parasitic worms invading child to obtain nutrients (and in some cases, means of reproduction). Common types of helminths seen in children are
   a. *Enterobius vermicularis* (pinworm)—white, threadlike worm transmitted by person-to-person contact (eggs lodged on skin around anus). Eggs hatch in duodenum. Adults migrate to cecum and appendix
   b. *Ascaris lumbricoides* (roundworm)—pencil-shaped worm, 6 to 15 inches long. Transmitted from eggs deposited in soil to child's fingers to mouth. Eggs hatch in duodenum. Larvae infest other organs as they penetrate the intestinal wall, mesenteric lymphatics, or venules
   c. *Necator americanus* (hookworm)—eggs hatch in damp soil. Larvae attach to and penetrate skin and enter bloodstream to lungs, exit in alveoli, migrate to upper respiratory tract, and are swallowed
4. Diagnosis is determined by symptoms (visual detection in feces or vomitus), stool examination (tape test), test for ova and parasites, and further investigation of severe symptoms (intestinal obstruction, anemia)
5. Treatment for helminthic infections is drug therapy with antihelmintics (piperazine [Antepar], pyrvinium pamoate [Povan], pyrantel pamoate [Antiminth])
6. Nursing care plan involves
   a. Preventing reinfestation and transmission of helminths to others
      (1) Institute enteric precautions
      (2) Treat child and family with prescribed medication
      (3) Disinfect and control environment (clothes, bed linens, toilet seats)
      (4) Educate child and family as to sources of eggs, means of transmission, and symptoms
   b. Observing child for complications resulting from heavy infestation of helminths

Fungal infections

A. Candidiasis
   1. In making additional assessment, observe mucous membranes of mouth for small white patches that resemble milk curds but that cannot be swabbed away, and check for a well-defined diaper-area rash
   2. Problems involve the following areas
      a. Vagina—itching and redness of perineal area
      b. Oral mucous membranes—painful; difficulty in swallowing and eating
      c. Diaper area—possible secondary infections from loss of skin integrity
   3. Candidiasis is caused by *Candida albicans* fungus. Fungus is transmitted by poor hand washing, contact with infected object, and, in neonates, from mother's vaginal tract
   4. Diagnosis is based on presenting symptoms and culture of mucous area
   5. Treatment involves topical application or oral administration of nystatin (Mycostatin)
   6. Nursing care plan involves
      a. Early detection to prevent systemic infection
      b. Application of medication as ordered by physician

B. Tinea (ringworm)
   1. In making additional assessment, look for circular lesion around hair follicle that gradually appears scaly and dirty (tinea capitis)
   2. Problems include
      a. Secondary infection
      b. Pruritus
   3. Tinea is skin infection caused by *Microsporum* (commonly the *M. audouini*). Fungus is transmitted from person to person and from animal to person
   4. Diagnosis is based on characteristic circular lesion and glowing of tinea capitis under Wood's lamp (glows green)
   5. Treatment is administration of oral griseofulvin (Fulvicin-U/F, Grifulvin V) and sometimes application of local antifungal agent
   6. Nursing care plan involves
      a. Relieving pruritus and preventing secondary infections
         (1) Dress lightly to prevent skin warming (increases pruritus)
         (2) Apply wet, cool compresses and soothing baths
         (3) Provide for good body hygiene
      b. Preventing transmission to others—educate child and parents as to potential fomites (hair brushes, community showers)

c. Determining type of tinea by presenting symptoms
   (1) Tinea capitis—lesions on scalp
   (2) Tinea corporis—round or oval scaling; erythematous patch on body
   (3) Tinea pedis (athletes's foot)

Common congenital and inherited conditions in children

INTRODUCTION

Conditions vary and may affect any system in the body. Conditions discussed are those most commonly occurring in children

ASSESSMENT

A. Information obtained from family history (familial tendencies) and parents' life-style (drug use—alcohol, stimulants—and tobacco use)
B. Information on social and environmental factors (nuclear radiation, x-ray, and pollution exposure)
C. Reaction of parents to knowledge of congenital problem
D. Parent-child relationship (interaction, habits)
E. State of grief reaction in parents (if applicable)

GENERAL NURSING CARE PLAN

A. Recognize parents' reaction to child and others
   1. Health professionals are to approach parents in a caring and concerned manner
   2. Assist parents to deal with grief/loss
   3. Provide opportunity for parents to express concerns and feelings
B. Educate parents on genetic screening and counseling
   1. Assist parents to understand cause and diagnosis
   2. Provide parents with options for dealing with risk of future births with same problem
   3. Assist in psychologic adjustment to disorder and to affected child

CONGENITAL CONDITIONS INVOLVING THE GASTROINTESTINAL TRACT

Cleft lip and/or palate

A. Problems include
   1. Feeding difficulty
   2. Child's body image
   3. Parental acceptance of child
   4. Speech difficulties
   5. Surgical care
   6. Difficulty in providing infant basic needs (sucking, socialization)
B. Cleft lip and palate are a result of failure of maxillary processes to fuse with the nasal elevations. Cleft may be unilateral or bilateral and may involve only the lip or palate (soft or hard or both) or can involve the lip and palate(s)
C. Diagnosis is made by visual detection of defect
D. Treatment is surgical intervention to correct defect
E. Preoperative nursing care plan involves
   1. Preparing infant and parents for surgery
      a. Introduce infant to lying on back (postoperative position) and elbow restraints
      b. Feed infant with rubber-tipped syringe or other device to be used after surgery
      c. Educate parents to mouth care and appliances used after surgery (Logan bar)
   2. Providing adequate nutrition
      a. Use suitable feeding device to allow infant to suck and feed (Nursettes, cleft palate nipple, long lamb's nipple)
      b. Encourage mother to feed infant, and allay anxiety by teaching method. Teach mother how to suction pharynx in case of aspiration
F. Postoperative nursing care plan involves
   1. Protecting operative site and promoting wound healing
      a. Prevent tension on suture line by attempting to keep infant from crying
      b. Apply elbow restraints to keep hands away from mouth
      c. Position on back or side to prevent rolling on stomach and rubbing face on sheet (cleft lip repair only)
      d. Cleanse sutures as prescribed by physician
      e. Rinse mouth after feedings with clear water
   2. Preventing aspiration and respiratory complications
      a. Gently aspirate mouth and nasopharynx
      b. Change position frequently (back to side, side to back)
      c. Elevate head of crib after feedings to prevent aspiration
      d. Feed slowly, and burp frequently

Esophageal atresia with tracheoesophageal fistula

A. In making additional assessment, observe for excessive salivation, frequent choking and coughing, and feeding returns through nose and mouth. Infant may also become cyanotic and stop breathing

B. Problems include
   1. Aspiration pneumonia
   2. Malnutrition
   3. Asphyxiation
   4. Dehydration

C. Esophageal atresia is structural anomaly in which the esophagus ends in blind pouch. Most commonly the esophagus has two blind pouches, one connecting by fistula with the trachea (tracheoesophageal fistula)

D. Diagnosis must be made early to prevent death. Symptoms and radiologic visualization confirm diagnosis

E. Treatment is directed toward surgical correction and prevention of secondary complications (aspiration pneumonia)

F. Preoperative nursing care plan involves
   1. Early detecting and preventing of complications
      a. Withhold feedings when infant demonstrates symptoms of drooling, choking, cyanosis, and respiratory distress associated with feedings
      b. Maintain clear upper respiratory passages by suctioning nasal and oral cavities
      c. Place patient in supine position with head elevated
   2. Emptying esophagus and trachea of mucus and saliva
      a. Maintain intermittent or continuous suction on small nasal catheter (indwelling)
      b. Observe aspirate for blood and excessive mucus

G. Postoperative nursing care plan involves
   1. Providing adequate oxygenation to all tissue cells
      a. Place infant in warm, humidified air
      b. Change position frequently to prevent pulmonary stasis
   2. Providing adequate nutrition
      a. Provide intravenous fluid to replace fluid and electrolyte losses
      b. Use gastrostomy tube for drainage until anastomosis has healed (10 to 14 days); then begin feedings as prescribed by physician
      c. Closely observe initial feedings for infant's ability to swallow without choking

Celiac disease (malabsorption syndrome/sprue)

A. In making additional assessment, observe nutritional state of child (skin color, nails, hair), bowel habits, nutritional intake, and behavior patterns (irritable, apathetic)

B. Problems include
   1. Fat, frothy, foul, and bulky stools
   2. Severe weight loss
   3. Abdominal distention
   4. Malnutrition of fat-soluble vitamins

C. Celiac disease is inability to absorb fats ingested in diet. Exact cause is unknown, but it is thought to be an inborn error in metabolism. Initially, child is unable to absorb fats (idiopathic steatorrhea), and later impairment in absorption of vitamins D, K, and B_{12}, calcium, iron, proteins, and carbohydrates occurs

D. Diagnosis is based on stool analysis for fat and serum studies for absence of essential nutrients (protein, iron). X-ray studies indicate signs of osteoporosis

E. Nursing care plan involves
   1. Promoting adherence to diet by educating parents and child
      a. Nutritional therapy is aimed at gluten-free diet (no foods containing wheat, rye, oats, or barley). A high-calorie, high-protein diet with simple sugars (fructose) is ordered
      b. Guide family in dietary planning, in food shopping (reading food labels) and in teaching child food restrictions (hot dogs, pizzas, bread)
   2. Assisting child and parents to adjust to chronic condition
      a. Encourage parents to discuss problems associated with child's diet restrictions (meal preparation, child offered foods by others)
      b. Encourage older child to participate in meal preparation and to cope with peer pressure
      c. Encourage parents to continue follow-up care (each developmental stage of child results in different dietary management problems)

Meckel's diverticulum

A. In making additional assessment, observations will depend on presenting symptoms (intestinal obstruction, diverticulitis—see Unit 5). Determine by history bowel and eating habits of child since birth

B. Problems include
   1. Rectal bleeding (possible hemorrhage)
   2. Infrequent to absence of stools
   3. Diverticulitis
   4. Intestinal adhesions, strangulation, or intussusception, which may cause intestinal obstruction
C. Meckel's diverticulum is failure of omphalomesenteric duct from terminal ileum to close, resulting in a diverticulum. Secretions of gastric mucosa cause irritation and ulceration in ileum or diverticulum
D. Diagnosis is determined by child's history and radiologic visualization of diverticulum or ulceration
E. Treatment is surgical removal of diverticulum
F. Preoperative nursing care plan (general care for child with abdominal surgery) involves
   1. Preparing child for surgery and educating child and parents on expectations of surgery and postoperative care
      a. Physical preparation (see Unit 4, Preoperative nursing care)
      b. Explain equipment to be used postoperatively (nasogastric tube, intravenous fluids, wound drains)
      c. Instruct and have child practice turning, coughing, and deep breathing
      d. Utilize play therapy to assist child in what to expect postoperatively (dressing, equipment)
   2. Continually observing child for acute symptoms of complications (perforation, hemorrhage)
G. Postoperative nursing care plan involves
   1. Relieving child of discomfort and decreasing parental anxiety
      a. Approach child slowly and carefully to prevent undue pain or discomfort
      b. Provide analgesic medications as ordered (child will not always ask for pain medication)
      c. Explain procedures to child and family
   2. Promoting wound healing
      a. Use aseptic technique in dressing changes and wound care
      b. Explain importance of preventing contamination of surgical site to child and parents
      c. Encourage eating after period of NPO by allowing child to select favorite foods

CONGENITAL CONDITIONS INVOLVING THE CENTRAL NERVOUS SYSTEM

Myelomeningocele

A. In making additional assessment, observe neurologic status, associated anomalies, and neuromuscular deficiencies (urine retention, immobility)
B. Problems include
   1. Infection of meningeal sac
   2. Extension of neuromuscular deficiencies
   3. Parental rejection and poor maternal-infant bonding
C. Myelomeningocele is a spina bifida occulta (failure of spinous processes to join) and protrusion of spinal meninges and spinal cord in sac outside of body. Condition results from failure of embryonic neural tube to form properly
D. Diagnosis is based on visual observation of myelocele on exterior surface of infant's back
E. Treatment is surgical placement of meninges and spinal cord in normal position and prevention of damage to major nerve pathways
F. Preoperative nursing care plan involves
   1. Preventing infection and harm to myelocele sac
      a. Observe for sign of cerebrospinal fluid leakage and infection
      b. Maintain infant in Trendelenburg's prone position (slightly) with legs in abduction
      c. Keep sac moist with antibacterial solution and sterile gauze covering
      d. Do not diaper infant; keep dry waterproof pad under area
      e. Provide meticulous skin care to prevent skin breakdown in immobile areas
   2. Assessing infant to determine extent of neuromuscular damage
      a. Observe movement of lower extremities
      b. Observe urine and bowel elimination; palpate bladder to express urine
G. Postoperative nursing care plan involves
   1. Preparing parents for habilitation of infant
      a. Utilize an interdisciplinary team plan for care and follow-up of infant
      b. Begin physical therapy exercises to prevent muscle contractures (as prescribed by physician)
      c. Explain necessity for long-term follow-up of infant, and encourage parents to express concerns and feelings
   2. Fostering infant-parent relationship
      a. Allow parents to hold infant as soon as possible

b. Encourage parents to participate in daily care of infant
c. Allow parents to proceed through chronic grief, and provide support to them
d. Encourage parents to facilitate developmental growth in infant (explain normal stages of development)

3. Preparing parents to care for infant at home
a. Instruct parents in daily care
b. Explain signs and symptoms of anticipated problems (urinary retention, infection, skin breakdown)
c. Provide resources from which parents can receive assistance (public health, financial aid)

4. Observing infant for complications (hydrocephalus, meningitis—see following section; urinary tract infections—see Unit 5; skin breakdown—see Unit 4)

Hydrocephalus

A. In making additional assessment, compare head circumference with normal ranges and previous measurements daily, assess infant's fontanelles (bulging), and observe for symptoms of increased intracranial pressure (vomiting, irritability, headache, neurologic deficits)

B. Problems include
1. Increased intracranial pressure
2. Impaired motor function
3. Increased susceptibility to infections caused by immobility

C. Hydrocephalus is symptom of excessive accumulation of cerebrospinal fluid in ventricles and subarachnoid spaces of brain and can be classified as follows
1. Communicating hydrocephalus—fluid flows freely from ventricles and subarachnoid space, but meningeal absorption of fluid does not occur; causes include subarachnoid hemorrhage, meningitis, and adhesions
2. Noncommunicating hydrocephalus—blockage exists between subarachnoid and ventricular spaces (partial or complete), causing accumulation of cerebrospinal fluid in ventricles; causes include stenosis and tumors

D. Diagnosis is made by presenting symptoms (increased head circumference, bulging fontanelles, and separated cranial sutures or signs of intracranial pressure in older child) and diagnostic studies (transillumination—flashlight held against infant's head in dark room, radiography, pneumoencephalogram, ventriculogram, brain scan)

E. Treatment is surgical intervention to relieve pressure (ventriculoarterial or ventriculoperitoneal shunt) and in the older child with noncommunicating hydrocephalus surgical removal of blockage (tumor)

F. Preoperative nursing care plan involves
1. Observing for signs of increasing intracranial pressure
a. Measure head circumference and fontanelles daily
b. Observe changes in behavior (irritability, lethargy, seizures)
c. Note frequency and character of vomiting
d. Evaluate vital signs (widening pulse pressure, decreased pulse rate, change in respiratory rate and pattern—Cheyne-Stokes, if brainstem pressure)

2. Providing maintenance of nutritional state
a. Because of frequent vomiting, infant needs to be fed small amounts frequently
b. Hold infant or child to support head for feedings

3. Preventing problems associated with immobility
a. Change position frequently
b. Encourage range of motion exercises
c. Observe for signs of upper respiratory problems (pneumonia)
d. Support head and neck when lifting or moving to prevent trauma

G. Postoperative nursing care plan involves
1. Observing for effectiveness and for complications of shunt placement
a. Observe for signs of increased intracranial pressure
b. Observe for signs of infection (meningitis)
c. Position on unoperated side
d. Maintain level of head elevation prescribed by physician
e. Measure head circumference daily
f. Observe neurologic status (level of consciousness, pupil size and reaction to light, reflexes)

2. Providing support to parents during hospitalization and preparing for home care
a. During child's hospitalization, support and clarify explanations of physician to parents for cause of hospitalization (diagnosis of hydrocephalus, infection, shunt repair/revision)
b. To allay anxiety, provide explanations for

medical and nursing activities (positioning, tests)
c. Demonstrate interest in listening to parents' concerns and feelings
d. Instruct parents to observe for signs of complications
e. Involve parents in care expected to be continued at home
f. Provide anticipatory guidance to parents to cope with problems (peer relationships, family adjustment, and physical limitations of child, if applicable)

CONGENITAL CONDITIONS CAUSING HEMATOPOIETIC DISORDERS

Sickle cell anemia

A. In making additional assessment, observe for weakness, joint and abdominal pain, fever, pallor, hematuria, and convulsions or sickle cell crisis. Physical changes in child noted as a result of disease are long, thin extremities, short trunk, and barrel-shaped chest
B. Problems include
 1. Anemia
 2. Sickle cell crisis
 3. Enuresis
C. Sickle cell anemia is inherited defect in synthesis of hemoglobin. A sickling appearance of hemoglobin is apparent after 4 months of age. With sickle cell trait, only 25% to 45% of total hemoglobin is sickled
D. Diagnosis is usually made when child is seen in sickle cell crisis. Sickle cell screening tests can verify presence of disease or trait in persons with family history
E. Treatment is specific to prevention (sickling phenomenon) and intervention (sickle cell crisis). No cure exists for the condition
F. Nursing care plan includes the following
 1. To prepare child for frequent laboratory tests
  a. Explain reason for tests at level appropriate for child's development
  b. Familiarize child with laboratory equipment
  c. Comfort child, and allow expression of feelings before and after procedures
 2. To prevent and observe for signs of infection, oxygen deficit, and transfusion reaction
  a. Limit child's contact with persons with signs of infection (upper respiratory, wound)
  b. Observe changes in vital signs
  c. Observe child's level of physical tolerance, and limit activities and environments requiring increased need for oxygen (exercise, high altitudes)
  d. Observe for signs of cardiac failure
  e. Observe benefit of oxygen administration
  f. Infuse blood transfusions slowly, and observe for signs of reaction (chills, fever, flank pain, shock, or renal failure)
 3. To prevent injury and promote safety
G. Sickle cell crisis care involves the following
 1. To promote hydration and prevent sickling
  a. Monitor prescribed intravenous fluid rate and explain importance of adequate oral fluid intake to parents and child
  b. Increase fluid intake during periods of increased activity, fever, and stress
  c. Observe for signs of dehydration (dry mucous membranes, weight loss)
 2. To prevent stress on child
  a. Increase awareness of precipitating stress factors (loss, hospitalization, enuresis)
  b. Instruct parents in normal growth and development (including toilet training)
  c. Allow expression of concerns and feelings and assist parents and child to cope with stress
 3. To provide comfort measures and decrease pain
  a. Administer analgesics as prescribed by physician
  b. Support joints during positioning for comfort
  c. Apply warmth to painful areas as prescribed by physician
  d. Encourage bed rest
  e. Assess benefit of oxygen administration
 4. To assist parents and child in adjusting to long-term life-threatening condition

Hemophilia

A. In making additional assessment, observe for increased bleeding time, bruising, and signs of hemorrhage
B. Problems include
 1. Hemorrhage
 2. Loss of joint mobility
 3. Death
C. Hemophilia is syndrome resulting in congenital defect of one or more blood coagulation factors. Various types of hemophilias exist, depending on type of blood factor involved

D. Diagnosis is made when symptoms of increased bleeding time are observed, usually in early infancy (bleeding from umbilical cord or after circumcision)
E. Treatment is directed at resolving complications and preventing hemorrhage (transfusions of blood factor defective in child)
F. Nursing care plan involves
   1. Instructing parents and child (if of appropriate developmental level) in long-term care
      a. Administer blood factor
      b. Control bleeding (direct pressure, immobilization above level of heart, application of cold to site)
      c. Decrease risk of injury (provide safe environment, limit physical activities, provide effective skin care and oral hygiene, control weight, and educate significant others)
      d. Assist parents in encouraging child to participate in intellectual pursuits rather than physical activities
   2. Fostering independence and normal growth and development in child
      a. Provide basic, motor, and physical needs appropriate to child's stage of growth and development
      b. Encourage child to learn self-help techniques
      c. Encourage child and parents to participate in group activities (hemophilia camps, group sessions)
   3. Providing supportive care for hemarthrosis
      a. Administer analgesics or sedatives
      b. Immobilize joint, and apply cold to area
      c. Prevent weight on affected joint (bed cradle, bed rest)
      d. Institute same care as for child with anemia (see Nursing care plan, p. 201)
   4. Observing for signs of critical sites of hemorrhage (intracranial, renal, arterial)

Thalassemia (Cooley's anemia)

A. In making additional assessment, observe signs of severe anemia (pallor, weakness), jaundice, abdominal distention, and cardiac failure
B. Problems include
   1. Stunted growth and enlarged flat bones
   2. Intraabdominal pressure
   3. Arrhythmias and cardiac failure
   4. Threat of death
C. Thalassemia is congenital deficiency in ability to synthesize mature hemoglobin
D. Diagnosis is based on clinical symptoms, family history (Mediterranean family), and hematologic studies
E. No cure for condition exists, and treatment is nonspecific and supportive
F. Nursing care plan involves the following (see also Nursing care plan, p. 201)
   1. Observe for complications of blood transfusion(s)
      a. Signs of transfusion reactions
      b. Signs of hemolysis (decreased circulating blood volume, renal shutdown, and shock)
      c. Signs of circulatory overload, electrolyte imbalance, and hypothermia
   2. Assist parents and child to adjust to life-threatening condition and effects
      a. Assist in adjustment to changes in body image (skeletal and skin)
      b. Support parents during critical developments in child's condition

CONGENITAL HEART DEFECTS

Assessment

Additional assessment of children with heart disease should include observation for the following
A. Cry—low pitch, weak, breathless
B. Color of skin—cyanotic (generalized; worse in supine position when crying; lessened slightly with administration of oxygen), pallor (may have mottled appearance on exertion)
C. Level of activity tolerance—seeks frequent rest periods; becomes restless or lethargic after activity, or cyanosis may worsen with minimal activity
D. Posture—assumes orthopneic position when in need of more oxygen; assumes knee-chest position; muscles are hypotonic
E. Heart rate—persistent bradycardia or tachycardia, respirations—tachypnea or dyspnea (with diaphoresis or grunting, gasping), retractions with nasal flaring
F. Feeding difficulties—anorexic, poor sucking ability, pulls away from nipple to catch breath

Cyanotic heart defects

A. Tetralogy of Fallot
   1. Problems include
      a. Polycythemia
      b. Anoxemia
   2. Tetralogy of Fallot is congenital defect associated with three conditions of heart: ventricular septal defect, pulmonary stenosis, and overrid-

ing aorta. As a result of these three defects, the right ventricle hypertrophies

3. Diagnosis is made on child's history and physical findings (clubbing of fingers, polycythemia, squatting after activity, and cyanosis)
4. Treatment is surgical intervention to increase pulmonary blood flow (infants—Waterston-Cooley shunt; children—Blalock-Taussig procedure)
5. Preoperative nursing care plan involves the following general procedures for child with heart surgery
   a. Familiarize child and family with equipment and expectations
      (1) Introduce staff to care for child after surgery (recovery room, intensive care unit)
      (2) Indicate equipment, noises, and lights with which child will come in contact after surgery
      (3) Utilize play therapy with dolls to demonstrate oxygen tents, endotracheal tubes, bandages, and tubes
      (4) Practice postoperative procedures (coughing and deep breathing, using blow bottles, using incentive spirometer, suctioning, turning, postural draining, and using bedpan or urinal)
   b. Collect data for comparison during postoperative period
      (1) Record vital signs (resting, following activity, signs of infection)
      (2) Monitor wake and sleep patterns, bowel habits, and normal fluid intake and preferences
   c. Prepare child for immediate preoperative procedures
      (1) Utilize explanations and play to prepare child for shave and preparation, nothing by mouth before surgery, and enemas
      (2) Demonstrate initial anesthetic preparation
6. Postoperative nursing care plan involves the following general procedures for child with heart surgery
   a. Decrease demand for oxygen by body cells
      (1) Provide maximum rest (plan care, analgesics, sedatives, and visiting hours)
      (2) Monitor vital signs with activity levels, and prevent overexertion of heart to meet oxygen demands
      (3) Maintain respiratory patency (suction, turn, cough, and deep breathe; ensure chest tube drainage; and report any sudden change in status)
      (4) Increase activity gradually (as ordered by physician)
   b. Provide adequate intake of fluids and nutrients
      (1) Maintain strict record of intake of all fluids during immediate postoperative period
      (2) Monitor daily morning weights
      (3) Monitor urine specific gravity, output, and bowel movements
      (4) Gradually increase diet by providing small frequent feeding of favorite foods (well-balanced diet as prescribed by physician)
   c. Provide comfort and emotional support
      (1) Observe child and family for appearance of anxiety, discuss precipitating factors, and allow expressions of feelings
      (2) Provide analgesics and position and support child when requesting child to perform painful procedures
      (3) Include parents in care, and encourage them to support child
   d. Observe for complications following heart surgery
      (1) Note change in vital signs, laboratory reports, and general condition (neurologic, cardiac, respiratory, renal)
      (2) Report all observations that indicate change in condition

B. Transposition of the great vessels
   1. Problems include
      a. Congestive heart failure
      b. Cardiomegaly
   2. Transposition of great vessels is several defects causing the pulmonary artery to exit from left ventricle and aorta to exit from right ventricle (unoxygenated blood sent to peripheral areas). Several defects may exist to support extrauterine life (atrial septa defect, patent ductus arteriosus, ventricular septal defect), but these also increase blood volume in heart and cause congestive heart failure
   3. Diagnosis is made soon after birth and is confirmed by cardiac catheterization

4. Treatment is palliative until child is old enough to tolerate extensive surgical repair
5. For nursing care plan, see Tetralogy of Fallot

C. Truncus arteriosus
1. Problems include
   a. Pulmonary congestion
   b. Anoxemia
   c. Congestive heart failure
2. Trunctus arteriosus is failure of pulmonary artery and aorta to separate in embryonic development. As a result, one vessel overrides both ventricles and sends blood to systemic and pulmonary areas simultaneously
3. Diagnosis is made soon after birth by clinical symptoms and distress of newborn
4. Treatment is palliative until infant is old enough for more extensive surgery. Palliative surgery is banding of pulmonary arteries to decrease blood flow to lungs
5. For nursing care plan, see Tetralogy of Fallot

Acyanotic heart defects

A. Coarctation of the aorta
1. Problems include
   a. Decreased blood pressure to areas distal to coarctation (insufficient renal circulation)
   b. Increased blood pressure to areas proximal to coarctation (intracranial hemorrhage)
2. Coarctation of aorta is narrowing of aorta. Type of coarctation depends on position of the narrowing (preductal-proximal to ductus arteriosus, or postductal-distal to ductus arteriosus)
3. Diagnosis of coarctation is based on clinical symptoms resulting in blood pressure differences in areas of body, depending on type of coarctation (early infancy after closure of ductus arteriosus—left ventricular hypertrophy; early adulthood when growth of aorta causes increased narrowing of aorta—decreased femoral pulses and muscle weakness and cramps in legs)
4. Treatment is surgical resection with end-to-end anastomoses or replacement of coarctation with graft
5. For nursing care plan, see Tetralogy of Fallot

B. Patent ductus arteriosus
1. Problems include
   a. Dyspnea on exertion
   b. Congestive heart failure
2. Patent ductus arteriosus is normal opening in fetal development to shunt circulating blood directly to systemic circulation and bypass lungs. The patent ductus arteriosus should close within a few hours or days after birth (except in prematurity when closure should occur at gestational maturity)
3. Diagnosis is made on auscultation of heart (machinelike murmur) and widening pulse pressure
4. Treatment is surgical division and ligation of the ductus
5. For nursing care plan, see Tetralogy of Fallot

C. Ventricular septal defect (VSD)
1. Problems with severe VSD include
   a. Retarded growth
   b. Pulmonary hypertension
   c. Cardiac failure
2. VSD is abnormal opening in septum between the ventricles
3. Diagnosis is made on auscultation of heart (loud, harsh murmur best heard at lower left sternal area)
4. Treatment is surgical closure of opening
5. For nursing care plan, see Tetralogy of Fallot

D. Atrial septal defect (ASD)
1. Problems with severe ASD include
   a. Cyanosis (if sinus venosus or endocardial cushion defect)
   b. Right atrial and ventricular hypertrophy
2. ASDs are abnormal openings in septum of the atriums. Three types of ASDs can occur: ostium secundum defect (failure of foramen ovale to close), ostium primum defect (inadequate development of endocardial cushions), and sinus venosus defect (superior section of atrial septum does not form)
3. Diagnosis is based on auscultation of murmur. Unless severe atrial septal defect exists, child is asymptomatic
4. Treatment is delayed (unless severe) until just before child enters school
5. For nursing care plan, see Tetralogy of Fallot

CONGENITAL CONDITIONS OF THE SKELETAL AND MUSCULAR SYSTEMS

Muscular dystrophy

A. Problems include
1. Contractures
2. Muscle atrophy

3. Infections
4. Cardiopulmonary complications
5. Obesity

B. Muscular dystrophy is believed to be metabolic disturbance not associated with nervous system
C. Diagnosis is made when child is noted to have progressive muscle weakness (delay in motor development) and difficulty with activities (changing position from sitting to standing)
D. Treatment is directed at maintaining function of muscles and prevention of complications (see problem list)
E. Nursing care plan involves
  1. Utilizing an interdisciplinary team to prepare child and parents in progressive, fatal disease
    a. Instruct parents and child in self-help techniques
    b. Instruct in observation of complications, especially signs of infections (pneumonia)
    c. Allow parents and child to express anticipatory feelings of grief and death
  2. Maintaining body function as long as possible
    a. Encourage range of motion exercises and physical therapy
    b. Control carbohydrates in diet to prevent obesity and undue exertion on muscles
    c. Encourage independence and social activity

Legg-Calvé-Perthes disease

A. Problems
  1. Immobility during treatment periods
  2. Loss of full range of motion in affected leg(s)
B. Legg-Calvé-Perthes disease is self-limiting aseptic necrosis of head of femur. Cause is unknown. Disease occurs in three distinct stages
  1. Avascular stage—decreased circulation and aseptic necrosis of femoral epiphysis
  2. Revascularization stage—circulation returns to area
  3. Regeneration stage—new bone formation and gradual reformation of femoral head
C. Diagnosis is based on child's history of leg pains, joint dysfunction, or inability to stand on affected leg(s)
D. Treatment is directed to allow stages to progress with no weight bearing on head of femur
E. Nursing care plan involves
  1. Providing child the opportunity to channel activities intellectually rather than physically during periods of immobilization
    a. During second and third stages of disease, child must be prevented from bearing weight on head of femur
    b. Instruct parents and child of need for continuing education, diversional activities, and range of motion exercises (except on affected limb, unless ordered by physician)
    c. Allow parents and child to express feelings and concerns of long periods of bed rest or restraints (traction, braces)
  2. Preparing parents for observing symptoms of recurrence of condition during next growth spurt
  3. Assisting child and parents to cope with physical limitations if treatment or conditions did not prevent flattening of head of femur (loss of range of motion in affected leg[s])

Scoliosis (structural)

A. In making additional assessment, have child bend downward and observe curvature of spine and muscle hypertrophy (rib and flank hump)
B. Problems include
  1. Change in body image
  2. Limitations on activity during treatment phases
  3. Interference in basic needs associated with psychosocial development (adolescent's identity development)
  4. Noncompliance with medical treatment by child
C. Structural scoliosis is an inherited or idiopathic lateral curvature of the spine, eventually causing alterations in appearance and physiologic aspects of spine, chest, and pelvis. Nonstructural scoliosis is differentiated from structural in that the curve in the spine is flexible
D. Diagnosis is based on clinical symptoms and radiologic examination of the spine
E. Treatment depends on type of scoliosis (nonstructural—bracing and exercises; structural—surgical spinal fusion followed by casting [body] to maintain alignment of spine)
F. Nursing care plan includes bracing and exercise
  1. Reinforce necessity of maintaining regimen
    a. Assist in measuring and maintaining alignment with Milwaukee brace
    b. Encourage child to practice daily exercises while in and out of brace

2. Allow child to express feelings of "being different"
   a. Assist child to cope with peer reactions
   b. Explain long-term benefits of wearing brace
   c. Assist child and parents with coping of long-term treatment regimen
3. Preoperative nursing care plan involves
   a. Preparing child and family for long period of immobilization during postoperative period
      (1) Explain and reinforce instructions provided by physician
      (2) Instruct in cast and hygienic care
      (3) Practice postoperative procedures (coughing, turning, voiding)
   b. Meeting child and family needs depending on type of preoperative treatments ordered (traction, brace)
4. Postoperative nursing care plan involves
   a. Observing for signs of infection and complications of immobilization
      (1) Monitor vital signs, "hot spots" on cast surface, and changes in pulmonary status
      (2) Encourage range of motion exercises to maintain muscle tone and prevent circulatory stasis
      (3) Observe for renal calculi and signs of urinary tract infection
   b. Providing diversional activity and supporting normal growth and development
      (1) Allow child to have choices in daily care routine
      (2) Permit peer interaction within institutional guidelines
      (3) Maintain and encourage interest in school activities
      (4) Encourage interest in activities within limitations of restrictions

Miscellaneous diseases occurring in children

INFECTIOUS DISEASES

Meningitis

A. In making assessment, note that symptoms can be influenced by age of child and bacteria causing infection
   1. Assessment in newborn—poor feeding, irritable, change in body temperature (hypothermia, fever), and cyanosis
   2. Assessment in infants and children—fever, vomiting, increasing irritability, and seizures
   3. Assessment in children (over 2 years of age) and adolescents—fever, chills, headache, vomiting, nuchal rigidity, and seizures

B. Problems include
   1. Peripheral circulatory collapse (more common in meningococcal meningitis)
   2. Hydrocephalus
   3. Behavioral changes
   4. Neurologic deficits (hemiparesis, deafness)

C. Meningitis can be caused by bacterial, viral, or tuberculous infection of the meninges

D. Diagnosis is determined by laboratory examination of cerebrospinal fluid, clinical symptoms, and culture and viral studies to determine cause of disease

E. Treatment is directed to reducing inflammatory response and complications and determining infecting organisms. Children with suspected meningitis should be isolated from others and maintained on intravenous fluids and electrolyte therapy, with control of seizure activity and drug therapy

F. Nursing care plan involves
   1. Preventing spread of infection (see Common infectious conditions in children, General nursing care plan)
   2. Monitoring and reporting neurologic status
      a. Make hourly neurologic assessment of pupil reaction and dilation, reflexes, level of consciousness, and behavior
      b. Observe for signs of complications (see problem list)
   3. Providing optimal care to unconscious child
      a. Maintain patent airway and pulmonary toileting (suctioning to prevent atelectasis)
      b. Maintain skin integrity and body hygiene
      c. Maintain muscle and joint condition by range of motion exercises (passive)
      d. Maintain nutritional state and hydration (diet and method of delivery as prescribed by physician)
      e. Observe for side effects of medications (antibiotics, steroids)
      f. Provide sensory stimulation (touch, sounds)
      g. Support parents by allowing parents to participate in care and to discuss fears and concerns
   4. Educating parents in need for follow-up care and observation of child's capabilities within normal stages of growth and development

Rheumatic fever

A. In making assessment, observe for presence of fever, epistaxis, weight loss, fatigue, signs of carditis (tachycardia, pericardial pain), migratory polyarthritis (joint inflammation and pain), and subcutaneous nodules
B. Problems include
   1. Pain (joint and pericardial)
   2. Fever and lassitude
   3. Cardiac involvement (rheumatic heart disease)
   4. Emotional reactions to long-term bed rest
C. Rheumatic fever is inflammatory disease most commonly related to group A beta-hemolytic streptococcal infections (more commonly follows throat infections). Susceptibility of individuals to rheumatic fever following streptococcal infections seems to be influenced by familial tendencies, overcrowded living conditions, lower socioeconomic level, and climate
D. Diagnosis is based on presentation of major manifestations (carditis, polyarthritis, chorea, subcutaneous nodules, and rash [erythema marginatum]) and laboratory tests (positive C-reactive protein, elevated erythrocyte sedimentation rate)
E. Treatment is antibiotic and steroid therapy, bed rest, and rheumatic process monitoring
F. Nursing care plan during acute phase involves
   1. Enforcing strict bed rest and decreasing workload on heart
      a. Provide comfort measures (back rubs, support of joints, turning)
      b. Discuss and reinforce necessity of bed rest (healing of heart)
      c. Provide diversional activities (appropriate to physician's orders on activities allowed), and promote continuing of education (as condition permits)
   2. Promoting comfort and relief of pain
      a. Position with care
      b. Provide hygiene and skin care to maintain integrity of skin
      c. Administer analgesics and sedatives (as ordered)
      d. Explain purposes and significance of frequent laboratory studies (inform child of the results as they pertain to increase in activities)
   3. Monitoring cardiac status and need for oxygen
      a. Record pulse and respirations when child is at rest and after activity
      b. Observe for signs of oxygen need (restlessness, fatigue, cyanosis)
      c. Monitor intake and output
   4. Maintaining nutritional state
      a. Encourage frequent small feedings of child's favorite food (child is usually anorexic)
      b. Provide food that can be easily chewed
      c. Offer fluids as child requires but not in excess
G. Nursing care plan during convalescent phase involves
   1. Providing activities to keep child entertained
      a. Select activities that encourage development and interests
      b. Select activities based on physical limitations
   2. Gradually increasing physical activity
      a. Follow physician's prescribed activity levels
      b. Explain to child and parents importance of adherence to regimen
   3. Preventing injury and infection
      a. Constant medical supervision is necessary
      b. Explain importance of prophylactic medications
      c. Prevent child from being exposed to persons with upper respiratory infections

Reye's syndrome

A. In making assessment, observe for signs of increased intracranial pressure, changes in level of consciousness, and respiratory distress
B. Problems include
   1. Coma
   2. Seizures
   3. Respiratory arrest
C. Reye's syndrome is acute encephalopathy of unknown cause. Clinical manifestations are identified in five stages, which proceed rapidly
   1. Vomiting and lethargy
   2. Acute change in behavior (delirium, combative)
   3. Decorticate rigidity and hyperventilation
   4. Fixed, dilated pupils, deep coma, and loss of ocular reflex
   5. Seizures and respiratory arrest
D. Diagnosis is based on history of recent influenza symptoms, laboratory tests (elevated liver enzymes) and clinical manifestation stages

E. Nursing care plan involves
  1. Providing critical care and observation of child
    a. Maintain patent airway
    b. Assist physician and other personnel to perform procedures and secure laboratory samples
    c. Monitor vital signs and neurologic status every 15 minutes
    d. Monitor intake and output of fluids
    e. Observe for signs of impaired liver function (increased bleeding time, jaundice, ascites)
  2. Supporting parents during critical stages of disease
    a. Inform parents of reason for intensive care nursing
    b. Reinforce information provided by physician to parents
    c. Assist parents to adjust and cope with crisis (see Unit 7, Crisis intervention)

Croup (acute spasmodic laryngitis)

A. In making assessment, observe child for "barking" sound to cough, cyanosis, and dyspnea
B. Problems include
  1. Parental anxiety
  2. Respiratory difficulty in child
C. Croup is acute infection of larynx. Croup can be precipitated by change in environmental temperature and viral infections (except in cases resulting from diptheria, pertussis, or acute epiglottis), and it is commonly seen in hyperactive children in early night hours
D. Diagnosis is based on presenting symptoms
E. Treatment is directed at decreasing laryngeal spasms (administration of syrup of ipecac, sedatives, and bronchodilators) and liquidizing secretions (humidified air)
F. Nursing care plan involves
  1. Providing rest and comfort to child
    a. Administer medications as ordered by physician
    b. Position in orthopneic or semi-Fowler's position under croup tent
    c. Reassure child, and calm anxiety resulting from strange environment and respiratory difficulty
    d. Supply quiet diversional activity
  2. Maintaining patent airway and observing for increased respiratory difficulty
    a. Have available tracheostomy tray and airway
    b. Administer humidified air (croup tent)
    c. Administer oxygen as ordered by physician
    d. Encourage liquids after laryngeal spasms have ceased
  3. Alleviating anxiety in parents
    a. Explain low communicability of croup
    b. Assure parents that child usually does have acute symptoms that will resolve when laryngeal spasms are gone
    c. Instruct parents in home measures to relieve laryngeal spasms (hot shower's steam to be inhaled by child)

NEUROLOGIC DEFICITS

Cerebral palsy

A. In making assessment, observe motor development for delayed or abnormal movements, abnormal posture, and presence of infantile reflexes past normal existence
B. Problems include
  1. Muscle weakness
  2. Difficulty with voluntary movements
  3. Possible mental disabilities
C. Cerebral palsy is condition of neuromuscular impairment resulting from brain trauma or various prenatal, perinatal, and postnatal factors (maternal anemia, pregnancy-induced hypertension, birth trauma, head trauma, meningitis). Brain pathophysiologic changes are nonspecific; occasionally neuromuscular dysfunctions will indicate anatomic location of brain dysfunction
D. Diagnosis is based on maternal and infant history, neurologic examination of child, and clinical manifestations
E. Treatment is directed at habilitating child to function as independently as possible with minimal limitations. Physical therapy is used to train child to use and control certain motor groups and to prevent contractures in spastic motor groups
F. Nursing care plan involves
  1. Detecting gross motor deficits in early development
    a. Determine from maternal-infant history if poor motor and/or muscular development have been noted
    b. Educate parents in normal growth and development
  2. Supporting parents in coping with emotional responses associated with having a handicapped child

a. Assist parents in establishing goals for daily management of child
b. Provide support and encouragement
c. Assist parents to cope with commonly observed behavior problems of children with cerebral palsy

Mental retardation

A. In making assessment, observe newborn for characteristics of inherited syndromes associated with mental retardation (Down's syndrome), and observe children for learning disabilities, delayed psychosocial development, and behavior problems
B. Problems include the following (depend on extent of retardation)
   1. Borderline—slow in academic abilities
   2. Mild—difficulty with social skills and daily life crises
   3. Moderate—difficulty in training to do home tasks
   4. Severe—impaired judgment, physical and social limitations
   5. Profound—immobility or limited ability to move, tendency for upper respiratory infections
C. Mental retardation is broad classification of varying degrees of social and intellectual dysfunction. Mental retardation can be a result of heredity or trauma to brain (infection, fevers, birth process, prenatal trauma)
D. Diagnosis can be determined by chromosomal studies for inherited conditions (Down's syndrome), psychologic testing, and academic capabilities (IQ tests)
E. Nursing care plan involves
   1. Encouraging child to learn self-help skills
      a. Teach child, and allow child opportunity to feed, bathe, dress, and groom self
      b. Instruct parents to continue skills learned by child in home
   2. Providing child opportunity to develop to optimal developmental level
      a. Allow child opportunity to play, communicate with others, and learn social skills
      b. Encourage parents to establish limits to child's behavior
   3. Protecting child from infection and communicable diseases by sound nutrition, immunizations, and environmental control

MATERNAL AND CHILD HEALTH REVIEW QUESTIONS

Read each question carefully, and consider all possible answers. When you have decided which answer is **best,** blacken the corresponding space on the answer sheet. There is only **one** best answer for each question.

Situation: Mrs. Mary Jones suspects she is pregnant. She has missed two menstrual periods and decides to go to the physician to confirm her suspicions.

1 From this time until term, the growing child in Mrs. Jones' uterus is called the
1. Embryo
2. Fetus
3. Gamete
4. Egg

2 Some positive signs of pregnancy that would be detected by the physician are
(A) Palpation of the fetus
(B) Feeling and seeing active movements
(C) Seeing the skeleton on x-ray film
(D) Cessation of menstruation
(E) Hearing the fetal heartbeat
1. B, C, and E
2. A, B, and E
3. B, C, and D
4. A, B, D, and E

3 In order to estimate delivery date, Mrs. Jones would
1. Count 300 days from the first day of the last menstruation
2. Count back 7 months from the first day of the last menstrual period and add 3 days
3. Count back 3 months from the first day of the last menstrual period and add 7 days
4. Count 200 days from the first day of the last menstrual period

4 Prenatal examination includes the following
(A) Routine physical examination
(B) Past medical history
(C) Urinalysis
(D) Temperature, pulse, and respiration
(E) Gallbladder series
1. B
2. B and C
3. B, C, D, and E
4. A, B, C, and D

5 Nausea and vomiting are common during the
1. First trimester
2. Second trimester
3. Third trimester
4. Entire pregnancy

6 Nausea and vomiting can be controlled by
(A) Liquid diet
(B) High-fat diet
(C) High-protein diet
(D) High-carbohydrate diet
(E) Frequent small feedings
1. B and D
2. B, C, and E
3. C, D, and E
4. A, B, and C

7 Backache is relieved by
1. Mustard plasters
2. Tight-fitting girdles
3. High-heeled shoes
4. Low-heeled shoes

8 The most acceptable theory at present maintains that labor is usually started by
(A) A cathartic
(B) Hormones
(C) Digestive juices
(D) Fetal movements
(E) A vaginal douche
1. B and D
2. A, B, and E
3. D
4. B

9 "Show" is
1. Enlarged abdomen
2. Fetal head in vagina
3. Pinkish vaginal discharge
4. Leaking bag of water

10 Charting during labor should consist of
1. Full note charting, including graphic sheets
2. Graphic charting only
3. Minimal notes with complete antepartal history
4. Medical record

11 During the first stage of labor the nurse should watch for
(A) Meconium in the discharge
(B) Change in blood pressure
(C) Appearance of the child's head
(D) Prolapsed cord
(E) Excessive bleeding
1. A, C, D, and E
2. A, B, D, and E
3. B, C, D, and E
4. A, B, C, and E

12 The period from the complete dilation of the cervix until the delivery of the child is called
1. First stage
2. Second stage
3. Third stage
4. Pregnancy

13 During the second stage of labor the mother should be encouraged to
(A) Bear down with contractions
(B) Relax with contractions
(C) Rest between contractions
(D) Bear down between contractions
(E) Breathe through mouth during contractions
1. A and E
2. B, D, and E
3. A and C
4. A

14 Episiotomy means
1. Forceps delivery
2. Incision of the perineum
3. Breech presentation
4. Version

15 Anesthetics that may be used during delivery are
(A) Inhalation
(B) Spinal or caudal
(C) Rectal
(D) Local
(E) Hypodermic
(F) Hypnosis
1. A, B, D, E, and F
2. A, B, C, E, and F
3. B, C, D, E, and F
4. A, B, C, D, and E

16 The purpose of massaging the uterus after delivery is to
1. Keep it contracted
2. Help it to relax
3. Quiet the patient
4. Follow hospital routine

17 The expression "afterpains" means
1. Contractions of the uterus after delivery
2. Uterine contractions occurring usually after the second delivery
3. Uterine contractions that usually stop 2 days after the delivery
4. Pain in the breasts after delivery

18 "Rooming-in" means that the
1. Newborn is in a crib at the mother's bedside
2. Mother is in a two- to six-bed ward
3. Mother does not see the infant until she goes home
4. Infant sleeps in bed with the mother

19 Birth registration is the responsibility of the
1. Father
2. Mother
3. Physician
4. Nurse

20 Instillation of drops in the newborn's eyes is
(A) A legal responsibility
(B) The responsibility of the physician
(C) Done 2 days after birth
(D) A 10% solution
(E) Wiped out after instillation
1. B
2. A
3. A, B, C, and D
4. A, B, C, D, and E

21 The best care of the umbilical cord stump is to
1. Leave it uncovered
2. Cover it aseptically
3. Pull it off when loose
4. Cauterize with phenol

22 Prematurity in a newborn is determined by
(A) Weight and gestational age
(B) Term of pregnancy
(C) General appearance and weight
(D) Low temperature
1. A
2. C and D
3. A, B, and C
4. A, B, C, and D

23 Some known facts about abortion are that it
(A) Means the interruption of pregnancy before the seventh month
(B) Always has legal implications
(C) Carries the danger of bleeding
(D) Carries the danger of infection
(E) Is best treated by prevention
1. A, B, and D
2. B, C, D, and E
3. A, C, D, and E
4. A, B, C, D, and E

24 A form of pregnancy-induced hypertension is
1. Hyperemesis gravidarum
2. Placenta previa
3. Preeclampsia
4. Abruptio placentae

25 In giving perineal care to the obstetric patient, the important points to remember are
(A) Solution ordered
(B) Steps of the procedure
(C) Cleanliness
(D) Temperature of the solution
1. A and B
2. A and C
3. A, C, and D
4. A, B, C, and D

26 The perineal pad is removed from
1. Front to back
2. Back to front
3. Right side
4. Left side

27 A sitz bath for the obstetric patient would be used to
1. Begin labor
2. Soothe and heal the perineum
3. Enhance uterine involution
4. Provide personal hygiene

28 The perineal light is used
1. Before the sitz bath
2. After the sitz bath
3. As ultraviolet radiation
4. For 1 hour

29 Tucks (astringent gauze) on stitches is applied
1. Routinely after the perineal light
2. Directly on the stitches as needed
3. On the stitches as ordered by the physician
4. Routinely before the perineal light

30 Mrs. Jones is having difficulty in voiding; the nurse can employ all of the following nursing measures to help her void except
1. Giving her more fluids to drink
2. Allowing water to run for her to hear
3. Catheterizing her
4. Having her blow bubbles in the water through a straw

31 Mrs. Jones asks the nurse, "What position can I use in bed now that I have had the baby?" The nurse answers
1. "It is best that you lie on your back."
2. "It is best that you lie on either side."
3. "Do not lie on your abdomen."
4. "You can lie in any comfortable position."

32 An abdominal binder is not put on after delivery because it
1. Displaces pelvic organs
2. Predisposes to involution
3. Encourages relaxation of abdominal muscles
4. Slips out of position and contaminates the perineal area

33 The nurse would inform Mrs. Jones that, unless specifically told to do so by her physician, she should not
1. Wash her hair
2. Take vaginal douches
3. Take a daily shower
4. Resume her housework

34 Routine breast care for Mrs. Jones would include
1. Daily cleansing with clear water
2. Cleansing the nipples with alcohol
3. Cleansing the nipples with boric acid
4. Massaging the breasts with cold cream

35 In getting Mrs. Jones up for the first time the nurse would
1. Lift her from the bed to the chair
2. Walk her to the bathroom
3. Let her dangle her feet for a few minutes
4. Ask a a nursing assistant to help her

36 In checking Mrs. Jones' fundus, the nurse should normally find the consistency
1. Boggy
2. Soft
3. Firm
4. All of these

37 Two days after delivery, Mrs. Jones is complaining of afterpains; the nurse should
1. Dismiss their importance
2. Give analgesic per standing order
3. Massage the abdomen
4. Apply a heating pad to the abdomen

38 The primary reason for identifying the newborn in the delivery room is that
1. It is required by law
2. It prevents a mix-up in the nursery
3. The mother and newborn have not yet been separated, and there is little chance of a mistake
4. The delivery room nurse has the equipment

39 A permanent method of identifying the newborn would be by
1. Ident-a-band
2. Wristlet and anklet
3. Footprints
4. Bead necklace

40 The head of the bassinet is slightly lower in order to
1. Stimulate circulation
2. Prevent aspiration
3. Prevent respiratory infection
4. Prevent shock

41 The principle underlying the concept of demand feedings for the newborn is
1. Maintaining a rigid 4-hour schedule to establish eating habits
2. Feeding every 3 hours to stimulate digestion
3. Fitting individual feedings to individual needs
4. Ensuring an adequate nutritional intake

42 After a protracted labor and a difficult delivery, the newborn's head has an elongated appearance. Which of the following statements would be true?
1. The newborn's head is molded during delivery and will return to normal in a few days
2. All newborns' heads are shaped this way
3. It will take 6 months for the head to return to normal
4. The head will remain in that shape

Situation: Mrs. Jones has just left the hospital and might ask the following questions. What should be the nurse's answer?

43 When can I go out to visit now that I am home?
1. "Go out right now if you wish."
2. "You should wait at least 1 week and then go out for only short intervals."
3. "You should wait 4 weeks and then just go to the neighbors."
4. "You should wait until your checkup."

44 When shall I see the doctor again?
1. "In 2 weeks."
2. "In 4 weeks."
3. "In 6 weeks."
4. "In 8 weeks."

45 When can I take my first tub bath?
1. "In 3 weeks."
2. "In 4 weeks."
3. "In 5 weeks."
4. "As instructed by the physician."

46 How long should I refrain from intercourse?
1. "For 2 weeks."
2. "Whenever you feel like it."
3. "After the physician examines you at his or her office."
4. "At least 1 year for birth control."

47 What should I eat?
1. "Continue essentially the same diet as during pregnancy."
2. "Eat a low-salt diet."
3. "Eat a high-carbohydrate diet."
4. "Eat a high-fat diet."

---

48 The chief reason that physicians recommend that new mothers refrain from sexual intercourse is to aid in preventing
1. Pregnancy
2. Subinvolution
3. Introduction of infection
4. Injury to the vagina

49 In a good knee-chest position
1. The thighs are perpendicular to the floor
2. The back is straight
3. The knees are slightly separated
4. All of these

Situation: A nurse studying the care of children needs to consider the following facts.

50 Knowledge of normal growth and development of the child is essential to the nurse because
1. It is basic to understanding the sick child
2. Most nurses have children
3. Most children do not get sick
4. It helps the nurse to be a good father or mother

51 Growth and development of the child
1. Occurs in an orderly process
2. Occurs in spurts and plateaus
3. Is influenced only by the environment
4. Is determined by a genetic code

52 Chronologically, infancy is that period
1. From birth to 6 months
2. From 4 weeks to 1 year
3. From birth to 2 years
4. From birth to 3 years

53 During the toddler years, the average child
(A) Learns his or her relationship to members of the family
(B) Obtains satisfaction by sucking and putting things in the mouth
(C) Becomes aware of the immediate environment
(D) Increases interest in personal appearance and the opposite sex
(E) Learns control of body elimination
1. A and E
2. B and C
3. A, C, and E
4. C and D

54 Normal desires of the adolescent include
(A) Recognition by family and friends
(B) Acceptance of sexual changes
(C) Help in making decisions about school or work
(D) Understanding of physical and emotional changes
1. B, C, and D
2. A, B, and D
3. A, B, and C
4. A, C, and D

55 The number of deciduous teeth is
1. Eighteen
2. Twenty
3. Twenty-two
4. Twenty-four

56 The nursery staff are the primary persons who control infection in a newborn nursery. This is best accomplished by
1. Wearing masks and gowns
2. A 10-minute scrub on arrival on duty
3. Hand washing between caring for each newborn
4. Routine nasopharynx cultures of staff

57 Techniques of feeding children include the following principles
(A) Have them eat all food on their plates
(B) Disguise the taste of one food with another
(C) Begin the use of the cup and spoon at 4 months of age
(D) Allow child to feed self after the age of 2
(E) Introduce a new food with each meal
1. A
2. B
3. C
4. D

58 Mrs. Hesse is inexperienced with children and nervous about handling her newborn. Which of the following approaches would be best?
(A) Allow her to handle her newborn and assist as needed
(B) Demonstrate proper bathing and handling techniques
(C) Tell her she will get used to her newborn after a while
(D) Suggest she attend infant care classes
1. A and C
2. A and B
3. A, B, and D
4. A, B, C, and D

59 The most effective toilet training includes the following principles
(A) Readiness of the child physically and emotionally
(B) Avoidance of tension
(C) Stimulation of interest in developing a habit
(D) Expression of approval when successful
1. C and D
2. B, C, and D
3. A, B, and D
4. A, B, C, and D

60 Children's books should possess the following
1. Emotional value
2. Suitability to the individual child's need
3. Educational value
4. A morale factor

61 In considering a child's recreation one should plan for
(A) At least two to play
(B) A party to top off each play period
(C) Activities in which the child can express him- or herself
(D) Activities from which the child obtains pleasure
(E) The proper use of toys
1. B and C
2. D and E
3. C and D
4. D and E

62 Sex education of the child
(A) Begins with a child's curiosity
(B) Should be explained at the child's level of understanding
(C) Is part of normal development
(D) Should imply guilt and shame
1. B, C, and D
2. A, C, and D
3. C
4. A, B, and C

63 Hospital procedures for a child are
1. The same in each hospital
2. Different in basic principles from those for adults
3. Entirely different for each age group
4. The same in principle as those for adults

64 The temperature of the child under 4 years of age should be taken by
1. Mouth
2. Rectum
3. Mouth or rectum
4. Axilla

65 Children are sometimes restrained during treatments; this is done in order to
1. Ensure that the child cannot see treatment performed
2. Keep the child in the proper position
3. Quiet the child
4. Comfort the child

66 A child with "growing" pains should be
1. Encouraged to forget them
2. Hospitalized at once
3. Given a thorough physical examination
4. Watched for a couple of weeks

67 A mother tells you that her 1-month-old infant sleeps most of the time and cries when awake. How best can you allay the mother's anxiety?
1. "Crying is the way your infant lets you know when she is uncomfortable. An infant needs a lot of sleep and is usually awake only 4 hours a day."
2. "Infants sleep 20 out of the 24 hours in a day. How do you comfort the infant when she cries?"
3. "Sleep is most important to an infant, and if you provide for all her basic needs, she will not cry."
4. "Infants need a lot of sleep. If you let her cry, she will get tired and stop."

68 Nursing care of croup includes
(A) Providing humidified air
(B) Holding the child during spasms
(C) Reporting the spasm to the charge nurse or doctor
(D) Giving fluids during the spasm
1. B, C, and D
2. A, C, and D
3. A, B, and D
4. A, B, and C

69 Rheumatic fever is caused by
1. A virus
2. Hemolytic streptococci
3. Staphylococci
4. An ameba

70 Convalescent nursing care of rheumatic fever consists of
1. Protection from colds and infections
2. Unlimited activity
3. Avoidance of mental fatigue
4. Daily reading of books to a child

71 In explaining an infant's diet and feeding schedule to a mother, the following principles are included. Which is the most important to emphasize?
1. New foods are introduced one at a time to observe for allergies.
2. Pureed fruits and cereals are added when formula no longer satisfies the infant.
3. Solid foods are added when the infant begins to chew.
4. Formula feedings are supplemented with plenty of water.

72 Nursing care of eczema includes
(A) Keeping the skin and clothing clean and dry
(B) Using warm soaks to soothe
(C) Preventing the child from scratching
(D) Helping to find the cause
(E) Leaving the patient in the same position
1. B, C, and E
2. A, C, and D
3. B and C
4. C, D, and E

73 The most important thing to remember about accidents is
1. Immediate treatment
2. Prevention
3. Obtaining a physician
4. Getting to a hospital

74 To prevent accidents when caring for children the nurse should remember to
1. Leave the crib sides up
2. Keep child in crib at all times
3. Have a gateway in door
4. Keep room tidy and environment safe

75 The adjustment of an infant to hospitalization depends on
1. The nurse's adeptness in caring for the infant
2. The nurse's personality
3. The parents' feelings and participation in care
4. The relationship of the parents and the nurse

76 Preschool children develop emotional satisfaction by
(A) Imitation
(B) Physical activity
(C) Attending the movies
(D) Developing complete independence
(E) Contacts with family and friends
1. A, C, and E
2. C, D, and E
3. A, B, and E
4. B, C, and E

77 In infant feeding the principle of allowing the infant to establish his or her own time schedule is called
1. Forced feeding
2. Demand feeding
3. Irregular feeding
4. Daytime feeding

78 You would position an infant for an enema by placing him or her
1. On the right side (give 100 ml solution)
2. On the left side (give only up to 100 ml solution)
3. The same as for an adult
4. In a semi-upright position on the bedpan

79 A child has become ill in a home where the nurse is caring for another member of the family. The physician has been called. Until he or she arrives the nurse should
(A) Keep the child in bed
(B) Take his TPR
(C) Save specimens of urine, feces, and vomitus
(D) Let other children help to keep him quiet
(E) Place a hot-water bottle on his abdomen
1. B, C, and E
2. A, B, and C
3. C, D, and E
4. A, C, and E

80 Five-year-old Johnny has chickenpox. Chickenpox is spread by
(A) The crust that scales off
(B) Discharge from the vesicles of the rash
(C) Secretions from the nose and throat
(D) Secretions from the eyes
1. A and C
2. B and C
3. B and D
4. C and D

81 It is difficult for Johnny to keep from scratching the lesions; therefore, the nurse should apply
(A) Old socks as mitts
(B) Restraints to hands and feet
(C) Jacket restraint
(D) Elbow restraints
1. A and D
2. B and D
3. A and C
4. C and D

82 Two-year-old Sheryl was found to have lead in her urine. She was admitted for observation and treatment with EDTA. In caring for her, which of the following is most important to her progress?
1. Close observation of intake and output
2. Weighing her daily
3. Forcing fluids
4. Giving the medicine on time

83 Three-year-old Tommy was admitted with the diagnosis of laryngotracheobronchitis. The most important concern of the nurse in caring for Tommy is
1. Removal of copious secretions
2. Maintaining a patent airway
3. Controlling the high fever
4. Close observation of vital signs

84 Tommy had a stool culture for ova and parasites that indicated pinworms. It is most important for his parents to
1. Have all family members treated with Antepar
2. Get rid of the two dogs in the family
3. Burn the contaminated linen and clothing
4. Treat the family with Antepar, and boil the linens and clothes

85 Roundworms differ from pinworms in that they are transmitted by
1. Contaminated food
2. Air
3. Cats
4. Contaminated soil

86 A goal of nursing care in the treatment of nephrosis is to
1. Prevent child from playing to allow for rest
2. Provide emotional support to child because of change in appearance
3. Isolate child to prevent transmission of nephrosis to other children
4. Encourage increased fluid intake

87 Frances is a 10-year-old neighbor's child. She spends many evenings talking with you about her interests. The best example of a 10-year-old child's interest is
1. An art museum
2. Imitation of activities of mother
3. A club of mixed sex
4. A heroine's life

88 A self-limiting necrosis of the head of the femur is
1. Slipped epiphysis
2. Osteoporosis
3. Rickets
4. Legg-Calvé-Perthes disease

89 Compared to an adult, the administration of medications (oral and injections) to an infant varies in that
1. Medicines must be diluted
2. Oral medicine is given crushed in liquid form, and injections are given in the anteriolateral thigh
3. All medicines are in prepared dosage form
4. Oral medicines are given in liquid form, and the deltoid muscle is preferred site for injections

90 Seven-year-old Linda has the measles. The symptoms of measles are
(A) Macular rash starting at the hairline and behind ears and neck and then spreading over the body
(B) Elevated temperature with running nose and sore throat
(C) Cough
(D) Koplik's spots
(E) Vomiting
1. A, B, D, and E
2. A, B, C, and E
3. A, C, D, and E
4. A, B, C, and D

91 If Linda's eyes become inflamed (conjunctivitis), the treatment would include
(A) Wearing colored glasses
(B) Rinsing her eyes with a 4% solution of boric acid
(C) Avoiding reading
(D) Putting drops in her eyes
(E) Avoiding bright lights in her room
1. A, C, and E
2. A, B, and E
3. B, D, and E
4. C, D, and E

92 When playing with other children, a toddler's play can best be described as
1. Parallel
2. Competitive
3. Cooperative
4. Sharing

93 In hospitalization of a toddler, the nursing staff should not take the responsibility for
1. Toilet training
2. Introducing new foods to diet
3. Preparing the child for hospitalization
4. Mediating in conflicts between child and family

94 The treatment of croup is
1. Highly humidified, cool oxygen and sedatives for rest
2. Vaporized oxygen and sedatives
3. Highly humidified, warm air and syrup of ipecac
4. Rest, antibiotics, and oxygen

95 When Mrs. Mallory went to the physician for prenatal care, her VDRL was positive. This indicates
1. Measles
2. Gonorrhea
3. Syphilis
4. Anemia

96 Because Mrs. Malloy was in the first trimester of pregnancy, she was given a massive dose of
1. Aureomycin
2. Benzathine penicillin G (Bicillin)
3. Vioform
4. Chloromycetin

97 Mrs. Malloy told the nurse she was always careful to bathe daily, so how could she possibly have syphilis. The best reply for the nurse to make is
1. "You should douche daily also."
2. "Perhaps you should use a stronger soap for bathing."
3. "You should always clean commode seats thoroughly."
4. "Syphilis is contracted by sexual intercourse and other intimate contact."

98 After careful examination, 10-year-old George was said to be a diphtheria "carrier." This means that he
1. Has a serious case of diphtheria and should be hospitalized immediately
2. Is recuperating from diphtheria
3. Carries the disease-causing organism but does not have the disease himself
4. Contracts diphtheria each time he is exposed

99 Mrs. Little complains that Alice, 24 months old, never takes time to eat and appears to be losing weight. It is important that you explain that
1. Alice's body needs less food, and she will grow out of it
2. Alice needs a balanced diet, but her body requires less amounts of food
3. Between meal snacks will help compensate for what she does not eat at meal time
4. Alice will eat what she needs and is now developing preferences for foods

100 The adolescent male patient with mumps must take precautions to avoid developing the complication of
1. Otitis media
2. Orchitis
3. Heart murmur
4. Calcification of the gland

101 The skin test given to determine susceptibility to diphtheria is
1. PPD test
2. Salk test
3. Dick test
4. Schick test

102 Mrs. Vincent is 4 months pregnant. The physician has asked her to keep her calories at 1800 per day. The best ways to do this will be to
(A) Omit breakfast
(B) Omit milk
(C) Use fresh fruits for desserts
(D) Omit gravies and sauces
1. A and C
2. B and C
3. C and D
4. B and D

103 Mrs. Vincent's supper exchange list has one milk exchange; she may use
(A) One cup fortified milk
(B) One-half cup evaporated milk
(C) One-fourth cup condensed milk
(D) One cup pasteurized milk
1. A, B, or C
2. B, C, or D
3. A, B, or D
4. Any of these

104 At bedtime Mrs. Vincent has one milk exchange and one bread exchange; she may have
1. Cornflakes and milk
2. Ice cream
3. Skim milk, crackers, and peanut butter
4. Soda and potato chips

105 When her friends stop at the drugstore for a soda, Mrs. Vincent may have
(A) Iced tea
(B) Hot coffee
(C) White soda
(D) Beer
1. A
2. C
3. A or B
4. B or D

106 Mrs. Green was told to use lactose in her baby's formula; she would
1. Use the sugar from the sugar bowl
2. Strain oatmeal
3. Purchase it at the drugstore
4. Use dry milk powder

107 Johnny is in the first grade and does not want to eat breakfast. The best ways to cope with the situation are
(A) Pay him 25 cents each time he eats breakfast
(B) Let him go without breakfast, but give him a candy bar to eat at recess
(C) Let him help decide his breakfast menu
(D) Make breakfast a family affair
1. C and D
2. A and B
3. B and D
4. A and C

108 Five-year-old Elsie does not like to eat; she can be helped most by
1. Demanding that she eat everything on her plate
2. Putting the timer on so that she will know when she must finish
3. Giving her small servings
4. Feeding her between meals instead of at the table

109 Mrs. Young's 6-year-old daughter has asthma. The physician wants her to omit eggs from her diet. For a bedtime snack she may have
(A) Cream puffs
(B) Cheese and crackers
(C) Cornflakes and milk
(D) Chocolate cake
1. A and B
2. C and D
3. B and D
4. B and C

110 Randy, 4 years old, has pneumonia. He receives antibiotics by injection every 6 hours. The nurse can best help Randy cope with his fear of injections by
1. Allowing him to use needle play with a doll
2. Asking physician to change the medicine to tablet form
3. Teaching Randy to give his own injections
4. Letting Randy save the used syringes without the needle

111 Sixteen-year-old Jim plays football every night after school. He becomes hungry between meals. The best foods for him to select are
1. Milk and fresh fruit
2. Candy bars
3. Potato chips and soda
4. Chile and crackers

112 Erythroblastosis fetalis is caused by
(A) ABO incompatibility
(B) Phenylpyruvic acid in urine
(C) Rh incompatibility
(D) Phenylalanine in blood
(E) Elevated bilirubin level in blood
1. A and B
2. B and D
3. A and C
4. A, B, C, D, and E

113 Early detection of possible erythroblastosis fetalis requires observation of
(A) Jaundice soon after birth
(B) Yellow-tinged vernix caseosa
(C) Susceptibility to eczema
(D) Neurologic disturbances
(E) Yellow-tinged cord
(F) PKU test
1. A
2. A and B
3. A, B, and E
4. C, D, and F

114 Treatment for erythroblatosis fetalis includes
1. Diet low in phenylalanine within 2 to 3 weeks after birth
2. Diet low in protein and high in fat
3. Replacement of 85% of infant's blood soon after birth
4. None of these

115 The years of adolescence are very difficult for the child and his or her family. This is characteristic of the age because the adolescent is attempting to
1. Become involved in romantic affairs
2. Make decisions about his or her future
3. Show need for help from parents
4. Discover self-identity

116 Adolescence is considered to begin when
1. Growth rate increases rapidly
2. Secondary sex characteristics appear
3. The child begins taking interest in his or her appearance
4. The child shows interest in the opposite sex

117 Karen has acute acne problems. In talking with her about this problem it is important to emphasize
1. Personal hygiene and diet low in fats and carbohydrates
2. Rest and routine administration of topical antibiotics
3. Sunlight, exercise, and high-carbohydrate diet
4. Balanced diet and limited exercise

118 At 24 hours of age, Roy Hesse appears jaundiced. He is irritable and not eating well. These symptoms could indicate
1. Phenylketonuria
2. Milk allergy
3. Physiologic jaundice
4. ABO incompatibility

119 Problems encountered by parents during the child-rearing stage of the family cycle are
(A) Adjustment to parental roles
(B) Allowing child to become dependent
(C) Avoiding using child to satisfy parents' own needs
(D) Balancing the needs of the children with the parents' personal and marital needs
1. A, C, and D
2. A, B, and D
3. A, B, and C
4. B, C, and D

120 Skills and attitudes important for the adolescent to acquire before leaving the family circle include
(A) Adequate skills for either beginning a job or entering a higher educational level
(B) Realistic attitude toward opposite sex
(C) Preparation for marriage and a family
(D) Emotional dependence on parents
1. B, C, and D
2. A, B, and D
3. A, B, and C
4. A, C, and D

121 Difficulties with adolescents encountered by parents may be the result of
1. Fear of independence
2. Immaturity or instability
3. Conflict in cultural value
4. Large family

122 Girl Adams, 2 days old, has excessive mucus and salivation. She has been diagnosed as having a tracheoesophageal fistula. In feeding her the nurse is responsible for
1. Adequate intake
2. Sucking before feeding
3. Preventing aspiration
4. Preventing vomiting

123 The first immunization given to an infant at 2 months of age is
1. DPT and rubella
2. Diptheria, pertussis, tetanus toxoid (DPT)
3. DPT and trivalent oral polio virus (TOPV)
4. Measles and mumps

124 Amenorrhea is
1. Painful menstruation
2. Abnormal menstrual flow
3. Bleeding irregularly
4. Absence of menstruation

125 Fertilization of the ovum usually takes place in the
1. Fallopian tubes
2. Ovary
3. Uterus
4. Abdomen

126 The region between the vaginal orifice and the rectum is called the
1. Cul-de-sac
2. Perineum
3. Peritoneum
4. Fourchette

127 The term "dystocia" means
1. Difficult labor
2. Diminished strength of contractions
3. Continuous uterine contractions
4. Short labor

128 In breech presentation the presenting part of the fetus is the
1. Shoulder
2. Face
3. Brow
4. Buttocks

129 One of the most important functions of the amniotic fluid is to
1. Provide nourishment to the fetus
2. Absorb waste products of the fetus
3. Act as a cushion for the fetus against injuries
4. Prevent the cord from wrapping around the fetus' neck

130 The most important principles for a mother to remember concerning diet in pregnancy are
(A) Basic Four foods
(B) Force fluids
(C) Feeding two
(D) Quality of food
(E) Dieting
1. A, B, and C
2. A and D
3. A, D, and E
4. A, B, C, D, and E

131 A pregnant woman who has a tendency toward varicose veins should be advised never to wear a
1. Foundation garment
2. Two-way stretch girdle
3. Round garter
4. Garter belt

132 If the newborn has difficulty grasping the nipple because of breast engorgement, the nurse should explain that
1. It would be best to omit breast feedings
2. It would be best to feed the baby less often
3. The baby is not going to be able to nurse
4. This is a common temporary condition that should not interfere with nursing

133 Breast-feeding is contraindicated if
1. The newborn is jaundiced
2. The newborn spits up milk with bubbling
3. The newborn was born by cesarean section
4. The mother has tuberculosis

134 The government agency that outlines standards for obstetric care is the Department of
1. Health and Human Services
2. Labor
3. Interior
4. Commerce

135 The greatest factor influencing decreased maternal mortality and morbidity is
1. Better hospital facilities
2. Healthier adult population
3. Improvement in prenatal care
4. New drugs and treatments

136 The majority of all deaths during the first year of life occur during the first
1. Twenty-four hours
2. Month
3. Six months
4. Nine months

137 The bone of the newborn most frequently fractured at delivery is
1. The humerus
2. The clavicle
3. The scapula
4. The femur

138 The average weight of the normal newborn is
1. From $5^1/_2$ to $6^1/_2$ pounds
2. From $6^1/_2$ to $7^1/_2$ pounds
3. From $7^1/_2$ to $8^1/_2$ pounds
4. From $8^1/_2$ to $9^1/_2$ pounds

139 The Moro reflex is important in newborn infants because it indicates
1. Life of the newborn
2. Awareness of equilibrium
3. Age of the newborn
4. None of these

140 Which of the following observations on a full-term newborn would suggest that an abnormality might be present?
1. Regurgitation of food after nursing
2. Lack of a sucking reflex
3. Engorgement of the breasts
4. A quiver of the lower jaw

141 The leading cause of infant death is
1. Accidents
2. Heart disease
3. Leukemia
4. Immaturity

142 Emotional problems in the preschooler are manifested by
(A) Thumbsucking
(B) Oliguria
(C) Negativism
(D) Aggressiveness
1. A, B, and D
2. A, C, and D
3. B, C, and D
4. A, B, and C

143 The periods of rapid growth are
(A) First 6 months
(B) Preschool age
(C) School age
(D) Adolescence
1. B and C
2. A and D
3. B and D
4. A and B

144 The nursing care plan of a child with scoliosis repaired by fusion includes
(A) Keeping the area clean
(B) Changing the dressing frequently
(C) Keeping the head lower than the body
(D) Changing position every 2 hours
1. A, C, and D
2. A, B, and D
3. B, C, and D
4. A, B, and C

145 In the nursing care of cerebral palsy, the nurse's function is primarily
1. Prevention
2. Observation
3. Habilitation
4. Anticipation

146 In preventing juvenile delinquency, emphasis should be placed on the study of the child's
1. Heredity
2. Environment
3. Personality
4. Psychologic development

147 Nursing care of heat rash includes
(A) Frequent bathing
(B) Keeping area open to air
(C) Applying cornstarch to area
(D) Avoiding sweats
1. A, B, and C
2. B, C, and D
3. A, C, and D
4. A, B, C, and D

148 The best way for a nurse to establish rapport with parents is to
1. Answer their questions honestly
2. Avoid contact
3. Ignore questions and talk to child
4. Refer them to the physician

7 MENTAL HEALTH NURSING

REFERENCES

Campbell, C.: Nursing diagnosis and intervention, New York, 1978, John Wiley & Sons, Inc.

Chapman, A.H., and Almeida, E.M.: The interpersonal basis of psychiatric nursing, ed. 2, New York, 1972, G.P. Putnam's Sons.

Crawford, A.L., and Buchanan, B.B.: Psychiatric nursing, ed. 4, Philadelphia, 1974, F.A. Davis Co.

Dugger, J.: The new professional: introduction for the human services/mental health worker, Monterey, 1975, Brooks/Cole Publishing Co.

Freedman, A.M., Kaplan, H.I., and Sadock, B.J.: Modern synopsis of psychiatry II, Baltimore, 1976, The Williams & Wilkins Co.

Grace, H.K., Layton, J., and Camilleri, D.: Mental health nursing: a socio-psychological approach, Dubuque, Iowa, 1977, William C. Brown Co., Publishers.

Kyes, J.J., and Hofling, C.K.: Basic psychiatric concepts in nursing, ed. 4, Philadelphia, 1980, J.B. Lippincott Co.

Lipkin, G.B., and Cohen, R.G.: Effective approaches to patient's behavior, New York, 1973, Springer Publishing Co., Inc.

Longo, D., and Williams, R.A.: Clinical practice in psychosocial nursing, New York, 1978, Appleton-Century-Crofts.

Manfreda, M.L., and Krampitz, S.D.: Psychiatric nursing, ed. 10, Philadelphia, 1977, F.A. Davis Co.

Mayers, M.G.: A systematic approach to the nursing care plan, New York, 1978, Appleton-Century-Crofts.

Mereness, D.A., and Taylor, C.M.: Essentials of psychiatric nursing, ed. 10, St. Louis, 1978, The C.V. Mosby Co.

Morgan, A.J., and Moreno, J.W.: The practice of mental health nursing: a community approach, Philadelphia, 1973, J.B. Lippincott Co.

Murray, R.B., and Zentner, J.P.: Nursing assessment and health promotion through the life-span, Englewood Cliffs, N.J., 1979, Prentice-Hall, Inc.

Rines, A.R., and Montag, M.L.: Nursing concepts and nursing care, New York, 1976, John Wiley & Sons, Inc.

Snell, H.: Mental disorders—an introductory textbook for nurses, London, 1977, George Allen and Unwin Ltd.

Stuart, G.W., and Sundeen, S.J.: Principles of psychiatric nursing, St. Louis, 1979, The C.V. Mosby Co.

Topalis, M., and Aguilera, D.C.: Psychiatric nursing, ed. 7, St. Louis, 1978, The C.V. Mosby Co.

INTRODUCTION

Mental health

A. Describes state of individual who has developed mature patterns for solving life's problems
B. Is the ability to perceive reality and act accordingly
C. Facilitates adjustment to environment in a socially approved manner
D. Allows consideration of future goals and movement toward them. Investment in living involves outside interests, relationships, concerns about occupation, ideas, and other factors
E. Is an individual matter. No one characteristic is evidence of mental health, nor is lack of any one characteristic evidence of mental illness

Mental illness

A. Definition is difficult but is usually based on what people think of as socially accepted behavior norms
B. Mentally ill describes state of individual who is unable to adequately adjust to life situations
C. Behavior is often considered abnormal and out of line with reality
D. It is easier to identify the extreme in mental illness; agreement is not as readily reached when symptoms are less obvious
E. Relationships with others are often affected

Psychiatry

A. Is branch of medicine dealing with the area of mental health and mental illness

B. Focuses on viewing how and why people become ill, how to prevent illness, and how to deal with patient's behavior

Care of the mentally ill, past and present

A. History bears evidence that social attitudes and viewpoints have always influenced care and treatment of mentally ill
B. Superstitions, ignorance, and mysticism contributed to past treatment
   1. Possession by demons as a punishment for sins was widely believed in by primitive peoples
   2. Some mental disorders were regarded as divine
   3. Patients were often locked in dungeons or jails
   4. Patients were often exhibited to the public for fees
C. Progress in humane treatment was very slow, and attitudes toward mentally ill have changed very gradually
D. Prevalent attitudes toward mentally ill (some still exist) included
   1. All mentally ill were dangerous
   2. Mental illness was incurable
   3. Mental illness was inherited
   4. Mental illness was shameful
   5. Mentally ill patients should not marry and have children
E. Twentieth-century reforms have contributed greatly toward a growing knowledge of prevention, cause, and treatment of mental illness
   1. Facilities are expanded, and emphasis is placed on treating patients before hospitalization is necessary
   2. Psychiatric units are located in general hospitals
   3. Community mental health facilities often provide impatient treatment, outpatient treatment, partial hospitalization, and 24-hour emergency care where crisis intervention is a major focus
   4. Day and night hospitals provide parttime treatment during day or night
   5. Halfway houses provide help for patient during transition from hospital to community
   6. Foster family care may be used as a substitute for hospitalization or as a transitional stage in the return to the community
   7. Nursing homes are often a potential source of help with the milder psychiatric patient and with aging person who has mental or emotional problems
   8. Sheltered workshops are workshops in which recovering mentally ill patients can be gainfully employed
   9. Expatient clubs provide social contacts and some active therapy
   10. Major focus of mental health care is on prevention, reduced length of hospitalization, and returning patient to the community as soon as possible

Significant needs

A. More and better prepared personnel to provide specialized care
B. Better education of public so it will seek early treatment
C. Proper financial support for mental health agencies
D. More and better hospital and clinic facilities
E. More positive community attitudes in efforts to rehabilitate patients

MENTAL HEALTH NURSING

Defined as a therapeutic relationship in which nursing activities are purposeful and goal directed and in which the patient is aided to become a more healthy, adequately adjusted human being

Introduction

A. It is important for nurse to be aware of own behavior and strive toward self-understanding
B. Nurse uses own personality as a therapeutic tool in providing patient with healthy interpersonal experiences
C. Empathy is used in making meaningful contacts with patients
D. Observational skills and knowledge of communication are applied to appropriately intervene in patient care
E. Nurse attempts to help patient make positive changes in behavior
F. Ultimate goal is achievement of appropriate and effective relationships between patient and others

Nursing in mental health settings

A. Nurse attempts to create and maintain a therapeutic environment (environment conducive to improvement and recovery)
B. Nursing subroles are
   1. Supportive role—provides assistance to patient as he or she attempts to cope with everyday experiences

2. Mothering role—uses activities that nurture and assist in restoring patient to health (bathing, dressing, feeding, soothing, comforting)
3. Technician role—uses skills that are scientifically accurate and are based on patient needs, such as administering medication and treatments
4. Teacher role—may be formal or informal and involves the communication of knowledge that may be helpful to the patient
5. Socializing role—assists in regaining or maintaining social skills necessary for living in society. Nurse provides opportunities for and encourages participation in social or group activities
6. Counselor role—involves a psychotherapeutic relationship in which special attention is paid to the communications exchanged between the patient and nurse

Basic principles of mental health nursing

A. Have self-awareness—an important therapeutic tool
   1. Nurse should seek to understand self
   2. Knowledge of own needs and motivations is very useful in better understanding patients
B. Accept patient as he or she is
   1. Display genuine interest
   2. Show patience and understanding
   3. Act in a nonjudgmental and nonpunitive manner
      a. Attitude does not necessarily mean approval of behavior
      b. Attitude demonstrates acceptance of patient regardless of behavior
C. Offer reassurance
   1. Demonstrate nursing competence
   2. Attempt to see the situation from the patient's point of view
   3. Do not minimize patient's fears and anxiety
   4. Show sincere interest in patient
D. Encourage reality experiences
   1. Do not support unrealistic ideas
   2. Encourage communication with staff and others that is healthy and appropriate
E. Promote a sense of security and provide consistency in experiences
   1. Consistency is useful in routines
   2. Attitudes of staff toward patients are important
   3. Patients are made to feel more comfortable by knowing what to expect
F. Avoid promoting unnecessary anxiety
   1. Limit demands made on patient
   2. Avoid use of unfamiliar, professional jargon
   3. Concentrate on patient's strengths, not weaknesses
   4. Be sincere
G. Maintain objectivity
   1. Do not allow personal needs and feelings to take precedence over those of the patient
   2. Be accurate and free of bias in reporting and recording observations
H. Maintain a realistic relationship
   1. Recognize difference between friendliness and being a friend, pal, or buddy to the patient
   2. Focus on patient's needs
   3. Offer warmth and understanding, not intimacy, in relationships

Nurse-patient relationship

A. Relationship consists of interactions between nurse and patient, with focus on patient and his or her needs
B. Relationship offers patient opportunity to modify behavior
C. Nurse's action is directed toward meeting needs of patient
D. Nurse uses healthy personality to promote mental health in others
E. Therapeutic relationship provides security for patient and enables him or her to grow and develop potential
F. Effective relationship does not necessarily denote doing what patient wants but does entail providing what patient needs

Communication skills

A. Communication involves all modes of behavior by which people influence one another. It is a two-way process in which the purpose is to promote understanding
B. Modes of communication are
   1. Verbal
      a. Spoken word
      b. Written language
   2. Nonverbal
      a. Gestures
      b. Mannerisms
      c. Voice tone

   d. Body movements
   e. Facial expressions
   f. Silence
C. Nonverbal component is always present when verbal communication takes place; for example, inflection of voice when statement is made carries feeling of message
D. Characteristics of successful communication are
   1. Feedback—opportunity for listener to respond. It may serve to clarify, extend, or alter the original idea contained in the communication
   2. Appropriateness—reply is fitting and relevant to the communication received; there is neither too much nor too little stimulation
   3. Efficiency—language used by the communicators is understood, and enough time between verbal responses is allowed for the listener to perceive and evaluate them
   4. Flexibility—undercontrol or overcontrol is absent. Undercontrol implies a disregard for the effects of feedback, appropriateness, and efficiency. Overcontrol occurs when there is too much checking and rechecking of communications exchanged
E. Techniques of communication are various devices or methods used to facilitate communication
   1. Listening—provides opportunity for other person to take the communication lead and allows for releasing and alleviating uncomfortable feelings; however, it requires much attentiveness on the part of the listener
   2. Silence—gives the opportunity for the communicators to reflect on what has been said
   3. Comment—involves interjecting appropriate comments during conversation to show interest and attentiveness (''Go on.'' ''Tell me more.'')
   4. Reflection (flashback)—involves repeating all or part of an individual's statement. It has a prompting and encouraging effect and aids in helping the person to focus on the topic (The person states, ''I feel worried about my condition.'' The responder may say, ''You feel worried?'')
   5. Open-end statements—involve referring back to a topic that has been previously mentioned in order to obtain more information. (''You were telling me about. . . .'')
   6. Questions—should be used carefully and appropriately. They are often helpful when there is need to clarify. (The patient consistently refers to ''they.'' It would be appropriate for the nurse to ask, ''Who do you mean by 'they'?'') Questions are also useful in eliciting necessary information
F. Blocks to effective communication are
   1. Persistent questioning or probing of information—avoid asking ''why'' and ''how'' questions since they place the patient on the defensive
   2. Failure to listen—intended message is not received
   3. Overloading or underloading the conversation or talking too much or too little
   4. Using cliches indiscriminately—this includes using pat answers and offering false reassurance (''Don't worry.'' ''You are going to be fine.'')
   5. Using value statements, such as ''good'' or ''nice,'' indiscriminately—find out how patient really feels
   6. Giving advice—this often indicates that patient is not capable of directing own activities and may also set nurse up for blame if he or she gives advice that does not work
   7. Changing the subject—this results in avoidance of discussions of interest to one communicator and is often done when the other is uncomfortable with the topic

Nursing assessment of the psychiatric patient

A. Observation involves deliberate overall viewing of the person and situation
   1. Involves all the sense organs, not just the eyes
   2. Is important for planning intervention
   3. Has legal ramifications as well
B. Important aspects to observe include
   1. Appearance—includes everything one can see about the patient
      a. Hair
      b. Eyes
      c. Facial expression
      d. Skin
      e. Mouth
      f. Clothing
      g. Posture
      h. Movements

2. Behavior—constitutes all of patient's actions (spontaneous actions, required behavior, habitual responses) in such areas as
   a. Sleep
   b. Appetite
   c. Hygiene
   d. Elimination
   e. Medications
   f. Treatment
   g. Social interaction
3. Conversation
   a. Relevant or irrelevant
   b. Loose or appropriate thought connections
   c. Possible hesitancy or refusal to speak
   d. Rapid or extremely slow speech

C. Aim of assessment is to identify psychologic and physiologic needs, keeping in mind patient's strengths and weaknesses

D. Assessment has following outcomes
   1. Enables nurse to plan care
   2. Enables nurse to anticipate needs
   3. Affords better understanding of patient

E. Patient should still be considered nurse's primary source of information

PERSONALITY DEVELOPMENT

Human personality

Somewhat predictable behavior response patterns that characterize the individual

A. Is all a person feels, is, and does, both consciously and unconsciously
   1. Intellectual and physical qualities
   2. Social behavior patterns
   3. Psychologic and emotional attributes
   4. Awareness of individual self

B. Is *not* the same as is referred to when stating that a person has a nice or nasty personality

Factors in personality development

A. Physical makeup
B. Early childhood experiences
C. Family attitudes, feelings, and values
D. Satisfaction of physical and emotional needs
E. Social environment

Influential theorists

A. Sigmund Freud—freudian theory
   1. Founded psychoanalytic movement
   2. Was most acclaimed for his work with neurotic patients
   3. Was responsible for developing the process of "free association," which allowed individuals in therapy to say anything that came into their minds
   4. Explored the unconscious part of the mind and developed dream theory
   5. Categorized human drives

B. Harry Stack Sullivan—sullivanian theory
   1. Was responsible for the interpersonal theory of psychiatry
   2. Emphasized the influence of growth and development and referred to "significant others" as important in child's growing into healthy or unhealthy adult
   3. Saw reduction in anxiety as major behavioral goal for the individual
   4. Elaborated on the role of "emphathic communication" from which a child's self-concept is formed
   5. Focused on communication and interpersonal behavior and their later impact on the transaction of behavior

C. Other theorists
   1. Alfred Adler
   2. Otto Rank
   3. Carl Jung
   4. Karen Horney
   5. Erich Fromm

D. Four basic concepts of personality development that almost all psychoanalytic groups agree on
   1. All behavior is meaningful and is not determined by choice
   2. The role of the unconscious is important in determining behavior
   3. All behavior is goal directed
   4. The foundation for later personality development is laid in the early years of life

Personality structure

A. Id
   1. Is bundle of promotive and pleasure-seeking instincts and is whole of personality at birth
   2. Is concerned with biologic drives
   3. Seeks immediate gratification of needs

B. Ego
   1. Begins to develop toward the end of the first year of life
   2. Develops from experience with external reality
   3. Is referred to as the "self" or "I"
   4. Guides and controls actions of the individual

5. Seeks to postpone immediate satisfactions until appropriate time
6. Preserves the sense of reality; that is its main function

C. Superego
1. Is referred to as conscience or sense of right or wrong
2. Begins to develop around the second year of life
3. Represents demands of society

Levels of awareness

A. Unconscious—anything concerning self of which the individual is unaware
B. Conscious—that of which individual is aware
C. Preconscious—that which may be called into awareness

Developmental stages of the personality

A. Oral phase (birth to 1 year of age)
1. Primary activity is gaining oral satisfaction
2. Relationship with mother is of prime importance
3. Love (fondling by mother) and satisfaction of physical needs help develop security
4. Weaning brings phase to an end
5. Good experiences set firm basis for future development

B. Anal phase (1 to 3 years of age)
1. Child learns pleasurable bodily sensations relating to passage of urine and feces
2. Period of conformity commences as toilet training is begun; child learns to give and take
3. Training should begin only after sphincter control develops, usually around 15 months of age
4. Child needs love and understanding during toilet training, which should be accomplished without punishment
5. Child begins to relate to others and use words to communicate
6. Motor skill and independence increase

C. Oedipal phase (3 to 6 years of age)
1. Child becomes aware of own body and differences between sexes
2. Curiosity about body results in self-exploration
3. Positive attitude of parents is important in handling situation
4. Boy becomes attached to mother and sees father as rival
5. Girl is antagonistic toward mother and desires to take mother's place with father
6. Conflicts produce anxiety and fear of loss of love
7. Conflict is resolved as child takes on characteristics of parent of same sex (identification)
8. This phase is the most crucial period of development for social and sexual adjustment; children need stable figures with whom to identify; superego formation with evidence of guilt feelings is apparent

D. Latency phase (6 to 12 years of age)
1. Energy is available for intellectual growth and socialization
2. Child learns to compete with others and to give and take and to compromise
3. Hero worship and identification with figures outside family take place
4. This is period when group becomes important; child has strong group loyalties, wants to be one of the gang, and seeks acceptance of the group
5. Companionship with members of own sex is outstanding characteristic of the phase

E. Adolescence (12 years of age to maturity)
1. This is a period of many conflicts; it begins with onset of physical maturity and ends with acquisition of patterns with which to handle conflicts
2. Physiologic changes include glandular changes, growth of pubic hair, voice changes, and changes in body shape
3. Desire for independence often leads to conflict with parents and to rebellion against rules, regulations, and family restrictions
4. Dating begins as adolescent expands socially and seeks heterosexual companionship
5. Group identification continues
   a. Adolescent conforms to group standards
   b. Group ideas tend to be idealistic
   c. Group offers security
6. Outcome of this phase is
   a. Selection of vocation
   b. Emancipation from parents
   c. Adjustment to opposite sex
   d. Integration of personality
7. If experiences have been successful throughout this stage, mature person emerges

F. Maturity—emotional maturity is an ideal state
   1. Has a working philosophy of life
   2. Is able to see own assets and limitations
   3. Is able to master environment in realistic way
   4. Is able to give and receive, enjoys and accepts lasting friendships, and is able to love
   5. Is able to learn and profit from mistakes and successes

Adjustment mechanisms

A. Need for mechanisms
   1. All humans experience conflict and tension; life is a constant struggle between desires and hindering forces
   2. When conflicts arise, individual must learn patterns to cope with them (adjustment)
   3. One way of handling increased tension is through ego defense mechanisms
B. Characteristics of defenses
   1. Ego defense mechanisms are intrapsychic processes employed to resolve emotional conflict and anxiety
   2. They usually operate without individuals conscious awareness
   3. They are utilized by all humans during periods of stress
   4. Main goal is to maintain personal worth of ego (through allaying or preventing anxiety)
C. Commonly used defenses
   1. Repression
      a. This is process whereby unacceptable thoughts and feelings are barred from consciousness
      b. Repression is way of excluding painful, unpleasant material from awareness
      c. Example is upsetting event in childhood that is pushed from awareness and may not be recalled at the will of the individual without assistance
   2. Suppression
      a. This is process of deliberately forgetting unpleasant thoughts and feelings
      b. Unlike repressed material, suppressed material can be recalled into awareness
      c. Example is student who chooses not to think about her assignment until tomorrow
   3. Reaction formation
      a. This is mechanism in which overt attitudes and behavior are opposite those of individual's repressed feelings
      b. Example is overly friendly, overly polite person who may have unconscious feelings of hatred toward others
   4. Projection
      a. This is process of attributing undesirable thoughts and feelings to others
      b. Individual fails to recognize own faults by finding them in others
      c. Example is wife who is frequently critical of husband saying that her husband is always finding fault with her
   5. Rationalization
      a. This is process by which attempt is made to explain or make excuses to self for unacceptable behavior
      b. Rationalization serves to hide real motives behind behavior
      c. Example is student who does not study for examination and fails and says poor teaching was the cause
   6. Displacement
      a. This is process whereby an emotion is transferred from original object onto another object
      b. Displacement occurs when it is unsafe to express feelings directly
      c. Example is employee who has a misunderstanding with the boss and goes home and is unpleasant to his or her family
   7. Sublimation
      a. This is mechanism in which energy associated with primitive drives is successfully utilized in constructive social activities
      b. Example is executive who pours energies into creative activity instead of choosing to get married
   8. Identification
      a. This is process whereby person adopts characteristics, feelings, or attributes of another
      b. Identification is necessary mechanism for child; it is method by which child becomes social being
      c. Examples are little boy who develops mannerisms like his father, and girl like her mother
   9. Conversion
      a. This is unconscious mechanism by which psychologic conflicts are expressed through physical symptoms
      b. Example is wife who develops deafness on hearing her husband demand a divorce

10. Regression
    a. This is process whereby individual utilizes patterns of behavior characteristic of earlier phase of life
    b. Regression helps person to temporarily escape painful reality
    c. Example is hospitalized person who cries easily or shows excessive dependency needs
11. Fantasy
    a. This is use of wishful and imaginative activity to relieve tension
    b. Fantasy is frequently used when no satisfaction can be found in reality
    c. Example is daydreaming

D. Coping devices
1. These are specific acts used to deal with stress, difficulties, and new situations without using adjustment mechanisms
2. Common acts include
    a. Talking problem over
    b. Drinking, eating, and smoking (oral activites)
    c. Sleeping or withdrawing from the situation
    d. Pacing or finger tapping (pointless activities)
    e. Laughing, crying, and swearing

MANIFESTATIONS OF MENTAL AND EMOTIONAL DISTURBANCE

Concepts of anxiety, frustration, and conflict

A. Mentally disturbed people attempt to alleviate anxiety through mental symptoms that are expressions of unbearable anxiety

B. Mental illness and mental symptoms are regarded as products of anxiety as well as defenses against it

C. Anxiety is defined as a subjective or feeling experience not necessarily confined to the mentally disturbed
1. Anxiety is an invisible form of energy
2. It is described as an unpleasant, diffuse, vague, and frequently unexplainable feeling of apprehension
3. It interferes with thinking and concentration
4. Mild anxiety may serve to alert an individual to protect self from threatening situations
5. Moderate and more severe degrees of anxiety may be incapacitating and therefore motivate defensive behaviors aimed at reducing or alleviating the discomfort
6. Observable signs of anxiety include
    a. Behavioral manifestations—changes in voice tone and rate of speech, preoccupation with thoughts, and feeling of powerlessness
    b. Physical manifestations—restlessness, fatigue, palpitations, tremors, frequent urination, vomiting, diarrhea, and perspiration
7. In severe anxiety, person may become immobilized in thought and action.
8. If defenses fail to work, a state of panic or terror may result
9. Temporary disintegration of personality may result if relief is not forthcoming

D. Theories of anxiety include the following
1. Psychoanalytic theory holds that anxiety is aroused by the emergence of formerly repressed drives, thoughts, feelings, wishes, and actions
2. Interpersonal theory postulates that anxiety is experienced as the anticipated disapproval or loss of love from significant others

E. Frustration is defined as anything that interferes with one's drive to attain a need or desired goal that would produce feelings of satisfaction and security
1. Frustrations are prevalent in a complex society
2. People must learn to cope with frustration in order to adapt
3. Anxiety is felt when frustrating experiences occur frequently
4. Defensive behavior is activated so that three common responses to frustration may occur
    a. Goal may have to be changed to one that the individual has a better chance of attaining
    b. Goal may be abandoned so that the individual withdraws
    c. Individual may try to work around the obstacle
5. When mechanisms fail to handle frustration, the individual may resort to pathologic behavior

F. Conflict is manifested by the existence of two opposing or incompatible drives
1. Individual experiencing conflict is required to make a choice between the possible responses
2. Opposing drives or actions may have negative or positive values
3. Difficulty in making the choice is the conflict that causes the person to hesitate or even be unable to decide
4. Conflicts are usually of a short duration
5. Resolution occurs when the individual makes the choice

Common disorders and symptoms

A. Introduction
  1. Mental illness is complex; it is impossible to define any one specific cause
  2. Psychiatry should not deal with diseases as such; emphasis should be placed on understanding why patient is ill and attempting to assist patient in returning to a more effective state of functioning
  3. Many factors are considered in determining why patient is ill; individual's total life experience, with consideration of genetic, physiologic, interpersonal, and cultural factors, must be examined

B. Psychoses
  1. Psychosis refers to type of mental disorder characterized by loss of contact with reality and disorganization of personality; mental functioning is impaired to the point of interfering with capacity to meet ordinary demands of life
  2. Psychoses are classified as
    a. Psychoses associated with organic brain syndromes (related to impaired brain tissue)
      (1) Symptoms include impairment of memory, orientation, intellectual functions, and judgment; lability (rapidly shifting emotions); and shallow affect
      (2) Examples are dementia, alcoholic psychosis, and cerebral arteriosclerosis
    b. Psychoses not attributed to physical conditions
      (1) Schizophrenia
        (a) Schizophrenia is a group of severe mental disorders characterized by disturbances in thinking, feeling, and acting
        (b) Patient has strong tendency to retreat from reality
        (c) This is largest group of behavior disorders; types, or subgroups, are simple, hebephrenic, catatonic, paranoid, and some childhood types
        (d) Age of onset is frequently adolescence through young adulthood
      (2) Affective disorders
        (a) Affective disorders are characterized by a disorder of mood, either extreme depression or elation; manic-depressive psychosis and involutional psychosis are examples
        (b) Age of onset is usually after 30 years of age

C. Neuroses (psychoneuroses)
  1. Neuroses are characterized by anxiety and minimal loss of contact with reality. Most frequently recognized reactions are anxiety, phobia, conversion, and obsessive-compulsive behavior
  2. Patient is usually aware of a disturbance in mental functioning
  3. No gross personality disorganization occurs, but patients can be extremely ill and require hospitalization in some cases

D. Personality disorders
  1. Personality disorders are characterized by ingrained maladaptive patterns of behavior
  2. Patients include antisocial individuals, sexual deviates, alcoholics, and drug addicts

E. Special terms
  1. Hallucination—an imaginary sensation without an external stimulus; person experiences a sensation without one being present
    a. Auditory (hearing)
    b. Olfactory (smelling)
    c. Visual (seeing)
    d. Tactile (feeling)
    e. Gustatory (tasting)
  2. Delusion—a false belief, not based on fact, which cannot be changed by reasoning
    a. Delusions of grandeur—feeling of greatness ("I am Christ.")
    b. Delusions of persecution—feeling of being mistreated ("Nobody cares about me. They are after me.")
    c. Delusions of sin or guilt—feelings that one has done something wrong or bad ("I am being punished for all my sins.")
    d. Flight of ideas—extreme distractibility; person goes quickly from one idea to another
    e. Anxiety—feeling of uneasiness, dread, apprehension, and tension
    f. Depression—feeling of dejection and hopelessness

CARING FOR THE PSYCHIATRIC PATIENT

Basic needs

A. Everyone has basic needs that are instinctive or have been acquired during the process of growth and development

B. Needs generate tension, which causes the individual to behave in certain ways

C. Basic needs include
   1. Acceptance
   2. Self-esteem
   3. Attention and recognition
   4. Love
   5. Security
   6. Understanding
   7. Communication
   8. Dependence
   9. Independence
   10. Interdependence

Frequent behaviors requiring nursing intervention

A. Anxiety
   1. Problems can be both physiologic and behavioral
      a. Tension and restlessness
      b. Fear (often)
      c. Difficulty in concentrating
      d. Feeling of inferiority (often)
      e. Indecisiveness
      f. Ritualistic behavior
      g. Tremors
      h. Sweating
      i. Palpitations
      j. Flushed face
      k. Nausea and vomiting
      l. Diarrhea
   2. Anxiety can be produced by any situation or event that is perceived to be threatening to an individual. It is a key factor in the development of emotional problems
   3. Diagnosis is made on the basis of data collection, which includes history, physical examination, and assessment of emotional and behavioral information
   4. The use of tranquilizing drugs has proved helpful in conjunction with such treatments as individual and/or group psychotherapy
   5. Nursing care plan involves
      a. Recognizing signs and symptoms of anxiety
         (1) Distinguish from fear, which is a response to a specific source. (Anxiety is an emotion without a specific object)
         (2) Identify level of anxiety (mild, moderate, severe, panic)
         (3) Be aware of own anxiety, and keep in mind that it is communicated interpersonally. Be calm
      b. Communicating in ways that will promote understanding
         (1) Speak slowly and distinctly
         (2) Do not overload—be brief and specific
      c. Recognizing the chief role is supportive
         (1) Do not offer false reassurances or give empty explanations ("Don't worry. Everything will be OK.")
         (2) Do not push or probe. Encourage ventilation of thoughts and feelings, but at the patient's own pace
         (3) Keep decision making to a minimum during periods of high anxiety
      d. Adjusting environmental stimulation as necessary
         (1) Adjust contacts with others as patient's condition permits
         (2) Allow sufficient time to accomplish activities
      e. Providing for safety
         (1) Allow for protection of patient's own defenses. Do not push into situations with which he or she cannot cope
         (2) Work with staff to identify anxiety-producing situations, and attempt to reduce them
         (3) Assume a quiet, calm manner to convey security to the patient
         (4) Minimize contact with other patients in which anxiety reaches a level where the patient becomes "out of control" or unduly upset by contact with others
      f. Assisting patient in learning to cope with anxiety in a more constructive way
         (1) Include the patient in the therapeutic plan of care insofar as possible
         (2) Identify short- and long-term goals
         (3) Help patient develop insight into his or her anxiety—assist patient in connecting present anxiety with what happened before he or she felt anxious
         (4) Assist in the development of more effective coping mechanisms

B. Depression
1. Problems include
   a. Predominately sad mood
   b. Inability to concentrate
   c. Insomnia
   d. Anorexia
   e. Weight loss
   f. Indecisiveness
   g. Feelings of guilt, worthlessness, and self-deprecation (often)
   h. Low self-esteem
2. Under certain conditions, depression may be considered ''normal'' (loss of a loved one, loss of body function or integrity, loss of job), but true depression is prolonged and often severe and becomes incapacitating. It is a destructive process in which anger is directed inward toward the self. Depressions are often ''reactive'' and are thus precipitated by stress caused by a loss. Other types of depression may be representative of a more severe mental illness
3. Diagnosis involves distinguishing depression from anxiety, since they may present similar behaviors. The presenting problem and related stressors are assessed, along with a history and physical examination
4. Treatment often includes hospitalization, antidepressant drugs (''mood elevators''), psychotherapy, and, depending on severity, electroconvulsive therapy (ECT)
5. Nursing care plan includes the following
   a. Chief nursing activities are supportive
      (1) Show sincere interest
      (2) Demonstrate kindness, patience, and understanding
      (3) Support patient in working through loss
      (4) Identify short- and long-term goals, allowing the patient to participate in therapeutic plan of care
   b. Communicate in ways that will promote understanding
      (1) Attempt to draw the patient into conversation, but at his or her own pace
      (2) Speak clearly, and allow time for response
      (3) Remember that overloading of conversation or demands for activity may result in regression
   c. Plan activities with the degree of depression in mind
      (1) Make tasks appropriate and simple
      (2) Give ample time to complete tasks
      (3) Give encouragement, and offer sincere compliments
      (4) Take the initiative; it is not always helpful to ask, ''Would you like to go for a walk?'' Rather, say, ''Let's go for a walk.''
   d. Encourage adequate diet
      (1) Offer nutritious and appetizing foods; include adequate bulk and fluids
      (2) Assist with feeding, if necessary (some patients may lack the initiative to eat or may feel unworthy to accept food)
      (3) Periodic attempts to offer food are generally more successful than expecting patients to eat three meals a day
   e. Offer assistance with personal hygiene and grooming, as necessary
      (1) Observe for condition of skin
      (2) Be alert for signs of physical illness or injury
      (3) Encourage regular use of toilet; constipation is a common problem
   f. Provide for adequate rest; insomnia is often a problem
      (1) Warm milk at bedtime may be helpful
      (2) Give medications as ordered
      (3) Offer support and reassurance during periods of wakefulness
   g. Provide a safe environment
      (1) Keep patient under observation since suicide is *always* a potential danger for depressed patients
      (2) Suicide is a particular risk when patient is *coming out* of a depression rather than when patient is deeply depressed, because he or she may have more energy to make an attempt
      (3) Maintain a safe environment
         (a) Keep objects that could be used in a suicide attempt away from patient
         (b) Observe closely
         (c) Be aware that visitors may bring in ''contraband''

C. Overactivity
1. Problems include the following
a. Mood is elated
b. Thought is accelerated, and motor activity ranges from mild to severe
c. Patient is easily distracted and often domineering and meddlesome
d. Judgment and insight are poor
e. Overactivity results in lack of sleep, indifference to body hygiene, and poor eating habits
2. Overactivity is thought to result from regression to earlier patterns of behavior. Patient is basically ambivalent and dependent. Some thought has also been given to possible hereditary predispositions
3. Overactive patient is readily observed by intensity of actions and conversation. A thorough assessment must be done, with particular emphasis on the patient's history
4. Drug therapy is the most common treatment for this disorder (sedatives, major tranquilizers, lithium). Group psychotherapy may be helpful when patient is calm enough. Individual psychotherapy may be employed also. ECT has also been employed in some cases
5. Nursing care plan involves the following
a. Be consistent, and set limits
b. Convey warmth, acceptance, patience, and understanding
c. Manipulate the environment; patient responds best to nonstimulating surroundings, such as single room with simple furnishings and quiet atmosphere
d. Protect from injury
(1) Allow for proper rest to avoid exhaustion
(2) Observe interactions with others. Intervene when necessary
(3) Avoid physical force or threats; if separation from others is necessary, have frequent contacts with patient
e. Provide activities that are noncompetitive and can be accomplished quickly and easily
f. Encourage adequate diet
(1) Provide foods that can be eaten "on the run," since patient often does not have "time" to eat
(2) Offer foods and fluids frequently
(3) Encourage regular use of toilet

D. Suspiciousness
1. Problems may include
a. Basic distrust of people (sometimes termed "paranoid")
b. Doubt about many things
c. Perception of the environment as hostile (may be expressed as resentfulness, sarcasm, and irritability)
d. Aggressive behavior (arrogant, demanding)
e. Expression of feelings by being passive and overly submissive
2. The roots of this problem are thought to be developed in the early stages of growth and development when excessive demands to achieve were placed on the child. Family and home relationships are commonly unpleasant and foster feelings of insecurity and suspiciousness
3. The suspicious patient often readily conveys a suspicous attitude by actions, conversations, and manner
4. Long-term treatment may be necessary to help the patient develop trust in others. Establishing a one-to-one relationship initially is helpful
5. Nursing care plan involves
a. Being aware of own behavior
(1) Do not whisper to others in the patient's presence, as patient may misinterpret and refer such action to him- or herself
(2) Be honest at all times; keep promises made to the patient
(3) Act calm, firm, and self-assured
b. Avoid becoming part of patient's delusional system. Listen, but do not encourage or support his or her false beliefs
c. Be aware of the positive and negative connotations of touch; physical contact may be misinterpreted
d. Wait until patient can handle interactions before introducing competitive activities, since they are not tolerated too well
e. If eating becomes a problem because of mistrust (patient thinks food is poisoned), use the following approach
(1) Have patient observe the preparation of food (if possible) or assist in serving the food
(2) Serve food in the original container
(3) Taste food in the patient's presence, or secure an identical serving

E. Antisocial behavior (sociopathic)
   1. Problems include the following
      a. On the surface patient may appear charming, intelligent, and genuine
      b. Behaviors often exhibited are inconsistency, untruthfulness, and insincerity
      c. Patient does not profit from experience
      d. Patient lacks insight and judgment
   2. While the exact cause of antisocial behavior is unknown, theories concerning problems arising during the formative years are thought to be important. A basic ego defect causes the individual to respond to primitive impulses rather than to employ social control. Often leads to problematic behaviors
   3. Antisocial patient often finds him- or herself in difficult legal situations because of lack of ego control and faulty judgment. Many authorities believe that institutionalization provides corrective experiences where there are firm, reasonable controls set on behavior
   4. Nursing care plan involves
      a. Using a kind, matter-of-fact, firm approach
      b. Encouraging consistency among staff in order to deal effectively with patient
      c. Being aware of attempts to take advantage of people and situations. Use limit setting as necessary

ADDICTIVE DISORDERS

Introduction

Two main categories of self-destructive behavior are alcoholism and drug abuse. Both have common causes with similar problems and can have disastrous results if left untreated. Both are contemporary problems that affect an overwhelming number of persons directly and many, many more indirectly

Alcoholism

A. Problems include
   1. Use of alcohol to decrease anxiety
   2. Usually low self-esteem and many unmet dependency needs
   3. Self-centeredness and difficulty relating on a mature level
   4. Physical complications—hepatitis, cirrhosis of the liver, anemias, pancreatitis, osteoporosis, peripheral neuropathy, and brain damage
   5. Psychologic behavior—depression, hostility, suspiciousness, and in some persons, aggressiveness

B. Persons who rely excessively on alcohol to the point of addiction are thought to have feelings of inadequacy that have arisen from conflicts or frustrations causing an inability to cope in healthy ways

C. Diagnosis is usually made on the basis of history, physical examination, and assessment of the pattern of drinking (including frequency, duration, and amounts)

D. Nursing care plan involves the following
   1. Maintain an objective manner
      a. An empathic and nonjudgmental approach is essential
      b. Be aware of own attitudes toward self-destructive behavior
   2. Provide for a safe environment
      a. Assess for suicidal potential, and observe closely
      b. Take dangerous objects away from patient
      c. Be aware that visitors may bring in "contraband"
   3. Identify short- and long-term goals—allow patient participation in therapeutic plan of care
   4. Treat patient fairly, but be alert for efforts to manipulate. Provide consistency and set limits when necessary
   5. In stages of withdrawal, patients require expert, skilled care with frequent monitoring of physical and mental condition

Drug abuse

A. Problems include the following
   1. Drug abuse can involve physical dependency, psychologic dependency, or both
   2. Person often becomes addicted to more than one drug
   3. Withdrawal from many drugs can be serious
   4. Drug addiction has become a great social problem because of frequent illegal measures to continue the habit

B. Drug addiction can be found in all age groups, although it is more frequently thought to be a problem of youth. This self-destructive behavior can result from any stress that is perceived to be overwhelming by the individual. Factors such as anxiety, anger, low self-esteem, and extreme dependency needs are thought to contribute to the development of this problem. Social conditions, such as those created by rapid social change, are also contributors

TREATMENT FOR THE MENTALLY ILL

Introduction

Many new areas of care for the psychiatric patient with improved facilities, therapies, and various treatment modalities have been developed

Types of treatment in current use

A. Psychotherapy
   1. Individual psychotherapy—process making use of the relationship between therapist and patient to identify, explore, and achieve understanding of patient's life situation
   2. Group psychotherapy—includes several patients and a therapist who meet regularly to achieve insight and support from one another; it is beneficial in that one patient may find that others have similar problems
   3. Family therapy—a form of psychotherapy focusing on the family as a system; work is aimed toward improving attitudes and behavior within the family unit
   4. Behavior therapy—a type of treatment based on learning theory (that all behavior is learned and can be unlearned). Specific programs may be set up for the patient using rewards or punishments

B. Chemotherapy—use of drugs to allow patients to become more accessible to therapy by relieving overt symptoms
   1. Drugs affect mood and behavior; they do not "cure"
   2. Classification of psychiatric drugs is as follows
      a. Tranquilizers—calm patient, reduce anxiety
         (1) Commonly used major tranquilizers are
            (a) Chlorpromazine (Thorazine)—first major tranquilizer to be used in psychiatry
            (b) Trifluoperazine (Stelazine)
            (c) Promazine (Sparine)
            (d) Thioridazine (Mellaril)
            (e) Haloperidol (Haldol)
         (2) Major tranquilizers are used primarily with psychotic patients
         (3) Possible side effects of major tranquilizers are
            (a) Drowsiness
            (b) Central nervous system involvement—parkinsonian symptoms
            (c) Dry mouth
            (d) Postural hypotension
            (e) Agranulocytosis—most serious complication; incidence is extremely rare
            (f) Dangerous side effects—rare
         (4) Commonly used minor tranquilizers are
            (a) Meprobamate (Equanil)
            (b) Diazepam (Valium)
            (c) Chlordiazepoxide (Librium)
         (5) Minor tranquilizers are more commonly used with neurotic patients; they are useful in mild to moderate anxiety states
         (6) Possible side effects of minor tranquilizers are
            (a) Ataxia
            (b) Fainting
            (c) Skin eruptions
            (d) Gastrointestinal upsets
      b. Antidepressants
         (1) Stimulants have effects on mood and behavior
         (2) Commonly used drugs are
            (a) Amitriptyline (Elavil)
            (b) Imipramine (Tofranil)
            (c) Nortriptyline (Aventyl)
            (d) Phenelzine sulfate (Nardil)
         (3) Common side effects are
            (a) Nervousness
            (b) Insomnia
      c. Lithium
         (1) Lithium is effective in treatment of manic or hypomanic phase of manic-depressive psychosis
         (2) Blood lithium levels must be checked frequently. Blood sodium must be adequate to lessen the incidence of toxicity
      d. Nurse's responsibilities in chemotherapy
         (1) Give medications as ordered, and record accurately
         (2) Know effects of drugs and side effects
         (3) Report any untoward reactions immediately

C. Electroconvulsive therapy (ECT, EST, or shock therapy)
   1. This therapy was introduced in 1937
   2. Its use depends on philosophy of psychiatrist and hospital
   3. It is useful in some cases of depression and agitation; number of treatments varies
   4. Therapy consists of application of electric currents by way of electrodes on patient's temples

5. Grand mal seizure is induced
6. Medications for anesthesia and muscle relaxation are most often used before treatment
7. Patient is usually given nothing by mouth before treatment
8. Patient usually sleeps following ECT and is usually confused and drowsy on recovery
9. Memory loss is common but usually clears up after treatments are discontinued
10. Patients are usually anxious, particularly before first treatment and need considerable reassurance and support

D. Adjunctive therapies
   1. Occupational and recreational therapy (OT, RT)
      a. Activities are correlated with treatment goals
      b. Approach is based on patient's needs and interests; patient is actively involved in plans
      c. Purposes include
         (1) Stimulation and maintenance of reality interest
         (2) Redevelopment of social skills, providing opportunity for developing positive interpersonal relations
         (3) Allowance for expression of feelings in constructive manner
         (4) Reestablishment of old skills and knowledge or initiation of new ones
   2. Other adjunctive therapies
      a. Industrial therapy—to identify patient's interests and abilities for employment
      b. Bibliotherapy—prescribed therapeutic reading
      c. Music therapy—provides for self-expression and socialization through group singing and rhythm bands
      d. Art and dance therapy

E. Hospitalization
   1. Psychiatric hospital
      a. Much like general hospital in that it provides for care and treatment of patients who are ill
      b. Viewed as therapeutic communication designed to meet patient's total needs and facilitate improvement
   2. Psychiatric hospital setting
      a. Patient
         (1) Is most often ambulatory
         (2) May resent being hospitalized
         (3) Frequently lacks insight
      b. Nurse—self-understanding is paramount to adequately care for patients
      c. Care and treatment
         (1) Diagnosis is relatively unimportant; rather treatment is dictated according to the predominate behaviors of the patient
         (2) Care and treatment often are not evident to the patient, who frequently feels that he or she is held without cause
         (3) Recovery may take considerable time

F. Crisis intervention
   1. Subject has become of great interest to all health professionals
   2. Techniques are used by a variety of persons with varying backgrounds and levels of training to assist those in immediate need
      a. Crisis is seen as a state of disequilibrium. Factors included are events that the person perceives as threatening or disturbing and for which his or her coping mechanisms are inadequate
      b. Resolution of the crisis is more likely to occur with appropriate intervention
   3. The stages of crisis are recognized by experts
      a. They include some of the following: denial, increase in tension, disorganization, reorganization attempts, and escape
      b. Acute phase of crisis is usually over within a 6-week period
   4. Techniques of crisis intervention include
      a. Thorough assessing of situation
      b. Attempting to define the event(s)
         (1) Person may be unaware and needs help to recall
         (2) Use appropriate interview skills to elicit information
      c. Helping person(s) develop plan for coping with the crisis situation
         (1) Resources (other persons, agencies, own strengths)
         (2) Follow-up to further assist and evaluate
   5. A mental status examination of the patient is usually required
      a. There is usually a time limit within which examination must be done
      b. Qualifications of one doing the examination may be specified by statutes
      c. Determination of patient's admission may be made by a court, physician, or some other designated person or body

G. Emergency admission
   1. This is provided for by almost all states
   2. It is considered for those thought to be harmful to self or others
   3. Limited goals are set
   4. There are statutes regarding who can file to admit another
   5. Limited time is allowed for confinement as well as for examination to be done
H. Court commitment—formal judicial hearing determines need for confinement

Discharges

A. Voluntary patients usually are discharged when sufficient improvement is noted
B. Voluntary patient who demands release before maximum benefit is noted must be released within specified time if court commitment process is not begun
C. Committed patients are often given conditional discharges
   1. Certain conditions are specified, such as returning for follow-up care
   2. Conditional discharges help make transition from hospital to home easier
D. Absolute discharge terminates legal relationship between patient and hospital; patients may not return to hospital without having a new admission procedure done
E. A judicial discharge may be sought if hospital does not approve of a patient's discharge; the patient or relatives may petition the court to allow discharge

Rights of patients

A. Civil rights
   1. Patient still retains power to enjoy certain privileges (right to vote; right to sell and maintain property; right to keep driver's license)
   2. Patients committed by court action retain all civil rights with exception of leaving the hospital or terminating treatment with court's consent
B. Habeas corpus proceedings
   1. Court action is sought by confined person who believes he or she has been illegally detained
   2. Purpose is to get release
   3. Patient is brought before court to determine sanity and whether hospitalization is necessary
C. Confidentiality
   1. In some states, confidential information exchanged between physician and patient during time of treatment cannot be used as evidence in court
   2. Staff members are under ethical and moral obligations to be discriminating in relating knowledge of patients
D. Records
   1. Records are legal documents and can be subpoenaed in court
   2. Nurse's notes may be placed in evidence in court, and nurse may have to testify that notes are based on observations of patient
   3. Records contain personal information about patient as well as therapeutic plans
   4. Revealing anything contained in patient's record other than what is necessary is not ethically sound

Responsibilities of the nurse

A. Should be familiar with laws of own state
B. Is expected to provide adequate protection for patients
   1. Suicide attempts
   2. Accidental injuries
   3. Improper use of restraints
   4. Elopement
C. Should know rules and regulations of hospital or agency
D. Should practice discretion in carrying out job responsibilities
E. Should practice nursing functions as defined by law

Negligence

A. Negligence is failure of a professional person to use kind of care and caution in treatment of patients that others in the same discipline use
B. In mental health nursing, negligence may involve such things as patients committing suicide or complications of ECT
C. Nurse must be very diligent in all aspects of care and treatment and strive to protect patient from harm to self or others

MENTAL HEALTH NURSING REVIEW QUESTIONS

Read each question carefully, and consider all possible answers. When you have decided which answer is **best,** blacken the corresponding space on the answer sheet. There is only **one** best answer for each question.

1 A mentally healthy individual
(A) Can perceive reality and act accordingly
(B) Has the ability to adjust to his or her environment in socially approved ways
(C) Has developed mature patterns for solving life's problems
(D) Considers future goals and movement toward them
1. A and B
2. C and D
3. A, B, and C
4. A, B, C, and D

2 Psychiatry is a branch of medicine concerned with
(A) Treatment of the mentally ill
(B) Intervention into patient's behaviors
(C) Hows and whys of mental illness
(D) Prevention of mental illness
1. A and B
2. A, C, and D
3. A and C
4. A, B, C, and D

3 Care and treatment of the mentally ill have included
(A) Actions based on superstition, ignorance, and mysticism
(B) Attitudes based on prevalent social attitudes and viewpoints
(C) The regarding of some mental illness as divine
(D) Humane treatment throughout history
1. A and B
2. A, B, and D
3. A, B, and C
4. A, B, C, and D

4 Twentieth-century reforms in the care and treatment of the mentally ill include
(A) Psychiatric units in general hospitals
(B) Day and night hospitals
(C) Crisis intervention
(D) Community mental health centers
1. A and B
2. A, B, and C
3. C and D
4. A, B, C, and D

5 Nursing subroles in the area of mental health may include
(A) Supportive role
(B) Socializing role
(C) Counseling role
(D) Mothering role
1. A and C
2. B and C
3. A, C, and D
4. A, B, C, and D

6 Basic principles of mental health nursing include
(A) Self-awareness
(B) Acceptance of patients
(C) Approval of behavior
(D) Reassurance
1. A, B, and C
2. A, B, and D
3. A, C, and D
4. A, B, C, and D

7 A statement that indicates a positive attitude in a practical nurse is
1. "Mr. Johnson is easy to work with; I feel so sorry for him."
2. "Mr. Johnson makes me feel good; I'm the only person who can get him to eat."
3. "I'd like to work with Mr. Johnson; his diagnosis is very interesting."
4. "I am interested in Mr. Johnson, and I'd like to help him if possible."

8 Characteristics of successful communication include
(A) Feedback
(B) Efficiency
(C) Appropriateness
(D) Flexibility
1. A and B
2. B and C
3. C and D
4. A, B, C, and D

9 When the nurse says to a patient during a conversation, "I'm not clear about what you said; go on," this is the communication technique known as
1. Reflection
2. Commenting
3. Clarification
4. Questioning

10 A communication technique that involves repeating all or part of an individual's statement is
1. Reflection
2. Silence
3. Clarification
4. Commenting

11 When a patient verbalizes anger about being hospitalized, the most appropriate response would be
1. "I'll get you a glass of juice; you'll feel better in a little while."
2. "You seem upset about being here."
3. "Something is bothering you; I'll come back later."
4. "I understand how you feel; all the patients feel this way at first."

12 Blocks to effective communication include
(A) Persistent questioning or probing
(B) Overloading or underloading the conversation
(C) Using value judgments
(D) Changing the subject
1. A and B
2. B and C
3. A and D
4. A, B, C, and D

13 In assessing the psychiatric patient, the nurse considers
(A) Appearance
(B) Behavior
(C) Conversation
(D) Past history
1. A, B, and C
2. B and D
3. B, C, and D
4. A, B, C, and D

14 Outcomes of a nursing assessment include
(A) Planning for care
(B) Assistance in anticipating needs
(C) Better understanding of the patient
(D) Early recovery
1. A and B
2. A, B, and C
3. A and C
4. A, B, C, and D

15 The type of therapy thought to be most commonly used in the treatment of mental illness today is
1. Electroshock therapy
2. Hydrotherapy
3. Insulin therapy
4. Chemotherapy (drugs)

16 Mr. Dean is very agitated, hyperactive, and combative. The physician would probably order
1. Antidepressants
2. Anticholinergics
3. Tranquilizers
4. Hypnotics

Situation: Mr. Jones is sad and depressed, showing little interest in activities around him. He states frequently, "Life is so empty, it's shameful for me to live."

17 If drug therapy is offered, the physician would probably order
1. Tranquilizers
2. Psychic energizers
3. Anticonvulsants
4. Anticholinergics

18 The most serious complication of a major tranquilizer is
1. Parkinsonian symptoms
2. Photosensitivity
3. Agranulocytosis
4. Hypotension

19 Mr. Jones verbalizes extreme fear of a treatment he is to receive for the first time. A probable supportive response is
1. "If you ask the doctor, he will be glad to explain the treatment."
2. "You need not be afraid; every precaution is taken during the treatment."
3. "I know you're apprehensive, Mr. Jones; let's talk about it."
4. "The doctor wouldn't order the treatment if he felt it was harmful; just trust him."

20 Before electroconvulsive therapy, the procedures are to
(A) Explain the treatment to the patient
(B) Withhold food and fluids
(C) Place the patient on strict bedrest
(D) Instruct patient to void before treatment
1. A and D
2. A, B, and D
3. B and D
4. A, B, C, and D

21 Mr. Jones has been pacing the halls and appears anxious and apprehensive. The most effective course is to
1. Permit him to pace as long as he does not disturb others
2. Secure the physician's permission to seclude him
3. Tell him that he must stop pacing at once
4. Insist that he sit down and work a picture puzzle

---

22 Mr. White is a depressed patient who has said, "I'm fed up. I don't intend to go on like this." The practical nurse should
1. Tell him he shouldn't say such things
2. Comment that others are worse off than he is
3. Report incident to charge nurse and record it in chart
4. Ignore the statement

23 In caring for a depressed patient, an important factor to consider is that he or she
1. Requires constant protection against suicide
2. Will always speak of suicide before an attempt
3. Will probably not attempt suicide if he or she talks about it
4. Is unlikely to attempt suicide for any reason

24 In caring for depressed patients, it is important to remember that
(A) Activity must be initiated for them since thinking and actions are considerably slowed
(B) Certain physical problems are likely to occur, such as constipation, edema, and skin infections
(C) Personal hygiene activities are often neglected
(D) Eating may be problematic because of frequent refusal of food
1. A and B
2. B, C, and D
3. A, B, and C
4. A, B, C, and D

25 A primary goal of nursing care for a withdrawn patient would be directed toward
1. Building his or her trust in all the staff initially
2. Gradually building trust by means of a one-to-one relationship
3. Encouraging numerous group activities
4. Insisting on patient's own management

26 When a depressed patient refuses food the explanation may be
1. Desire for attention
2. Feelings of unworthiness and guilt
3. Fear of being poisoned
4. Not enough energy to eat

27 To effectively motivate a withdrawn patient to engage in activity, the nurse might say
1. "Do you mind coming with the group today, Mr. Mann?"
2. "It is time for occupational therapy, Mr. Mann."
3. "Would you like to go to OT today, Mr. Mann?"
4. "I'll be waiting on you in the OT department, Mr. Mann."

28 In planning nursing care for the elated patient, a primary aim is
1. Encouraging interpersonal contact
2. Providing a nonstimulating environment
3. Demanding that the patient follow rules
4. Accepting and understanding behavior

29 A characteristic symptom of the elated patient is
1. Retarded speech
2. Increased motor and thought activity
3. Delusions of sin and guilt
4. Depressed mood

30 Nursing care of the elated patient will often include
(A) Frequently offering small amounts of easily handled food and fluids that can be eaten "on the run"
(B) Encouraging participation in competitive activities
(C) Providing a calm, nonstimulating environment
(D) Maintaining a permissive, sympathetic attitude
1. A and B
2. A and C
3. B, C, and D
4. A, B, C, and D

31 The most important factor to consider if mechanical restraints are used to control aggressive behavior is
1. The amount of the patient's aggressive behavior
2. The attitude of the staff in applying restraints
3. The type of restraints used
4. The need for written orders of the physician

Situation: Mr. Zayre was brought to the hospital by the police. Reports indicated that he assaulted a neighbor with an ice pick. He accused the neighbor of being a communist and repeatedly said that "the Lord told me to do away with you people."

32 On Mr. Zayre's admission, your *first* nursing action would be to
1. Search Mr. Zayre for a weapon
2. Show Mr. Zayre to his room
3. Introduce yourself
4. Begin immediately to interview the patient

33 While in a group painting a wall mural, Mr. Zayre began to throw his paint and paint brushes around the day room, shouting, "Get those communists away from me." The best course of action would be to
1. Discontinue the painting session until later
2. Remove Mr. Zayre from the group and remain with him
3. Allow Mr. Zayre to remain if he promises to behave
4. Remove the patient from the group and seclude him in his room

34 Nursing intervention for Mr. Zayre must first be directed toward
1. Long-range planning for care and treatment
2. Developing a trusting relationship
3. Elimination of all overt symptoms before making frequent contact
4. Obtaining a complete history on the patient

35 In attempting to cope with the delusions of the paranoid patient, the nurse should
1. Ask for explanations of the delusions
2. Go along with the delusions, since to disagree would upset the patient
3. Listen to the patient, indicating neither agreement nor disagreement
4. Disagree with the delusions any time he brings them up

36 The behavior of the patient who is anxious is characterized mainly by
1. Complete withdrawal from reality
2. Apprehension, fears, and worries
3. Confusion and hallucinations
4. Impaired judgment and lack of insight

37 Mr. Smith has been attending occupational therapy daily, but one morning he refuses to go. The most therapeutic approach would be to
1. Offer a reward on returning if he will go
2. Tell him he does not have to go
3. Inform him that he must go anyway
4. Attempt to find the reason for his refusal

38 If a patient refuses to eat, the practical nurse should first
1. Attempt to discover his reasons for not eating
2. Discontinue all nourishment between meals
3. Discontinue all privileges until he begins to eat
4. Tell him that if he does not eat he will be tube fed

39 Mr. Kay is a 62-year-old confused patient. At mealtime he is observed eating rapidly with his hands. The most helpful course of action is to
1. Comment, "You shouldn't eat with your hands, Mr. Kay."
2. Place a spoon in his hand, saying "Here, Mr. Kay, use your spoon."
3. Remove him to a corner where he is alone
4. Send him back to the ward until he learns to eat correctly

40 In the oedipal stage of growth and development, a child will often experience
(A) Peer rejection
(B) Curiosity about sex differences
(C) Separation anxiety
(D) Intense feelings toward the parent of the opposite sex
1. B and D
2. A and C
3. A, C, and D
4. A, B, C, and D

41 When Ethel learned that her physical condition would prohibit active involvement in her favorite sport, she studied hard to join the debate team. This behavior is an example of
1. Reaction formation
2. Displacement
3. Compensation
4. Identification

42 A patient has just had a session with his therapist and returns to the unit noticeably upset. When he pounds his pillow, cries, and gets his suitcase out, the nurse decides to
1. Reassure him by saying "You'll be alright in a few minutes."
2. Leave him alone to calm down
3. Encourage him to talk and release his feelings
4. Closely observe him but not attempt to get him to talk at this point

43 During the anal period of growth and development, a child is most likely to be concerned with
1. Peer relationships
2. Curiosity about sex differences
3. Separation from parents
4. Toilet training

44 Tommy, aged 3 years, is reacting to the birth of a baby brother. His parents can best help Tommy through his period of adjustment by
(A) Giving him special attention
(B) Sending him to a relative's home for a few days
(C) Ignoring his actions toward his new brother
(D) Allowing Tommy to help with simple tasks in caring for the baby
1. A and B
2. B
3. A and D
4. A and C

45 Typical characteristics of the adolescent phase of development are
(A) Conformity to peer group standards
(B) Desire for independence
(C) Looking to group for security
(D) Rebellion against authority figures
1. B and D
2. C and D
3. A, B, and C
4. A, B, C, and D

46 A patient refuses to get out of bed after repeated urgings from the nurse assigned to him. This behavior would best be charted
1. "Patient uncooperative. Refuses to get out of bed."
2. "Patient apparently withdrawn. Will not cooperate by getting out of bed."
3. "Did not get out of bed even after repeated urgings."
4. "States he wants to stay in bed. Will not abide by unit rules."

47 If group therapy has been successful, an individual will most likely be expected to
1. Be free from all emotional problems
2. Be more understanding of the behavior of others
3. Gain personal insights into his or her own behavior
4. Be free from anxiety

48 An initial assessment of a depressed patient observed by the nurse would best be charted
1. "Apparently depressed; not talking with others."
2. "Sat in chair, gazed at floor, did not respond to questions or comments."
3. "Appears sad; does not communicate."
4. "Unresponsive; has depressed expression."

49 When a nurse-patient relationship is ending, the patient may react by
(A) Rejecting the nurse
(B) Becoming angry
(C) Regression and withdrawal
(D) Acceptance
1. A and B
2. B and C
3. A, C, and D
4. A, B, C, and D

50 Mrs. Smith frequently is seen to lean her head to one side, cup her ear, and move her lips when no one is present. She is most likely experiencing a(n)
1. Illusion
2. Hallucination
3. Delusion
4. Obsession

51 The best source of information in conducting a nursing assessment is
1. The patient's chart
2. Family members
3. The patient
4. Staff comments

52 Methadone is a drug used in the treatment of
1. Alcoholism
2. Drug addiction
3. Neuroses
4. Psychoses

53 The first step in dealing with a crisis situation is
1. Defining the event
2. Assessing the situation
3. Suggesting appropriate resources
4. Determining how the person perceives the event

8 VOCATIONAL ASPECTS

REFERENCES

American Nurses' Association: Facts about nursing. Published annually by the American Nurses' Association, New York, N.Y.

Becker, B.G., and Fendler, D.T.: Vocational and personal adjustments in practical nursing, ed. 3, St. Louis, 1978, The C.V. Mosby Co.

Bush, C.H.: Personal and vocational relationships for practical nurses, ed. 2, Philadelphia, 1966, W.B. Saunders Co.

Cafferty, K.W., and Sugarman, L.K.: Steppingstones to professional nursing, ed. 5, St. Louis, 1971, The C.V. Mosby Co.

Creighton, H.: Law every nurse should know, ed. 3, Philadelphia, 1975, W.B. Saunders Co.

Sarner, H.: The nurse and the law, Philadelphia, 1968, W.B. Saunders Co.

Smith, E., and Huber, B.: Concepts in leadership for the licensed practical nurse, St. Louis, 1973, The C.V. Mosby Co.

CODE OF ETHICS FOR THE LPN

The following is paraphrased from the code of ethics that was adopted by the National Federation of Licensed Practical Nurses as a principle of conduct by which and through which its members, all licensed practical nurses, shall govern their private lives and nursing careers.

This digest of principles is designed to guide the nurse in and out of the profession—as an individual and as a nurse. It shall serve to guide the relationships—to the patient, to the physician, to the patient's family, to the employer, to fellow nurses, and as a member of the community.

1. The licensed practical nurse shall practice the profession with integrity.
2. The licensed practical nurse shall be loyal—to the physician, to the patient, and to the employer.
3. The licensed practical nurse strives to know the limitations and to stay within the bounds of these limitations.
4. The licensed practical nurse is sincere in the performance of duties and generous in rendering service.
5. The licensed practical nurse considers no duty too menial if it contributes to the welfare and comfort of the patient.
6. The licensed practical nurse accepts only that monetary compensation which is provided for in the contract employed, and does not solicit gifts.
7. The licensed practical nurse holds in confidence all entrusted information.
8. The licensed practical nurse shall be a good citizen.
9. The licensed practical nurse participates in and shares responsibility of meeting health needs.
10. The licensed practical nurse faithfully carries out the orders of the physician or registered nurse.
11. The licensed practical nurse refrains from entering into conversation with the patient about personal experiences, personal problems, and personal ailments.
12. The licensed practical nurse abstains from administering self-medication and, in event of personal illness, takes only those medications prescribed by a licensed physician.
13. The licensed practical nurse respects the dignity of the uniform by never wearing it in a public place.
14. The licensed practical nurse respects the religious beliefs of all patients.
15. The licensed practical nurse abides by the Golden Rule in daily relationships with all people.
16. The licensed practical nurse is a member of the National Federation of Licensed Practical Nurses, Inc., and the state and local membership associations.
17. The licensed practical nurse may give credit to a commercial product or service but does not identify with advertising, sales or promotion.

VOCATIONAL RESPONSIBILITIES

To the patient

A. The following is paraphrased from the Patient's Bill of Rights adopted by the American Hospital Association and published in *Modern Hospital*

The patient should

1. Be given considerate and respectful care
2. Obtain from the physician complete current information concerning diagnosis, treatment, and prognosis in terms he or she can be reasonably expected to understand
3. Receive from the physician information necessary to give informed consent prior to the start of any procedure or treatment
4. Be allowed to refuse treatment to the extent permitted by law and be informed of the medical consequences of that action
5. Be given every consideration of privacy concerning his or her own medical care program
6. Expect that all communications and records pertaining to his or her care be treated as confidential
7. Expect that within its capacity a hospital must make reasonable response to the request of a patient for services
8. Obtain information as to any relationships of the patient's hospital to other health care and educational institutions insofar as his or her care is concerned
9. Be advised if the hospital proposes to engage in or perform human experimentation affecting the patient's care or treatment
10. Expect reasonable continuity of care
11. Examine and receive an explanation of the bill regardless of the source of payment
12. Know what hospital rules and regulations apply to the patient's conduct

B. The practical nurse must always keep the patient's rights in mind when implementing patient care

To self

A. Keep abreast with what is going on in health field by reading and by participating in continuing education
B. Join and actively participate in professional associations
C. Maintain good physical and mental health
D. Maintain an attractive appearance

To profession

A. Support local, state, and national nursing organizations
B. Conform to ethics and standards set up by organizations

To the employing agency

A. Uphold policies and standards
B. Direct complaints through proper channels of authority
C. Conform to institutional regulations
D. Be loyal to employer

LEGAL ASPECTS

Definition of legal terms

A. Abortion—the U.S. Supreme Court has ruled that a woman may obtain a legal abortion during the first 3 months of pregnancy provided it is performed by authorized medical personnel; the states may decide whether abortion is to be allowed during the second trimester; despite this ruling, abortion is still being discussed and contested, both morally and legally, in the United States
B. Assault—threat or attempt to contact body of another person without privilege of doing so and without consent
C. Battery—act of making an unauthorized contact with another person's body
D. Crime—act against the whole of society; any offense perpetrated against public interest
   1. Felony—a more serious crime; it carries penalties ranging from imprisonment in the state penitentiary to death
   2. Misdemeanor—misbehavior; it is a less serious form of crime
E. Defamation—a wrongful act meaning to injure the reputation of another person
   1. Slander—oral defamation
   2. Libel—written defamation
F. Defendant—party against whom a legal proceeding is instituted
G. Euthanasia—mercy killing (under much discussion morally and legally)
H. False imprisonment—unwarranted restriction of freedom
I. Homicide—to cause death of another person unlawfully (justifiable homicide—when death is incurred in attempt to prevent atrocious crime or in defense of oneself or one's close relatives)
J. Manslaughter—killing of another without malice aforethought
   1. Voluntary—occurs as a result of a temporary loss of emotion control
   2. Involuntary—occurs as result of offense no greater than misdemeanor

K. Murder—killing of another with deliberate intent and malice aforethought
L. Negligence—failure to do what a person of ordinary judgment or prudence would do or doing what a reasonable person would not do
M. Plaintiff—party who institutes and commences a civil proceeding
N. Press code rules—information that legally may be given concerning a patient
   1. Name, address, sex, marital status, approximate age, occupation, employer, and name and address of nearest relative
   2. Condition of patient (good, fair, serious, critical, DOA)
O. Reciprocity (endorsement) (interstate licensure)—the formal recognition by a state of the qualifications of a nurse from another state
P. Tort—wrongful act committed by one person against another

Incident report

A. This is a factual statement about an error made by the nurse or about a patient's or visitor's accident occurring on hospital premises
B. Nurse should be familiar with procedure dictated by employing agency

Nurse Practice Act

A. This defines limitations of nursing practice; it varies from state to state
B. Employing agencies, hospitals, and physicians further define the duties and limitations of the practical nurse

Accountability

A. Practical nurses must exercise reasonable care at all times and be willing to assume full responsibility for their actions
B. Standard for care for practical nurses is that degree of care ordinarily exercised by nurses of similar training and experience in the same or similar situation

Legal documents and nurse

A. Contracts
   1. Contract is an agreement between two or more people for a consideration (legal term meaning some recompense, such as a fee)
   2. Services of practical nurse may be contracted for by physician, registry, patient, or patient's family
   3. When employed by hospital or agency, practical nurse must accept decision of employing agency and perform only those duties outlined in the job description
   4. Private duty nursing contract with patient and family is arranged when registry or hospital obtains private duty nurse, usually at patient's, physician's, or family's request
   5. Patient or family is responsible for paying practical nurse
   6. In special cases a hospital may employ a private duty nurse and is responsible for fee
B. Wills
   1. Will is legal declaration of a person's wishes as to the disposition of his or her property after death
   2. Practical nurse may be asked to witness will
   3. Nurse should consent only in an emergency and if no one else is available
   4. Nurse should suggest to family and attorney that someone else witness; if will is contested, nurse may be called to court
   5. Types of wills are
      a. Written will—most common
      b. Noncupative, or oral, will—recognized as valid in most states under certain circumstances
   6. Essential parts of a will are
      a. Testator
      b. Executor for estate
      c. Disposal of property (real, personal, mixed)
      d. Date and signature
      e. Witnesses
         (1) Witnesses should not be persons named in will
         (2) There are age requirements in some states
   7. If practical nurse is called to court in regard to will or anything else, competent legal aid should be obtained. The professional registry or nursing organization may be able to give advice

LICENSURE AND NURSE

Purposes

A. To limit and control admission into health care occupations
B. To provide protection for the practical nurse and the general public from unqualified practitioners

Obtaining a license

A. All states have laws licensing practical nurses
   1. Mandatory law—everyone practicing must have license
   2. Permissive law—anyone may do work of practical nurse provided he or she does not represent self as a Licensed Practical Nurse

B. Information can be obtained from State Board of Nurse Examiners (official agency responsible for administering nurse practice laws), which is usually located in state capital

C. State Board of Nurse Examiners in each state is primarily responsible for setting minimum standards and granting approval for schools of practical nursing

D. In most states licensing of both practical and professional nurses is under the same board; both professional and practical nurses are appointed to the board

E. Practical nurse becomes licensed by meeting requirements set up by states, including taking examination at time and place specified by state board

F. When practical nurse wishes to nurse in a state other than that in which registered, he or she
   1. Writes for information and requirements to State Board of Nurse Examiners in new state
   2. Obtains this information before moving or accepting position in another state to be sure qualifications are met

G. *American Journal of Nursing,* January issue, carries complete directory of international, national, and state boards of nursing and their addresses

SEEKING EMPLOYMENT

Selecting position

A. Consider preference of
   1. Kind of nursing
   2. Location of employment
   3. Institutional or private duty
   4. Salary
   5. Fringe benefits
   6. Distance to drive
   7. Opportunity for advancement

B. Discuss with instructors and director of school before completing course in practical nursing

C. Be realistic regarding abilities, personality, health, and achievement in nursing

Applying for position

A. At local hospitals or agencies, apply to personnel department or in some instances to nursing office

B. Take Civil Service Examination; this is necessary in certain governmental hospitals and agencies; obtain information from local, city, or state offices

C. Apply to professional registry
   1. Some now place practical nurses; investigate what is done in your locality
   2. Inquire whether liability insurance is provided by the agency or whether it is the responsibility of the practical nurse

D. Answer advertisements in newspapers and nursing or hospital magazines

E. Make sure that employing individual, hospital, or agency is recognized and in good standing

F. Apply to commercial registry; many exist throughout United States
   1. Standing of registry can be obtained from practical nursing association; find out standing before registering with it
   2. Many do very good work and can place practical nurses in interesting positions

G. Be prepared for the following steps in applying for a position
   1. It is usually necessary to fill in an application blank; it may be sent by mail or obtained in local employing office
   2. Applicant should make sure all information requested is complete and accurate
   3. Personal resumé, photograph, birth certificate, draft status or service record, and verification of naturalization may be requested
   4. Usually names of persons who will recommend you are requested; these are character references, such as those from minister or teacher (ask permission to use their names), and work references, such as those from director of school, instructor, and previous employers
   5. Applicant should never make false or misleading statements; most information can be checked if necessary

Personnel policies

A. Booklets or pamphlets outlining personnel policies are available in most hospitals and employing agencies

B. Nurse should ask for a copy and be familiar with them before accepting position

C. Nurse should know terms of employment
D. Personnel policies should include
   1. Hours of work, time for meals, and whether straight or broken shifts
   2. Day, afternoon, or night assignments required
   3. Sunday and public holiday requirements
   4. Vacation—length with pay, time of year taken, eligibility for, and after how many months of employment
   5. Sick leave—length with pay
   6. Maternity leave
   7. Medical care
      a. Beginning and routine annual physical examination
      b. Health department or clinic for minor illnesses and accidents
      c. Hospitalization—cost and under what conditions given
      d. Health, medical, or hospital insurance available
   8. Promotion plan in work and wages
   9. Licensure as for practical nurses in state
   10. Social Security coverage
      a. Nurse should obtain Social Security number from local office
      b. Under Social Security program of social insurance, practical nurse may qualify for unemployment insurance, old age and survivor's insurance, or Medicare
      c. Provisions under Social Security are constantly changing and vary in different states; check with local Social Security office for information or assistance

Resigning from position

A. Resignation should be in writing if required by institution; reason is usually requested
B. It is customary to give 2 to 4 weeks' notice, depending on responsibilities of position, so that replacement can be obtained
C. Nurse should follow instructions given in personnel policies of institution
D. Nurse should thank employer for courtesies extended during employment in the letter of resignation
E. Letter of resignation is a permanent record; do not make unkind statements

NATIONAL ORGANIZATIONS

National Association for Practical Nurse Education and Services, Inc., 122 East 42nd Street, New York, New York 10017

A. NAPNES was organized in 1941 to promote development of sound practical/vocational nursing education and to promote advancement and recognition of the licensed practical/vocational nurse as a member of the health team
B. Membership includes
   1. Individual members—licensed practical/vocational nurses, practical nursing educators, other registered nurses, general educators, physicians, hospital and nursing home administrators, practical nursing students, and interested lay persons
   2. Per capita members—licensed practical/vocational nurses who are members of state-licensed practical/vocational nurse associations that are affiliated with NAPNES and pay dues to it on a per capita basis
   3. Student members—students in state-approved schools of practical/vocational nursing
   4. Agency members—hospitals, nursing homes, schools of practical nursing, alumni groups, civic organizations, and other institutions or groups in harmony with NAPNES' objectives
C. Functions and activities, as listed by the National Association for Practical Nurse Education and Services, Inc., are
   1. Serves as clearing house for information about practical/vocational nursing, including information about functions and roles of licensed practical/vocational nurses
   2. Publishes *Journal of Practical Nursing*, a monthly magazine
   3. Maintains national accreditation service for educational programs in practical/vocational nursing, which was established in 1945 and is recognized by U.S. Office of Education
   4. Maintains consultation service for those conducting or contemplating establishment of educational programs in practical/vocational nursing
   5. Prepares publications useful to faculties in schools of practical/vocational nursing
   6. Sponsors workshops and seminars for licensed practical/vocational nurses and practical nursing educators in conjunction with state LPN/LVN associations, universities, and national organizations

7. Conducts annual convention for exchange of ideas and experiences among those concerned with practical/vocational nursing
8. Disseminates information about practical/vocational nursing and schools of practical/vocational nursing to prospective students and career counselors
9. Provides scholarships to students of practical/vocational nursing in both basic programs and programs of continuing education for LPNs/LVNs
10. Engages in activities aimed at protecting and strengthening position of LPNs/LVNs and cooperates with state LPN/LVN associations in activities of this kind
11. Provides consultation to state LPN/LVN associations on matters relating to their organization and programs

National Federation of Licensed Practical Nurses, Inc., 250 West 57th Street, New York, New York 10019

A. NFLPN was organized in 1949 to foster high standards in practical nursing and to further practical nurses' welfare
B. Membership includes licensed practical nurses and student practical nurses
C. There are state associations in most states
D. Functions as listed by National Federation of Licensed Practical Nurses, Inc., are
   1. To preserve and foster the nursing ideal of comprehensive care for the ill and aged
   2. To associate together all licensed practical/vocational nurses and licensed nurses having an equivalent title
   3. To promote the economic and general welfare of all licensed practical/vocational nurses
   4. To secure continued recognition of all licensed practical/vocational nurses
   5. To uphold the standards and ethics of all licensed practical/vocational nurses and to interpret them to the public
   6. To promote the continued effective use of all licensed practical/vocational nurses
   7. To promote the efficient functioning of constituent state licensed practical/vocational nurse associations
   8. To cooperate with all members of health groups and with organizations interested in better patient care
   9. To collect and distribute information on practical/vocational nursing
   10. To further the continuing nursing education of all licensed practical/vocational nurses
   11. To promote, support, and speak for all licensed practical/vocational nurses in regard to legislative action
   12. To represent and serve as the spokesman for licensed practical/vocational nurses with allied health and governmental groups and the public
E. *Nursing Care,* the official publication of NFLPN, is published bimonthly
F. A scholarship program was established in 1962; conferences, institutes and workshops were provided for LPNs.

National League for Nursing, 10 Columbus Circle, New York, New York 10019

A. NLN was organized in 1952 by combining the National League for Nursing Education and six other national nursing organizations
B. Membership includes
   1. Registered professional nurses
   2. Qualified practical nurses
   3. Members of allied professions
   4. Consumers of nursing service and interested lay persons
   5. Agencies of nursing service or nursing education
C. Functions are
   1. Defining and furthering good standards for all nursing service
   2. Defining and promoting good standards for institutions giving nursing education on all levels
   3. Helping to extend facilities to meet these services when necessary
   4. Helping in proper distribution of nursing education and nursing service
   5. Working to improve organized nursing services in hospitals, public health agencies, nursing homes, and other agencies; accrediting community public health nursing services; developing criteria and other self-evaluation tools
   6. Working to improve nursing education programs; acting as an accrediting agency for nursing education
   7. Constructing and processing professional and practical nurse licensing examinations; providing preadmission, achievement, and qualifying tests
   8. Gathering and publishing information about trends in nursing, personnel needs, community nursing services, and schools of nursing
D. Official magazine is *Nursing Outlook*
E. NLN cosponsors with American Nurses' Association a national nursing careers program, a film service, and the magazine *Nursing Research*

F. Other factors are
   1. NLN employed consultants in practical nursing in 1956
   2. Council on Practical Nursing of NLN formed in 1957
   3. Council became Department of Practical Nursing in 1961
   4. Council on Community Planning for Nursing formed in 1969
   5. Title III grant of Public Law 911 since 1956 has enabled schools for practical nurses to expand and new ones to be organized from public funds

VOCATIONAL ASPECTS REVIEW QUESTIONS

Read each question carefully, and consider all possible answers. When you have decided which answer is **best,** blacken the corresponding space on the answer sheet. There is only **one** best answer for each question.

1 The activities of the practical nurse today are defined by
1. Physician
2. Professional nurse
3. Law
4. Custom and accepted practice

2 When caring for a patient in the home, the nurse should dispose of any unused narcotics by
1. Giving them to the patient for future use
2. Returning them to the physician
3. Keeping them for administration to a future patient
4. Giving them to the health department

3 The term most commonly applied to the practical nurse who has passed the state board examination is
1. Vocational nurse
2. Practical nurse
3. Licensed practical nurse
4. Trained practical nurse

4 The nurse is caring for a patient in his home and is asked to witness the patient's will by his lawyer; the nurse should
1. Comply with the request without question
2. Tell him that you will do so only if the registry approves
3. Suggest to the family and attorney that someone else witness it
4. Tell the family that a witness is not necessary

5 Malicious statements expressed orally are called
1. Slander
2. Libel
3. Gossip
4. Heresy

6 The practical nurse can obtain information about licensing from the
1. State health department
2. Local Social Security office
3. State Board of Nurse Examiners
4. American Nurses' Association

7 When a nurse resigns from a position in hospital nursing, it is customary to give a written notice of
1. 1 to 2 weeks
2. 2 to 4 weeks
3. 3 to 6 weeks
4. 6 to 8 weeks

8 The practical nurse may belong to the following national nursing organizations
(A) National Association for Practical Nurse Education and Services, Inc.
(B) American Nurses' Association
(C) National Federation of Licensed Practical Nurses, Inc.
(D) National League for Nursing
1. A, B, and C
2. A, C, and D
3. A and C
4. A, B, C, and D

9 Before accepting any position, the practical nurse should consider the
(A) Personnel policies of the employing agency
(B) Kind of nursing preferred
(C) Locality preferred
(D) Qualifications necessary
(E) Type of nursing done best
1. A, B, and C
2. A, B, and D
3. A, B, and E
4. A, B, C, D, and E

10 Reasons for licensing the practical nurse are to
(A) Safeguard the public
(B) Ensure higher wages

(C) Protect the practical nurse
(D) Enable employing agencies to obtain qualified personnel
1. A, C, and D
2. A, B, and C
3. A, B, and D
4. A, B, C, and D

11 Personnel policies usually include
(A) The length of the work week
(B) Vacation time and other leave with pay
(C) Medical care
(D) Promotion plan in work and wages
(E) State registration requirements
1. A, C, and E
2. B, D, and E
3. A, B, C, and D
4. A, C, D, and E

12 The practical nurse should be told about the personnel policies in any hospital or employing agency
1. Verbally by other employees
2. Verbally by the head nurse
3. In writing by the physician
4. In writing by the hospital administration and nursing service

13 Members of NAPNES include
(A) Licensed practical nurses
(B) Registered nurses
(C) Educators
(D) Physicians
(E) Citizens
1. A, B, D, and E
2. A, B, C, and E
3. A, B, C, and D
4. A, B, C, D, and E

14 In private duty nursing, the licensed practical nurse has a contract with the
1. Hospital
2. Patient or family
3. Superintendent of nurses
4. Physician

15 If a licensed practical nurse performs duties so that people or property are injured, the nurse is described as being
1. Emotionally incapable
2. Negligent
3. Malicious
4. Illegal

16 In practical nursing the licensed practical nurse should have legal knowledge of
(A) Licensing laws
(B) Controlled Substances Act
(C) Contracts
(D) Wills
(E) Hill-Burton Act
1. A, C, D, and E
2. A, B, D, and E
3. A, B, C, and D
4. A, B, C, D, and E

17 The national organization that limits individual membership to licensed practical nurses is the
1. National League for Nursing
2. National Federation of Licensed Practical Nurses, Inc.
3. State Board of Nurse Examiners
4. American Nurses' Association

18 Setting minimum standards and approving schools for practical nursing are done primarily by the
1. American Nurses' Association
2. National League for Nursing
3. Individual State Boards of Nurse Examiners
4. National Association for Practical Nurse Education and Services, Inc.

19 The registration of the practical nurse is the responsibility of the
1. State Department of Health
2. State Nurses' Association
3. State Hospital Association
4. State Board of Nurse Examiners

20 An oral will declared by a dying person before witnesses is known as
1. Probate
2. Testate
3. Intestate
4. Nuncupative

21 Vocational responsibilities of the licensed practical nurse include
(A) Continuing education
(B) Participating in professional associations
(C) Regular church attendance
(D) Conformance to institutional standards
(E) Keeping the community informed about hospital problems
1. A, B, and D
2. A, B, C, and D
3. A, B, D, and E
4. A, B, C, D, and E

22 Practical nurses are considered part of the health team today because
(A) Varied levels of skill are needed in team assignments
(B) Specialization in nursing has resulted in certain tasks being carried out by licensed practical nurses
(C) Practical nurses are now licensed
(D) It results in better utilization of all nursing personnel
1. B, C, and D
2. A, C, and D
3. A, B, and C
4. A, B, C, and D

23 In the nurse's code of ethics the fundamental responsibility is to conserve life and to promote health. The nurse can solve almost any ethical problem that might arise by following the
1. Patient's Bill of Rights
2. Nightingale pledge
3. Golden Rule
4. Hospital personnel policies

24 Practical nursing has expanded greatly since World War II because
1. It is required by law
2. Infant mortality has increased
3. The need for all nursing has increased
4. There are fewer opportunities for professional nurses

25 If you are having difficulty working with another nurse, the best remedy would be to
1. Report it to the head nurse
2. Resign
3. Ask to be transferred to another division
4. Discuss the problem with the person involved

26 The practical nurse should be familiar with the basic laws governing the
(A) Sale and use of narcotics
(B) Licensing of practical nurses
(C) Witnessing of wills
(D) Making and breaking of contracts
1. A and B
2. A, B, and C
3. A, B, and D
4. A, B, C, and D

27 Trends in nursing theory and procedures are changing constantly. The nurse can stay abreast of latest developments by
(A) Reading current professional magazines and newspapers
(B) Attending refresher classes
(C) Participating in inservice programs
(D) Joining professional organizations and participating
1. A, B, and C
2. A, C, and D
3. B, C, and D
4. A, B, C, and D

28 Confidential information is called
1. Privileged communication
2. Justifiable homicide
3. Negligence
4. Deposition

29 Included in a written application should be
(A) Desired days off
(B) Preference of hours on duty and type of nursing
(C) Date available
(D) Friends as references
(E) Relatives as references
1. A, B, and C
2. B, C, and D
3. A, C, and D
4. A, B, C, D, and E

30 The best policy when resigning is to
(A) Leave without notice
(B) Give 2 to 4 weeks' notice
(C) Discuss dissatisfaction with immediate supervisor
(D) State your regret at leaving
(E) Work at your best until leaving
(F) Explain tactfully your reasons
1. A, C, and E
2. B, E, and F
3. C, D, and E
4. B, D, E, and F

31 A criminal abortion is classified as
1. Felony
2. Manslaughter
3. Homicide
4. Suicide

32 In order to become licensed in another state, the LPN
(A) Must take the State Board Examination again
(B) May be eligible by endorsement or reciprocity
(C) Should write to the State Board of Nurse Examiners in the particular state
(D) Should write to the National Federation of Licensed Practical Nurses, Inc.
1. B and D
2. A and B
3. B and C
4. C and D

33 State Nurse Practice Acts are
(A) Carried out by the State Board of Nursing
(B) To protect the nurse as well as the patient
(C) Enforced by the ANA
(D) Uniform from one state to another
(E) Mandatory in nature
1. B and D
2. A and B
3. A, C, and D
4. A, B, and D

34 According to the Code of Ethics for the LPN, the nurse should
(A) Be a good citizen
(B) Never gossip about patients
(C) Not solicit gifts
(D) Never wear his or her uniform in a public place
(E) Identify products to promote sales
1. A, B, C, and D
2. B, C, D, and E
3. A, B, D, and E
4. A, B, C, D, and E

35 The practical nurse should keep the patient's rights in mind when
1. Implementing patient care
2. Signing a contract
3. Charting
4. Filling out application for state boards

36 Euthanasia is
1. A form of hypnosis
2. Information that may legally be given concerning a patient
3. Mercy killing
4. Unwarranted restriction of freedom

37 Accountability refers to
1. Reporting to work on time
2. Limitations of nursing practice
3. Formal recognition by a state of the qualifications of a nurse from another state
4. Assuming responsibility for actions

38 *Nursing Care* is published by
1. NLN
2. NFLPN
3. NAPNES
4. ANA

39 Mrs. Jones, LPN, instructed an aide to apply a hot-water bottle to a patient's leg. The patient received a burn. Mrs. Jones could be sued for
1. Defamation
2. Negligence
3. Felony
4. Assault

In questions 40 through 45 you are to decide whether or not an incident report is required.

40 Mr. Smith climbs over the side-rails and falls out of bed
1. A report is required
2. A report is not required

41 Mrs. Jones' mother sneaked into the hospital to see her
1. A report is required
2. A report is not required

42 Baby Brown develops a body rash
1. A report is required
2. A report is not required

43 Mrs. White, RN, gives aspirin (ASA) to the wrong patient
1. A report is required
2. A report is not required

44 Sally Blue, SN, gave a sitz bath to the wrong patient
1. A report is required
2. A report is not required

45 Mrs. Jarvis refuses her breakfast
1. A report is required
2. A report is not required

SAMPLE EXAMINATION 1

This examination contains several paragraphs concerning patients/clients. Following each such paragraph is a series of questions concerning the patient and the situation described in that paragraph. Read each situation carefully. Read each question carefully, and consider all possible answers. When you have decided which answer is **best,** blacken the corresponding space on the answer sheet. There is only **one** best answer for each question.

Situation: Mrs. Sara Lent has been an insulin-dependent diabetic for 20 years. Now at age 68 she has begun to notice that her right foot and leg get numb and the skin is shiny. She is admitted to your unit because last week she bumped her right leg while making her bed. The injured area has not healed but has worsened. Questions 1 through 20 refer to this situation.

1 During your initial assessment of Mrs. Lent, you discover that she is wearing garters. It would be appropriate for you to
1. Make a note of this on Mrs. Lent's chart
2. Notify the physician immediately
3. Explain that garters retard circulation to the lower extremities and should not be worn
4. Explain that garters are much better than wearing a girdle because they are not as restricting to circulation as a girdle

2 Which of the following descriptions of the injured area on Mrs. Lent's right leg would be most appropriate to chart?
1. "Large excoriated area on anterior aspect of the shinbone"
2. "50-cent size elongated area on anterior aspect of lower leg, with moderate amount of serous drainage"
3. "5-cm abraised lesion with small amount of serous drainage noted on right lower leg"
4. "I have an injury on my right lower leg where I hit it against my bed at home"

3 Mrs. Lent's right lower leg is taut and shiny. This is significant because
1. These symptoms indicate the diabetes is worsening
2. This indicates the circulation to this extremity may be compromised
3. Taut, shiny skin indicates edema of the extremity
4. These symptoms are consistent with a positive Homan's sign

4 During admission Mrs. Lent asks for assistance to the bathroom to void. You would
1. Assist her to use the bedpan; perform sugar and acetone test
2. Assist her to use the bedpan; collect admission BUN
3. Call for help to walk Mrs. Lent to the bathroom; perform sugar and acetone test
4. Call for help to walk Mrs. Lent to the bathroom; collect admission BUN

5 You would notify the physician immediately if the
1. Right pedal pulse was bounding; admission FBS, 168
2. Right femoral pulse was difficult to palpate; urine sugar and acetone, 0.5%
3. Right pedal pulse was not palpated; FBS, 320
4. Right pedal pulse was thready; sugar and acetone, 1%

6 In order to protect the affected extremity from further injury you would
1. Promote mobility and apply antiembolism stockings
2. Administer anticoagulants and apply warm moist compresses
3. Wrap the leg tightly with elastic bandage and administer antibiotics
4. Apply a bed cradle and heel protectors

7 Symptoms of diabetic ketoacidosis are
1. Hypotension, hypoglycemia, and thirst
2. FBS, 400; Kussmaul's respirations; and fruity odor on breath
3. Polyuria, polydipsia, and polyphagia
4. Hypertension, convulsions, and diaphoresis

8 Mrs. Lent is receiving 30 units of NPH insulin q. a.m. at 7:30. You might expect a hypoglycemic reaction at
1. 1 PM
2. 4 PM
3. 12 midnight
4. 3 AM

9 Mrs. Lent's leg worsens. Objective data to support this conclusion would be
1. FBS, 420; sugar and acetone, 1% to 2% daily, and BUN 16
2. Purulent drainage, cool right foot, and temperature of 101.6°F orally
3. Polyuria, polydipsia, and polyphagia
4. Ability to dorsiflex *both* feet and FBS, 300

10 Diabetes is a predisposing factor to peripheral vascular disorders because diabetes is a(n)
1. Mendelian recessive trait common to persons with poor venous integrity
2. Endocrine disorder that stimulates the kidneys to raise the blood pressure
3. Metabolic disorder of CHO metabolism in which accelerated fat metabolism leads to changes in arterial walls
4. Disorder in which the administration of insulin causes inhibition of blood supply to the lower extremities

11 Mrs. Lent's physician tells her she has decided to perform an above-the-knee amputation. After the physician leaves Mrs. Lent's room, she turns her head away from you and begins to cry. You would
1. Leave the room quietly and allow her to cry without embarrassment
2. Stay with Mrs. Lent and encourage her to talk about postoperative coughing and deep breathing
3. Leave the room and call her husband to come to the hospital to console her
4. Stay with Mrs. Lent; hold her hand

12 After Mrs. Lent leaves her room to go to OR, you begin readying the area for her return. Equipment most appropriate to obtain would be
1. IV pole, tourniquet, and extra pillows
2. Bed boards, Buck's traction equipment, and emergency drug box
3. Sandbags, extra pillows, and emesis basin
4. Booklet explaining phantom pain, IV pole, and extra elastic bandages

13 Symptoms exhibited immediately postoperatively that would necessitate emergency action would be
1. B/P, 100/70; pulse, 110; respirations, 26; and large amount of red drainage on posterior aspect of dressing
2. Continued flexion of the hip and urine output of 100 ml 2 hours postoperatively
3. B/P, 150/90; pulse, 86; and moderate amount of red drainage on anterior of dressing
4. Hgb level, 12.6; B/P, 140/90; and complaints of pain

14 To prevent hip contractures, you would position Mrs. Lent (postoperatively) with her stump
1. Flexed on a pillow
2. Extended
3. Externally rotated using pillows
4. Internally rotated using a trochanter roll

15 As a result of surgery Mrs. Lent's insulin requirements would be
1. Increased
2. Decreased
3. Met only by the intravenous route
4. Unchanged

16 Insulin administered intravenously is
1. NPH
2. Ultralente
3. PZI
4. Regular

17 Since surgery you notice Mrs. Lent has become increasingly demanding. Today when you enter her room, Mrs. Lent yells at you, "Get out of my room. Can't you see I am sleeping?" Your response would be
1. "Sorry, Mrs. Lent, but I have to get the baths done before noon."
2. "Are you having trouble sleeping at night?"
3. "You seem angry, Mrs. Lent. Would you like to talk?"
4. "Oh, excuse me. I'll come back later."

18 To prepare the stump for a prosthesis device you should encourage
1. Gluteal sitting exercises and straight leg raises and wrap the stump with elastic bandages
2. Upper extremity push-ups and active range of motion exercises
3. Massaging of the stump and irrigation of the suture line with Betadine solution
4. Placing the stump in a dependent position constantly to promote blood supply to the area

19 Considering Mrs. Lent's hospital stay, it would be most appropriate for you to
1. Review diabetic foot care before discharge
2. Send Mrs. Lent to a nursing home
3. Teach her to administer her own insulin
4. Ask Mr. Lent to hire a maid so this type of accident will not be repeated

20 One day Mrs. Lent asks if she may have beets on her diabetic diet. Your response would be
1. "No, they contain too much natural sugar."
2. "Yes, they are on the diabetic exchange list."
3. "Yes, you could. I'll call the dietitian, and you two can review the exchange list."
4. "I don't know. Ask your doctor. Your diet is too important in your treatment to change very much."

Situation: Janet Goldberg, aged 21, has recurrent ulcerative colitis. She is admitted to your unit because of increasing frequency of her diarrheic stools. She is to be graduated from college in 2 months. Questions 21 through 40 refer to this situation.

21 Because Janet's chief complaint is frequent diarrheic stools you would include which of the following in your initial assessment?
1. Symptoms of fluid and electrolyte imbalance
2. Urinalysis for presence of urobilinogen
3. Pupil check
4. Clinitest and Acetest

22 Ulcerative colitis is
1. Obstruction of the bowel resulting from electrolyte imbalance
2. Inflammation of the stomach
3. Inflammation of the mucosa of the small intestines
4. Electrolyte imbalance resulting from diarrhea

23 The diagnosis of ulcerative colitis is confirmed by
1. Upper GI series and liver biopsy
2. Lower GI series and sigmoidoscopy
3. Test of stool specimen for ova and parasites and upper GI series
4. Gastroscopy and signs and symptoms

24 During this acute phase of her disease you would plan Janet's care to include
1. Complete bed bath and frequent back care
2. Walks in the hall after a shower and bland diet
3. Bath with assistance in bed and forced fluids
4. Walks when she prefers and diet as desired

25 Recording bowel status in the nursing notes is essential. An appropriate notation might be
1. "Frequent diarrheic stools noted this shift"
2. "Six diarrheic stools since lunch today"
3. "Five mucoid diarrheic stools this AM"
4. "8 AM, 150-ml stool—liquid with bloody mucus"

26 Janet requests medication for her stools. Assuming all were ordered PRN, which would be appropriate?
1. Keflex
2. Azulfidine
3. Lomotil
4. ASA

27 Which of the following symptoms would indicate Janet suffers from electrolyte imbalance secondary to diarrhea?
1. Serum K of 3 and muscle weakness
2. Serum Na of 135 and convulsions
3. Serum K of 3.8 and diarrhea
4. Serum Na of 120 and edema of feet

28 Janet's hemoglobin level is 8.6 g. Her symptoms might be
1. Increased energy and pulse rate of 100
2. Decreased energy and pulse rate of 60
3. Weakness and pulse rate of 120
4. Increased muscular strength and pulse rate of 80

29 Which of the following foods should Janet be allowed on a low-residue diet?
1. Orange juice
2. Fried chicken
3. Cream of wheat cereal
4. Creamed corn

30 Janet has been placed on a high-protein, high-carbohydrate, low-fiber diet. An appropriate meal plan would be
1. Grapefruit, waffles with syrup, and Canadian bacon
2. Applesauce, chicken, and tossed salad

3. Sautéed chicken in cream sauce and carrot salad
4. Fresh bran bread, pecan pie, and broiled steak

31 Which complaint, if voiced by Janet, would indicate a potentially life-threatening complication of prednisone administration?
1. "I can't get my rings off."
2. "My stomach hurts."
3. "My face is swollen."
4. "I have hair on my chin."

32 Janet's urine is orange-yellow. The nurse recognizes this as a side effect of
1. Penicillin
2. Lomotil
3. Prednisone
4. Azulfidine

33 Janet's stools increase in frequency, and she had had a very restless day. Her blood pressure is 90/50, pulse rate is 120, and respirations are 22, and she is complaining of abdominal pain. Which of the following laboratory tests would be ordered by the physician if perforation is suspected?
1. Arterial blood gases
2. Barium enema
3. Hemoglobin and hematocrit levels
4. GB series

34 The physician decides to perform a colectomy and permanent ileostomy. This is the accepted procedure because
1. The small intestine will not heal effectively to provide adequate nutritional absorption
2. Patients with ulcerative colitis are more prone to colonic malignancy
3. Perforation leads to peritonitis
4. Ulcerative colitis is characterized by remissions and exacerbations

35 Immediately postoperatively you would expect the stoma to appear
1. Edematous and velvety red
2. Flush with the skin and pale pink
3. Edematous and dark brown
4. Flush with the skin and bluish

36 The aide complains that Janet's ileostomy bag needs changing again. "Won't it ever stop draining?" she asks. Your response would be
1. "Perhaps, if the surgery was successful."
2. "After several weeks she will learn to control the drainage."
3. "No, the drainage will always be constant and liquid."
4. "No, I don't think Janet will ever adjust well enough to control the drainage."

37 The physician orders potassium chloride, 20 mEq IV push every 8 hours. You would
1. Notify the RN that Janet's potassium chloride is IV push, and as an LPN you may not give IV push medication
2. Administer the medication since your hospital provided you with certification to give potassium chloride IV push
3. Clarify the order with the physician as this dosage is excessive
4. Clarify the order with the physician. Potassium chloride is not administered IV push

38 Janet refuses to talk to any of her visitors and looks out the window during the times you are caring for the ileostomy. An appropriate response would be
1. "I'll be finished in a moment, Janet, and then you can look inside at TV again."
2. "Why don't you watch me Janet; you'll need to learn how to do this soon."
3. "Do you want me to teach your mother to care for your ileostomy?"
4. "I notice when I change your ileostomy you always look out the window. What seems to be bothering you?"

39 In order to prevent irritation to the skin around the stoma you would
1. Change the bag frequently, cleansing the skin with soap and water
2. Release the bottom of the bag to empty it and apply Betadine to protect the skin
3. Cover the stoma with gauze during the day so that clothes fit appropriately
4. Change the bag when full and apply aluminum paste

40 Janet has been caring for her ileostomy and is making plans for graduation. Your evaluation is that
1. Janet has accepted her altered body image
2. Janet is denying her condition
3. Janet's behavior is false and she is potentially suicidal
4. Janet is a healthy normal 21-year-old

Situation: Mr. Douglas, aged 59, has been divorced recently and lives alone. All his recent efforts have been focused on making a success of his advertising agency. Mr. Douglas was admitted to the hospital because he vomited blood yesterday. Questions 41 through 60 refer to this situation.

41 During your assessment of Mr. Douglas he admits that his meals recently have been hurried and of the "fast food" variety. Your best understanding as to why Mr. Douglas has chosen this type of meal pattern would be
1. He lacks cooking skills
2. He believes these meals to be nutritious
3. He lives alone; therefore, meals are not a time of socialization
4. These foods do not produce any epigastric distress

42 Mr. Douglas denies any hobbies except his business. He states that he never gets angry with clients because "You can't get ahead in advertising making enemies." An appropriate response from you might be
1. "Tell me how you feel when you get angry."
2. "You must release the anger some way."
3. "I envy your control. How do you do it?"
4. "That sounds unhealthy to me."

43 You understand that repressed anger can cause
1. Increase in secretions and motility of the GI tract
2. Hypotension with a resultant CVA
3. Alopecia and steatorrhea
4. Decrease in gallbladder function and jaundice

44 Patient preparation for an upper GI series includes
1. Enemas until clear
2. NPO after midnight
3. Weighing the patient to determine the number of Oragrafin capsules to administer
4. An acid-free meal before blood being drawn

45 Mr. Douglas is also to have a gastric analysis. After insertion the nasogastric tube bubbles when submerged in water, and Mr. Douglas is unable to speak. Your nursing action would be based on the fact that these symptoms indicate
1. The tube is correctly positioned to obtain the specimens
2. Improper placement of the tube in the lungs
3. Correct positioning to obtain duodenal specimens
4. A tracheoesophageal fistula probably exists

46 The diagnosis of peptic ulcer has been confirmed. The physician orders cimetidine (Tagamet). The action of this drug is to
1. Reduce stress
2. Reduce gastric motility
3. Control gastric acidity
4. Relax the patient

47 Which of the following statements would indicate a side effect of the anticholinergic drugs used in Mr. Douglas's treatment?
1. "I don't have constipation anymore."
2. "I'm having trouble urinating."
3. "My feet are swollen."
4. "My skin is yellow."

48 Which of the following meal plans would be appropriate for Mr. Douglas?
1. Cream of potato soup, baked chicken, and vanilla custard
2. Bran cereal, orange slices, and skim milk
3. Country fried steak, broccoli with cream sauce, jello, and milk
4. Cream of asparagus soup, liver, stewed tomatoes, and coffee

49 Your next encounter with Mr. Douglas is the night before discharge when he summons you to his room. You find Mr. Douglas diaphoretic and complaining of severe abdominal pain. Your first nursing action would be to
1. Administer his antacid medications
2. Ask him if he ate food not on his diet
3. Check his vital signs
4. Ask him if he is fearful of the impending discharge in the morning

50 Mr. Douglas has a gastric resection. To promote wound healing in the immediate postoperative period you would
1. Administer milk to coat the stomach lining and neutralize acid
2. Maintain nasogastric suction
3. Administer pain medication to allow painless ambulation
4. Begin oral fluids only after bowel sounds are audible

51 Mr. Douglas is receiving an intravenous infusion. On checking the drip rate you discover it is dripping at 25 gtts per minute. He is to receive 150 ml per hour (10 gtts per milliliter is delivery rate of

infusion set). The most appropriate nursing action would be to
1. Readjust the rate to 30 gtts per minute
2. Reduce the rate to 20 gtts per minute
3. Procede with your assessment; the rate is correct
4. Fill out an incident report so that an accurate record of the mistake is made

52 Eight hours postoperatively Mr. Douglas develops hiccoughs. You would
1. Call the physician to obtain an order for Thorazine
2. Reposition Mr. Douglas and irrigate the nasogastric tube
3. Check vital signs, note drainage in nasogastric suction, and check dressings
4. Give him a paper bag to allow him to rebreathe carbon dioxide and thus stop hiccoughs

53 Frequent oral hygiene during gastric intubation will
1. Enhance comfort and tolerance of the tube
2. Increase Mr. Douglas's ability to talk with the tube in place
3. Prevent surgical mumps
4. Aid in tube patency

54 Mr. Douglas's nasogastric tube has been discontinued. He is to be placed on a progressive diet. Which of the following would be an indication that he could tolerate oral feedings?
1. Stable vital signs
2. Audible bowel sounds
3. Hunger pangs
4. "Good" results from an enema

55 Mr. Douglas is progressing nicely, tolerating oral feedings. Suddenly he complains of weakness and palpitations 30 minutes after eating supper. You would suspect that Mr. Douglas was suffering from
1. Malabsorption
2. Acute gastric dilation
3. Dumping syndrome
4. Postoperative infection

56 To accurately evaluate Mr. Douglas's incisional wound healing you might record
1. "Dressing dry and intact
2. "Suture line intact; no drainage noted"
3. "Tolerating diet well; large brown stool"
4. "Audible bowel sounds throughout abdomen; no jaundice noted"

57 You notice as Mr. Douglas gets stronger he spends much time pacing the floor and "calling the office." The most appropriate nursing action would be to
1. Administer the ordered tranquilizer early
2. Encourage Mr. Douglas to develop a hobby
3. Plan to spend time with Mr. Douglas, allowing him to talk
4. Suggest a psychiatric consultation

58 Mr. Douglas says his physician told him that during surgery they clipped a nerve leading to his stomach. Your understanding of this procedure is that
1. A vagotomy reduces gastric acid secretion
2. A vagotomy must be done to provide access to the site of the ulcer
3. This was probably a surgical error and questions about the procedure are best answered by the physician
4. This is a new procedure and as yet effects are not understood, although ulcer recurrence is inhibited

59 Mr. Douglas requests aspirin for a headache. The physician's standing orders state ASA gr x for headache. You would
1. Give the aspirin and get the charge nurse to indicate the order on the physician's order form
2. Tell Mr. Douglas the headache is probably caused by inappropriate control of stress and seek to question him about his stress
3. Notify the physician for a less acetic headache remedy
4. Give the ASA as ordered but would not chart it

60 When teaching Mr. Douglas preparatory to discharge, you would be assured that he knew the symptoms of ulcer recurrence if he
1. Verbalized a need to report hematemesis or melanaemesis
2. Demonstrated proper diet selection
3. Verbalized symptoms of toxic effects of anticholinergics
4. Asked you to recommend a good psychiatrist

Situation: Mr. Arthur, aged 62, is admitted to the hospital for a cataract extraction. He also has been previously diagnosed as having rheumatoid arthritis. Questions 61 through 80 refer to this situation.

61 During your initial assessment of Mr. Arthur, which of the following symptoms would be indicative of a cataract?

1. Gradual vision loss and opacity of lens
2. Loss of a portion of the visual field and severe pain in the affected eye
3. Intermittent blindness and lens opacity
4. Pupil dilation and decreased movement of the eye

62 Mr. Arthur gets up at night to void. In anticipation of these activities you would
1. Leave the bathroom light on (insist that the family provide a sitter)
2. Restrain Mr. Arthur from 10 PM through 6 AM (catheterize intermittently during the night)
3. Leave the bathroom light on and remove obstacles that are between the bed and the bathroom
4. Instruct Mr. Arthur to call for help so you could release the chest restraint and assist him to the bathroom

63 Patients frequently suffer from both rheumatoid arthritis and cataracts. The reason for both disorders is
1. A deficiency of vitamin A in the diet
2. Connective tissue disease
3. Secondary to the aging process
4. A result of infections from beta-hemolytic streptococci

64 Eye drops are ordered preoperatively for Mr. Arthur. The mydriatics ordered will
1. Dilate the pupils
2. Constrict the iris
3. Anesthetize the eye
4. Sterilize the eye for surgery

65 Postoperatively Mr. Arthur is nauseated. Appropriate nursing actions would be to
1. Apply a cool cloth to Mr. Arthur's forehead; do not administer antiemetics until you can be certain he has a gag reflex
2. Allow Mr. Arthur to vomit, making certain his head is turned to the side to prevent aspiration
3. Administer the ordered antiemetic even though Mr. Arthur has not vomited
4. Notify the physician, as nausea is a symptom of increased intracranial pressure

66 The morning after surgery Mr. Arthur wants to feed himself even though he has an eye patch over the eye that was operated on. As his nurse you would
1. Insist that he be fed to avoid sudden movements
2. Prepare his tray and allow him to feed himself so that he maintains his independence
3. Explain that he will still be NPO and therefore allowed no breakfast
4. Compromise and allow his wife to feed him

67 While assisting Mr. Arthur with his bath he tells you his arthritis is "acting up." A contributing factor to this exacerbation might be
1. Drugs used during surgery and a postoperative liquid diet
2. Postoperative inactivity and the stress of surgery
3. An allergic reaction to eye drops used preoperatively and a low fluid intake
4. The administration of whole blood during surgery and the stress of hospitalization

68 To reduce strain on the arthritic joints you would
1. Apply splints, especially at bedtime; allow rest periods
2. Encourage walking frequently and standing rather than sitting
3. Encourage aggressive active range of motion exercises and bed rest
4. Hyperextend affected joints to prevent flexion deformities and provide paraffin baths to relieve pain

69 Mr. Arthur's physician orders ASA gr xv PO q.i.d. You would
1. Refuse to give the medication because it far exceeds recommended dosage
2. Give this medication; this is the therapeutic dosage range for arthritis
3. Notify the physician about your concerns and revalidate the order
4. Give only gr V—you are certain this is what the physician meant to write

70 Which of the following statements by Mr. Arthur would be indicative of aspirin side effect?
1. "My hands are swollen."
2. "I still can't see with my eye where the cataract was removed last week."
3. "My arm is still bleeding where the lab drew blood an hour ago."
4. "I sure have gained a lot of weight recently."

Several weeks after discharge Mr. Arthur is readmitted for a total hip replacement secondary to rheumatoid arthritis.

71 Before the hip replacement Mr. Arthur signs a surgical consent form. His signature on the consent is legally interpreted as
1. Understanding what procedure is to be done and the risks involved

2. Agreeing to receive a general anesthetic
3. Assuming expenses incurred by the surgery
4. Willingness not to sue the hospital if postoperative complications result

72 Mr. Arthur's preoperative medication is M. SO_4 8 mg. You have ampules containing M. SO_4 10 mg per milliliter. You would give
1. 0.8 ml
2. 1.2 ml
3. 0.8 mg
4. 1.2 mg

73 Mr. Arthur gets up to void in the bathroom after his preoperative medication has been administered. He falls while getting back to bed. To prevent such occurrences you should have
1. Restrained Mr. Arthur and stayed with him
2. Administered the preoperative medication only after he was on the stretcher to go to surgery
3. Assisted Mr. Arthur to void before administering the preoperative medication, telling Mr. Arthur not to get up
4. Given the preoperative medication PO to avoid the side effect of drowsiness

74 In responding to Mr. Arthur's calls for help, your first action on entering the room would be to
1. Call for help to put Mr. Arthur back to bed
2. Assess for injuries to the eye previously operated on
3. Put Mr. Arthur back to bed
4. Stay with Mr. Arthur and call for charge nurse to assess injuries

75 As Mr. Arthur's nurse you could be sued for
1. Negligence
2. Assault
3. Battery
4. Manslaughter

76 Postoperatively Mr. Arthur has a Hemovac in place. The purpose of the Hemovac is to
1. Provide a means whereby the wound may be irrigated
2. Suction drainage from the wound
3. Maintain homeostasis
4. Maintain the hip in abduction

77 After 24 hours Mr. Arthur is allowed to turn to the unaffected side. To accomplish this you would
1. Place a triangular pillow between Mr. Arthur's legs and logroll him
2. Tape Mr. Arthur's legs together and logroll him
3. Ask Mr. Arthur to perform straight leg raises while turning him to the unaffected side
4. Ask Mr. Arthur to flex both knees, move his hips to the side opposite you, and then logroll him toward you

78 Mr. Arthur, 5 days postoperatively, spills the urinal in his bed, soaking his dressing. Your nursing actions would be based on the fact that
1. Dressing changes are not done without a physician's order
2. Urine is sterile so a bed change is in order but no dressing change
3. Changing the dressing may prevent wound infection
4. Reinforcing the dressing may prevent wound infection

79 Mr. Arthur can be up in the chair. Remembering he has had a right total hip replacement and is to have no weight bearing on that side, you would place the wheelchair on the patient's
1. Right side at the head of the bed
2. Right side at the foot of the bed
3. Left side at the head of the bed
4. Left side at the foot of the bed

80 Mr. Arthur is ready to return to bed. You would position the wheelchair
1. With his left leg closest to the bed
2. With his right leg closest to the bed
3. At right angles to the bed
4. On either side since returning to bed is best accomplished by lifting the patient

---

Situation: Mrs. Mary Simmons, 28 years old, is admitted to the hospital with a history of right parietal headaches over a period of 2 years. The pain has become increasingly severe in the last month and has been followed by episodes of nausea and vomiting. Physical and neurologic examinations reveal vital signs within normal limits. Some decreased sensation in the left upper extremity and papilledema are noted. Pupils are equal and reactive to light. No further neurologic symptoms are present. Questions 81 through 102 refer to this situation

81 From the history and physical examination it is obvious that Mrs. Simmons has
1. Symptoms of a malignant brain tumor
2. Three cardinal signs of increased intracranial pressure
3. Symptoms of intracerebral aneurysm
4. Cranial nerve damage

82 For the past 2 years Mrs. Simmons has been taking ergotamine tartrate for migraine headache attacks. It is believed that the physiologic cause of migraine is
1. A sudden rise in blood pressure resulting from stress
2. An inherited defect in cerebral function
3. Constriction of the cerebral vessels followed by dilation of the vessels
4. Increased intracranial pressure resulting from a structural defect

83 If given early in the migraine process, ergotamine tartrate may provide relief by
1. Promoting vasoconstriction of the cranial arteries
2. Relieving muscle spasms of the neck and scalp
3. Promoting vasodilation of the cranial arteries
4. Reversing the inflammatory process

84 On admission to the hospital Mrs. Simmons is scheduled for a lumbar puncture. Nursing care after a lumbar puncture includes
1. Keeping the patient in semi-Fowler's position
2. Applying a pressure dressing to the puncture site
3. Helping the patient to turn, cough, and deep breathe every 2 hours
4. Encouraging fluid intake

85 A brain scan may be useful in diagnosing intracranial tumors because
1. It detects abnormal brain waves in a region occupied by a tumor
2. It will reveal bone calcification or destruction
3. Tumors generally absorb large amounts of radioactive material
4. It demonstrates displacement of structures away from the midline of the brain

86 In preparing Mrs. Simmons for a CAT scan (computerized axial tomography), you should
1. Shave and prepare the inguinal areas, maintain the patient NPO, and administer the prescribed sedative
2. Reassure Mrs. Simmons that the examination is painless, requires no special preparation, and causes virtually no side effects
3. Explain the procedure to Mrs. Simmons, maintain NPO, and prepare her for the postexamination headache
4. Maintain Mrs. Simmons NPO and administer a soapsuds enema and her prescribed analgesic

87 Following a series of diagnostic tests Mrs. Simmons is scheduled for a craniotomy to remove a parietal tumor. Routine preoperative care for Mrs. Simmons will include
1. Soapsuds enema until clear the evening before surgery
2. Morphine, plus atropine 1 hour before surgery
3. A mild sedative the evening before surgery
4. Forcing fluids intravenously to increase hydration

88 In assessing Mrs. Simmons the most reliable indication of her neurologic status is
1. Pulse rate and blood pressure
2. Level of consciousness
3. Pupillary activity
4. Respiratory rate

89 In positioning Mrs. Simmons following her supratentorial craniotomy you should consider which of the following?
1. If a large tumor has been removed, the patient should be kept off the operative side
2. The patient should be placed in Trendelenburg's position to facilitate cerebral circulation
3. If a large tumor has been removed, the patient should be positioned on the operative side
4. The patient should be kept off her back and turned only side to side

90 The most important nursing measure to consider immediately when Mrs. Simmons returns from the recovery room is
1. Check the operative area for bleeding
2. Check IV tube patency and puncture site
3. Assess the level of consciousness
4. Establish an adequate airway

91 Mrs. Simmons's corneal reflex should be tested by
1. Applying pressure against the supraorbital ridge
2. Stroking the cornea lightly with a cotton wisp
3. Brushing the eyelashes with a cotton-tipped applicator
4. Shining a flashlight into the eye

92 The cranial nerve that controls pupil movement is cranial nerve
1. I
2. II
3. III
4. IV

93 A purposeful response to pricking Mrs. Simmons's right foot with a pin would be
1. Dorsiflexion of the right foot and flexion of the right knee

2. Tonic contractions of both arms and both legs simultaneously
3. Frowning, grimacing, and shaking the head back and forth
4. Rapidly alternating flexion and extension of all four limbs

94 The earliest signs of increasing intracranial pressure is
1. Projectile vomiting
2. Dilated pupils
3. Lethargy
4. Cheyne-Stokes respirations

95 Changes in the vital signs indicative of increasing intracranial pressure include
1. Decreasing blood pressure
2. Widened pulse pressure
3. Increased pulse deficit
4. Decreased temperature

96 You would be most helpful to Mrs. Simmons during a grand mal seizure by
1. Helping the patient to a sitting position to open the airway
2. Restraining her arms and legs to prevent injury
3. Raising the bed siderails and removing her pillows
4. Placing a waterproof pad under her to prevent urine or stool from soiling the bed

97 In placing a padded tongue blade between the patient's teeth it is important to insert it
1. Before the aura
2. Before the tonic stage
3. During the tonic stage
4. During the clonic stage

98 Following a convulsion, observations you should chart include all *except*
1. TPR and B/P during the seizure
2. Presence or absence of an aura
3. Progression, extent, and duration of the movements
4. Level of consciousness during and after the seizure

99 Immediately following the IV administration of mannitol during intracranial surgery, you can expect a
1. Large urine output with low specific gravity
2. Decreased urine output with high specific gravity
3. Large urine output with high specific gravity
4. Decreased urine output with low specific gravity

100 The normal range for specific gravity is
1. 1.001 to 1.005
2. 1.005 to 1.025
3. 1.015 to 1.025
4. 1.015 to 1.050

101 Excessive urine output after a craniotomy may indicate
1. Brainstem involvement
2. Swelling around the medulla oblongata
3. Swelling around the pituitary gland
4. Acute renal failure

102 Important nursing measures for patients with diabetes insipidus include
1. Keeping an accurate intake and output record
2. Teaching the patient proper foot care
3. A low-carbohydrate diet
4. A low-sodium diet

Situation: Mr. Hanson, a 46-year-old certified public accountant, visited his family physician for an annual checkup. Mr. Hanson is 5 feet 8 inches tall and weighs 220 pounds. He has a history of hypertension. He smokes 1½ packs of cigarettes per day, has two cocktails before dinner each evening, and states his main hobbies are watching television and reading professional magazines. Mr. Hanson's family history includes a brother who died from a myocardial infarction at the age of 42 and a mother who died at the age of 54 from complications of diabetes. On examining Mr. Hanson, the physician reports the following results:

ECG	Normal sinus rhythm
Serum cholesterol	325 mg/100
Blood pressure	210/130
Hemoglobin	16.2
Hematocrit	49%
Blood glucose	100
Weight	220 pounds

All other physical findings were normal. Questions 103 through 122 refer to this situation.

103 From the assessment of Mr. Hanson, you should determine that the patient will need
1. Activity restriction
2. Instructions in regard to diabetes
3. Genetic counseling
4. Sodium restriction

104 In teaching Mr. Hanson about a cholesterol restricted diet, you should encourage a limited intake of
1. Citrus fruits and fresh vegetables
2. Egg yolks and dairy products
3. Enriched breads and cereal
4. Caffeine and corn oil

105 To begin Mr. Hanson's health promotion plan it would be *most* important to
1. Find out what is most important to Mr. Hanson
2. Provide nutrition education to reduce his weight
3. Provide instructions on diabetes to reduce his blood glucose
4. Provide instructions on the risks of hypertension

Approximately 3 months after visiting his physician, Mr. Hanson, while mowing the lawn, suddenly experienced a severe type of squeezing pain under his sternum that rapidly spread to his left shoulder. The pain subsided after approximately 10 minutes when Mr. Hanson sat down to rest.

106 The discomfort experienced by Mr. Hanson was most likely caused by
1. Necrosis of the myocardium caused by a blood clot in a coronary artery
2. Necrosis of the myocardium caused by overexertion
3. Temporary lack of oxygen to the myocardium resulting from a sudden increased demand
4. Temporary lack of circulating oxygen because of overexertion

After seeking medical attention, Mr. Hanson was admitted to the hospital for further workup.

107 Following Mr. Hanson's coronary arteriography examination, it is most important during the first 12 hours to
1. Immobilize the patient with restraints and sandbags
2. Check the pulse rate distal to the puncture site every hour
3. Measure and record the intake and output every 2 hours
4. Have the patient dangle his feet several times before ambulation

108 In teaching about the use of nitroglycerin tablets, you should instruct Mr. Hanson to
1. Seek medical attention if chest pain is not relieved after three tablets taken 5 minutes apart
2. Seek medical attention if transient headache and light-headedness follow
3. Seek medical attention if pain is not relieved after one tablet
4. Allow at least a 4-hour interval between tablets to prevent side effects

109 Mr. Hanson should be instructed to prevent deterioration of nitroglycerin tablets by storing the medication in a(n)
1. Airtight container near a source of heat
2. Airtight container in the refrigerator
3. Cool airtight metal box
4. Dark, airtight container

110 The physician encourages Mr. Hanson to pursue a regular, mild exercise program with the overall goal of
1. Increasing the size of the left ventricle
2. Increasing musculoskeletal production of oxygen
3. Reducing the heart and blood pressure rates with exercise
4. Increasing the regularity of the heartbeat

Approximately 6 weeks after his initial hospitalization, Mr. Hanson was suddenly awakened in the middle of the night with a severe, crushing substernal pain that radiated into his left arm and up his neck into the jaws. Mrs. Hanson notified the family physician, who sent an ambulance for Mr. Hanson. On admission to the coronary care unit, Mr. Hanson was dyspneic, pale, and covered with perspiration. His blood pressure was 90/70, his pulse weak and rapid. He complained of nausea. The physician made an immediate diagnosis of myocardial infarction.

111 The pain of myocardial infarction typically differs from that of angina pectoris in that the former is always
1. More severe
2. More prone to radiate into the arm and neck
3. Less responsive to rest and vasodilating drugs
4. More often provoked by overexertion

Following Mr. Hanson's admission to the coronary care unit, the physician writes the following orders:

Complete bed rest
Light diet as tolerated
Blood pressure and pulse q. 30 minutes
Keep accurate intake and output record
Oxygen, 6 L, per mask
Lanoxin, 0.25 mg IV b.i.d.
Morphine, 15 mg IV q. 3 to 4 hours PRN for pain
Heparin, 5000 units subcutaneously q. 4 hours
Lasix, 40 mg IV q. 8 hours

112 In providing care for Mr. Hanson, it will be important for you to
1. Anticipate and provide for his needs
2. Discourage all visitors
3. Assist him to the bathroom frequently
4. Provide diversional activities

113 In assessing Mr. Hanson for signs of left ventricular failure you should look for
1. Increased blood pressure and widening pulse pressure

2. Irregular and slow bounding pulse
3. Decreased blood pressure and narrowing pulse pressure
4. Increased blood pressure and narrowing pulse pressure

114 In administering heparin to Mr. Hanson you will
1. Administer the prescribed dose promptly at the specified time
2. Monitor the daily prothrombin time to determine effectiveness of the drug
3. Massage the injection site following administration
4. Administer protamine within 30 minutes of heparin injection

115 While taking Lasix, Mr. Hanson should be encouraged to increase his intake of
1. Fluids
2. Sodium
3. Calcium
4. Potassium

116 Three days after admission to the coronary care unit Mr. Hanson suddenly develops symptoms of pulmonary edema. The best immediate action of the practical nurse is to place the patient in
1. Trendelenburg's position; administer prescribed doses of oxygen and morphine
2. Place in an upright position; administer prescribed doses of oxygen and morphine
3. Place in Trendelenburg's position; administer a decreased dose of oxygen and hold the morphine
4. Place in orthopneic position; administer a decreased dose of oxygen and hold the morphine

117 Following treatment of Mr. Hanson's condition with rotating tourniquets you will discontinue therapy by removing
1. All tourniquets at one time
2. One tourniquet every hour
3. The two leg tourniquets and follow 15 minutes later with removal of the arm tourniquets
4. One tourniquet every 15 minutes

118 In administering Mr. Hanson's daily dose of Lanoxin you will
1. Withhold the drug until the physician is notified if the apical pulse rate is less than 60 beats per minute
2. Administer the drug and notify the physician if the apical pulse rate is less than 60 beats per minute
3. Withhold the drug until the physician is notified if the apical pulse rate is over 90
4. Withhold the drug until the next day if the pulse rate is less than 60

119 Mr. Hanson is to receive morphine, 15 mg IM. The medication available is morphine, 10 mg per milliliter. The correct amount to administer is
1. 0.5 ml
2. 0.75 ml
3. 1 ml
4. 1.5 ml

Ten days after admission, following his transfer from the critical care unit, Mr. Hanson becomes very irritable and demanding. He insists that his briefcase be brought from work and stays on the phone continuously, making business calls. He has become very cool toward his wife and expresses resentment when she attempts to assist him in any way.

120 Depression often follows health disorders such as those Mr. Hanson experienced. Which of the following statements *best* describes such a state of depression?
1. Depression is caused by guilt over not having taken better care of himself
2. Depression is anger turned inward toward the self
3. Persons with infarcts are classified as having depressive personalities
4. Most depressive states are the result of interpersonal conflict

121 When Mr. Hanson's behavior causes the nursing staff to want to avoid him as much as possible, they decide to hold a conference to plan an approach to his care. Which of the following suggestions is *most* understanding of his present needs?
1. Use a direct, consistent approach. Be firm and unrelenting of your expectations
2. Allow Mr. Hanson some freedom in decision making, even for minor aspects of his care
3. Avoid unnecessary time spent with him. It only reinforces dependence
4. Insist that a counselor be called in to deal with this crisis

122 Mr. Hanson's reaction to his wife sends her to the nurse in tears: "We've always been so close and have never had trouble talking before. He just shuts me out. I don't know what to do!" The best response from you would be

1. "He'll snap out of it. All our patients act that way. It's to be expected."
2. "It must be very upsetting for you to have him treat you this way. I'll arrange for the doctor to talk with him."
3. "This must be a very difficult time for you right now. Let's talk about it."
4. "Your husband needs all the support from you that he can get. Try to ignore how he acts. It will pass."

SAMPLE EXAMINATION 2

This examination contains several paragraphs concerning patients/clients. Following each such paragraph is a series of questions concerning the patient and the situation described in that paragraph. Read each situation carefully. Read each question carefully, and consider all possible answers. When you have decided which answer is **best,** blacken the corresponding space on the answer sheet. There is only **one** best answer for each question.

Situation: Mr. Raymond Jenner, 59 years old, is brought to the emergency room after collapsing at work. A friend reports that he complained of a severe headache and then fell to the floor. Mr. Jenner exhibits right-sided weakness that includes drooping of the mouth on the right side. His vital signs are as follows: blood pressure, 200/120; pulse rate, 118; respirations, 16; and temperature 99.6°F. On his admission, Mr. Jenner's wife reports that her husband has complained of headaches and has had three blackout spells in the past 6 months. He has complained of numbness and tingling on his right side at intervals but has refused to see his physician since the symptoms have subsided. Questions 1 through 20 refer to this situation.

1 Previous symptoms experienced by Mr. Jenner are indicative of transient ischemic attacks (TIAs), which are caused by a
1. Complete obstruction in oxygen supply to the brain, resulting in necrosis
2. Decreased amount of circulating oxygen
3. Complete obstruction in the afferent nerve tracts
4. Temporary lack of oxygen to an area of the brain

2 Coumadin is a common drug of choice in the treatment of TIAs. Patients taking Coumadin should be instructed to
1. Increase their intake of vitamin K
2. Use razors and sharp instruments with care
3. Massage and exercise their legs daily
4. Take aspirin four times daily

3 The effects of Coumadin on the patient can best be assessed by monitoring the
1. Lee-White clotting time
2. Prothrombin time
3. Platelet count
4. Partial thromboplastin time

4 In caring for patients taking Coumadin it is important to
1. Change the IV site every 48 hours
2. Record intake, output, and daily weight
3. Observe mucous membranes, urine, and stools
4. Observe skin texture and turgor

5 Emergency nursing care of a suspected cerebrovascular accident patient includes
1. Placing the patient on the unaffected side to prevent aspiration
2. Elevating the head slightly to promote venous drainage
3. Encouraging the patient to talk to maintain level of consciousness
4. Lowering the head to increase circulation to the brain

6 Physical examination revealed that Mr. Jenner was suffering from systemic hypertension. Possible causes of hypertension include
1. Loss of fluid and electrolytes
2. Overstimulation of the sympathetic nervous system

3. Decreased elasticity of the arterioles
4. Decreased blood volume

7 Normal blood pressure for a man of Mr. Jenner's age would be
1. 100/40
2. 140/90
3. 160/100
4. 200/120

8 Rehabilitation of the CVA patient must begin on the day of admission. The *immediate* nursing goal in addition to saving Mr. Jenner's life during the acute stage is to
1. Retrain the paralyzed side
2. Ambulate with assistance
3. Encourage PO fluid intake
4. Prevent deformities and complications

9 CVA patients with expressive aphasia will benefit *most* if you
1. Speak more slowly and louder
2. Use gestures and facial expressions
3. Provide the patients with a tablet and pencil
4. Remove unnecessary items from the environment

10 In caring for Mr. Jenner, who has exhibited dysphagia, it is most important that you *first*
1. Gear verbal communication techniques to compensate for the patient's deficits
2. Assess the gag reflex
3. Use simple pictures to retrain the patient in the identification of objects
4. Offer small sips of water and progress as tolerated

11 Correct positioning for Mr. Jenner will include
1. Keeping him flat on his back as much as possible
2. Maintaining the upright position for long intervals
3. Keeping him on the affected side for long intervals to promote circulation
4. Assisting him to the prone position several times daily

12 When positioning Mr. Jenner on his back, the lower arm and hand of the affected side should be placed
1. Across the chest
2. Parallel with the body, with the elbow extended
3. Elevated on a pillow beside his chest and trunk
4. Extended above the head

13 To promote retraining of his affected side and a faster return to independence, Mr. Jenner should be encouraged to
1. Comb his hair, wash his face, and brush his teeth
2. Participate actively in physical therapy
3. Perform daily push-ups
4. Use a pen with the affected hand

14 Mr. Jenner cannot close his eye completely. Nursing measures to be employed to protect his eye include
1. Irrigating the eye daily with sterile water
2. Keeping the lights dim in the room
3. Instilling artificial tears and covering the eye with a patch
4. Applying an antibiotic ointment to the lower eyelid

15 When feeding Mr. Jenner you should
1. Place food on the affected side so it can be swallowed easily
2. Provide foods with minimal texture and viscosity
3. Provide mouth care immediately after meals
4. Provide only liquids

16 Mrs. Jenner tells you, "Every time I go into the room Raymond cries. I am afraid I have done something to upset him." The best response is
1. "Mr. Jenner is trying to get your sympathy. You must ignore the crying and talk about other things."
2. "Mr. Jenner has no control over his crying. It is a symptom of his illness and does not mean that he is unhappy."
3. "Mr. Jenner needs some time alone to sort out his feelings. You should consider staying away for a few days."
4. "Mr. Jenner might benefit from a psychiatric consultation. Perhaps you could talk to your doctor."

17 While bathing Mr. Jenner, you notice a reddened area on his right hip. The appropriate nursing action is to
1. Massage the area every 2 hours and keep him off his right side
2. Cleanse with alcohol and apply a sterile dressing
3. Apply warm moist compresses intermittently
4. Apply lotion and powder before turning him on the right side

18 To prevent constipation you should encourage Mr. Jenner to
1. Take daily enemas
2. Use a daily laxative
3. Increase fruits and fluids in his diet
4. Plan his bowel movement for early morning

19 In order to avoid urinary complications associated with decreased mobility you should encourage Mr. Jenner to
1. Increase intake of citrus fruits
2. Decrease intake of fluids
3. Decrease intake of dairy products
4. Increase urine acidity

20 To *best* assist Mr. Jenner to prepare for ambulation you should
1. Dangle the patient's legs and swing them back and forth daily
2. Have him push his popliteal space against the bed to the count of five several times daily
3. Perform passive range of motion exercises three times daily
4. Have him perform push-ups and use the bed trapeze bar as much as possible

---

Situation: Mr. Luke Gabriel, aged 48, is admitted to the hospital because of weight loss, weakness, and ascites. He has had a 10-year history of chronic alcoholism. The admitting diagnosis is Laennec's cirrhosis.

21 Often alcoholic patients find rejection by hospital personnel just as they find in society. When a nurse cannot help but convey disgust when working with such patients, it is best to
1. Seek reassignment to another area or other patients
2. Inform the patients of his or her attitude but continue to care for them
3. Seek assistance in determining his or her reaction to such patients
4. Ignore the situation and carry out his or her duties as usual

22 The primary treatment aim for alcoholic patients is to
1. Assist individuals to learn to drink in moderation
2. Aid them in meeting life's responsibilities without using alcohol as an escape
3. Encourage them to enter psychoanalysis to discover insights into their total responsibility
4. Encourage further dependency on you as a helper rather than returning to alcohol

23 Many alcoholic patients are described as having
1. Anal personalities
2. Oral personalities
3. Oedipal conflicts
4. Latency problems

24 Aversion therapy has been successful in the treatment of some alcoholic patients. Which of the following drugs have been used for this purpose?
1. Mellaril
2. Antabuse
3. Methadone
4. Thorazine

25 Treatment of Laennec's cirrhosis includes
(A) Frequent monitoring of vital signs
(B) Anticonvulsant drugs
(C) IV fluids
(D) Vitamin therapy and high-protein diet
1. A, B, and D
2. A, C, and D
3. A and C
4. A, B, C, and D

26 Nursing care of patients with this condition includes
(A) Keeping room lighted
(B) Always using restraints
(C) Explaining all procedures in detail before administering them
(D) Disregarding reality orientation since the patient's condition is too serious
1. A, B, and C
2. B and C
3. A
4. A, B, C, and D

27 Clinical manifestations of this condition include
(A) Tremulousness, agitation, and insomnia
(B) Visual, tactile, and auditory hallucinations
(C) Autonomic underactivity—bradycardia, hypothermia
(D) Anxiety and uncontrollable fear
1. A, B, and C
2. B and C
3. A, B, and D
4. A, B, C, and D

28 An acute psychotic state that follows a prolonged bout of steady drinking or a decrease in or cessation of alcohol intake is known as
1. Korasakoff's psychosis
2. Delirium tremens
3. Pathologic intoxication
4. Organic brain syndrome

29 Alcoholics Anonymous requires its members to *first*
1. Have a physician's order to join
2. Submit to hospitalization for treatment
3. Admit to being an alcoholic
4. Bring a family member to meetings

30 Nurses working with alcoholic patients must be aware that most patients have a tendency to become
1. Overly dependent
2. Overly independent
3. Interdependent
4. Passive

31 Laennec's cirrhosis is most often associated with
1. Biliary obstruction and alcoholism
2. Viral hepatitis and alcoholism
3. Viral hepatitis and nutritional deficiencies
4. Nutritional deficiencies and alcoholism

32 In the early stages, the chief signs of liver cirrhosis include
1. Jaundice, GI disturbances, and hepatomegaly
2. Jaundice, fever, ascites, and GI disturbances
3. GI disturbances, hobnail liver, fever, and purpura
4. Spider telangiectasis, jaundice, fever, and hepatomegaly

33 A nursing measure to help Mr. Gabriel overcome severe anorexia might include
1. Withholding all PO feedings
2. Giving parenteral fluids as ordered
3. Offering small frequent feedings
4. Administering prescribed vitamin K

34 In view of Mr. Gabriel's ascites it will be most important to
1. Keep the head of the bed elevated
2. Restrict PO intake
3. Provide frequent mouth care
4. Offer small frequent feedings

35 To assess the effect of diuretic therapy on Mr. Gabriel's ascites you will monitor
1. Blood pressure, pulse rate, and respirations
2. Intake and output, daily weight, and electrolytes
3. Temperature and white blood cell count
4. Abdominal girth and hemoglobin and hematocrit levels

36 In view of Mr. Gabriel's diseased liver, you must be particularly alert for signs of
1. Incontinence
2. Weight loss
3. Fatigue
4. Blood in the urine or stools

37 The most important nursing goal for Mr. Gabriel on admission is to provide
1. Diet instructions
2. Education on the danger of alcohol
3. Rest and supportive measures
4. Hepatotoxic drugs

38 Because Mr. Gabriel's liver has decreased production of prothrombin it is most important to
1. Provide a high-protein, high-calorie diet
2. Apply gentle pressure to injection sites
3. Restrict sodium intake
4. Carefully control IV drip rate

39 Mr. Gabriel should be observed for signs of impending hepatic coma, with the earliest manifestation being
1. Increased temperature
2. Decreased blood pressure
3. Cold clammy skin
4. Mental confusion

40 In preparing Mr. Gabriel for discharge you should stress avoidance of alcohol and encourage
1. A well-balanced diet
2. Fluid restriction
3. Increased physical activity
4. Involvement in community activities

Situation: Mrs. Kate Murphy, aged 40, is admitted to the hospital after several episodes of right upper quadrant abdominal pain and intolerance to fatty and gas-forming foods. She also reports episodes of light-colored stools and slight jaundice with the more actue episodes of her pain. After diagnostic studies a diagnosis of biliary colic is made. Questions 41 through 60 refer to this situation.

41 The ingestion of fatty foods will precipitate the pain of biliary colic because
1. Increased fat in the stomach increases peristalsis
2. Fat in the duodenum initiates contraction of the gallbladder
3. Fat in the duodenum increases abdominal distention
4. Increased fat intake may result in a gallbladder obstruction

42 Diet instructions for Mrs. Murphy should encourage the restriction of
1. Breads and cereals
2. Poultry, rice, and skim milk
3. Lima beans, cabbage, and onions
4. Cooked fruits, lean meats, and caffeine

43 In preparing Mrs. Murphy for surgery, which of the following laboratory values would concern you enough to call the physician?
1. WBC, 10,000
2. Hemoglobin, 9 g
3. Urine pH, 8.5
4. Hematocrit, 42%

44 Following insertion of a nasogastric tube before surgery you ascertain that the tube is properly placed by
1. Placing the end of the tube in a glass of water to make sure bubbles appear in the water on expiration
2. Injecting 10 ml of air into the tube and palpating for abdominal distention
3. Listening for the sound in the stomach with a stethoscope as 5 ml of air is injected into the tube
4. Feeling the end of the tube for the passage of air from the stomach

45 As a preoperative medication, you are to give 75 mg of Demerol intramuscularly. Demerol injection contains 50 mg per milliliter. How much of the solution should be administered?
1. 0.5 ml
2. 0.75 ml
3. 1 ml
4. 1.5 ml

46 You are to give 1/100 gr of atropine intramuscularly. Atropine injection contains 1 mg per milliliter. How much should be injected?
1. 0.01 ml
2. 0.4 ml
3. 0.6 ml
4. 1 ml

47 Following her cholecystectomy, Mrs. Murphy returns to her room from recovery in stable condition. Fluids are being given intravenously. She has a T--tube to BSD, a Foley catheter to BSD, and a nasogastric tube to low suction. Once settled in her bed she complains of nausea and looks like she is gagging. Your initial response in this situation is to
1. Administer ordered antiemetic
2. Check the nasogastric tube for patency
3. Check the wound for bleeding or dehiscence
4. See whether the T-tube has been dislodged

48 Mrs. Murphy has a Penrose drain for the purpose of
1. Rerouting bile flow to the reconstructed bile duct
2. Draining bile while the common duct is edematous
3. Removing bile and blood spilled in the operative area during surgery
4. Preventing bile from causing contamination and infection of the cystic duct

49 In order to prevent the most common complication following a cholecystectomy, it would be most important for Mrs. Murphy to
1. Have the abdominal dressing changed frequently and PRN for heavy drainage
2. Increase fluid intake and decrease fat intake
3. Receive pain medication at intervals ordered
4. Cough and deep breathe every 2 hours and fully expand her lungs

50 Following the first dressing change, the physician's order is to change the abdominal dressing every 8 hours and PRN. In changing Mrs. Murphy's dressing, it is particularly important to place sterile 4 × 4s around the Penrose drain because
1. Leakage of bile from the Penrose can cause severe skin irritation
2. The evacuated bile is normally high in bacteria and should not contact the abdominal incision
3. Absorption of bile by 4 × 4s aids in accurate measurement
4. The suture line must be protected from moisture

51 While Mrs. Murphy is being turned, her nasogastric tube becomes dislodged and falls on the bed. You should
1. Notify the physician and fill out an incident report
2. Leave the tube out since this indicates no further need for one
3. Obtain a new tube from central supply and replace it
4. Administer Mrs. Murphy's prescribed medication for nausea

52 In order to carry out good body mechanics when moving Mrs. Murphy, you should
1. Have a wide base of support
2. Bend her right knee
3. Extend her elbows out away from her body
4. Stoop over as close to the patient as possible

53 During the first 24 hours after surgery, Mrs. Murphy may require several doses of the prescribed analgesic in order to prevent
1. Pooling of respiratory secretions from limited inspiration
2. Excessive movement in bed
3. Accumulation of gas in the GI tract
4. Excessive coughing

54 Mrs. Murphy is to receive 1000 ml of IV fluids every 8 hours. Her IV set delivers 10 drops per milliliter. The drip rate should be set at
1. 10 drops per minute
2. 21 drops per minute
3. 36 drops per minute
4. 42 drops per minute

55 In administering Mrs. Murphy's IM analgesic, you should insert the needle at a
1. 15 degree angle
2. 45 degree angle
3. 60 degree angle
4. 90 degree angle

56 Mrs. Murphy's abdomen feels distended, and she complains of nausea. The nasogastric tube appears to be in place. Your first action would be to
1. Notify the physician
2. Administer the prescribed antiemetic
3. Irrigate the tube with 10 ml of sterile normal saline, if ordered
4. Inject 50 ml of air into the tube to check for patency

57 Mrs. Murphy complains of tenderness at her IV puncture site. On assessment you note redness and swelling. You should first
1. Discontinue the IV fluids, and report this to your head nurse
2. Notify the physician, and fill out an incident report
3. Elevate the arm, and apply warm compresses to the puncture site
4. Change the dressing over the puncture site using sterile technique

58 While changing Mrs. Murphy's abdominal dressing it is most important for you to
1. Use forceps
2. Touch sterile articles with sterile articles only
3. Replace all unused 4×4s in their package for future dressing changes
4. Apply ice packs to the incision to decrease swelling

59 A postoperative symptom that should be reported to the physician immediately is
1. A temperature of 101°F
2. An incisional pain
3. A productive cough
4. Audible bowel sounds

60 Mrs. Murphy asks you, "Will I have to stay on a fat-free diet for the rest of my life?" The best response would be
1. "You need to talk to your doctor about that."
2. "A fat-free diet will always be necessary if you wish to stay well."
3. "After you have completely recovered you will probably be able to eat a normal diet without excessive fat."
4. "Complications of this type of surgery might cause you to have to abstain from all fats."

Situation: Mr. Powell, aged 40, is a watch repairman. Recently he has been unable to work because of hand tremors. He has also noticed an increase in appetite, fatigue, and irritability. His physician suspects hyperthyroidism and is admitting Mr. Powell for diagnosis and treatment. Questions 61 through 80 refer to this situation.

61 Symptoms associated with hyperthyroidism are a result of
1. Underproduction of the thyroid gland
2. Overproduction of the thyroid gland
3. Underproduction of the parathyroid glands
4. Overproduction of the parathyroid glands

62 Mr. Powell is admitted to a semiprivate room. As yet he is the only patient in the room. Because of his diagnosis you would
1. Encourage Mr. Powell to take the bed next to the air-conditioning vent
2. Give Mr. Powell extra blankets
3. Notify admission personnel of the communicability of the disease and ask for a private room
4. Allow Mr. Powell to choose the bed he wants and make no comment

63 Hyperthyroidism initiates altered oxygen needs. Oxygen needs
1. Are increased
2. Are decreased

64 Diagnosis of hyperthyroidism is confirmed by
1. T_3 and T_4 tests
2. An upper GI series
3. A physical examination
4. A chest x-ray examination

65 Mr. Powell may have trouble sleeping. In anticipation of this you would plan to
1. Limit visitors after 8 PM and give a hypnotic at that time
2. Ask him to turn off the television by 9 PM and give him a glass of warm milk
3. Administer a hypnotic on request and give back care
4. Give him a cup of coffee and back care at 10 PM

66 An appropriate meal plan for Mr. Powell might include
1. Beef tips, spinach casserole, carrot salad, and coffee
2. Roast beef, macaroni and cheese casserole, vanilla custard, and milk
3. Waffles with syrup, grapefruit, doughnut and coffee
4. Roast pork, green beans, tossed salad, and tea

67 Mr. Powell will be sent home on propylthiouracil. The purpose of this drug is to
1. Control the systemic effects of the hormone production
2. Reduce the vascularity of the thyroid gland
3. Ready the gland for surgical removal
4. Reduce production of the hormone

68 When taking propylthiouracil, Mr. Powell should report which of the following symptoms?
1. Sore throat
2. Intolerance to cold
3. Headaches
4. Increased urinary output

Mr. Powell was readmitted several months later. His original symptoms had not subsided, and the physician decided to perform a subtotal thyroidectomy.

69 Preoperatively Mr. Powell is given an iodine preparation. This is done because iodine will
1. Anesthetize the throat
2. Provide an antimicrobial action on the throat to lessen the chance of postoperative infection
3. Reduce the vascularity of the thyroid gland
4. Reduce the overproduction of thyroid hormone

70 Following surgery, the best position for Mr. Powell would be
1. Prone
2. Trendelenburg's
3. Semi-Fowler's
4. Lithotomy

71 An appropriate immediate postoperative nursing action would include
1. Asking Mr. Powell to speak every hour
2. Turning Mr. Powell to the supine position to assess for hemorrhage
3. Assessing exophthalmos
4. Assessing Mr. Powell's ability to consume a regular diet

72 Mr. Powell is complaining of fullness in his neck. After inspecting the side and back of the neck dressing for bleeding, you would consider which of the following most significant?
1. Urinary output of 150 ml in the last 2 hours
2. B/P, 90/60; pulse, 108; and respirations, 24
3. Hoarseness of the voice
4. Pain at the surgical site

73 Which of the following complaints would indicate the need for a tracheostomy?
1. Pain in the surgical site and spasms of the hands
2. Increased temperature and widening pulse pressure
3. Restlessness and noisy breathing
4. Infiltration of the IV fluids and nausea

74 The surgeon is summoned, and a tracheostomy is performed on Mr. Powell. During the first 24 hours after the tracheostomy it is most important for you to
1. Evaluate patency of the tube
2. Evaluate patient response to altered body image
3. Turn him prone to promote drainage
4. Administer pain medication

75 Mr. Powell's tracheostomy tube needs suctioning. The first nursing action would be to
1. Turn on suction machine
2. Explain to Mr. Powell what you are going to do
3. Notify the physician
4. Remove the inner cannula

76 During suctioning of the tracheostomy, you would
1. Ask Mr. Powell to cough forcibly
2. Humidify the oxygen to reduce drying of mucous membranes
3. Ask Mr. Powell to speak
4. Wear sterile gloves

77 To avoid irritation and trauma, suction is applied to the catheter during
1. Insertion of the catheter
2. Removal of the catheter
3. Spasms of coughing only
4. The time Mr. Powell asks you to, since he can sense the obstruction's position

78 While changing the strings securing the tracheostomy tube, you would
1. Instruct Mr. Powell to cough forcibly
2. Suction his trachea
3. Instruct Mr. Powell to hold the edges of the tracheostomy tube
4. Remove the outer cannula for cleansing

79 Tetany may be a complication postthyroidectomy. This is a complication resulting from
1. Removal of the thyroid gland
2. Removal of the parathyroid glands
3. Excessive calcium intake postoperatively
4. Electrolyte imbalance

80 Increased temperature, widening pulse pressure, and tachycardia would indicate which of the following complications of thyroidectomy?
1. Tetany
2. Laryngeal edema
3. Hypothyroidism
4. Thyroid storm

Situation: Karen Green, a 16 year old, had an argument with her parents and moved in with her boyfriend, much to her parents' dismay. Karen, her younger brother, and her parents had taken part in family counseling for the past six months. Mr. Green's alcoholism, Timmy's acting out problems, and Mrs. Green's depression "caused me to leave home," Karen told the counselor. "I'm better off with Tom. He understands me."

Shortly after moving in with Tom, Karen appeared in the emergency department of the county hospital complaining of aching in her abdomen, nausea, vomiting, and a fever of several days duration. On examination, the physician discovered a purulent discharge. The blood sample showed leukocytosis.

Karen was hospitalized for treatment of acute pelvic inflammatory disease, and further testing revealed gonococcus to be the infecting organism. Questions 81 through 100 refer to this situation.

81 Diagnosis of the presence of gonococci in women is determined by
1. Urethral and pharyngeal smears
2. Urinalysis
3. Blood samples
4. Cervical, urethral, and anal smears

82 Which of the following statements are true of gonorrhea?
(A) Gonorrhea is introduced from the outside; it passes upward from cervical canal to uterus
(B) It can involve cervix, urethra, and rectum
(C) Spontaneous resolution can occur within 2 weeks, although this does not mean a cure
(D) Many women may be asymptomatic carriers of the disease
1. A, B, and C
2. A, B, and D
3. B, C, and D
4. A, B, C, and D

83 Which of the following is *not* a typical clinical manifestation of gonorrhea?
1. Swollen Bartholin's glands
2. Groups of chancres
3. Anemia
4. Jaundice

84 Acute gonorrhea symptoms most commonly occur
1. During or immediately after a menstrual period
2. Near the time of ovulation
3. Just before the menstrual period
4. During pregnancy

85 Which of the following drugs is more frequently used for treatment of gonorrhea?
1. Aqueous procaine penicillin
2. Garamycin
3. Streptomycin
4. Chloromycetin

86 When Karen receives this drug for the first time, you should be alert to the possibility of
1. Hypertensive crisis
2. Anaphylactic shock
3. Excessive bleeding from injection sites
4. Nausea and vomiting

87 Treatment of Karen's disorder would include
1. Cold applications to the abdomen
2. Semi-Fowler's position
3. An indwelling catheter
4. Vaginal packs

88 In caring for patients with gonorrhea, you must remember to
1. Wash your hands before and after coming in contact with the patient
2. Wear isolation attire (gown, gloves)
3. Double bag all articles that come from the room for proper disposal
4. See that visitors are restricted during the hospital stay

89 Karen was reluctant to divulge the names of her sexual partners. You could best handle this situation by
1. Explaining the seriousness of the disease and that her sexual partners could be in need of medical attention also
2. Reminding her that she is obligated by law to divulge the names of her partners
3. Telling her that you will report this to a case finder at the public health department
4. Explaining that you will have to contact her parents if she doesn't cooperate

90 In planning for discharge, you should stress the importance of
1. Birth control
2. Follow-up visits
3. Regular vaginal douching
4. Cleansing the perineum

91 One of the first symptoms in men who have contracted gonorrhea is
1. Burning on urination
2. Purulent discharge from the anus
3. Nausea and vomiting
4. Swelling of the penis

92 The most serious complication of pelvic inflammatory disease is
1. Organic brain syndrome
2. Sterility
3. Chronic cystitis
4. Peritonitis

93 Karen tells you that she couldn't have VD: ''I have an IUD, and I've been taking birth control pills. These are supposed to keep people protected from such things.'' Karen begins to cry and tells you that she wants to go home ''right now.'' You could best show your concern and support for Karen by
1. Telling her firmly that she has to remain in the hospital until the doctor releases her
2. Calling in another nurse to bring Karen a sedative
3. Telling Karen you will call her boyfriend to come stay with her
4. Quietly remaining with Karen and allowing her to cry

94 While Karen is in the hospital you note that she seems to yawn frequently, has a runny nose and teary eyes, and perspires heavily. While giving Karen a bath you discover what appears to be needle tracks in both arms. You suspect that Karen might be undergoing withdrawal from
1. Sedatives
2. Narcotics
3. Hallucinogens
4. Hypnotics

95 Karen says to you, ''Please don't tell anybody. I know I can trust you. I promise not to get messed up with drugs again.'' Which response would be most appropriate?
1. ''Karen, you know that I must report this. What you were doing is unlawful.''
2. ''Karen, I must report this. You are beginning to experience withdrawal, and we must help you through this time.''
3. ''Karen, I must report this. Hospital policy requires nurses to document all their observations.''
4. ''Karen, I must report this. Your doctor will know what to do.''

96 Karen is overwhelmed by all that has happened to her over the last few weeks. She becomes depressed, cries easily, won't eat, and says over and over, ''I want to die.'' One morning you find Karen in a much better mood. Her voice has a cheery tone, and she has bathed and put on clean pajamas. The nurse considers this change in behavior and appearance to be a(n)
1. Sign that the depression has lifted
2. Clue that she may be planning suicide
3. Chance to call her family and tell them that she's improved
4. Indication that she is showing some much needed maturity

97 Karen's mother comes to visit for the first time and demands to know what is wrong with her daughter. ''I'll go to your supervisor,'' she threatens. Your best response would be
1. ''You sound very angry, Mrs. Green. I'm sure you've been very worried about Karen. Let's sit down and talk.''

2. "Go ahead, Mrs. Green. She won't tell you any more than I have."
3. "That's your prerogative, Mrs. Green. May I give you my supervisor's name?"
4. "If you insist, Mrs. Green. But I think you are just feeling guilty yourself about the mess Karen is in."

98 Drug-dependent persons are often determined to maintain their habit at all costs. What preventive measures can be taken to keep Karen away from drugs while she is in the hospital?
1. Post a "no visitors" sign on her door
2. Keep her and visitors under close observation
3. Call the security force to search her room
4. Restrain her while she is alone

99 Karen is placed on an MAO inhibitor for her depression. Her diet must be monitored to prevent
1. Heartburn
2. Hypertensive crisis
3. Drowsiness
4. Blurred vision

100 While in the psychiatric unit, Karen appears to be moving her lips and cupping her ear when no one else is around. She is most likely experiencing
1. Delusions
2. Illusions
3. Halluciantions
4. Mirages

Situation: Mrs. Jane Adams, a 40-year-old mother of four boys, visits her physician after discovering a lump in her breast 2 days earlier. She is quite anxious, since her mother died of carcinoma of the breast several years ago.

The physician feels a small, movable lump, approximately 5 cm wide in the upper quadrant of the right breast. He sends Mrs. Adams to the outpatient x-ray department for a mammogram. The test results come back positive. Mrs. Adams is admitted to the hospital the next day for a biopsy. Questions 101 to 120 refer to this situation.

101 Some common early clinical manifestations of breast cancer include
(A) A nontender lump that may be movable and isolated
(B) Pain in the early stages
(C) Retraction or dimpling over the skin where the mass is noted
(D) Asymmetry
1. A, B, and C
2. A, C, and D
3. B, C, and D
4. A, B, and D

102 On examining the breast, it is important for the physician to manipulate the mass
1. Firmly, in no particular pattern
2. Gently, in different directions
3. Firmly, in the same direction
4. Gently, in no particular pattern

103 Mrs. Adams's breast biopsy revealed invasive adenocarcinoma. A radical mastectomy was performed. A radical mastectomy involves
1. Removal of the breast, pectoral muscles, and axillary contents
2. Removal of the breast
3. Removal of the breast and pectoral muscles
4. Removal of breast and axillary node

104 Mrs. Adams awakens in the recovery room grabbing at the operative site and moaning, "It's gone. It's all over." She pleads with you to "let me die." Even though Mrs. Adams was prepared by the surgeon for the possible removal of her breast, you must be aware that it is common to react with anger, withdrawal, depression, or other emotions. The next day when Mrs. Adams cries during her morning care, you say
1. "Don't cry. You're not going to help yourself by doing this."
2. "Go ahead and cry. Get it all out. You'll feel better afterward."
3. "It must be very upsetting for you right now. Let me get your husband."
4. "It must be very upsetting for you right now. Would you like me to stay with you awhile?

105 Initial postoperative care includes
(A) Monitoring vital signs
(B) Inspecting dressings for excessive bleeding
(C) Encouraging turning and deep breathing
(D) Positioning patient in Fowler's position with affected arm flat
(E) Exercising affected arm immediately
1. A, B, and C
2. A, B, C, and D
3. A, B, C, and E
4. A, B, C, D, and E

106 The Hemovac device
1. Is a portable suction unit used to prevent fluid collection under the skin
2. Should be emptied only according to institutional policy
3. Is applied 1 to 2 days after surgery
4. Is always applied after any breast surgery

107 Postoperative exercises for the mastectomy patient are done primarily to
1. Aid in healing of the wound
2. Help prevent shoulder motion limitation and deformities
3. Aid in recovering sufficiently to resume home-making activities
4. Assume self-care

108 Prevention of lymphedema may be aided by
(A) Proper exercise of the affected arm
(B) Regular massage of the affected arm
(C) Avoidance of carrying heavy objects
(D) Keeping the arm in an ''across-the-chest'' position as much as possible
(E) Wearing nonrestrictive clothing and jewelry
1. A, C, and E
2. A, B, C, and E
3. B, C, and E
4. A, B, C, and D

109 The nurse may promote the mastectomy patient's psychosocial recovery by
(A) Listening to her when she wants to talk
(B) Correcting any misconceptions regarding recovery
(C) Insisting that she meet with a Reach to Recovery volunteer as soon as possible
(D) Soliciting the support of the spouse or other family members even if the patient objects
(E) Showing the patient prosthetic devices as soon after surgery as possible
1. A, C, and D
2. A, B, C, D, and E
3. A and B
4. A, B, D, and E

110 Common early postoperative exercises for the mastectomy patient to do at home include
(A) Closing and opening window draperies
(B) Broom sweeping
(C) Vacuuming
(D) Hanging clothes on the line
(E) Playing tennis
1. A, B, and D
2. B, C, and D
3. A, B, C, and D
4. A, B, D, and E

111 Major treatment modalities for breast cancer include
(A) Radiotherapy
(B) Endocrine therapy
(C) Chemotherapy
(D) Immunotherapy
1. A, C, and D
2. A and C
3. A, B, and C
4. A, B, C, and D

112 Breast irradiation often produces which of the following side effects?
1. Pain
2. Dysphagia
3. Alopecia
4. Pyrexia

113 The single most valuable tool in the early detection of breast cancer is routine
1. Mammography
2. Xeromammography
3. Individual breast self-examination
4. Thermography

114 In performing breast self-examination, the most effective pattern to follow is to begin in the
1. Lower inner quadrant
2. Lower outer quadrant
3. Upper outer quadrant
4. Upper inner quadrant

115 Breast self-examination should
1. Be done once a month, just before the menstrual period
2. Be done once a month, just after the menstrual period
3. Be done every 6 months
4. Not be necessary if menses has ceased

116 Instructions to prepare Mrs. Adams for going home would include cautioning her against
1. Wearing loose rubber gloves when washing dishes
2. Allowing blood to be drawn from the affected area
3. Wearing a thimble when sewing
4. Allowing pulse to be taken in affected area

117 Reach to Recovery volunteers can be especially helpful to mastectomy patients because they are
1. Nurses trained to deal with crisis situations
2. Women who have had successful recoveries from mastectomies themselves
3. Volunteers who have undergone a 6-month training course
4. Salespersons who can fit the patient with a prosthesis

118 Discharge teaching for the mastectomy patient should include
(A) Exercising
(B) Care of the wound
(C) Recognizing signs of infection
(D) Maintaining proper posture
(E) Selection of a proper prosthesis
1. A, B, C, and D
2. B, C, D, and E
3. A, B, C, D, and E
4. A, C, D, and E

119 It is thought that cancerous cells in the breast are rather slow growing. It is likely for a lump to be present for how long before being large enough to be discovered?
1. 1 year
2. 10 months
3. 10 years
4. 3 years

120 The factor thought *most* likely to be a cause of breast cancer is
1. Age
2. Non-breast-feeding practices
3. Genetic predisposition
4. Hormone activity

SAMPLE EXAMINATION 3

This examination contains several paragraphs concerning patients/clients. Following each such paragraph is a series of questions concerning the patient and the situation described in that paragraph. Read each situation carefully. Read each question carefully, and consider all possible answers. When you have decided which answer is **best,** blacken the corresponding space on the answer sheet. There is only **one** best answer for each question.

Situation: While the Wellon's were driving to the park for a family picnic, they were hit in the back by a speeding car. The resulting explosion and fire killed both parents of 3-year-old Bill. Bill sustained a fractured left femur and second- and third-degree burns over 43% of his body. The emergency medical technician communicated to the hospital that Bill was burned on both anterior and posterior aspects of his torso, arms, and hands. Questions 1 through 20 refer to this situation.

1 As part of the emergency team, you would help prepare for Bill's arrival by obtaining a
1. Tracheostomy tray
2. Stretcher with sterile sheets
3. Cardiac defibrillator
4. Sterile dressing tray

2 On arriving at the emergency room, Bill is semiconscious, whining and calling for his mother. Once transferred to the trauma room, you begin to obtain baseline data. Bill's radial pulse is 160 per minute, respirations, 32 per minute, and blood pressure, 60/30. Based on the initial data, you would report vital signs to the physician and assist as ordered in initiation of
1. Removal of clothing
2. Central venous line
3. IV fluids
4. Antibiotics

3 Immediate physical observations of Bill would most importantly include
1. Physical development
2. Head circumference
3. Height and weight
4. Quality of respirations

4 The physician chooses the closed method of dressing the burned area. On the pediatric ward, Bill's room would be set up to provide which type of isolation?
1. Enteric
2. Strict
3. Reverse
4. Respiratory

5 During the first 24 hours of treating Bill for burns, you can assist in assessing fluid replacement needs by monitoring hourly
1. Urine specific gravity
2. IV fluid rate
3. Vital signs
4. IV fluid intake

6 On the second day of hospitalization, Bill becomes more fretful and cries continuously for his mother. To provide emotional support to Bill, you would
1. Plan care so that you can spend as much time in his room as possible
2. Frequently administer phenobarbital elixir as ordered

3. Tell Bill not to cry because "brave boys don't cry"
4. Explain to Bill that his grandmother is coming to stay after supper

7 Bill keeps tugging at the pulley ropes on the Russell's traction. To help Bill cope with being immobilized, you can
1. Play Chinese checkers with Bill as a diversional activity
2. Apply Russell's traction to Bill's favorite teddy bear
3. Place mitten restraints on his hands
4. Retie the pulley ropes out of Bill's reach

8 Bill's grandmother tells you she is concerned about Bill wetting the bed at night. The best response would be
1. "Bill will probably need to be toilet trained again after his discharge from the hospital."
2. "Don't worry about Bill wetting the bed at night. We change his sheets frequently."
3. "Bill has had a traumatic experience. When he gets used to being hospitalized, he will stop wetting the bed."
4. "Wetting the bed is not unusual for children Bill's age. Children will regress in some behaviors during hospitalization."

9 Frequent assessment of Bill's left leg would include maintaining proper alignment and
1. Checking sensation and circulation in the leg
2. Increasing the weight of traction as necessary to maintain countertraction
3. Taking the apical pulse every 2 hours
4. Checking temperature and range of motion in his right leg

10 Before changing the burn dressing, Bill is to receive 20 mg of Demerol elixir. The elixir has 50 mg of Demerol per teaspoon. How many milliliters of the elixir would Bill be given?
1. 1 ml
2. 2 ml
3. 4 ml
4. 6 ml

11 When changing the burn dressing, you would help Bill control his feelings of fear and pain by
1. Having another nurse restrain Bill until the treatment is over
2. Explaining firmly what is to be done and how he can help
3. Allowing Bill to cry until he is tired and less combative
4. Repeating administration of the prescribed pain medication

12 Bill's burned areas have healed sufficiently to receive skin grafts. After skin grafting, the most important nursing action to promote acceptance of the graft is to
1. Debride the outer edge of the recipient site to facilitate healing
2. Immobilize or restrict movement of the graft site to prevent dislodging of the graft
3. Apply a heat light to decrease drainage
4. Change the Vaseline gauze dressings daily

13 Because of the long period of immobilization, you would encourage Bill to drink fluids to prevent
1. Renal calculi resulting from urinary stasis
2. Dehydration and diuresis
3. Fluid and electrolyte imbalance
4. Anemia and weight loss

14 Normal nutritional requirements of a preschooler include food from the Basic Four food groups. As a result of the burns Bill would need a diet
1. High in proteins, carbohydrates, and calories
2. High in proteins, iron, and calcium
3. Low in sodium and cholesterol
4. Low in calcium and high in carbohydrates

15 Normally preschoolers have little interest in eating, and the anorexia associated with burns presents a problem of nutrition. Bill would most likely eat better if
1. Other children ate with him
2. His grandmother ate with him
3. You would feed him
4. Tube feedings were given when he did not eat

16 Bill has not had a bowel movement in 3 days. You can promote elimination by encouraging Bill to eat
1. Eggs and cheese toast
2. Popsicles and oranges
3. Apples and carrot sticks
4. Chicken and whole grain cereal

17 Bill is put in a spica cast several days before discharge from the hospital. Following drying of the cast, you can check the cast for tightness by
1. Inserting fingers between the skin and cast
2. Pulling the cast up and down to determine movement
3. Inserting a coat hanger as far down the cast as possible
4. Standing Bill on his feet to determine any pressure areas

18 Bill's grandmother is to be instructed in caring for the cast and Bill at home. You would emphasize
1. Protecting the cast from fecal smears
2. Providing Bill with vitamin supplements
3. Cleaning the cast weekly with cleanser
4. Changing Bill's position frequently

19 Several weeks following Bill's discharge from the hospital, his grandmother calls the unit. She is concerned about Bill because for the first time after the accident he is asking where his parents are. You would suggest the grandmother respond as follows
1. "Bill, what do you think happened to Mommy and Daddy?"
2. "Come here, Bill. Let me tell you a story about what happened to Mommy and Daddy."
3. "What do you remember about the accident that you were in with Mommy and Daddy?"
4. "Do you remember when Aunt Jessie died?"

20 Bill begins to cry when his grandmother talks about the accident. The best response to Bill's crying is to
1. Leave Bill alone in the room to cry
2. Continue discussing the accident
3. Hold Bill closely while he cries
4. Tell Bill not to cry and that everything will be alright

Situation: Cheryl Bader, the oldest of five children, is 12 years old. Her family lives in a small bungalow in a multicomplex housing project. Four weeks after beginning a new school year, Cheryl comes home complaining of her left knee hurting. Two days before, she had complained of her right knee hurting. Questions 21 through 40 refer to this situation.

21 When the school nurse called Cheryl's mother to suggest the child be seen by a physician, Cheryl's mother said, "It's just growing pains." The nurse explained that migratory joint pains could be a symptom of
1. Rheumatic fever
2. Rheumatoid arthritis
3. Legg-Calvé-Perthes disease
4. A prepuberty growth spurt

22 Cheryl is sent by her teacher to the school nurse. Cheryl is short of breath, complaining of precordial pain, and has a pulse rate of 150 per minute. The school nurse calls Cheryl's mother and has Cheryl
1. Collect a urine specimen
2. Cough and deep breathe
3. Swallow a nitroglycerin tablet
4. Lie down and rest

23 Cheryl is admitted to the hospital with a diagnosis of rheumatic fever. Important data to obtain from her medical history would be a recent illness of
1. Glomerulonephritis
2. "Strep" throat
3. Osteomyelitis
4. Measles

24 Characteristic of the child with rheumatic fever, Cheryl's home environment is most likely a
1. Rural housing project
2. Suburban housing development
3. Large industrial employee housing project
4. Crowded urban development

25 A nursing care objective in Cheryl's case would be the prevention of heart damage. This can be best accomplished by
1. Limiting activity 2 to 3 hours daily
2. Sedating Cheryl every 4 hours
3. Complete bed rest until resting pulse rate is 80 per minute
4. Allowing unlimited activity and reducing the stress of hospitalization

26 To gain Cheryl's cooperation in the treatment and nursing care plan, you would need to establish
1. Limitations and expectations of behavior, based on Cheryl's developmental level
2. Limited visiting hours for Cheryl's school friends and family
3. A rapport with Cheryl similar to that of a friend or peer
4. A data base to determine Cheryl's psychosocial and motor development

27 Which of the following criteria must Cheryl meet in order to be allowed to ambulate?
1. Normal temperature 30 minutes after taking aspirin and normal erythrocyte sedimentation rate
2. High C-reactive protein and normal temperature 30 minutes after taking aspirin
3. Resting pulse rate of 80 per minute and normal sedimentation rate
4. High C-reactive protein level and increased erythrocyte sedimentation rate

28 You can best prevent Cheryl from becoming frustrated and bored during the long period of bed rest by

1. Playing checkers and card games with her
2. Assisting Cheryl to decorate her hospital room with cards and pictures from friends
3. Providing Cheryl with her own television
4. Encouraging Cheryl to make needlework objects

29 Cheryl is anorexic during the acute stage of her illness. You can encourage her to obtain adequate nutrients by
1. Offering small, frequent liquid or soft feedings
2. Ordering Cheryl pizza and hamburgers with fries
3. Allowing Cheryl to skip meals and eat when she wants to
4. Feeding Cheryl her meals

30 Cheryl becomes very angry at the nursing staff for telling her what she can and cannot do. She yells, "I take care of my little brothers and sisters and myself. Leave me alone!" The best response to Cheryl would be
1. "That may be true at home, Cheryl, but this is a different situation. We know what is best for you."
2. "I'll leave you alone, Cheryl. Just remember that I'm here when you need me."
3. "What's going on, Cheryl? I want you to talk to me. Let it out."
4. "It must be hard to be here and take orders from others after you've been so independent. How can we help you feel better about that?"

31 To protect Cheryl from injury during chorea movements, you can
1. Pad bedrails and assist Cheryl with out-of-bed activities
2. Restrain Cheryl's arms and legs until the chorea movements subside
3. Administer Dilantin intravenously every 2 hours
4. Place Cheryl in an empty room until the movements subside

32 Cheryl is admitted to the hospital two times within 18 months for rheumatic fever. On the third admission, Cheryl is in critical condition, with evidence of cardiac decompensation. The physician orders Digoxin, 0.125 mg PO, and Lasix, 20 mg PO b.i.d. Important nursing observations to assess the therapeutic effects of these drugs are signs of
1. Increased blood pressure and oliguria
2. Decreased pulse rate and increased urine output
3. Increased pulse rate and decreased urine output
4. Increased blood pressure and increased urine output

33 While Cheryl is receiving Digoxin you would obtain a(n)
1. Radial pulse
2. Femoral pulse
3. Carotid pulse
4. Apical pulse

34 Immediately following administration of the Digoxin elixir, Cheryl vomits. You would
1. Administer another dose
2. Estimate the amount of medicine vomited and readminister that amount
3. Notify the physician and follow his or her instructions
4. Chart that the medicine was vomited

35 To reduce Cheryl's respiratory distress, you will place her in
1. Fowler's position with legs elevated
2. Semi-Fowler's position
3. Contour position for comfort
4. Jackknife position with head elevated

36 Most useful in determining the amount of fluid loss Cheryl has as a result of the Lasix is monitoring
1. Daily weight
2. Urine specific gravity
3. Fluid intake
4. Urine output

37 Several months later, Cheryl is scheduled for open heart surgery to replace the mitral valve damaged by the rheumatic fever. Preoperative preparation of Cheryl would include
1. Demonstration of equipment she will see after surgery
2. Sedating Cheryl at bedtime to decrease her anxiety
3. Explaining procedure by discussing a patient education booklet on open heart surgery
4. Tour of the recovery room area to introduce her to persons working in that area

38 Postoperatively, you observe bright red blood draining in the chest tubes. You would
1. Notify the physician immediately
2. Monitor hourly the fluid level in the chest bottle
3. Clamp the chest tube until the physician arrives
4. Check Cheryl's blood pressure more frequently than every 4 hours

39 Cheryl wakes up in ICU with an endotracheal tube. She becomes frightened with the equipment and is unable to talk. The best response to her fright would be
1. "Cheryl, remember the tube I told you about before surgery? That's why you can't talk. But we're right here if you need us. We will be close by. Just press this button, and someone will come."
2. "Cheryl, the doctor ordered that tube. It won't be in long. Don't worry, we're here."
3. "Cheryl, just don't fight it. That only makes you more afraid. We will take care of you."
4. "Cheryl, see that other girl over there? She has a tube just like you. She's not afraid."

40 When transferred to the floor, Cheryl is frightened something will happen to her while in the room alone. You can reassure her by explaining
1. Where the call light is in the room
2. A nurse will be assigned to her continuously
3. A family member must stay with her if she is scared
4. You will frequently be with her these first few days

Situation: Sam East began walking at 14 months of age. As a normal toddler, he explored energetically everything in his home. Now at the age of $2^1/_2$ years, Sam has had a cold for several months. He is irritable and less energetic. Because of the change in Sam's behavior and the bruises on his legs, his mother takes him to his physician. The pediatrician admits Sam to the hospital for diagnostic tests. Questions 41 through 61 refer to this situation.

41 Sam's mother takes a soda from him to allow you to take Sam's temperature. Sam throws himself on the floor in a temper tantrum. You would
1. Tell Sam you will take his temperature when you come back
2. Ask another nurse to hold Sam while you take his temperature
3. Tell Sam to stop and have his mother spank him if he does not
4. Ask Sam's mother to hold him down to take his temperature

42 Following the temper tantrum, Sam is short of breath and fatigued. To provide Sam with the needed rest, you could
1. Administer phenobarbital elixir and elevate the crib rails
2. Ask Sam's mother to leave until Sam goes to sleep
3. Place Sam in his crib with his favorite toy or blanket
4. Give Sam a bath and change the linens to help him rest

43 A bone marrow aspiration is scheduled for Sam later in the afternoon. To prepare Sam and his mother for the test, you would explain the test by
1. Drawing a diagram of the iliac crest and indicating where the needle will be inserted
2. Describing each step of the procedure and what Sam will feel
3. Simulating the procedure on Sam's favorite teddy bear and describing what the bear will feel
4. Explaining the procedure to Mrs. East so she can describe it to Sam

44 The diagnostic tests indicate that Sam has acute lymphocytic leukemia. Mrs. East says to the physician, "You are wrong! It's a mistake; there is nothing wrong with Sam!" You recognize Mrs. East's comments as
1. Anger directed at the physician
2. Blaming herself for Sam's condition
3. Unrealistic and immature for an adult
4. The first stage of the grief process, denial

45 Because of the leukemic process and the effects of the chemotherapy, Sam must be protected against
1. Secondary infections by instituting reverse isolation
2. Viral infections by restricting visitors
3. Overdosage of drugs because of hepatic failure
4. Anemia by encouraging foods high in iron

46 One of the chemotherapeutic drugs used in treatment of leukemia is cyclophosphamide (Cytoxan). Before and 2 days after administration of the drug, you have Sam
1. Void in bedpan to measure all output
2. Stop eating any protein foods to avoid proteinuria
3. Drink plenty of fluids to prevent chemical cystitis
4. Exercise twice a day to facilitate drug absorption by the cancer cells

47 Sam develops small mouth ulcerations. To provide oral hygiene for Sam, you can
1. Swab his mouth with a soft sponge toothbrush or cotton-tipped applicator

2. Give Sam an astringent mouthwash to gargle and rinse his mouth
3. Rinse Sam's mouth with a Water-Pik and hot water
4. Apply a water-soluble ointment to the ulcerations with a tongue depressor

48 Sam is anorexic and refuses to eat any of the foods on his diet tray. Sam can be encouraged to eat by allowing him to
1. Choose the foods he wants when marking the menu
2. Eat any foods he likes and can tolerate
3. Play with the food on his diet tray
4. Drink water or milk before and after each meal

49 Small areas of alopecia are noticeable after the drug and radiation therapy. Sam's mother expresses her concern that Sam will be embarrassed about his appearance. You can best reply by explaining
1. Sam will not notice the alopecia as much as his mother
2. Sam's friends are too young to be concerned or to tease Sam
3. Sam's hair will grow back, and until then he can wear a cap
4. Normal growth and development of a toddler and how the child is not concerned with appearance until adolescence

50 Sam's mother leaves to go home for awhile. Sam cries continuously for his mother. You can
1. Plan your care to spend as much time as possible with Sam
2. Ignore Sam until he stops crying
3. Call Mrs. East and ask her to return to the hospital
4. Take Sam out of his isolation room and walk him in the hall

51 Ritualism is a behavior the toddler exhibits to help him feel more secure in his environment. To minimize conflicts in Sam adjusting to his mother's absence you should have
1. A list of Sam's rituals from his mother
2. Sam perform his favorite ritual activities
3. A method of rewarding Sam's good behavior
4. An understanding of the family and child's background and rituals

52 Sam is becoming dehydrated as a result of vomiting and diarrhea in the past few days. His eyes appear dull, and he has lost 3 pounds. The physician orders IV fluids at 60 ml per hour and hourly intake and output. The data you would record about the stools are
1. Weight and color
2. Frequency, color, consistency, and odor
3. Color, amount, and odor
4. Number and type of specimens collected

53 Sam is receiving IV fluids from a "minidrip" set that delivers 60 gtts per milliliter of fluid. How many drops per minute would you need to administer 60 ml per hour?
1. 10 gtts per minute
2. 25 gtts per minute
3. 50 gtts per minute
4. 60 gtts per minute

54 To obtain a stool specimen to test for ova and parasites, you would need
1. Tongue blade and specimen cup
2. Syringe, needle, and sterile container
3. Bedpan and emesis basin
4. Sterile tongue blade and plastic container

55 To prevent excoriation of Sam's skin from the diarrhea, you could apply which of the following to the buttocks after each stool?
1. Baby powder
2. Benzoine spray
3. Vaseline
4. Betadine solution

56 Sam is diagnosed as having a *Salmonella* infection. To prevent spreading the diarrhea to the staff and other patients, you must
1. Wash hands before and after caring for each child
2. Institute enteric isolation on the entire unit
3. Place Sam in respiratory isolation
4. Notify county health department officials of the incident

57 Sam's condition improves, and he is ready for discharge from the hospital. Important for you to emphasize in discharge instructions is
1. Sam's need for foods from the Basic Four food groups
2. The need for Sam to wear his hat to hide the alopecia
3. A follow-up examination of Sam by his physician
4. Isolation of Sam from persons other than the immediate family

58 Mrs. East asks your advice in buying Sam a new toy to take home from the hospital. An appropriate toy for a toddler is a
1. Game
2. Stuffed animal
3. Music box
4. Pull toy

59 Sam's mother comes to pick him up from the hospital. Sam clings to you and pushes away from his mother. The best approach to this situation would be for you to
1. Take Sam and his mother to a private room to allow Sam time to begin interacting with his mother
2. Force Sam to go to his mother and leave them quickly
3. Explain to Mrs. East that Sam is very attached to the nurses
4. Ask Mrs. East to come back tomorrow when Sam is less tired

60 Sam has nightmares resulting from bone marrow aspirations and frequent blood drawing. You would advise his mother,
1. "Immediately take Sam into your bed. He'll only get more frightened if he fully wakens during the nightmares."
2. "Take Sam to a child psychologist. Nightmares that continue more than a week or two are pathologic."
3. "Hold Sam until he is calmer; talk calmly to him; leave the night-light on, and see if he will go back to sleep."
4. "Let Sam go into your bed; then when he is asleep take him back to his bed, and repeat as necessary."

61 After Sam leaves, you notice the dirty teddy bear he clung to during his hospitalization. You would
1. Discard the teddy bear since his mother bought Sam a new toy
2. Wash the teddy bear and save it for other children on the unit
3. Call Mrs. East and save the teddy bear for her to pick up later
4. Give the bear to the pediatrician for Mrs. East to get when she brings Sam in for an office visit

---

Situation: Sarah and Dick Stark anxiously awaited the birth of their first child. During the delivery Dick stayed beside his wife until he saw something was wrong with their new baby girl. The infant was born with a myelomeningocele. Questions 62 through 81 refer to this situation.

62 Dick leaves the delivery room and sits in the area of the nurse's station. The best way to approach Dick is to
1. Offer him a cup of coffee and leave him alone
2. Sit down beside him and ask if he needs help
3. Tell him that the infant is deformed but she can live a normal life
4. Ask him several questions about the delivery to encourage Dick to talk

63 Dick asks, "What is that horrible thing I saw on my baby's back?" In response, you would include
1. The term "myelomeningocele" and a simple description of the anomaly
2. A description of the long-term care the infant will need
3. The complications of a myelomeningocele, such as paraplegia, hydrocephalus, and urine retention
4. Conversation that would direct Dick's attention from the fact his daughter was born with a congenital anomaly

64 An important nursing objective in caring for the newborn with a myelomeningocele is to
1. Maintain the newborn in a prone position
2. Observe the lower extremities for movement
3. Promote wound healing
4. Prevent infection and harm to the meningocele sac

65 To keep the meningocele sac moist, you should
1. Place the newborn in an Isolette in high humidity
2. Pour sterile normal saline every 2 hours over the sac
3. Apply sterile gauze soaked with an antibacterial solution
4. Keep a diaper wet with sterile water over area

66 You must observe closely the newborn's
1. Urine and bowel elimination
2. Moro reflex
3. Relationship with mother
4. Hematocrit and hemoglobin levels

67 You can assist the physician in determining the extent of neuromuscular damage by
1. Observing for movement of extremities

2. Testing response to deep pain
3. Checking tendon reflexes every hour
4. Recording type of cry heard from infant

68 Because of the length of hospitalization and separation of the parents from their infant, the nursing staff, to foster the child-parent relationship, would
1. Encourage both parents to see the child during the specified visiting hours
2. Explain the process of parent bonding and how the parents should treat the child at home
3. Encourage the parents to touch and hold the newborn as much as possible
4. Ignore the parents' statements indicating their grief of not having a normal baby

69 Following repair of the myelomeningocele, you would daily observe for signs of hydrocephalus by
1. Palpating anterior and posterior fontanelles
2. Maintaining strict intake and output
3. Weighing newborn each morning
4. Measuring head circumference

70 Signs of increased intracranial pressure you may observe are
1. Increased blood pressure and pulse and decreased pulse pressure
2. Bulging fontanelles, high-pitched cry, and separated cranial sutures
3. Cheyne-Stokes respirations, hypotension, and increased pulse pressure
4. Decreased reflexes, bulging fontanelles, weak cry, and hypotension

71 Sarah tells you that her daughter vomits frequently. To promote adequate nutrition, you would advise the mother to
1. Hold the infant while supporting the head and offer small frequent feedings
2. Withhold feedings until the baby stops vomiting; then thicken the feedings
3. Increase carbohydrates in each feeding by adding sugar to the formula
4. Insert a nasogastric tube to give the formula and instruct the mother in the proper technique

72 Sarah's baby is scheduled for insertion of a ventriculoperitoneal shunt to decrease accumulation of cerebrospinal fluid causing hydrocephalus. Postoperatively the infant would be placed
1. On the operative side
2. In Trendelenburg's position
3. On the nonoperative side
4. In high Fowler's position

73 The initial postoperative check of the infant's pupils indicated the pupils to be equal and reactive to light. Four hours later, the right pupil dilated and fixed. You would
1. Decrease the IV flow rate to keep the vein open
2. Notify the charge nurse to administer any IV push medications
3. Change the infant's position to reduce intracranial pressure
4. Check pupil reaction in 1 hour to validate the problem

74 Sarah asks you, "Why do you keep measuring my baby's head every day? I thought after the shunt was put in, everything would be alright." In response, you would say,
1. "The baby's head size should have decreased immediately after surgery. I am checking to see if the shunt helped your baby."
2. "By measuring the baby's head, I will know if there is an increase in intracranial pressure."
3. "As the cerebrospinal fluid drains from the ventricles of the brain, the baby's head circumference will gradually decrease."
4. "You need not be concerned with what we are doing. Your baby is alright and will be going home soon."

75 Two days after the infant is discharged from the hospital, Sarah brings her to the emergency room. The infant has a rectal temperature of 104°F and a high-pitched cry and has had seizure activity. The infant is admitted with the diagnosis of meningitis. The physician has ordered urine for U.A., blood cultures, and preparation of infant for lumbar puncture. To prepare the infant for a lumbar puncture, you would
1. Restrain the infant in a side-lying position with the head hyperextended during the procedure
2. Administer 10 mg of IM Demerol to sedate infant before the procedure
3. Obtain infant lumbar puncture set and hold infant in sitting position with head flexed during the procedure
4. Place infant in a mummy restraint and hold neck flexed during the procedure

76 To obtain a urine specimen from the infant, you would
1. Cleanse and dry genitalia, perineum, and skin; apply a self-adhesive plastic bag (urine strap)
2. Cleanse and dry perineum; catheterize infant with sterile infant feeding tube
3. Apply disposable diaper; aspirate urine from diaper with needle and syringe
4. Place infant on small fracture pan; pour urine into specimen container

77 Following puncture for collection of blood cultures, you would immediately
1. Take the specimen to the laboratory
2. Apply direct pressure to the area until bleeding stops
3. Apply a warm compress to decrease pain and ecchymosis
4. Obtain an arterial blood specimen for comparison

78 Sarah asks you how long her infant will be in isolation. Your response would be based on the knowledge that
1. Isolation will be maintained until a negative bacterial growth culture is returned on spinal fluid specimens
2. 24 hours after antibacterial therapy, isolation is not necessary
3. Preventing the spread of infection is the primary objective in care of the infant
4. Isolation is maintained until completion of 7 days of IV antibiotics

79 During seizure activity you would protect the infant by
1. Holding the infant's extremities tightly to prevent injury
2. Placing clove-hitch restraints on all extremities
3. Placing blankets over the infant to keep her warm
4. Placing pillows or padding along the sides of the crib

80 While providing daily care to the infant you would observe for
1. Skin redness and breakdown and check the IV tube site for inflammation and infiltration
2. Urine specific gravity increase, rise in body temperature, and decreased urine output
3. Change in vital and neurologic signs and increased urine output
4. Frequent bowel movements, signs of nuchal rigidity, and hypothermia

81 The physician has ordered the infant to receive 125,000 units of aqueous penicillin q.6h. intravenously. Before each administration of the medicine, you would
1. Check the IV tube site for signs of phlebitis and infiltration
2. Flush IV line with 30 ml of IV fluid to test patency of line
3. Verify with pharmacist the amount of reconstituted solution of penicillin to be administered
4. Ask Sarah to leave her infant's room during the procedure

Situation: The Gatlin's adopted Harry when he was 6 months old. Mrs. Gatlin was informed that the pediatrician was concerned about Harry's frequent respiratory infections, large foul-smelling stools, and the baby's failure to gain weight and height. Harry was admitted to the hospital for diagnostic evaluations of "failure to thrive." Question 82 through 101 refer to this situation.

82 In preparing a nursing care plan for Harry, you would include observations and interventions directed at establishing the diagnosis. In addition to preparing the family and infant for diagnostic tests, you would assess the family's
1. Social and economic factors that may influence infant's failure to thrive
2. Daily interactions with Harry to determine parent-child relationship(s)
3. Intellectual ability to understand complexity of diagnostic tests
4. Hereditary tendencies to congenital malabsorption syndromes

83 After Harry undergoes invasive diagnostic tests, you would encourage Harry's mother to
1. Keep the infant still in his crib for 1 hour after the test
2. Force the infant to eat, since food intake had been restricted before the test
3. Hold and cuddle the infant to provide comfort after a painful procedure
4. Allow Harry to cry in his crib because crying will increase pulmonary infusion

84 Harry is scheduled for a palmar sweat test. You understand this test is to determine
1. The quantity of sweat produced in one area following electrode stimulation of the glands
2. The level of potassium on the surface of the palm

3. Presence of electrolyte concentration in sweat
4. Enzyme concentration in sweat of the palm

85 Harry is diagnosed as having cystic fibrosis. The clinical symptoms manifested by Harry resulted from
1. Poor nutrition, maternal deprivation, and inadequate immunologic defenses
2. Inadequate care in the orphanage and incomplete maternal bonding
3. Physiologic anorexia, high cholesterol levels in formula, and absence of pancreatic enzymes
4. Obstruction of pancreatic ducts and air passages by thick mucus and inability to absorb fats

86 Chronic obstructive pulmonary disease occurs in children with cystic fibrosis because of the inability of the lungs to
1. Exchange oxygen and carbon dioxide in the alveoli
2. Remove thick mucus, causing hyperaeration of alveoli and emphysema
3. Resist bacterial growth in lower lung segments
4. Receive unoxygenated blood via the pulmonary arteries

87 The respiratory and physical therapy teams instruct the Gatlins in chest physiotherapy. The instruction would include how to perform
1. Chest vibration, percussion, and postural drainage
2. Endotracheal intubation and nasal suctioning
3. Passive range of motion exercises, postural drainage, and home humidification
4. Postural drainage, active range of motion exercises, and the setting up of a mist tent at home

88 Following treatment with pancreatic enzymes, Harry would be on a diet
1. High in protein and low to moderate in fat, with liberal amounts of salt
2. High in residue, with vitamin supplements and no fat
3. Low in residue, high in fat, and high in calories
4. Moderate in fat and protein and high in salt, with vitamin supplements

89 Harry is ordered to receive Viokase, a pancreatic enzyme replacement. Harry is to receive the Viokase
1. 30 minutes after meals and snacks
2. 30 minutes before meals and snacks
3. Once a day in the early morning hours
4. At bedtime every other night

90 Mrs. Gatlin would be instructed to protect Harry in the summer from
1. Otitis media infections from swimming in public pools
2. Overheating and salt depletion
3. Sunburn and dehydration
4. Children with influenza and other communicable diseases

91 While Harry is under a mist tent, you would be sure to
1. Regulate flow meter to administer a high concentration of oxygen
2. Have the tent edges secured to prevent air leakage
3. Keep Harry dry and comfortable while checking his respiratory status frequently
4. Keep the air cool and regulated to deliver large water droplets

92 While caring for children with a chronic disease, the parents are encouraged to
1. Deal with their feelings of guilt and to forget about death of the child
2. Permit the child to have a home environment that encourages free rein and limitless activity
3. Provide the child with objects that stimulate play and development of self-esteem
4. Promote normal growth and development and the child's self-image

93 At the age of 3 years, Harry has developed obstructive emphysema. In patients with chronic obstructive pulmonary disease, the physiologic stimulation to breathe is the
1. Concentration of oxygen in the blood
2. Hormonal levels affecting the hypothalmus
3. Autonomic nerve stimulation of the diaphragm
4. Concentration of carbon dioxide in the blood

94 Harry is seen by the pediatrician for a slight fever, skin macules and papules, and rhinitis. The pediatrician tells Mrs. Gatlin that Harry has the chickenpox. Chickenpox is communicable as long as
1. Harry has a fever
2. Vesicles are "weeping"
3. Skin rash is present
4. Rhinitis is present

95 Initially Mrs. Gatlin thought Harry has red measles. Rubeola can be differentiated from rubella by the
1. Number of days the rash is present
2. Characteristic color and formation of the rash
3. Presence of Koplik's spots on the buccal mucosa
4. Evidence of muscular weakness

96 By the age of 12 months, Harry would have received the following immunizations
1. Measles, rubella, and mumps
2. Pertussis, measles, and polio vaccine
3. Diphtheria, mumps, and pertussis
4. Diphtheria, tetanus, pertussis, and trivalent oral polio vaccine

97 The most common GI complication of cystic fibrosis is
1. Rectal prolapse
2. Diverticulitis
3. Hirschsprung's disease
4. Chronic diarrhea

98 Caring for the child with cystic fibrosis involves a team approach. Parents are encouraged to
1. Refrain from becoming involved in the technical aspects of care
2. Convert one room in their home to a hospital-type room
3. Participate in care and regimen to be continued at home
4. Seek financial assistance to pay for expenses incurred as a result of the illness

99 By the age of 8 years, Harry is taught to
1. Position himself for chest physiotherapy
2. Cook the special foods needed in his diet
3. Protect himself from communicable diseases
4. Administer self-injections of pancreatic enzymes

100 Harry is again admitted to the hospital for an acute pulmonary infection. Following admission, you would
1. Explain hospital routines to Harry
2. Limit Harry's activities and behaviors according to his age
3. Allow Harry to make choices about his foods and bath time
4. Assess and compare Harry's growth and development with the last admission's data

101 When Harry's condition improves, you instruct him in good dental, physical, and general health habits. Your action is based on the understanding that schoolchildren
1. Have poor health habits because of peer pressures
2. Are interested in their physical appearance
3. Are very active and take little time to care for themselves
4. Prefer to learn from nonfamily adult role models

Situation: Bill Jones, 14 years old, dived into a shallow pond while on a camping expedition. Friends rescued him from drowning when they saw he was in difficulty. Questions 102 through 121 refer to this situation.

102 When the emergency team arrived, they placed Bill on a stretcher, being especially careful *not* to
1. Move extremities unnecessarily
2. Flex his head
3. Put pressure on the diaphragm
4. Strap him to the stretcher too tightly

103 Diagnosis of spinal cord injury is most often done as soon as possible by x-ray studies on arrival at the hospital. The reason for this is to
1. Detect the presence of edema around the cord
2. Lessen movement of the spinal column at a critical period
3. Detect spinal shock
4. Check for hemorrhage into the spinal activity

104 The most critical level for a spinal cord injury to occur is at the
1. Sacral level
2. Cervical level
3. Lumbar level
4. Thoracic level

105 Following upper cervical cord injury, the patient almost always requires immediate
1. Relief from excruciating pain
2. Respiratory assistance
3. Crisis intervention
4. Immobilization

106 A common type of stabilization maneuver in such injuries is
1. Steinmann's pins
2. Crutchfield tongs
3. Kirschner wires
4. Harrington rod

107 You must take care that skeletal traction is being put to its intended use. Which of the following actions is appropriate?
1. Elevate the head of the bed
2. Place sandbags above the patient's shoulders
3. Make certain that weights barely touch the floor
4. Allow for rest by releasing traction periodically

108 When first feeding patients in hyperextension who are lying on their back, you should
1. Use suction on the patients first
2. Offer sips of liquid to prepare them for solid food
3. Raise the head of the bed to facilitate swallowing
4. Offer soft food

109 The patient who is immobilized because of spinal cord injuries should have a diet high in
1. Calories
2. Carbohydrates
3. Fats
4. Proteins

110 The best means of preventing urinary infection is
1. High fluid intake and clean intermittent catheterizations
2. High fluid intake and continuous bladder irrigations
3. Lower fluid intake and indwelling catheterizations
4. Lower fluid intake and continuous bladder irrigations

111 Which liquid would be *less* apt to cause the formation of urinary calculi?
1. Cranberry juice
2. Coffee
3. Milk
4. Tomato juice

112 Regardless of the level of the injury, the patient must begin early mobilization. This can begin with
1. Active or passive turning movements and range of motion exercises
2. Wheelchair or bracing exercises
3. Resistive exercises
4. Turning every hour

113 Prevention of respiratory complications can be accomplished by
(A) Encouraging frequent deep breathing
(B) Frequent turning and positioning
(C) Use of incentive spirometers
(D) Coughing (if not contraindicated by physician)
1. A, B, and C
2. A and B
3. B, C, and D
4. A, B, C, and D

114 Long-term nursing measures for the patient with a cervical cord injury include
1. Meticulous skin care
2. Weekly exercise programs
3. Taking vital signs every 2 hours
4. Daily catheter care

115 Rehabilitation depends on which of the following factors?
(A) Extent and level of the cord injury
(B) Age
(C) Emotional factors
(D) Sex
1. A, B, and C
2. A, C, and D
3. A and C
4. A, B, C, and D

116 Psychologically, the patient experiencing a spinal cord injury has a loss that he or she mourns. It is not uncommon for the patient to experience shock, denial, anger, and depression before adjustment. One morning as you enter Bill's room, you note that he is crying. He turns his head away from you and says, "Get out, leave me alone! I don't need anybody!" Your initial response might be
1. "Okay, Bill, cut this out. You're just feeling sorry for yourself."
2. "Sure, Bill. But I'll be back in a few minutes."
3. "Would you like to talk, Bill?"
4. "I'll give you something to calm you down."

117 A sudden extreme elevation in blood pressure, a throbbing headache, nasal stuffiness, sweating and flushing, and chills and pallor in the spinal cord–injured patient are indicative of a(n)
1. Urinary tract infection
2. Autonomic dysreflexia
3. Transient ischemic attack
4. Septicemia

118 An action by which you could quickly lower the blood pressure would be to
1. Get the patient to a sitting position
2. Call the physician
3. Administer oxygen
4. Put the patient in Trendelenburg's position

119 Which of the following symptoms would alert you to possible spinal cord compression?
1. Severe headaches
2. Changes in motion or sensation of the extremities
3. Unconsciousness
4. Convulsions

120 A drug used frequently in the management of head or neck injuries is
1. Solu-Medrol
2. Decadron
3. Diamox
4. Diuril

121 Patients often have a great deal of pain with some spinal cord injuries. Narcotics are contraindicated for long-term use, however, because of the possibility of
1. Development of respiratory complications
2. Addiction
3. Abscesses from frequent injections
4. Development of circulatory complications

SAMPLE EXAMINATION 4

This examination contains several paragraphs concerning patients/clients. Following each such paragraph is a series of questions concerning the patient and the situation described in that paragraph. Read each situation carefully. Read each question carefully, and consider all possible answers. When you have decided which answer is **best,** blacken the corresponding space on the answer sheet. There is only **one** best answer for each question.

Situation: Mrs. Flynn is admitted to your unit with a diagnosis of a uterine tumor. She states that she has been tired and depressed in the last 8 or 9 months and has had painful menstruation and a heavy flow. Mrs. Flynn is 33 years old and tells you that she is concerned that this tumor may prevent her from having more children. Question 1 through 10 refer to this situation.

1 Mrs. Flynn's laboratory reports show a hemoglobin level of 9.8. This is most likely associated with
1. Severe dysmenorrhea
2. Poor dietary habits
3. Excessive menstrual flow
4. Lower abdominal pain and stress

Mrs. Flynn's physician tells you that he suspects a malignancy and that he has told Mrs. Flynn that a total abdominal hysterectomy will be necessary.

2 When you enter Mrs. Flynn's room she is sitting on the bed crying. "I won't let him do it," she mutters between sobs. It would be best for you to
1. Leave the room and come back in a few hours
2. Call her husband and tell him his wife needs his support
3. Explain to her the severe consequences of such a decision
4. Sit beside her and hold her hand

3 You may best reduce Mrs. Flynn's preoperative anxiety by
1. Instructing her in coughing and deep breathing
2. Explaining the purpose and administration of preoperative treatments
3. Suggesting she begin to investigate adoption agencies with her husband
4. Explaining the purpose and possible complications of her planned surgery

4 Following her surgery, you may best assess Mrs. Flynn for a possible hemorrhage by
1. Monitoring vital signs closely
2. Changing the dressing to note bleeding
3. Observing perineal pads for bleeding
4. Observing skin color and temperature

5 If Mrs. Flynn had a vaginal hysterectomy rather than an abdominal approach, you would observe her closely for which common problem?
1. Hemorrhage
2. Atelectasis
3. Urinary retention
4. Paralytic ileus

6 Following the total abdominal hysterectomy, Mrs. Flynn is susceptible to the development of thrombophlebitis. You may best help prevent this by
1. Making certain the knee gatch is down
2. Encouraging active leg exercises and ambulation
3. Encouraging increased fluid intake
4. Having her turn, cough, and deep breathe every 2 hours

7 Mrs. Flynn is discharged with instructions to return for radiation therapy in 8 weeks. She asks you when it would be alright to douche. The best response would be
1. ''You won't need to douche now as you have no uterus.''
2. ''You should discuss this with your physician.''
3. ''In 6 weeks your wound will be healed, and it should be safe.''
4. ''I don't see any value in douching. The vagina maintains a carefully balanced flora that should not be disturbed.''

8 Mrs. Flynn returns in 2 months for vaginal insertion of a radium implant. She is to have this treatment for 6 days and then will be allowed to return home. Which of the following is true?
1. Radium is less radioactive than other radioactive materials
2. When radium is implanted into a body cavity, the gamma rays will not affect other people near the patient
3. The radium will destroy healthy cells as well as malignant cells
4. Internal radium can selectively destroy disease cells, sparing healthy ones

9 Three things to consider when caring for the patient with a radium implant in terms of protecting one's self from radiation effects are
1. Type of implant, duration, and strength
2. Time, distance, and shielding
3. Distance, contamination, and exposure
4. Type of implant, time, and strength

10 Mrs. Flynn is discharged by her physician. She is concerned about contaminating her friends with radiation. Your response to this would be
1. ''Only persons who touch you or have close contact are susceptible.''
2. ''Your family and friends will receive no harmful effects.''
3. ''It will not be a problem if you limit the time you spend with each person.''
4. ''You may purchase a lightweight shield to wear under clothing to protect others.''

---

11 Mrs. Bart has had endometriosis for 4 years. She has had an increase in severity of symptoms and has been admitted for evaluation. The problem occurring in patients with endometriosis that most often limits the patient's activity is
1. Amenorrhea
2. Severe depression
3. Severe dysmenorrhea
4. Dyspareunia

12 Problems of the patient with endometriosis are a result of
1. Low hormone levels
2. Hormonal influence on seeded endometrium
3. Changes in hormone levels occurring at menopause
4. Previous episodes of venereal disease

13 June Ford is admitted with retroversion and prolapse of the uterus. Treatment that is generally used when the condition is first discovered includes
1. Surgical correction of the prolapse
2. Synthetic oral hormones
3. Placement of a pessary to maintain correction
4. Manual manipulation and placement of a diaphragm

14 Which of the following factors is *not* associated with uterine displacement?
1. Poor posture
2. Congenital malposition of uterus
3. Endometriosis
4. Irregular bowel patterns

15 Following surgical intervention for the patient having a rectocele, you may best reduce pressure on the operative site and promote wound healing by
1. Observing the incision and changing dressings every 8 hours
2. Administering ordered stool softeners and instructing patient not to strain with bowel movements
3. Administering ordered antibiotics and providing perineal care
4. Carefully positioning catheters and observing for fecal contamination of wound

Situation: Tom Robins is admitted to the nephrology unit complaining of fatigue, anorexia, and scanty urinary output. He is accompanied by his wife, who is constantly pacing around the room during her husband's admission interview. Mr. Robins tells you that he was hospitalized last month with streptococcal pneumonia. Mrs. Robins adds that it was a very long and unpleasant experience. Questions 16 through 32 refer to this situation.

16 Mr. Robins's physician tells you that he suspects acute glomerulonephritis to be the source of Mr. Robins's problems. Other findings characteristic of the patient with this diagnosis are
1. Gastrointestinal bleeding and anemia
2. Mild hypertension and generalized edema
3. Dysuria and weight loss
4. Diarrhea and malnutrition

17 Acute glomerulonephritis is primarily the result of
1. An infectious process
2. An inflammatory process
3. An inherited nephron defect
4. Poor medical management of hypertensive disease

18 Although acute glomerulonephritis is commonly seen following an upper respiratory tract infection, the responsible organism is most frequently
1. Herpes simplex
2. *Escherichia coli*
3. Beta-hemolytic streptococci
4. Alpha streptococci

19 Diagnostic tests that indicate the ability of the kidneys to filter out toxic waste products from the body are
1. IV pyelogram and KUB x-ray examination
2. KUB x-ray examination and urinalysis
3. Urine culture and cystoscopy
4. Creatinine clearance and BUN

20 Mr. Robins throws a piece of paper across the room as you enter to check his blood pressure. "Writing down every stupid drop I drink makes no sense! I don't see what this has to do with my getting well," he exclaims. The best response would be
1. "Your doctor wouldn't have ordered it if it weren't important."
2. "Your doctor uses this intake of oral fluids to evaluate needed fluid and electrolyte replacement."
3. Leave the room until his anger subsides
4. "Writing down every drink can be annoying, but your doctor needs this information to evaluate your kidneys' functioning."

21 Which of the following would *not* be a dietary restriction for Mr. Robins?
1. Carbohydrates
2. Sodium
3. Protein
4. Fluids

22 The antiinflammatory agent commonly given to pediatric patients with glomerulonephritis is
1. Butazolidin
2. Prednisone
3. Inderal
4. Acetylsalicylic acid

23 Mr. Robins must be weighed daily. In order to be accurate this should be done
1. Before meals
2. At bedtime only for accuracy
3. At the same time each day
4. In the morning and at night to ensure accuracy

24 Which of these nursing actions known to reduce complications of bed rest would be contraindicated for Mr. Robins?
1. Turn him every 2 hours
2. Encourage fluids
3. Encourage range of motion exercises every 8 hours
4. Massage bony prominences

25 When recording on Mr. Robins's chart at the end of your 8-hour shift, which of the following factors should be reported to the physician immediately?
1. Blood pressure, 140/94
2. A 200-ml urinary output
3. Apical pulse, 94
4. Bilateral dependent edema in feet

26 Mr. Robins's blood pressure continues to increase daily, and he becomes confused and irritable. These problems most likely indicate
1. Increasing renal failure
2. Development of another infection
3. A pending stroke
4. Cardiac failure is imminent

27 The electrolyte commonly retained in patients with renal failure that has toxic effects on the myocardium is
1. Sodium
2. Chloride
3. Phosphorus
4. Potassium

28 Mrs. Robins comes to the desk demanding to see the head nurse. When questioned about her reasons for seeing the head nurse she replies, "It's none of your business!" You would
1. Tell her it might be something that is your business
2. Direct her to the head nurse's office
3. Go to get the head nurse
4. Tell her that you may have a solution to the problem that is obviously upsetting her

29 Mr. Robins is being prepared to start routine hemodialysis. This means
1. His prognosis for survival is poor and his wife should be prepared
2. An artificial kidney machine will be used to cleanse his blood
3. A trocar will be inserted into his abdomen for peritoneal dialysis
4. His medical problems will soon be resolved

30 Skin care is of particular importance to Mr. Robins because of the following factor associated with renal failure
1. Elevation of BUN
2. Prolonged bed rest for dialysis patients
3. Presence of uremic frost
4. Proteinuria and hematuria

31 The dialysis patient will be most likely to follow ordered diet and treatments if
1. The nurse explains them well
2. They can be adapted to the patient's daily living patterns
3. A family member can monitor the patient's behavior and correct errors
4. The patient can correctly repeat all directions

32 You may best help prevent renal failure in patients by
1. Encouraging less use of salt
2. Using an aseptic technique in catheter insertion and management
3. Accurately monitoring vital signs on all patients
4. Monitoring weight daily

---

33 Malignant tumors of the urinary tract are frequently characterized by the presence of
1. Proteinuria
2. Painless hematuria
3. Hypertension
4. Arteriosclerosis

34 Mr. Cook has returned to his room from recovery following a left nephrectomy. In order to prevent atelectasis, often associated with flank incisions, it would be most helpful to
1. Splint the diaphragm with a pillow
2. Administer his pain medication before he coughes and deep breathes
3. Change saturated dressings frequently
4. Clamp the nephrostomy tube when he is coughing and deep breathing

35 For a patient having a pyelolithotomy the critical observation to report to the physician postoperatively would be
1. A large amount of pink drainage from the nephrostomy tube
2. Diaphoresis; blood pressure, 90/60; phosphorus, 110
3. Chest pain on deep inspiration
4. Abdominal distention

Situation: Lisa Newby is a gravida 1, para 0, admitted to the labor unit in beginning labor. She is accompanied by her husband who appears to be very excited about the upcoming delivery. He tells you that they have been attending Lamaze classes in preparation for childbirth. Questions 36 through 70 refer to this situation.

36 Mrs. Newby tells you that her EDC is January 5. This means that this is
1. The first day of her last menstrual period
2. Her expected delivery date
3. The date her pregnancy was confirmed by her physician
4. The day her labor will begin

37 Mrs. Newby's presumptive signs of pregnancy most likely included
1. Urinary frequency, Chadwick's sign, and quickening
2. Fatigue, positive Grav-index, and nausea and vomiting
3. Amenorrhea, fatigue, and urinary frequency
4. Chadwick's sign, breast enlargement, and fetal movement felt by an examiner

38 Mrs. Newby probably first felt her fetus move during which month of pregnancy?
1. Third
2. Fourth
3. Fifth
4. Sixth

39 A recent trend in parent-child nursing that has benefited all expectant families, including the Newbys, is
1. Improved quality and availability of prenatal care
2. Having the father present in labor and delivery
3. The use of birthing rooms in most hospitals
4. The increased knowledge and use of antibiotics

40 During their childbirth classes the Newbys probably learned that the fetus is fully developed in the
1. Third month
2. Fourth month
3. Fifth month
4. Sixth month

41 Mrs. Newby's pregnancy could have been positively confirmed by
1. A palpable enlargement in uterine size and shape
2. A positive Grav-index test
3. Fetal heart tones heard by examiner
4. Amenorrhea for 2 months

42 Tests routinely performed on expectant mothers on their initial prenatal visit include all of the following *except*
1. Hemoglobin and hematocrit
2. Abdominal ultrasound
3. Maternal blood type and Rh factor
4. Urinalysis

43 During her pregnancy, Mrs. Newby's weight was carefully monitored. The maximal weight gain usually recommended for an entire pregnancy is
1. 15 pounds
2. 20 pounds
3. 25 pounds
4. 30 pounds

44 During the first trimester of her pregnancy Mrs. Newby most likely would have found nausea and vomiting best controlled by
1. Moderate exercise and Bendectin
2. Plenty of fluids and a well-fitting girdle
3. Increasing bulk in her diet and restricting salt
4. Rest periods and a high-carbohydrate diet

45 Mrs. Newby's physician informs you that she is dilated 3 cm and that the fetus is in cephalic presentation. This means that the
1. Cervix is 3 cm thick and the head of the fetus is high in the pelvis
2. Fetal head is against the cervix and the cervix is thinned
3. Cervix has opened 3 cm and the fetal head will present first
4. Fetal head is 3 cm above the ischial spines of the pelvis

46 True labor is best characterized by which of the following?
1. Braxton Hicks' contractions and a pinkish vaginal discharge
2. Regular, forceful contractions and cervical dilation
3. Spontaneous rupture of the amniotic membrane and abdominal pain
4. Descent of the presenting part into the pelvis

47 As this is Mrs. Newby's first labor, the infant will be delivered in approximately
1. 14 hours
2. 16 hours
3. 18 hours
4. 20 hours

48 Mrs. Newby is having contractions 2 minutes apart, of 45 seconds duration, and of moderate intensity. Fetal heart tones at this time should be monitored
1. During contractions
2. Simultaneously with the mother's vital signs
3. Between contractions, every 30 minutes
4. Immediately following each contraction

49 Mrs. Newby's fetal heart tone rate is 150. This rate is
1. High, and oxygen should be administered to her by mask
2. Within normal limits
3. High, and her physician should be notified
4. Expected during contractions but should decrease afterward

50 Mr. Newby tells you that he has learned how to count fetal heart tones in childbirth classes, and he will record them for you on the labor record. Your best response would be to
1. Provide him with paper to record FHTs and check his accuracy at intervals
2. Tell him that this is your job and would only increase his anxiety about the infant's condition
3. Explain that you must monitor the FHTs and ask him to assist in timing contractions
4. Explain that childbirth classes don't teach you everything you need to know about monitoring FHTs

51 Mrs. Newby's physician informs you that she is completely dilated and effaced. The fetal heart tones and maternal vital signs are within safe limits. Mrs. Newby says she feels the urge to push with contractions. The most important nursing action to perform at this time is to
1. Prepare the delivery room and equipment
2. Increase frequency of monitoring fetal heart tones and maternal vital signs
3. Place Mrs. Newby's legs in stirrups and apply wrist restraints
4. Assist the physician to gown and glove

52 Accompanied to the delivery room by her husband, Mrs. Newby delivers a female infant with an Apgar rating of 9 at 1 minute after birth. The infant's identity is legally recorded by
1. Placing ID bracelets on mother and infant
2. Attaching laboratory slips of the mother to the infant's record to verify blood type
3. The signature of the R.N. and physician on the ID sheet
4. Obtaining the infant's footprints and the mother's fingerprint on the delivery record

53 Mrs. Newby's labor is complete when the
1. Infant is delivered
2. Cord is cut
3. Placenta is delivered
4. Uterus is involuted

54 The infant is taken to the nursery, and Mrs. Newby's legs are removed from the stirrups. Her physician had performed a midline episiotomy to facilitate a safe delivery. The perineum is cleansed, and a pad is applied. When checking Mrs. Newby you note that the fundus is boggy and soft. The nursing action of critical importance at this time is to
1. Notify the R.N. immediately
2. Check the perineum for vaginal bleeding
3. Check her blood pressure and pulse
4. Massage the fundus

55 In charting the passage of the neonate's first stool, which of the following descriptions would most likely be accurate?
1. Sticky dark brown stool
2. Blackish green and tarry
3. Soft consistency and greenish brown
4. Reddish brown and sticky

56 In observing baby Newby the first 12 hours after delivery, you note that her eyelids are puffy and red. The appropriate nursing action is to
1. Notify the pediatrician
2. Culture any exudate noted at the inner canthus
3. Gently clean any exudate with warm sterile water
4. Review the labor record to see if any trauma to the head or eyes is noted

57 Baby Newby should be "bubbled" during and after feeding to prevent
1. Regurgitation of feeding
2. Gas pains and colic
3. Pneumonia
4. Pneumaturia

58 Baby Newby is admitted to the newborn nursery in good condition. On assessment, the respirations of the normal neonate will be
1. Regular, 24 to 36 per minute
2. Irregular, 28 to 40 per minute
3. Regular, 30 to 44 per minute
4. Irregular, 32 to 48 per minute

59 Baby Newby has acrocyanosis. This means
1. The skin is reddish, changing to pink
2. Initially her extremities are bluish
3. The skin has a mottled appearance
4. The skin is coated with vernix caseosa

60 When baby Newby's cheek is stroked, she turns her head in the direction of the stroked cheek. This reflex, present at birth, is known as
1. Rooting
2. Moro
3. Tonic neck
4. Sucking

61 Mrs. Newby is breast-feeding her new daughter. She is using the demand feeding method. This means baby Newby will be fed
1. Whenever she cries
2. Approximately every 4 hours
3. At the time and in the amount she wishes
4. Whenever Mrs. Newby's breasts feel full

62 On the second day postpartum Mrs. Newby says that her breasts feel tight and are tender to touch. The correct nursing action in response to this information would be to
1. Offer to feed her baby in the nursery for the next several feedings
2. Notify the physician as this may be a sign of mastitis

3. Apply a breast binder and ice packs to the breasts
4. Tell her that this is probably a result of her milk "coming in" and nursing her baby may provide some relief

63 The third day postpartum Mrs. Newby's lochia is red and of moderate amount. This is known as
1. Lochia rubra
2. Lochia serosa
3. Lochia alba
4. Lochia puerpura

64 Because she is breast-feeding, Mrs. Newby's nutritional requirements will increase. This increase includes
1. An additional 1000 ml of fluids daily and increased protein
2. An additional $^1/_2$ quart of milk and an additional 1000 calories daily
3. Additional vitamin supplements and protein
4. An additional $^1/_2$ quart of milk daily and forced fluids

65 You may best facilitate the return of normal bladder and bowel elimination for Mrs. Newby by
1. Providing perineal care and administering sitz baths as ordered
2. Encouraging ambulation and a well-balanced diet
3. Obtaining orders for simple catheterization PRN and a cathartic PRN
4. Recording intake and output accurately and instructing Mrs. Newby in perineal care

66 Mrs. Newby has decided to try "rooming-in." This means that
1. Mr. Newby will be allowed to stay in the room and assist in caring for his new daughter
2. A private duty nurse will care for Mrs. Newby for the first few days
3. Mrs. Newby will be sharing her room with another postpartum mother who is more experienced in infant care
4. Mrs. Newby's infant will be at her bedside so that she may care for her as she is able and desires to do so

67 The newborn is considered to be premature when he or she
1. Is large for gestational age
2. Has a gestational age of 37 weeks or less
3. Weighs under 6 pounds at birth
4. Has a deficiency of surfactant in alveolar spaces

68 The most important sign of possible hemolytic disease of the newborn that is noted on assessment by the nurse is
1. Difficult grunting respirations
2. Appearance of jaundice at birth or soon after
3. Persistent watery or frequent greenish stools
4. Lethargy or hyperirritability

69 When assessing the premature newborn, which of the following characteristics would you *not* expect to see?
1. Shallow irregular respirations
2. Thin transparent skin
3. Flaccid movements and poor muscle tone
4. Thick eyelashes and eyebrows

70 Oxygen therapy for the newborn must be administered with caution to prevent
1. Ophthalmia neonatorum
2. ABO incompatibility
3. Respiratory distress syndrome
4. Retrolental fibroplasia

Situation: Mr. B.O. Cowper, a 60-year-old white man, has been admitted to the hospital complaining of burning on urination, hesitancy, and nocturia. He says that he "just hasn't felt like doing anything lately." Questions 71 through 90 refer to this situation.

71 You understand that the problem of burning on urination is most often associated with
1. Tumors of the urinary tract
2. Infections of the urinary tract
3. The aging process
4. Venereal diseases

72 You would expect the following diagnostic tests to be ordered initially
1. Renal arteriogram and urinalysis
2. X-ray examination of kidneys, ureter, and bladder
3. BUN and creatinine
4. Urinalysis and culture and sensitivity

73 Mr. Cowper develops nausea and vomiting the evening of admission. You understand that this is probably caused by
1. His state of dehydration
2. Renointestinal reflexes and anatomic proximity
3. The severity of his abdominal pain
4. Embarrassment and his anxiety over his diagnosis

74 The most common causative organism of infections of the urinary tract is
1. *Escherichia coli*
2. Beta-hemolytic *Streptoccocus*
3. *Pneumoccocus*
4. *Monilia*

75 Treatments ordered for care of the patient with a urinary tract infection include
1. Cold applications to the perineum and encouraging ambulation
2. Administering Demerol and maintaining bed rest
3. Administering pyridium and giving sitz baths three times a day
4. Performing perineal care and applying scrotal support

Mr. Cowper's fatigue increases, and he develops headaches and anorexia. His urine culture reveals a colony count of 200,000, *Escherichia coli*. His physician orders ampicillin, 500 mg four times a day; strict bed rest; 1000 ml D_5W every 8 hours; and IVP in AM.

76 You understand that Mr. Cowper may have developed pyelonephritis. Pyelonephritis may be caused by
1. An obstruction of urinary drainage
2. An antigen-antibody reaction
3. Dehydration
4. Associated respiratory tract infections

77 In preparing Mr. Cowper for his intravenous pyelogram in the morning, it would be *most* important to
1. Force fluids to tolerance
2. Determine if he has an allergy to shellfish or iodine
3. Have him sign an operative permit
4. Administer ordered Oragrafin

78 In assisting the physician to determine adequate renal function you would perform the following nursing action
1. Force fluids to 3000 ml daily
2. Encourage ambulation
3. Monitor intake and output
4. Monitor IV fluid intake

79 Your assessment that Mr. Cowper is unlikely to develop glomerulonephritis is based on the understanding that
1. He is elderly and retired
2. He is a nonsmoker
3. He has no history of strep throat
4. He has had frequent urinary tract infections

Mr. Cowper's physician tells you that Mr. Cowper probably has benign prostatic hypertrophy. You are instructed to prepare Mr. Cowper for a cystoscopic examination.

80 Cystoscopic examination will allow the physician to
1. Identify causative organisms and prescribe appropriate antibiotic therapy
2. Inspect the urethra, bladder, and lower ureters
3. Resolve all of Mr. Cowper's present problems
4. Reduce the incidence of Mr. Cowper's infections

81 You know that benign prostatic hypertrophy occurs most often in the
1. Adolescent male
2. Second and third decades of life
3. Third and fourth decades of life
4. Fourth and fifth decades of life

Mr. Cowper is scheduled for a transurethral prostatectomy in the morning. The physician orders an operative permit for transurethral prostatectomy, soapsuds enemas until clear in the morning, and no foods by mouth past midnight. Preoperative medication includes Demerol, 50 mg IM, and atropine, 0.4 mg IM, on call to operating room. Dalmane, 30 mg PO h.s., is also prescribed.

82 When Mr. Cowper is asked to sign his operative permit he becomes fidgity and hesitant. When asked why he is reluctant to sign, he states, "I've heard that this surgery can make you impotent, and I'm not so sure it's worth the risk." Your best response is
1. "Your doctor wouldn't operate if it weren't an absolute necessity."
2. "Impotence is rare, and most people adjust."
3. "Have you discussed this with your doctor?"
4. "Your wife will understand that the surgery is necessary, and she will adjust."

83 After signing the operative permit Mr. Cowper is medicated for sleep. When the orderly enters his room to administer the enemas as ordered, Mr. Cowper refuses, saying he has "been up most of the night with diarrhea." Your initial nursing action would be to
1. Check the nurses' notes and question Mr. Cowper regarding his diarrhea
2. Call the operating room and cancel surgery
3. Notify the physician immediately
4. Reassure Mr. Cowper that the enemas are necessary and will not affect his surgical success

Mr. Cowper has his surgery as scheduled. He returns to the nursing unit with an IV in progress, a three-way Foley catheter to bedside drainage, and 2000-ml normal saline genitourinary irrigant flowing at 30 gtts per minute.

84 Mr. Cowper complains of lower abdominal pain and a grabbing sensation in his lower abdomen. Your initial nursing action would be to
1. Increase the flow of the GU irrigant
2. Notify the physician
3. Check the catheter tubing for kinks
4. Take his vital signs

85 The drainage from Mr. Cowper's Foley is dark red and contains numerous clots. You would
1. Milk the catheter tubing
2. Notify the physician
3. Check the tubing for kinks
4. Stop the GU irrigant immediately

86 In order to promote wound healing and detect infection it would be most important to
1. Change dressings frequently
2. Observe Mr. Cowper's bladder for distention
3. Monitor his temperature every 4 hours
4. Accurately describe Foley drainage

87 For relief from bladder spasms not caused by catheter obstruction, you would expect to administer the following medication
1. Demerol
2. Pro-Banthine
3. Phenergan
4. Thorazine

88 Which of the following actions would be contraindicated in caring for Mr. Cowper postoperatively?
1. Turning him side to side every 2 hours
2. Administering narcotics
3. Having him ambulate with assistance
4. Taking rectal temperatures

89 The restoration of bladder tone and continence can be promoted by
1. Limiting fluid intake
2. Performing perineal exercises
3. Avoiding sexual activity
4. Taking Pyridium three times a day

90 You review the activities prescribed for Mr. Cowper after his discharge. You know that he has learned how to care for his problems when he is able to
1. Repeat all your instructions verbally
2. Perform hygienic functions without assistance
3. Demonstrate exercises and self-care activities
4. Follow all directions given by his wife

Situation: Mr. Alt is admitted to the hospital with a diagnosis of hepatitis A. His sclera have been jaundiced for 4 days, and he says he has not "felt like eating or doing anything." Mr. Alt is placed on enteric isolation. Questions 91 through 100 refer to this situation.

91 According to the known incubation period for hepatitis A, Mr. Alt may have been exposed to the viral organism
1. 1 week ago
2. 4 weeks ago
3. 2 months ago
4. 5 months ago

92 Which of the following mechanisms of transmission is least likely to have been the source of Mr. Alt's illness?
1. Contaminated food
2. Blood transfusion in the past
3. Contaminated water
4. Eating shellfish caught locally

93 Which of the following diagnostic tests would specifically confirm the diagnosis of hepatitis B?
1. Elevated serum bilirubin level
2. Elevated urine urobilinogen level
3. Decreased serum gamma globulin level
4. Presence of Australian antigen in serum

94 In maintaining enteric isolation precautions with Mr. Alt it is most important to
1. Wear a gown and mask while providing nursing care
2. Restrict his visitors to his immediate family
3. Wear gloves when emptying his bedpan and urinal
4. Avoid staying in his room for long periods of time

95 Serum hepatitis B and infectious hepatitis A are different in that
1. Gamma globulin will prevent hepatitis A
2. Isolation is not necessary for hepatitis B
3. The incubation period is longer for hepatitis B
4. Jaundice is more severe with hepatitis A

96 Nursing care for Mr. Alt is primarily centered on
1. Maintaining enteric isolation
2. Maintaining bed rest and adequate nutrition
3. Identifying carriers and administering gamma globulin to family members
4. Providing diversional activities and reducing anxiety

97 Vitamin supplements of primary importance to Mr. Alt at this time are
1. B-complex vitamins
2. A and D vitamins
3. Minerals and iron
4. Vitamin C

98 Mr. Alt's dietary needs (in addition to vitamin supplements) include
1. A low-protein, high-carbohydrate diet and forced fluids
2. A high-protein, high-carbohydrate diet and forced fluids
3. A low-fat, high-calorie, low-protein diet
4. A high-protein, high-carbohydrate diet with fluids restricted

99 Mr. Alt's urine is brownish. This change is caused by
1. An increased hemoglobin level
2. Anorexia and dehydration
3. Vitamin deficiencies
4. The presence of bilirubin

100 When assessing Mr. Alt for signs of hepatic coma, which of the following would be characteristic of progression of liver failure?
1. He refuses to eat his evening meal
2. He is having heartburn after eating
3. He cannot remember if he ate any breakfast
4. He tires easily and says he needs an afternoon nap

Situation: This is Sue Park's first pregnancy, and she is admitted to the labor and delivery area with vaginal bleeding and cramplike pain in the lower abdomen. She is 5 months pregnant and has had no problems with her pregnancy until now. Questions 101 through 105 refer to this situation.

101 Mrs. Park's physician informs you that Mrs. Park is threatening to abort. Should an abortion occur, would it be classified as
1. Therapeutic
2. Induced
3. Incomplete
4. Spontaneous

102 Had Mrs. Park elected to have an abortion at this point in her pregnancy, it would be classified as
1. Legal, because it is past the third month
2. Illegal, because it is past the third month
3. Socially unacceptable
4. Legal, according to individual state laws

103 Mrs. Park's blood loss can be best monitored for the physician by which nursing action?
1. Monitoring vital signs every 4 hours
2. Counting used perineal pads
3. Ordering a test for hemoglobin level
4. Monitoring intake and output

104 Mrs. Park is having frequent contractions of moderate intensity. As the contractions increase in strength she tells you she just cannot stand the pain anymore. You would best help Mrs. Park by
1. Slowing down the IV infusion containing Syntocinon
2. Positioning her for comfort
3. Administering ordered Demerol
4. Sitting with her and holding her hand

105 Mrs. Park talks continuously and mentions frequently that she was taking some medication for a sinus infection and had not told this to her gynecologist. You understand that she is
1. Expressing feelings of grief
2. Having feelings of guilt
3. Nervous and needs to chatter awhile
4. Handling her anxiety well

Situation: Mrs. Donna Center is admitted to the labor and delivery area with painless vaginal bleeding. Her baby is due in 1 week. She says she has had some mild contractions throughout the day, but they have been irregular. Questions 106 through 120 refer to this situation.

106 Mrs. Center's physician tells you that he suspects a placenta previa. This means that the placenta
1. Is attached to the lower part of the uterus
2. Is not functioning properly to support the fetus
3. Has separated from the uterine wall prematurely
4. Has stimulated the uterus to contract prematurely

107 Placenta previa is characterized by the following problems
1. Painless vaginal bleeding and boardlike rigidity over the abdomen
2. Vaginal bleeding and fetal distress
3. Severe sudden abdominal pain and shock
4. Hidden or vaginal bleeding and severe abdominal pain

108 The primary difference in problems of patients with placenta previa and abruptio placentae is that
1. Shock is more severe with abruptio placentae
2. Fetal distress occurs less frequently with abruptio placentae

3. Sudden severe abdominal pain occurs with abruptio placentae
4. Bleeding is usually hidden with placenta previa

109 Mrs. Center is scheduled for an emergency cesarean section. Which of the following preoperative orders would you question?
1. Shave and prepare abdomen and perineum
2. Give Demerol, 35 mg, and atropine, 0.4 mg IM, on call to operating room
3. Provide a Fleets enema before preoperative medication
4. Give no foods by mouth; insert nasogastric tube if patient has eaten in last 6 hours and connect to low suction

110 Anesthesia for Mrs. Center will most likely be in the form of
1. A paracervical block
2. Scopolamine
3. Nitrous oxide
4. A pudendal block

111 A major difference in Mrs. Center's care after delivery, as opposed to someone who has a normal spontaneous delivery, will be
1. Observing for vaginal bleeding
2. Monitoring vital signs every 4 hours
3. Having her turn, cough, and deep breathe every 2 hours
4. Observing closely for adequate urinary output

112 Following delivery Mrs. Center will most likely be primarily concerned about her
1. Condition and recovery
2. Infant's condition
3. Husband's condition
4. Future childbearing ability

113 Three days postoperatively Mrs. Center complains of gas pains and a feeling of fullness. It would be most helpful to
1. Administer ordered Demerol, 50 mg IM, PRN pain
2. Obtain an order for a laxative
3. Encourage her to eat fresh fruit and drink gingerale
4. Assist her to ambulate as frequently as tolerated

114 Mrs. Center is 4 days postpartum. Which of the following developments would necessitate notifying the physician?
1. Abdominal tenderness
2. Temperature of 101°F
3. Breast tenderness
4. Lochia serosa

115 The most common organism responsible for the development of puerperal infection is
1. Escherichia coli
2. Staphylococci
3. Pneumococci
4. Enterobacteria

116 Mrs. Center's new son weighed 7 pounds at birth. Four days after birth he weighs 6 pounds, 12 ounces. This weight loss
1. Is excessive
2. Will increase even more before he starts to gain
3. May be indicative of a congenital metabolic defect
4. Is within the acceptable range of physiologic weight loss

117 Mrs. Center asks you why her son did not have a funny elongated head, as her mother told her to expect. You reply,
1. "Your baby was lucky not to have a traumatic delivery."
2. "Sometimes temporary changes occur in the shape of the infant's head as it passes through the birth canal in vaginal deliveries."
3. "Don't be concerned about that. You had a cesarean section."
4. "Your mother is probably remembering an unpleasant situation from her past that has nothing to do with your baby."

118 Parent-infant bonding is best facilitated by the nurse who
1. Teaches childbirth preparation classes
2. Provides skilled nursing care to the newborn and mother
3. Encourages parents to hold their infant and participate in care
4. Reads current nursing journals to stay up to date

119 A medication frequently used to stimulate and regulate uterine activity of the labor patient is known as
1. Deladumone
2. Methergine
3. Magnesium sulfate
4. Syntocinon

120 The newborn receives an injection in the delivery room to help prevent hemorrhage until the liver is able to form prothrombin. This medication is
1. AquaMephyton
2. Protamine sulfate
3. Silver nitrate, 1%
4. Thrombin

ANSWERS AND RATIONALES

REVIEW QUESTIONS

Introduction

1. (4)
2. (2)
3. (2)
4. (4)
5. (4)
6. (3)
7. (4)
8. (1)
9. (1)
10. (4)

The practical nurse

1. (1)
2. (4)
3. (4)
4. (3)
5. (3)
6. (1)
7. (3)
8. (1)
9. (2)
10. (4)
11. (4)
12. (4)
13. (1)
14. (1)
15. (3)
16. (3)
17. (2)
18. (1)
19. (3)
20. (1)
21. (3)
22. (2)
23. (1)
24. (4)
25. (3)
26. (4)
27. (3)
28. (3)
29. (2)
30. (1)
31. (1)
32. (3)
33. (2)
34. (4)
35. (1)

Basic science

1. (2)
2. (4)
3. (1)
4. (4)
5. (4)
6. (1)
7. (4)
8. (2)
9. (3)
10. (4)
11. (2)
12. (4)
13. (2)
14. (1)
15. (1)
16. (3)
17. (1)
18. (3)
19. (4)
20. (1)
21. (3)
22. (4)
23. (3)
24. (3)
25. (3)
26. (2)
27. (1)
28. (2)
29. (2)
30. (3)
31. (2)
32. (1)
33. (2)
34. (4)
35. (3)
36. (4)
37. (3)
38. (4)
39. (2)
40. (2)
41. (4)
42. (3)
43. (1)
44. (4)
45. (1)
46. (2)
47. (1)
48. (1)
49. (4)
50. (2)
51. (1)
52. (4)
53. (3)
54. (4)
55. (4)
56. (3)
57. (2)
58. (2)
59. (3)
60. (4)
61. (2)
62. (4)
63. (3)
64. (2)
65. (1)
66. (1)
67. (1)
68. (4)
69. (4)
70. (4)
71. (2)
72. (3)
73. (2)
74. (1)
75. (4)
76. (1)
77. (3)
78. (4)
79. (4)
80. (4)
81. (2)
82. (4)
83. (2)
84. (2)
85. (3)
86. (2)
87. (4)
88. (2)
89. (1)
90. (1)
91. (4)
92. (2)
93. (2)
94. (4)
95. (1)
96. (3)
97. (4)
98. (1)
99. (2)
100. (2)
101. (4)
102. (1)
103. (2)
104. (3)
105. (4)
106. (2)
107. (2)
108. (4)
109. (4)
110. (1)
111. (3)
112. (4)
113. (3)
114. (4)
115. (3)
116. (3)
117. (2)
118. (3)
119. (4)
120. (2)
121. (1)
122. (4)
123. (4)
124. (2)
125. (1)
126. (1)
127. (2)
128. (3)
129. (3)
130. (3)
131. (1)
132. (4)
133. (3)
134. (1)
135. (4)
136. (2)
137. (1)
138. (4)
139. (1)
140. (4)
141. (4)
142. (2)
143. (4)
144. (3)
145. (2)
146. (2)
147. (3)
148. (4)
149. (1)
150. (3)
151. (1)
152. (4)
153. (3)
154. (2)

Fundamentals of nursing

1. (2)
2. (1)
3. (1)
4. (2)
5. (4)
6. (3)
7. (4)
8. (2)
9. (1)
10. (4)
11. (1)
12. (3)
13. (2)
14. (1)
15. (4)
16. (4)
17. (1)
18. (1)
19. (1)
20. (1)
21. (2)
22. (3)
23. (4)
24. (1)
25. (2)
26. (1)
27. (2)
28. (4)
29. (1)
30. (3)
31. (2)
32. (2)
33. (3)
34. (2)
35. (1)
36. (3)
37. (1)
38. (3)
39. (2)
40. (3)
41. (2)
42. (2)
43. (1)
44. (2)
45. (3)
46. (4)
47. (1)
48. (3)
49. (2)
50. (1)
51. (2)
52. (1)
53. (3)
54. (3)
55. (4)
56. (2)
57. (3)
58. (2)
59. (4)
60. (3)
61. (1)
62. (1)
63. (2)
64. (1)
65. (1)
66. (4)
67. (2)
68. (2)
69. (2)
70. (3)
71. (2)
72. (4)
73. (1)
74. (2)
75. (1)
76. (2)
77. (3)
78. (2)
79. (4)
80. (1)
81. (1)
82. (4)
83. (1)
84. (3)
85. (2)
86. (2)
87. (1)
88. (4)
89. (2)
90. (4)
91. (3)
92. (1)
93. (1)
94. (2)
95. (1)
96. (2)
97. (4)
98. (1)
99. (3)
100. (3)

Nursing the adult patient

1. (4)
2. (2)
3. (3)
4. (1)
5. (1)
6. (2)
7. (3)
8. (2)
9. (2)
10. (2)
11. (1)
12. (2)
13. (1)
14. (4)
15. (1)
16. (4)
92. (2)
93. (2)
94. (3)
95. (2)
96. (2)
97. (3)
98. (3)
99. (1)
100. (2)
101. (1)
102. (4)
103. (3)
104. (2)
105. (1)
106. (2)
107. (4)
183. (4)
184. (1)
185. (3)
186. (2)
187. (4)
188. (1)
189. (1)
190. (4)
191. (3)
192. (2)
193. (1)
194. (4)
195. (3)
196. (3)
197. (3)
198. (2)

17. (2)
18. (2)
19. (1)
20. (3)
21. (2)
22. (2)
23. (1)
24. (2)
25. (1)
26. (2)
27. (4)
28. (1)
29. (4)
30. (3)
31. (1)
32. (3)
33. (1)
34. (3)
35. (4)
36. (2)
37. (2)
38. (3)
39. (1)
40. (2)
41. (2)
42. (4)
43. (4)
44. (3)
45. (1)
46. (3)
47. (2)
48. (1)
49. (1)
50. (2)
51. (1)
52. (1)
53. (2)
54. (1)
55. (4)
56. (3)
57. (4)
58. (1)
59. (3)
60. (3)
61. (2)
62. (3)
63. (2)
64. (4)
65. (1)
66. (2)
67. (4)
68. (3)
69. (1)
70. (4)
71. (2)
72. (4)
73. (3)
74. (4)
75. (3)
76. (3)
77. (1)
78. (3)
79. (1)
80. (3)
81. (3)
82. (4)
83. (2)
84. (4)
85. (1)
86. (1)
87. (4)
88. (4)
89. (1)
90. (1)
91. (3)
108. (3)
109. (1)
110. (1)
111. (2)
112. (3)
113. (3)
114. (3)
115. (2)
116. (1)
117. (1)
118. (2)
119. (4)
120. (4)
121. (3)
122. (3)
123. (3)
124. (3)
125. (2)
126. (1)
127. (4)
128. (2)
129. (3)
130. (2)
131. (1)
132. (1)
133. (2)
134. (1)
135. (3)
136. (4)
137. (3)
138. (3)
139. (1)
140. (2)
141. (2)
142. (1)
143. (3)
144. (3)
145. (1)
146. (2)
147. (3)
148. (4)
149. (4)
150. (2)
151. (4)
152. (2)
153. (2)
154. (1)
155. (4)
156. (3)
157. (4)
158. (2)
159. (2)
160. (3)
161. (3)
162. (1)
163. (3)
164. (3)
165. (1)
166. (1)
167. (3)
168. (3)
169. (3)
170. (4)
171. (3)
172. (4)
173. (1)
174. (2)
175. (2)
176. (3)
177. (1)
178. (2)
179. (3)
180. (2)
181. (3)
182. (3)
199. (4)
200. (3)
201. (4)
202. (1)
203. (2)
204. (1)
205. (2)
206. (2)
207. (3)
208. (2)
209. (3)
210. (1)
211. (1)
212. (4)
213. (2)
214. (3)
215. (2)
216. (4)
217. (1)
218. (1)
219. (3)
220. (2)
221. (3)
222. (4)
223. (4)
224. (4)
225. (3)
226. (3)
227. (4)
228. (1)
229. (4)
230. (4)
231. (4)
232. (3)
233. (4)
234. (1)
235. (4)
236. (3)
237. (4)
238. (3)
239. (3)
240. (3)
241. (1)
242. (4)
243. (4)
244. (2)
245. (3)
246. (4)
247. (3)
248. (4)
249. (1)
250. (1)
251. (4)
252. (1)
253. (3)
254. (4)
255. (2)
256. (4)
257. (3)
258. (2)
259. (4)
260. (3)
261. (3)
262. (3)
263. (1)
264. (3)
265. (4)
266. (2)
267. (2)
268. (2)
269. (1)
270. (3)
271. (4)
272. (1)

Maternal and child health

1. (2)
2. (1)
3. (3)
4. (4)
5. (1)
6. (3)
7. (4)
8. (4)
9. (3)
10. (1)
11. (2)
12. (2)
13. (3)
14. (2)
15. (4)
16. (1)
17. (4)
18. (1)
19. (3)
20. (2)
21. (1)
22. (3)
23. (3)
24. (3)
25. (4)
26. (1)
27. (2)
28. (2)
29. (3)
30. (3)
31. (4)
51. (4)
52. (2)
53. (1)
54. (4)
55. (2)
56. (3)
57. (4)
58. (3)
59. (4)
60. (2)
61. (3)
62. (4)
63. (4)
64. (2)
65. (2)
66. (3)
67. (1)
68. (4)
69. (2)
70. (1)
71. (1)
72. (2)
73. (2)
74. (4)
75. (3)
76. (3)
77. (2)
78. (4)
79. (2)
80. (2)
81. (1)
100. (2)
101. (4)
102. (3)
103. (4)
104. (1)
105. (3)
106. (3)
107. (1)
108. (3)
109. (4)
110. (1)
111. (1)
112. (3)
113. (3)
114. (3)
115. (4)
116. (2)
117. (1)
118. (4)
119. (1)
120. (3)
121. (2)
122. (3)
123. (2)
124. (4)
125. (1)
126. (2)
127. (1)
128. (4)
129. (3)
130. (2)

32. (3)	82. (3)	131. (3)
33. (2)	83. (2)	132. (4)
34. (1)	84. (4)	133. (4)
35. (3)	85. (4)	134. (1)
36. (3)	86. (1)	135. (3)
37. (2)	87. (4)	136. (2)
38. (3)	88. (4)	137. (2)
39. (3)	89. (2)	138. (2)
40. (2)	90. (4)	139. (2)
41. (3)	91. (1)	140. (2)
42. (1)	92. (2)	141. (4)
43. (2)	93. (1)	142. (2)
44. (3)	94. (3)	143. (2)
45. (4)	95. (3)	144. (2)
46. (3)	96. (2)	145. (3)
47. (1)	97. (4)	146. (2)
48. (3)	98. (3)	147. (4)
49. (4)	99. (2)	148. (1)
50. (1)		

Mental health nursing

1. (4)	19. (3)	37. (4)
2. (4)	20. (3)	38. (1)
3. (3)	21. (1)	39. (2)
4. (4)	22. (3)	40. (1)
5. (4)	23. (1)	41. (3)
6. (2)	24. (4)	42. (4)
7. (4)	25. (2)	43. (4)
8. (4)	26. (2)	44. (3)
9. (3)	27. (2)	45. (4)
10. (1)	28. (2)	46. (3)
11. (2)	29. (2)	47. (3)
12. (4)	30. (2)	48. (2)
13. (4)	31. (2)	49. (4)
14. (2)	32. (3)	50. (2)
15. (4)	33. (2)	51. (3)
16. (3)	34. (2)	52. (2)
17. (2)	35. (3)	53. (2)
18. (3)	36. (2)	

Vocational aspects

1. (3)	16. (3)	31. (3)
2. (2)	17. (2)	32. (3)
3. (3)	18. (3)	33. (2)
4. (3)	19. (4)	34. (1)
5. (1)	20. (4)	35. (1)
6. (3)	21. (1)	36. (3)
7. (2)	22. (1)	37. (4)
8. (2)	23. (3)	38. (2)
9. (4)	24. (3)	39. (2)
10. (1)	25. (4)	40. (1)
11. (3)	26. (4)	41. (2)
12. (4)	27. (4)	42. (2)
13. (4)	28. (1)	43. (1)
14. (2)	29. (2)	44. (1)
15. (2)	30. (4)	45. (2)

SAMPLE EXAMINATION 1

1. (3) Garters and girdles restrict the circulation to lower extremities.
2. (3) Size, location, and character of drainage should be noted on the chart. This provides a reference for future evaluation of wound progress.
3. (2) Trophic change (taut shiny skin, loss of hair) indicates circulation is poor.
4. (1) Assisting Mrs. Lent to use the bedpan to obtain a specimen for admission urinalysis would be appropriate. Since she is also diabetic, checking the urine for sugar and acetone would also be appropriate.
5. (3) Absence of the pedal pulse on the affected leg indicates lack of circulation. FBS of above 120 mg per liter is abnormally high and should be reported to the physician.
6. (4) A bed cradle would prevent the sheets from irritating the injured area. Heel protectors would guard the heels from friction on the sheets, which could lead to breakdown of the heels.
7. (2) Diabetic ketoacidosis is manifested by elevated blood glucose levels; deep, blowing, rapid respirations (Kussmaul's respirations); and excessive protein and fat metabolism, which results in acidosis. Fruity breath odor results when excessive acetones are excreted during respiration.
8. (2) Peak action from NPH insulin is 8 to 12 hours.
9. (2) Purulent drainage indicates the exudative stage of inflammation; coolness of the affected extremity signals increasing circulatory compromise distal to the injury. Temperature elevation is a symptom of systemic infection.
10. (3) Excessive fat metabolism causes changes in the arterial walls (atherosclerosis), causing inability to dilate and constrict, and arteriosclerosis, which is a narrowing of the lumen through which blood must pass to nourish distal tissues.
11. (4) Crying is a normal response. Mrs. Lent needs to vent her grief. Holding her hand is a nonverbal method to communicate understanding and empathy.

12. (1) Postoperatively the stump may be elevated on a pillow for the first 24 hours. Pillows will also be needed to reposition Mrs. Lent comfortably on her side. IV fluids will be ordered to maintain fluid balance and to provide route for medication administration. A tourniquet, as a safety measure, should be in the room in case there is hemorrhage from the stump.
13. (1) Hypotension, tachycardia, and tachypnia, accompanied by a large amount of red (bloody) drainage dependent to the wound, are indicative of shock—an emergency situation requiring prompt attention.
14. (2) Extension of the hip prevents hip flexion contracture.
15. (1) Stressful events such as surgery increase blood glucose levels. Consequently higher dosages of insulin are required.
16. (4) Regular insulin is administered intravenously because it is rapidly acting insulin and is chemically ready for utilization by the body very soon after administration.
17. (3) Overt displays of anger about hospital routines are common in persons going through the grieving process. An accepting, nonjudgmental attitude by the nurse will facilitate resolution of the process.
18. (1) Gluteal setting and straight leg raises will strengthen muscles necessary for walking. Wrapping the stump with elastic bandages encourages a cone shape that prevents prosthetic pressure at the distal point of the stump.
19. (1) Foot care for the diabetic patient is essential because of the vascular changes that occur secondary to diabetes. Mrs. Lent's symptoms preceding the amputation indicate vascular changes have occurred; therefore injury to the feet may result in poor healing.
20. (3) Beets are allowed on the diabetic exchange list. Her question indicates that further explanation of the exchange list is needed. The dietitian is the apppropriate health team member to provide this information.
21. (1) Frequent diarrheic stools result in loss of essential electrolytes, especially potassium.
22. (3) Ulcerative colitis is an inflammation of the mucosa of the large intestine or colon.
23. (2) The diagnosis of ulcerative colitis is confirmed by a lower GI series (barium enema), sigmoidoscopy, and patient history of signs and symptoms.
24. (3) During the acute phase of ulcerative colitis, the patient is encouraged to rest. Diarrhea is prevalent; therefore fluids should be forced to replace lost water.
25. (4) Time, amount, and character of stools should be noted. This information is necessary in assessment of disease progression.
26. (3) Lomotil is an antidiarrheic drug.
27. (1) Normal serum potassium level is 3.5. Symptoms of hypokalemia are muscle weakness and paralysis.
28. (3) Hemoglobin levels of below 10 g indicate anemia or reduction of oxygen-carrying ability of the blood. Symptoms indicative of anemia include tachycardia, tachypnea, weakness, and pallor.
29. (1) Orange juice is considered to be low in fiber.
30. (1) Other foods listed contain a high fiber content and not as much carbohydrate as waffles and syrup. Canadian bacon is broiled and high in protein.
31. (2) Gastric ulceration is a side effect of oral prednisone administration. Frequently, antacids (Maalox) are ordered concurrently.
32. (4) Azulfidine administration causes urine to become red-orange.
33. (3) Hemoglobin and hematocrit are valid laboratory tests to indicate blood loss as might be expected in perforation with bleeding into the peritoneal cavity.
34. (2) Research statistics show that patients with a history of ulcerative colitis are at risk to develop cancer of the colon.
35. (1) Postoperatively the stoma should appear edematous (because of the trauma of surgery) and velvety red (indicating adequate blood supply to the stomal tissue).
36. (3) Ileostomies are openings into the ileum or small intestine. Control at this point is impossible, and the consistency of the contents is always liquid. Liquid is not reabsorbed until the contents reach the large intestine.
37. (4) Potassium chloride is never administered by IV push. This medication is always diluted in a large volume of fluid.
38. (4) Janet's behavior reveals nonacceptance of the ileostomy. You should "open the door" for Janet to discuss her feelings. Then acceptance will be fostered.
39. (2) Constant changing of the bag irritates skin around the stoma. Bags constructed with open ends allow for emptying and thus prevent irritation. Betadine toughens the skin, preventing further breakdown and irritation.
40. (1) Active participation in self-care and planning for the future indicate Janet has accepted the alteration in her body image caused by the ileostomy.
41. (3) In the United States, mealtimes are times of socialization. Mr. Douglas is living alone; therefore, socialization is not possible during meals at home.
42. (1) Mr. Douglas is venting his anger inward. To deal with or control this, he first must learn to identify how he feels during times of stress.
43. (1) Studies show that persons who do not vent their anger outwardly have increased acid secretions in the stomach as well as increased motility of the GI tract.
44. (2) The only preparation required for an upper GI series is for the patient to be NPO. After an upper GI series, some type of cathartic is usually required to assist in evacuation of the barium.

45. (2) Bubbles emanating from a submerged nasogastric tube and the patient's inability to speak indicate incorrect tube placement in the lungs.
46. (3) The pharmacologic action of Tagamet is to control gastric acidity.
47. (2) A side effect of anticholinergic drug administration is urinary retention, as evidenced by "I'm having trouble urinating."
48. (1) Patients with active ulcers are placed on a bland diet. Foods to avoid include food high in fiber, fried foods, and stimulants such as coffee and tea.
49. (3) Diaphoresis and severe abdominal pain may indicate Mr. Douglas's ulcer has perforated and is bleeding into the peritoneal cavity with resulting shock. Vital sign assessment is necessary to evaluate the occurrence of this complication. The physician should be notified immediately.
50. (2) During the immediate postoperative period, nasogastric suction is maintained to prevent overdistension of the stomach (applying pressure to suture line) and to keep stomach secretions minimal to decrease their irritation on the suture line.
51. (3)

$$\frac{\text{Total amount} \times \text{gtts/ml}}{\text{Total time} \times 60 \text{ (minutes in 1 hr)}} = \text{gtts/min}$$

$$\frac{150 \text{ ml} \times 10 \text{ gtts/ml}}{1 \text{ hr} \times 60 \text{ min}} = \frac{1500}{60} = 25 \text{ gtts/hr}$$

52. (3) Hiccoughs are caused by pressure on the diaphragm. This may indicate bleeding into the peritoneal cavity. Consequently checking vital signs and noting drainage in the nasogastric tube and dressing would be appropriate methods to assess for bleeding.
53. (3) During nasogastric intubation the patient is receiving nothing by mouth. Stimulation of the parotid glands is dependent on the presence of food. Lack of this stimulation causes the glands to swell, or "surgical mumps." The causation of surgical mumps is not the same as the childhood disease.
54. (2) Audible bowel sounds indicate return of peristalsis. Peristalsis is necessary for food to pass through the GI tract.
55. (3) The Dumping syndrome is characterized by weakness and palpitations soon after eating. Foods high in carbohydrates absorb fluid from the bloodstream, causing the symptoms.
56. (2) Evaluation of wound healing must include comments regarding the integrity of the suture line and the presence or absence of drainage.
57. (3) "Pacing the floor" and calling the office indicate anxiety and stress. Planning to spend time with Mr. Douglas to allow him to talk may provide a productive problem-solving opportunity for him. Anxiety and stress led to the ulcer occurrence.
58. (1) Vagus nerve innervation to the stomach increases secretion in the stomach. Clipping this nerve reduces the amount of acid in the stomach.
59. (3) Aspirin is highly acid and would irritate the stomach. Nonaspirin headache remedies are indicated.
60. (1) Vomiting of blood or black tarry stools indicate bleeding along the GI tract and should be reported immediately.
61. (1) Cataracts are manifested by gradual vision loss and opacity of the lens.
62. (3) Mr. Arthur should be encouraged to be independent. You should provide a safe uncluttered environment.
63. (2) Cataracts and rheumatoid arthritis both are diseases of connective tissue.
64. (1) Mydriatics dilate the pupils.
65. (3) Vomiting increases intraocular pressure and may cause rupture of suture line within the eye.
66. (2) Preparing Mr. Arthur's tray would diminish the chance for sudden movements, which would be contraindicated. Allowing him to feed himself would foster independence.
67. (2) Inactivity and stress seem to activate the symptoms of rheumatoid arthritis.
68. (1) Splints at bedtime are used to provide support during the immobility during sleep. Rest periods coupled with an exercise program prevent deformities.
69. (2) The plasma salicylate level for a therapeutic range is 15 mg per 100 ml. To obtain this level, as much as 100 gr or more may be given.
70. (3) Aspirin side effects may include prolonged prothrombin time.
71. (1) Signature on the surgical consent means that Mr. Arthur has been informed of the risks involved and understands the procedure to be done. This is also known as informed consent.
72. (1) $\frac{10 \text{ mg}}{1 \text{ ml}} = \frac{8 \text{ mg}}{x \text{ ml}}$

$$10x = 8$$

$$x = \frac{8}{10}$$

$$x = 0.8 \text{ ml}$$

73. (3) Before administering the preoperative medication you should assist the patient to void and record this information on the chart. Mr. Arthur should be cautioned that the medication will make him drowsy and therefore he should not try to get up. Siderails should be raised and bed height lowered.
74. (4) Before moving the patient, an assessment for injuries must be done. Always stay with the patient to protect him from further injury.

75. (1) Negligence is failure to do what a person of ordinary judgment or prudence would do or doing what a reasonable person would not do.
76. (2) A Hemovac is a wound suction device that exerts gentle, even, negative pressure to evacuate wound drainage.
77. (1) To prevent dislocation of the new prosthesis, the patient's leg must be maintained in abduction by a triangular pillow. Logrolling also promotes proper alignment while turning.
78. (3) Urine is a medium in which bacteria may grow well. Sepsis is a main complication of total hip replacement, and therefore all efforts to maintain sterility of the dressing must be enforced.
79. (3) You would place the wheelchair on the patient's unaffected side. Since he will pivot on the unaffected or left leg, the wheelchair should be placed at the head of the bed.
80. (1) You want to pivot the patient in the direction of the unaffected side, which necessitates positioning him with his left leg closest to the bed.
81. (2) The three cardinal signs of increased intracranial pressure are headache, projectile vomiting, and papilledema.
82. (3) The typical migraine attack begins with vasoconstriction affecting the arteries of the scalp and cerebrum. The patient appears pale and may experience sensory, motor, and mood alterations. Pain and discomfort result from dilation of extracerebral and intracerebral vessels.
83. (1) Ergotamine preparations may be effective if taken early in the attack by acting on smooth muscle and causing prolonged constriction of cranial blood vessels.
84. (4) A liberal fluid intake is encouraged following lumbar puncture to aid in the establishment of a normal amount of cerebrospinal fluid, which is lost during the procedure.
85. (3) Normal brain tissue is relatively impermeable. There is increased uptake of radioactive material at the site of pathologic conditions.
86. (2) Computerized axial tomography is a noninvasive procedure that is painless and has a high degree of sensitivity for detecting pathologic conditions.
87. (3) Mild sedatives and mild analgesics are used with patients having increased intracranial pressure. Enemas and increased IV fluids may increase intracranial pressure. Strong narcotics are avoided since they depress respiration and mask neurologic status.
88. (2) The earliest sign of increasing intracranial pressure is lethargy, manifested by slow speech, delayed response, or difficulty in arousing patient from sleep.
89. (1) If a large tumor has been removed, the patient should be kept off the operative side to prevent shifting of brain tissue into the evacuated space.
90. (4) Establishing an airway will ensure adequate cerebral oxygenation.
91. (2) When the cornea is touched lightly with clean cotton, blinking denotes normal function of cranial nerves V (trigeminal) and VII (facial).
92. (3) Cranial nerve III, the oculomotor, regulates pupil size.
93. (1) A prompt, purposeful withdrawal of only the injured part denotes normal functioning of spinal motor reflexes.
94. (3) Lethargy (see rationale 88).
95. (2) As intracranial pressure rises, the circulatory system attempts to compensate for decreased circulation to the brain by increasing pulse and respiratory rates and increasing systolic blood pressure. This physiologic reaction causes the pulse pressure (difference between the systolic and diastolic pressures) to increase.
96. (3) The major nursing objective during a seizure is to protect the patient from injury by placing him flat, loosening tight clothing, and removing obstacles from the area. Soft pillows under the head may result in suffocation. If the patient is in bed, siderails, preferably padded, should be put up.
97. (2) Any attempt to place a tongue blade or other protective device after the tonic stage may result in injury to the patient, such as broken teeth or injury to the lips and tongue.
98. (1) It is not possible to take accurate pulse, blood pressure, or respiratory rates during the grand mal seizure. Taking a temperature during seizure could result in serious injury to the patient. The remaining options are important observations that should be documented.
99. (1) Mannitol is an osmotic diuretic that induces diffusion of water from body tissues into the plasma to be eliminated through the kidneys.
100. (2) 1.005 to 1.025.
101. (3) Swelling around the pituitary gland may result in the condition diabetes insipidus, which is the inadequate secretion of vasopressin. Vasopressin promotes reabsorption of water in the kidneys by the renal tubules. Inadequate amounts of vasopressin cause an excessive output of water from the body.
102. (1) Monitoring intake and output is critical with diabetes insipidus in order to determine whether the patient is losing dangerous amounts of fluid.
103. (4) Sodium and water retention in the kidneys increases the electrolyte concentration in the blood vessels to a level that enhances vasoconstrictor response of the blood vessels to sympathetic stimulation.
104. (2) Egg yolks and dairy products contain a high amount of cholesterol.
105. (1) Involvement of the patient in the establishment of goals and priorities serves the purpose of getting him involved and getting him to take some of the responsibility for learning.

106. (3) Angina pectoris is a clinical symptom characterized by pain or pressure in the chest resulting from inadequate oxygen supply to the myocardium. The pain of angina is generally associated with exertion and is relieved by rest.
107. (2) Arteriography involves injecting dye into the vascular system to outline the heart and coronary blood vessels for examination. In addition to checking the puncture site for bleeding and hematoma, it is important to check the distal extremity for color and intact pulses.
108. (1) Nitroglycerin tablets may be taken every 5 minutes times three tablets. Taking more tablets than necessary may further decrease coronary blood flow by producing systemic hypotension. Pain not relieved after 15 minutes may denote acute myocardial infarction.
109. (4) Nitroglycerin is extremely sensitive to time, heat, air, and moisture. Tablets lose considerable potency in containers made of plastic, metal, or cardboard.
110. (3) Exercise is encouraged to improve cardiac efficiency and enhance the patient's ability to perform work at reduced heart and blood pressure rates.
111. (3) The pain of mycardial infarction is a heavy, viselike pain that occurs in the chest and may radiate into the neck, shoulder, and arms. Unlike angina, it may begin spontaneously, is not associated with stress, and is not relieved by rest or nitroglycerin.
112. (1) The most important therapeutic consideration in care of the myocardial infarction patient is provision of complete physical and emotional rest. Anticipating needs will relieve anxiety about having to make requests that may contribute to the patient's feelings of helplessness and dependency.
113. (3) The underlying mechanism of heart failure involves decreased contractibility of the heart muscle. Low cardiac output results in a low systemic arterial blood pressure.
114. (1) The action of heparin is prompt and predictable. Peak effect is reached in 5 to 10 minutes. Clotting time returns to normal within 2 to 6 hours.
115. (4) Lasix increases the excretion of potassium.
116. (2) The orthopneic position allows blood to pool in dependent portions of the body, decreases blood return to the heart, and improves lung volume and vital capacity. Oxygen is administered in high concentrations to relieve high hypoxia and dyspnea. Morphine is given to reduce anxiety and dyspnea.
117. (4) Simultaneous removal of more than one tourniquet at a time causes a sudden rush of too much blood back to the heart and could precipitate a recurrence of pulmonary edema.
118. (1) Lanoxin is a cardiotonic drug that slows and strengthens cardiac contraction. If the apical pulse rate is less than 60 beats per minute, the physician should be notified before proceeding with the drug administration.
119. (4)

$$\frac{10 \text{ mg}}{1 \text{ ml}} = \frac{15 \text{ mg}}{x \text{ ml}}$$
$$10x = 15$$
$$x = 1.5 \text{ ml}$$

120. (2) This defines depression.
121. (2) Patients who have some control in their care usually are more cooperative. This approach also promotes independence rather than dependence.
122. (3) This response acknowledges the wife's feelings and allows her the opportunity to ventilate them.

SAMPLE EXAMINATION 2

1. (4) Transient ischemic attacks (TIAs) are temporary neurologic disturbances manifested by sudden loss of motor, sensory, or visual function and lasting a few minutes to several hours. The cause is a temporary lack of blood flow to the area.
2. (2) Coumadin interferes with blood clotting mechanisms by blocking the synthesis of vitamin K in the liver. Even minor injuries may result in hemorrhage in the patient taking Coumadin.
3. (2) Clotting factor II–prothrombin is dependent on the adequate synthesis of vitamin K. The one-stage prothrombin time test is used to monitor Coumadin therapy. The usual aim of therapy is to maintain prothrombin time 1 to $1\frac{1}{2}$ times normal.
4. (3) Patients taking Coumadin should be monitored for any signs of bleeding. The mucous membranes, intestines, and urinary tract are common sites.
5. (2) Emergency nursing care of the CVA patient includes placing the patient on the affected side to promote drainage of saliva, elevating the head slightly to promote venous drainage, and keeping the patient as quiet as possible.
6. (2) High blood pressure is a hereditary disease that is caused by increased vasoconstrictor activity as a result of increased stimulation of sympathetic nerve fibers on the blood vessels.
7. (2) The normal blood pressure range is 100/60 to 140/90.

8. (4) Prevention of contractures, decubitus, and other physiologic complications will speed up the eventual rehabilitative process.
9. (3) Expressive aphasia results from damage to Broca's speech area. The patient understands what is said to him and knows the words he wishes to say, but he cannot form the words verbally. Many times he may still be able to write words.
10. (2) Dysphagia is defined as difficulty in swallowing. If the patient has lost the gag reflex, he may easily aspirate oral fluids.
11. (4) Positioning the patient prone for 15 to 30 minutes several times daily will promote hyperextension of the hip joints, which is essential for normal gait and helps drain bronchial secretions.
12. (3) Elevation of the arm helps prevent edema and fibrosis, which will interfere with normal range of motion.
13. (1) These activities will put the arm through range of motion as the patient assumes some responsibility for personal care.
14. (3) Artificial tears and a patch will protect the cornea from drying, trauma, and ulceration.
15. (3) Food particles tend to become trapped in the paralyzed side and could be aspirated.
16. (2) Depression is a natural response to catastrophic illness. Other psychologic problems manifested by cerebral damage include emotional lability, hostility, frustration, and noncooperation.
17. (1) Massaging the area and avoiding repeated pressure will enhance circulation.
18. (3) An increase in fruits in the diet will increase bulk in the intestines. Increasing bulk and fluids in the intestines will promote normal elimination.
19. (3) Ingestion of dairy products increases calcium intake. Excessive calcium in the body during periods of decreased mobility increases the chance of kidney stone formation.
20. (2) Quadriceps setting exercises improve the strength of muscles needed for walking.
21. (3) The nurse shows more potential for change by attempting to develop insight into his or her own behavior.
22. (2) Part of rehabilitation is assisting with the development of new coping skills.
23. (2) According to freudian theory, the roots of alcoholism are developed in the first stage of growth and development when oral needs are most predominant.
24. (2) Antabuse is the only drug used for this purpose.
25. (4) All are correct.
26. (3) Keeping the room lighted reduces the incidence of visual hallucinations.
27. (3) Autonomic overactivity, tachycardia, profuse perspiration, and fever are the clinical manifestations.
28. (2) Delirium tremens is the psychotic state following withdrawal from heavy drinking.
29. (3) Alcoholics Anonymous is based on the theory that you cannot help yourself until you admit you have a problem.
30. (1) The alcoholic is thought to be very dependent, and an aim of rehabilitation is to increase independent functioning.
31. (4) Nutritional deficiency results from decreased protein intake and alcohol.
32. (1) The liver becomes enlarged with excessive fat cells, jaundice is caused by failure of liver function, and gastrointestinal disturbances result from obstruction of the portal circulation.
33. (3) Small frequent feedings might help Mr. Gabriel overcome anorexia.
34. (1) Elevating the head of the bed will assist in elevating the diaphragm and facilitating respiration.
35. (2) Intake and output measurement and daily weight will indicate the effect of the diuretic. Diuretics may result in depletion of electrolytes, which may cause other complications.
36. (4) Since liver disease may interfere with the production of clotting factors, patients may exhibit bleeding tendencies.
37. (3) Patients with active liver disease require rest and supportive measures to permit the liver to reestablish its functional ability.
38. (2) Decreased prothrombin production may result in bleeding tendencies.
39. (4) Mental confusion could result from brain dysfunction caused by the accumulation of ammonia and other toxic metabolites in the blood.
40. (1) A well-balanced diet will enhance healing and functioning of the liver.
41. (2) Pain is caused by contracture of the gallbladder, which has been stimulated by fat in the duodenum and is having difficulty releasing bile because of obstruction.
42. (3) Lima beans, cabbage, and onions are gas-forming foods.
43. (2) The normal hemoglobin level for women is 12 to 16 g.
44. (3) This procedure is the correct technique to ensure the nasogastric tube is in the stomach.
45. (4) $\frac{50 \text{ mg}}{1 \text{ ml}} = \frac{75 \text{ mg}}{x \text{ ml}}$

$$50x = 75$$

$$x = 1.5 \text{ ml}$$

46. (3) $\frac{60 \text{ gr}}{1 \text{ ml}} = \frac{1/100 \text{ gr}}{x}$

$$60x = \frac{1}{100}$$

$$x = 0.6$$

47. (2) Collection of fluids in the stomach may cause nausea and vomiting.
48. (3) Penrose drains are used to remove bile and blood from the operative area.
49. (4) Location of the incision associated with cholecystectomy makes the patient prone to pulmonary complications.
50. (1) Bile is very irritating to the skin.
51. (3) The new tube should be ordered and replaced.
52. (1) A wide base of support will provide balance and prevent strain on the back.
53. (1) Providing analgesics, especially before turning, coughing, and deep breathing, will facilitate movement and respiration.
54. (2) $\frac{125\text{ml}}{60} \times 10 = 21$ gtts
55. (4) Insert at a 90-degree angle.
56. (3) Irrigating the tube will ensure patency.
57. (1) Discontinue the IV fluids to prevent further swelling, and report to charge nurse.
58. (2) A principle of surgical asepsis states sterile objects only touch sterile objects.
59. (1) A temperature may be indicative of a postoperative infection, which requires initiation of treatment.
60. (3) Following cholecystectomy, most patients can return to a normal diet as long as they avoid excessive fat intake.
61. (2) Hyperthyroidism results from overproduction of the thyroid gland.
62. (1) Patients with hyperthyroidism have an intolerance to heat and can be made more comfortable by placing them near air-conditioning.
63. (1) The metabolic rate of patients with hyperthyroidism is greatly increased. This elevated rate requires increased oxygen.
64. (1) Diagnosis of hyperthyroidism is confirmed by T_3, T_4, PBI, and I_{131} uptake.
65. (3) Measures to promote sleep include hypnotics, back care, and warm drinks. Caffeine should be avoided. Diversional activities should be encouraged.
66. (2) Diet should be high in carbohydrates and proteins. Caffeine should be avoided.
67. (4) Propylthiouracil is an antithyroid medication that reduces thyroid production.
68. (1) Toxic effects of propylthiouracil are leukopenia, fever, skin rash, and sore throat.
69. (3) Iodine reduces the vascularity of the thyroid gland.
70. (3) Semi-Fowler's position prevents hyperextension of the neck and undue pressure on the suture line.
71. (1) To assess for laryngeal edema, you should ask the patient to speak one or two words every hour.
72. (2) Hypotension, tachycardia, and tachypnea with the symptoms complained of by the patient may indicate hemorrhage.
73. (3) Restlessness indicates diminished oxygen supply to the brain. Noisy respirations indicate mechanical obstruction (edema of the glottis) in which the patient is unable to inspire oxygen adequately.
74. (1) Keeping the tracheostomy tube patent is of utmost importance since lack of adequate oxygen may lead to more severe complications.
75. (2) To lessen Mr. Powell's apprehension, you should explain what you are going to do. This may be done simultaneously with preparing the equipment.
76. (4) Suctioning of the tracheostomy must be done as aseptically as possible to prevent introducing bacteria into the lungs.
77. (2) The catheter suction is applied during withdrawal from the trachea.
78. (3) Mr. Powell can assist by holding the edges of the tracheostomy to prevent dislodgment should he cough. Changing the strings should be accomplished quickly.
79. (2) The parathyroid glands may be injured or removed during a thyroidectomy. Altered parathyroid function results in lowered calcium plasma levels causing irritability of the nerves, especially those of the hands and feet.
80. (4) Thyroid storm results from stress, infection, or surgery. Large amounts of thyroid hormone are released into the bloodstream, resulting in symptoms of increased metabolic rate (elevated temperature, pulse, and respirations and irritability).
81. (4) These are the most common procedures. The cervix, urethra, and anus are the locations where the organism is usually found.
82. (4) All describe this disorder.
83. (2) Other symptoms are associated with syphilis.
84. (1) Symptoms commonly occur before the menstrual period because of greater vulnerability of the uterine cavity to gonorrheal invasion at time of menstrual desquamation.
85. (1) Some other drugs (streptomycin, tetracycline, chloramphenicol) may be used if the patient is allergic to penicillin.
86. (2) Each year a number of deaths occur from such allergic reactions.
87. (3) An indwelling catheter would encourage dependent drainage and prevent spread.
88. (1) Gonorrhea is spread by direct contact. Proper hand washing is the most effective method of controlling this disease.
89. (1) Work to offer appropriate information and demonstrate concern for others with whom you have come in contact. Threats are often blocks to cooperation.
90. (2) The patient can become easily infected again if she does not continue treatment.

91. (1) The organism has a fast incubation period once the penis has come in contact with it. The organism travels up the urethra to cause infection with the common symptoms: burning on urination, nausea and vomiting, purulent discharge from anus, and swollen penis.
92. (2) Pus forms in the fallopian tubes so that when adhesions develop, sterility often is the result.
93. (4) This allows time for Karen to express emotion and treats her as an adult.
94. (2) These are common clinical symptoms of narcotic withdrawal.
95. (2) This is a firm, but kind statement, and it assures Karen that your aim is to help, not harm, her.
96. (2) Beware of sudden mood changes in depressed states. It only means that the patient may now have enough energy to carry out suicidal intentions.
97. (1) Acknowledgment of feelings also allows for ventilation.
98. (2) Even under the best of measures, people who are addicted can somehow manage to get drugs. Watching her closely, along with those who come in contact with her, is less severe than the other choices yet affords some measure of protection.
99. (2) In combination with certain foods containing tyramine, hypertensive crisis may occur.
100. (3) Hallucinations are sensory perceptions in the absence of external stimuli. Karen is obviously ''hearing'' things.
101. (2) All may be present with the exception of pain; they are usually present in late stages.
102. (2) The breast should be manipulated gently to avoid unnecessary seeding of tumor cells and to widen the search for nodes.
103. (1) Others describe simple and modified approach.
104. (4) The nurse offers him- or herself—not cliches, advice, or others who might not be wanted at that time.
105. (1) A, B, and C are common postoperative measures. D and E would not take care of prevention of edema and might harm the operative site.
106. (1) This is the only true statement.
107. (2) Because of the removal of important muscles, the patient must keep others active.
108. (2) D would only encourage edema and could also result in motion deformities.
109. (3) Other approaches might be taken as too ''pushy.'' The patient should set the pace.
110. (3) Tennis would be too strenuous and could cause injury to the operative site.
111. (4) All are present therapies.
112. (2) The esophagus is close to the chest and becomes irritated during this treatment.
113. (3) About 95% of women discover this condition through breast self-examination.
114. (3) Most lesions occur in this quadrant.
115. (2) Most growths occur during the active ovarian period.
116. (2) Drawing blood could lead to serious infection and increased swelling.
117. (2) A woman who has experienced anxiety disabilities, and pain associated with surgical intervention usually can anticipate a patient's needs more effectively than those who have not.
118. (3) All are appropriate for patient teaching.
119. (4) A lump can be present for as long as 3 years or more; it is hard to palpate if it is less than 1 cm wide, and it grows slowly.
120. (3) Women may be not only predisposed genetically to the development of breast cancer, but they may develop it earlier (10 to 12 years) than women without a history of breast cancer.

SAMPLE EXAMINATION 3

1. (1) The tracheostomy tray is obtained in the event that Bill develops an obstructed airway. Tracheal edema results from the inhalation of smoke and heat.
2. (3) In assisting the physician you would prepare an IV fluid administration set and fluids (as ordered) for the immediate replacement of fluids lost from the burn site(s).
3. (4) An immediate physical observation of a person burned in the area of the face is assessment of respiration (difficulty, rate, sound).
4. (3) Reverse isolation protects the patient and the burned areas from infections transmitted by others.
5. (1) Urine specific gravity is monitored to assess filtration capabilities of the renal glomerulus. Urine output and urine specific gravity provide data to determine fluid replacement needs and the status of renal function.
6. (1) Nurturing Bill and spending time with him will decrease his fears of the unknown, anxiety about separation from his parents, and pain (injury).
7. (2) To help Bill cope with immobility, you can use play therapy and diversional activity to decrease his anxiety. Preschoolers describe objects as real, and by simulating application of Russell's traction on Bill's favorite toy you can lessen his feelings of aloneness.

8. (4) Your response informed Bill's grandmother that bed-wetting is normal in children Bill's age and that hospitalized children frequently regress into some behaviors that would not normally be seen at home.
9. (1) Circulation and sensation are periodically assessed to determine the presence of pressure areas that may obstruct circulation and nerve pathways.
10. (2) To administer 20 mg of Demerol elixir, you would convert teaspoon measurement of milliliters and give 2 ml.
11. (2) Informing Bill as to what is expected of him during the procedure will lessen his anxiety and increase his capability to control his feelings.
12. (2) Immobilization of the recipient site prevents the possibility of dislodging the graft and destroying the tissue-building process.
13. (1) During long periods of immobilization, calcium from bones and other tissues enters the circulatory system to be filtered and excreted by the kidneys. The increased level of calcium and urinary stasis in the renal pelvis predisposes to renal calculi.
14. (1) The diet provides essential nutrients that encourage tissue repair and replacement, energy for increased metabolic demands, and carbohydrates to prevent utilization of protein for energy.
15. (2) A preschooler enjoys the close family relationship of mealtimes. Parents are the significant persons in the preschool years.
16. (2) Increasing fluids, cellulose, and bulk in the diet will facilitate bowel elimination.
17. (1) Swelling and edema of the injured limb may increase after application of a cast. The tightness of the cast is determined to be sure pressure areas that may constrict circulation are not present.
18. (4) Changing of position increases circulation to the area and prevents pressure areas from developing.
19. (3) The grandmother should try to determine how much information he has and build on that.
20. (3) Physical contact offers much needed security at this time.
21. (1) The nurse's response corrects the misinformation that ''growing pains'' are normal in children.
22. (4) Placing Cheryl in a recumbent position decreases the oxygen demand by body cells and reduces the workload of the heart.
23. (2) The group A beta-hemolytic *Streptococcus* organism is the most frequently observed cause for the inflammatory process that may predispose to rheumatic fever.
24. (4) Rheumatic fever is most commonly seen in children from urban, crowded environments where external stressors are multiple (low income, poor nutrition).
25. (3) Resting decreases the workload on the heart. A therapeutic resting pulse rate is 80 per minute in most school-aged children.
26. (1) Defining limitation and expectations to the school-aged child assists the child to cope with the treatment and care during hospitalization. School-aged children are encouraged to have choices in certain aspects of care (bath time, activities for diversion) to foster their sense of industry.
27. (3) Resolution of the inflammatory response in rheumatic fever is determined by a resting pulse rate of 80 per minute, normal erythrocyte sedimentation rate, absence of serum C-reactive protein, and normal body temperature.
28. (2) A developmental characteristic of the school-aged child is the enjoyment of collecting objects, especially from friends. Also, school activities and friends are significant at this age.
29. (1) The child is encouraged to eat small frequent meals and drink liquids to prevent fatigue and to decrease the workload of the heart.
30. (4) This response acknowledges her feelings, gives an OK to how she feels, and asks for participation in her care.
31. (1) Chorea movements are uncontrolled movements of the extremities. Protecting the child from objects and falls is essential in preventing injury.
32. (2) With the increased pumping action of the heart ventricles, more blood is circulated in the body, causing excretion of excessive fluid. This combined with the diuretic effect of Lasix increases the urine output, slows the apical pulse, and causes a decrease in body weight.
33. (4) The apical pulse is monitored because a pulse deficit may be present from the inability of the heart ventricles to pump effectively.
34. (3) The physician must determine the dose of the medication if it is to be administered again.
35. (2) Placing the patient in a semi-Fowler's position (orthopneic) allows for full expansion of the lungs.
36. (1) Daily weight is monitored to determine amount of weight loss caused by fluid excretion. A sudden increase in weight can be indicative of fluid retention.
37. (3) The schoolchild is at a developmental level in which simple explanations of procedures can allay anxiety and decrease postoperative problems.
38. (2) Bloody drainage from the pleural space is expected immediately after surgery. The amount of drainage in a period of time and a change in appearance and/or amount are reported to the physician.
39. (1) This response reinforces preoperative teaching, offers security by stating availability and proximity of staff, and offers the call button as a means of summoning help.
40. (4) The change from intensive and frequent contact by nurses helped Cheryl feel insecure. You can initially plan care to reduce Cheryl's anxiety.

41. (1) Preparing Sam for the procedure and allowing him to ventilate his feelings before taking the temperature prevents future problems with temperature taking. The child having a temper tantrum is not reinforced for the behavior but is taught more acceptable methods of controlling feelings.
42. (3) Disturbing the child by performing nursing procedures does not meet the child's need for rest. If placed in a crib with an environment conducive for rest the child will sleep.
43. (3) Children Sam's age learn about the adult world through play and play objects. Demonstrating and explaining what he should expect will gain his cooperation and trust.
44. (4) The patient and the family in crisis initially express disbelief and denial of the situation causing the crisis.
45. (1) The leukemic process and chemotherapeutic drugs depress bone marrow production. The child is anemic and has increased amounts of immature white blood cells that are ineffective in resisting infection; therefore reverse isolation (protection from others) is prescribed.
46. (3) The cellular destruction and irritation of the drug can cause chemical cystitis if urine is allowed to be concentrated and retained in the bladder.
47. (1) Oral hygiene can prevent the mouth ulcerations caused by normal flora when the body is unable to combat the infecting organisms. Soft applicators, mild mouthwash, and gentleness in providing oral hygiene can prevent breaks in buccal mucosa and subsequent infections.
48. (2) Physiologic anorexia is a normal occurrence in the toddler years. The normal anorexia is intensified by the illness and sde effects of cancer therapy.
49. (3) The alopecia results from the affinity of cancer drugs for rapidly growing cells (hair follicles, epithelial cells). Once excretion of chemotherapeutic drugs occurs, hair growth will return.
50. (1) Separation anxiety is the major problem in the hospitalized child under 6 years of age. Reaction to separation is frequently described in stages (protest, despair, and denial). If the parent does not return, the child turns to staff for support and affection. Establishing a trusting relationship between you and Sam will decrease his fear of permanent maternal separation.
51. (4) Ritualism is a mechanism the toddler uses to feel secure in a growing and complex adult world. Familiarity with rituals allows you to provide, if possible, the same routines to assist the child in feeling more secure in the hospital environment.
52. (2) Information about frequency and character of the stool helps the physician to determine diagnosis and method of treatment.
53. (4) The "minidrip" set delivers 60 gtts per milliliter. You would regulate the set to run at 60 gtts per minute.
54. (1) The tongue blade is used to scrape the stool from a diaper or bedpan. The specimen cup is water repellent and can be sealed.
55. (3) After each stool the infant's buttocks and perineum are cleaned to prevent excoriation and skin breakdown. The Vaseline is used because of its water-resistant properties, which would prevent acidic stools from irritating the diaper area.
56. (1) To prevent spread of infection you routinely wash your hands before and after caring for each child. Bacterial infections of the bowel are communicable, and enteric precautions prevent transmission of bacteria to others.
57. (3) Discharge follow-up by the physician is essential in evaluating resolution of the illness.
58. (4) Selection of play objects is determined by the developmental level of the child. Toddlers enjoy pull toys because pulling the toy gives them a feeling of control over the object.
59. (1) Once the child reaches the stage of despair from parental separation, the child clings to others for emotional needs. Allowing the mother, the child, and the nurse to have time in a relaxed environment helps the child regain confidence in the mother and reestablishes their relationship.
60. (3) Physical security (holding him) is important. Nightlights lessen anxiety, as do your own calmness and self-assuredness.
61. (3) At this age such an object serves as a measure of security.
62. (2) Your assuming a sitting position beside the father communicates concern and a willingness to help the person in emotional crisis.
63. (1) When responding to a person in crisis, you simply respond to questions and provide only the information asked for by the person.
64. (4) Any trauma to the meningocele sac can cause further neurologic damage and infection.
65. (3) The meningocele sac is kept moist to prevent drying of the meninges from exposure to air.
66. (1) A complication of myelomeningocele is neurologic dysfunction at and below the site of the spina bifida. The parasympathetic and sympathetic nerve damage results in the atonia of the bladder and bowel.
67. (1) Preoperatively and especially postoperatively the infant is observed for movement in the extremities and functioning of bowel and bladder to determine the extent of neurologic dysfunctions.
68. (3) Parent-child bonding can be impeded by separation of the ill neonate from the parents. The bonding process can be encouraged by allowing the parents to touch, hold, and talk to the neonate. The neonate receiving proper stimulation will thrive more quickly than the neonate deprived of stimulation.

69. (4) Hydrocephalus results from the obstruction in cerebrospinal fluid caused by the myelomeningocele. Daily measurement of head circumference that indicates increasing size, (bulging) fontanelles, and high-pitched cry are some of the symptoms of increased intracranial pressure.
70. (2) As the cerebrospinal fluid accumulates, the neonate's or infant's head increases in size (noted by separation of cranial sutures and increased head circumference), and intracranial pressure increases.
71. (1) Vomiting (projectile) is a result of increased intracranial pressure. The infant is fed small frequent meals to decrease possibility of aspiration of feeding. The hydrocephalic head must be supported to prevent trauma to the neck from the head's weight.
72. (3) The postoperative position of the head is on the nonoperative side to prevent fluid and brain shift, which would traumatize the operative area of the brain.
73. (2) Change in neurologic status (pupil reaction and/or size, level of consciousness, movement ability) needs to be reported to institute treatment to reduce the cerebral edema.
74. (3) Measuring the head circumference provides data to determine change over a period of time.
75. (3) The young child is placed in a sitting position with the neck flexed to separate the spinous processes to ease insertion of the needle. While in this position the child must be observed for breathing difficulties from poor lung expansion.
76. (1) To be adhesive and to seal, the self-adhesive plastic bag must be applied to a clean, dry area.
77. (2) Direct pressure is applied immediately for 1 to 2 minutes to stop bleeding.
78. (2) Bacterial infections treated with antibiotics for 24 hours are not considered communicable.
79. (4) During seizure activity the patient is never restrained, as injury may occur. The bed or crib sides are padded to protect the child from injury.
80. (3) You make periodic comparative observations to note differences in vital signs, neurologic status, and renal function. Accurate intake and output measurements are essential to determine fluid replacement needs and detect cerebral edema.
81. (1) Maintenance and care of the IV site is primary in caring for the child with meningitis who receives medications intravenously. The long-term fluid and antibiotic therapy increases the child's susceptibility to phlebitis and fluid infiltration at the site.
82. (2) Definitive etiologic factors in failure to thrive are difficult to determine because of the interrelationship of emotions and biologic effects on growth. Primary known contributing factors are a poor maternal-child relationship and malabsorption.
83. (3) Following a painful or uncomfortable procedure, the child must be comforted to decrease distrust and fear. Children with failure to thrive because of emotional deprivation gain weight and grow when loved and stimulated and their needs are met.
84. (3) In cystic fibrosis the sweat glands, pancreas, and lungs are involved. The palmar test indicates the amount of sodium, chloride, and potassium excreted in sweat. High levels of these electrolytes support a diagnosis of cystic fibrosis.
85. (4) Symptoms occur because of mechanical obstruction by viscous mucus.
86. (2) The pulmonary mucus is thick and obstructs normal air exchange in the lungs.
87. (1) Chest physiotherapy is essential to dislodge and move the thick mucus from the lungs. Aerosol medications are administered to lower the surface tension of the mucus to ease removal from the lungs.
88. (1) The pancreatic enzyme deficiency results in improper digestion of fats and utilization of proteins by the body. The child develops malnutrition unless pancreatic enzymes are administered. To correct the nutritional state of the child, a diet high in protein, low to moderate in fat, and with a liberal amount of salt (sodium and chloride are lost in large amounts in sweat) provides the nutrients needed for the child to grow.
89. (2) The pancreatic enzymes are given 30 minutes before eating so digestion of foods occurs normally and nutrients (fats, vitamins) are not lost.
90. (2) Because large amounts of fluid and electrolytes are lost from perspiration, the child can suffer heat prostration more quickly.
91. (3) Humidified air or mist is administered to liquefy the pulmonary secretions. The child is changed frequently to prevent chilling and skin irritation from the constant dampness.
92. (4) Children with chronic conditions must be protected from overprotective parents that do not allow the child to accomplish developmental tasks successfully, thus impairing the child's psychologic development.
93. (1) The consistent higher level of carbon dioxide desensitizes the medulla. Consequently the medulla becomes sensitized to higher levels of oxygen.
94. (2) The serous fluid from the vesicles is communicable.
95. (3) Rubella and rubeola have similar rashes, clinical manifestations, and communicability. The presence of Koplik spots in the mouth is definitive for a diagnosis of rubeola.
96. (4) Children 18 months and under are inoculated against diphtheria, polio, tetanus, and pertussis, with booster injections given periodically until the age of 18 years.
97. (1) The large, bulky stools associated with cystic fibrosis decrease muscle tone in the colon.

98. (3) Cystic fibrosis is a chronic condition requiring continuous intensive care to prevent pulmonary complications (pneumonia). Parents are instructed in care of the child at home to continue the therapy regimen instituted in the hospital.
99. (1) The school-aged child is developed intellectually and is able to actively participate in care and therapy. Many times the child develops new methods of performing chest physiotherapy himself.
100. (3) The school-aged child enjoys the independence of an expanded environment (school, clubs, church) and needs guidance in developing acceptable behaviors and solutions to problems. The hospitalized schoolchild loses independence and the autonomy desired at this level. To gain cooperation and promote normal development, the staff permit the child to decide certain aspects of care by offering the child several options.
101. (4) The school-aged child identifies him- or herself with adult role models and heros (Superman, teacher, coach). Influence by adults outside the family is great during these years; therefore the nurse is often viewed as a person with identifiable qualities attractive to the child.
102. (2) Improper handling may result in further cord damage.
103. (2) Frequent or improper handling may result in further cord damage.
104. (2) Injury at the cervical level causes paralysis of all four extremities and the trunk. Respiratory failure and death may result.
105. (2) Respiratory assistance is required because of lack of diaphragm innervation.
106. (2) Crutchfield tongs lessen pressure on the spinal cord.
107. (2) Sandbags prevent slipping, thus rendering traction useless.
108. (4) Fluids tend to flow into the nasopharynx easily, with the danger of aspiration.
109. (4) A diet high in proteins decreases the incidence of decubiti.
110. (1) High fluid intake and intermittent catheterizations keep the kidneys active and initiate voiding.
111. (1) Cranberry juice promotes acidic urine and cuts down on stone formation.
112. (1) These help to prevent pressure sores and contractures and can be done without danger of further injury.
113. (4) All are appropriate.
114. (1) Decubiti can form very easily without proper attention.
115. (1) Sex has not been statistically as important as the other factors.
116. (3) You should offer Jim the opportunity to verbalize his feelings rather than internalize them.
117. (2) Autonomic dysreflexia can occur in 85% of all spinal cord–injured patients with lesions at T6 level or above. This response can happen even years after injury.
118. (1) Elevating the head of the bed 45 degrees or helping the patient sit up usually remedies the situation automatically.
119. (2) Changes in motion or sensation of the extremities are the most reliable determination of the presence of edema of the cord. Edema causes trauma to motor and sensory nerves.
120. (2) Decadron prevents and alleviates spinal cord edema.
121. (2) Addiction to narcotics can develop over a short period of time. Other measures must be found to alleviate pain caused by long-term problems.

SAMPLE EXAMINATION 4

1. (3) Prolonged excessive menstrual flow for 8 or 9 months, as in this patient's case, will significantly lower the hemoglobin level regardless of the underlying pathologic condition.
2. (4) Other options do not acknowledge the patient's feelings or offer an immediate opportunity for her to express them.
3. (2) You may best relieve the patient's anxiety by providing information about treatments you are to perform. Option 1 is less complete. Options 3 and 4 are not within the realm of the nurse's responsibility.
4. (1) Following a total abdominal hysterectomy, hemorrhage will be best indicated by signs of shock manifested in an increase in pulse and respirations and a decrease in blood pressure. Bleeding may be internal and would be visually undetected.
5. (3) Other problems are not common, and proximity of the urinary bladder and urethra to the operative area often requires insertion of a Foley catheter for several days postoperatively.
6. (2) Venous stasis and pelvic congestion may be best reduced by active movement of the pelvis and lower extremities.

7. (2) Questions the patient may have regarding self-administered treatments and sexual activity should be answered by the physician.
8. (3) Radium is non–cell specific and will destroy all cells within its prescribed range of effect.
9. (2) Regardless of the source of radiation, the time of exposure, the distance from the source, and the shielding present are factors you must consider in protecting yourself from radiation effects.
10. (2) Vaginal radium implants are usually removed before the patient's discharge, and the patient is no longer a source of contamination.
11. (3) Pelvic pain and a dragging sensation often immobilize the patient with endometriosis.
12. (2) Endometrial tissue present in the pelvic cavity of the patient with endometriosis responds to hormonal influence during menstruation, as does endometrial tissue inside the uterus.
13. (3) Manual manipulation and placement of a pessary are often done by the physician until such time as surgery is indicated for permanent correction. Endometriosis is not commonly associated with this disorder.
14. (3) Poor posture, congenital malposition of the uterus, and irregular bowel patterns are all associated with uterine displacement.
15. (2) It is necessary to prevent any strain on suture sites that may result from hardened feces in the rectum or from straining at stool. Instructing the patient and administering stool softeners help to prevent this.
16. (2) Edema and hypertension result from protein losses and impaired glomerular filtration in the patient with glomerulonephritis.
17. (2) Glomerulonephritis is an inflammatory disease of the glomeruli thought to be the result of an antigen-antibody response.
18. (3) The antigen-antibody response causing an inflammation of the glomeruli is commonly associated with a beta-hemolytic streptococcal infection (strep throat).
19. (4) Creatinine clearance and BUN are the renal function studies that most accurately measure glomerular filtration.
20. (4) This response acknowledges the patient's feelings as well as providing an explanation for the ordered intake and output.
21. (1) Sodium, protein, and fluids may be restricted for the patient with glomerulonephritis, according to the degree of edema and renal damage.
22. (2) Children with glomerulonephritis and nephrosis often respond to treatment with prednisone. The use of steroids in treatment of adults with this disease is less effective.
23. (3) Daily weights must be taken at the same time each day in order to ensure accuracy. Patient activities and routines should be considered in selecting the time.
24. (2) Fluids should not be forced for the patient with glomerulonephritis, as fluid retention and edema are common problems.
25. (2) A patient having a urinary output of less than 30 ml per hour is experiencing serious loss of renal function, and the physician should be notified.
26. (1) Confusion and irritability result from retention of toxic materials in the bloodstream (urea, creatinine, and so on). These problems, as well as an increasing blood pressure, indicate decreasing renal function.
27. (4) Potassium is known to directly affect the conduction system of the heart. (Ventricular fibrillation and cardiac arrest may occur with hyperkalemia.)
28. (3) Contacting the head nurse first may prevent interruption of a conference in progress, treatment of another patient, or failure of the family member to find her.
29. (2) Only statement number 2 is true. Hemodialysis is done by use of the artificial kidney. The patient's blood is circulated through the machine, cleansed of toxic materials, and returned to the patient's vascular system.
30. (3) Deposits of urea (uremic frost) form on the skin of the patient with renal failure. This causes pruritus and an unpleasant odor. Frequent cleansing and the avoidance of use of lotions containing alcohol help to relieve this problem.
31. (2) The patient who can adapt ordered treatment regimens to his or her usual living habits will be more successful in adjusting to necessary restrictions. Providing good patient instruction cannot by itself guarantee follow-through.
32. (2) Preventing urinary tract infections and resultant renal damage begins with proper aseptic technique in catheter insertion and management. Option 1 has not been validated, and options 3 and 4 are less preventive.
33. (2) Painless hematuria is commonly associated with malignancies of the urinary tract.
34. (2) With a flank incision, pain is intense when coughing and deep breathing. This pain causes the patient to splint the diaphragm in order to decrease the discomfort. Administration of pain medication will reduce pain and facilitate the patient's cooperation, thus achieving full inspiration and helping to prevent atelectasis.
35. (2) These signs indicate possible hemorrhage and shock. Options 1 and 3 are not highly unusual. Option 4 is not life threatening.
36. (2) EDC, or estimated date of confinement, is the estimated delivery date and is calculated by Nagel's rule.
37. (3) Presumptive signs of pregnancy include amenorrhea, fatigue, and urinary frequency. Chadwick's sign and pregnancy tests are probable signs of pregnancy. Fetal movements felt by an examiner are a positive sign.
38. (2) In the fourth month of antepartal growth and development, muscles are developed, and movements of the fetus may be felt by the mother.

39. (1) Improved quality and availability of prenatal care have had greater impact on reducing maternal and infant morbidity and mortality for the population than other options listed.
40. (3) In the fifth month of growth and development the fetus is fully developed, and the fetal heart rate is heard by the examiner using a fetoscope.
41. (3) Fetal heart tones heard by an examiner are a positive sign of pregnancy. Other options listed are probable or presumptive signs.
42. (2) Abdominal ultrasound is not a routinely ordered examination. It may be used to confirm suspected pregnancy at an early date, to evaluate fetal development, or to investigate problems (placental placement).
43. (3) Most physicians recommend a weight gain of 20 to 25 pounds for an entire pregnancy. Greater gains are thought to contribute to problems, but dieting to achieve weight loss during pregnancy may be harmful to fetal development.
44. (4) "Morning sickness" is a frequent problem for patients during the first few months of pregnancy. Receiving adequate rest and increasing carbohydrates in the diet help to reduce this problem.
45. (3) The physician is referring to the degree of dilation (or opening) of the cervix as expressed in centimeters. The term "cephalic presentation" refers to the part of the fetus (in this case the head) that is against the cervical opening and will be delivered first.
46. (2) True labor is characterized by regular forceful contractions, dilation and effacement of the cervix, and descent of the presenting part into the pelvis. Other options refer to signs of impending labor.
47. (1) The duration of labor for the first infant is approximately 14 hours. For subsequent pregnancies it may be shorter.
48. (3) Fetal heart tones are most accurately measured between contractions. During the early stages of labor, monitoring is generally done every 30 minutes.
49. (2) The normal range for fetal heart tones is 120 to 160 per minute. Rates higher or lower may indicate fetal distress.
50. (3) A prepared father (or other support person) should be allowed to assist in the mother's care. You, however, are responsible for monitoring the fetal heart tones and validating the pattern of contractions. Other options may be interpreted as discounting the father's preparation or avoiding assuming nursing responsibilities.
51. (2) This patient is now in the second stage of labor. All options listed include nursing responsibilities done during this time. Increasing the frequency of monitoring FHTs and maternal vital signs is most critical to maternal-infant well-being.
52. (4) Identification is legally validated by recording infant footprints and the mother's fingerprint. Other options listed may leave room for error.
53. (3) The third stage of labor is completed with the delivery of the placenta.
54. (4) A soft, boggy uterus must be massaged immediately to prevent postpartum hemorrhage. Other options lose time and may allow for greater blood loss.
55. (2) The first stool of the newborn is known as meconium and is blackish green and tarry.
56. (3) The eyes of the newborn may initially be puffy and red as a result of the delivery and instillation of silver nitrate solution. Gentle cleansing of exudate is sufficient intervention at this time. Purulent or odoriferous drainage should be reported.
57. (1) Air swallowed during feeding most frequently causes regurgitation, and the infant should be burped during and after feedings.
58. (4) Respirations in the newborn may be irregular and range from 32 to 48 per minute. Respiratory distress evidenced by abnormal rate, cyanosis, substernal retraction, and flaring of nares should be reported.
59. (2) Following birth the newborn's extremities may be bluish. This is known as acrocyanosis.
60. (1) The rooting reflex is demonstrated when the infant turns his or her head in the direction of the stroked cheek.
61. (3) Demand feeding is popular and allows the newborn to be fed at the time and in the amount he or she wishes.
62. (4) The nursing mother may have some breast engorgement as her milk comes in. Nursing the newborn will help to reduce this congestion.
63. (1) Lochia rubra occurs in the first few days postpartum. It is bright red and may have small clots.
64. (2) Lactation requires the same diet as is required during the latter half of pregnancy plus an additional ½ quart of milk and an additional 1000 calories daily.
65. (2) Normal elimination patterns may be reestablished by encouraging a well-balanced diet and ambulation. These actions help to reduce constipation and restore normal patterns.
66. (4) Rooming-in is a plan whereby the mother may have her infant at the bedside to care for as she is able to do.
67. (2) The gestational age of the premature newborn is 37 weeks or less. The low birth weight newborn is 5.516 pounds or less at birth. Option 1 is incorrect, as a normal newborn may be large for its gestational age. Option 4 refers to the newborn with a respiratory distress syndrome.
68. (2) The appearance of jaundice at birth or soon after is usually the initial sign to support suspected diagnosis of erythroblastosis fetalis.
69. (4) The premature newborn is covered in lanugo (fine downy hair), and eyelashes and eyebrows may be thin or absent at birth.

70. (4) Oxygen therapy for the newborn must be administered with great caution in order to prevent retrolental fibroplasia. This condition is caused by toxic levels of oxygen concentration and may result in blindness.
71. (2) Dysuria, or burning on urination, frequently is seen in patients with urinary tract infections. Options 1, 3, and 4 are less frequently associated with this problem.
72. (4) Diagnostic tests initially ordered to identify the cause of a patient's dysuria will include a urinalysis and culture and sensitivity. These would confirm presence of an infection, which is the most common cause.
73. (2) Renointestinal reflexes and anatomic proximity often cause the patient with disorders of the urinary tract to have gastrointestinal symptoms.
74. (1) *Escherichia coli* is the most common causative organism of infections of the urinary tract. This is associated with fecal contamination of the urinary meatus.
75. (3) Pyridium is a urinary antiseptic with analgesic properties commonly used in treatment of urinary tract infections. Sitz baths are often ordered to provide relief from dysuria.
76. (1) Pyelonephritis, an infection of the kidney, is commonly associated with obstruction of urinary drainage (stones, strictures), ureterovesical reflux, and ascending infections of the lower urinary tract.
77. (2) The dye used in performing an IVP is iodine based. The patient should be questioned concerning allergies to prevent an anaphylactic reaction during the test.
78. (3) Accurate monitoring of the patient's intake and output by the nurse is the response most complete in providing assessment data to the physician concerning renal infection.
79. (3) The patient has no history of strep throat, a condition which is frequently associated with glomerulonephritis. Frequent urinary tract infections are not known to cause glomerulonephritis. Options 1 and 2 are not related to this disease.
80. (2) Cystoscopic examination of the lower urinary tract allows the physician to inspect the structures as well as perform certain procedures (urethral dilation, removal of some stones, biopsy).
81. (4) Benign enlargement of the prostate is known to occur most frequently in men during the fourth and fifth decades of life.
82. (3) Patients having surgery involving the reproductive system are frequently anxious about possible loss of sexual functioning. The physician should discuss this with the patient before surgery.
83. (1) You should first obtain additional data to validate this patient's statement, as hypnotics may cause confusion and forgetfulness in the older persons.
84. (3) Obstruction of urinary drainage is frequently a cause of pain and bladder spasms in the patient following prostatic surgery. You should initially check the drainage system for patency.
85. (2) The presence of dark red drainage with numerous clots indicates postoperative bleeding and should be reported immediately.
86. (3) Signs of postoperative infection that would interfere with wound healing may initially be indicated by a temperature elevation (above 101°F or 38.2°C).
87. (2) Pro-Banthine is an anticholinergic agent used for its antispasmodic effects on the bladder.
88. (4) Rectal temperatures may cause trauma to the operative site and should be avoided in patients having prostatic surgery.
89. (2) Perineal exercises are known to increase muscle tone and help to restore continence. These are ordered by the physician.
90. (3) Learning can be validated by correct performance of the desired activity. Patients frequently can repeat directions but may not fully understand them.
91. (2) The incubation period for hepatitis A is 2 to 7 weeks. Other options indicate an incubation period that is either too brief or too long.
92. (3) Transmission of the hepatitis A virus is most frequently the result of ingestion of contaminated food, water, shellfish, and/or by close contact with carriers.
93. (4) The presence of the Australian antigen is found in the serum of patients with hepatitis B.
94. (3) The virus may be acquired by direct contact with urine and stools of infected persons. Gloves must be worn when handling excreta of infected persons.
95. (3) The incubation period for hepatitis B is 2 to 5 months. This is much longer than the 2 to 7 weeks incubation period for type A. Other options are false statements.
96. (2) Nursing care for hepatitis A is primarily supportive by encouraging optimal nutrition (high-carbohydrate, high-protein diet; forced fluids) and maintaining bed rest.
97. (1) B-complex vitamins are necessary for oxidation of food and energy production and are therefore essential for normal cell metabolism. B-complex vitamins are not stored in the body in the same manner as A and D vitamins. Options 3 and 4 indicate nutrients less critical to liver function and recovery.
98. (2) The diet for the patient with hepatitis is high in carbohydrates and high in proteins, with forced fluids. Vitamin supplements are also needed.
99. (4) The presence of bilirubin in the urine of patients with hepatitis causes it to appear brownish.
100. (3) Forgetfulness and other signs of confusion or disorientation may indicate progressing liver failure.
101. (4) This patient's abortion would be classified as spontaneous, as it is the result of physiologic processes and not manual or medical intervention.
102. (4) The legality of abortions performed after the third month of pregnancy is determined by individual state laws.

103. (2) Keeping an accurate count of saturated perineal pads can provide the most useful data for the physician to estimate blood loss. Option 4 is not a nursing action.
104. (3) Narcotics may be needed for pain relief. Effects on the fetus are not considered when the abortion is induced or inevitable.
105. (2) The patient experiencing an abortion often has feelings of guilt and blame herself for its occurrence. These feelings need to be expressed, and the nurse may provide reassurance and support.
106. (1) Placenta previa is a condition in which the placenta is attached to the lower portion of the uterus. It may be classified as complete or partial.
107. (2) Vaginal or hidden bleeding and fetal distress are problems seen in patients with placenta previa.
108. (3) Sudden severe abdominal pain occurs more frequently in patients with abruptio placentae. It is rare in placenta previa.
109. (3) Administration of an enema may stimulate uterine contractions and increase bleeding.
110. (3) General anesthesia for cesarean section is usually in the form of nitrous oxide. First and fourth options are regional forms of anesthesia. Scopolamine is no longer recommended and is not a form of general anesthesia.
111. (3) A cesarean section is abdominal surgery; thus the patient must be encouraged to turn, cough, and deep breathe to prevent atelectasis.
112. (2) Each mother awakening in the recovery room is usually initially concerned about the health of her baby and wants to know its gender.
113. (4) Early and frequent ambulation helps to stimulate the return of peristalsis and expulsion of flatus. Narcotics may reduce peristalsis. Carbonated beverages may increase gas formation.
114. (2) A temperature elevation to 101°F or 38.2°C may indicate an infection.
115. (2) Staphylococci and streptococci are the organisms most frequently associated with postpartum (puerperal) infection.
116. (4) Normally occurring (physiologic) weight loss is expected but should not exceed 9% of birth rate. This infant's weight loss is within acceptable limits.
117. (2) Response number 2 provides an explanation to the patient and does not discount this mother's inquiry.
118. (3) Parent-infant bonding occurs as a result of contact between the infant and parents. The nurse may facilitate this bonding by encouraging parents to hold and care for their infant.
119. (4) Syntocinon is a synthetic form of Pitocin and is used to induce labor as well as promote contracting of the uterus following delivery.
120. (1) AquaMephyton is a medication administered to prevent hemorrhage in the neonate until the liver is able to form prothrombin.

GLOSSARY

The practical nurse needs to learn many new words in order to intelligently understand the physician, the professional nurse, and others. This can be done by adding some new vocabulary words every day and by finding out the meaning of every unfamiliar word or phrase. The nurse should have access to a nursing or medical dictionary as well as to a general dictionary. As a rule, these books are found on every ward.

The following list of prefixes (forms at the beginning of words) and suffixes (forms at the end of words) should help in understanding new scientific words.

The vocabulary that follows is not intended to take the place of a dictionary but is planned for quick reference and includes the most common words with which the practical nurse should be familiar.

PREFIXES

adeno- glandular (adenoma, glandular tumor)
auto- self (autoinfection, infecting one part of body from another)
brady- slow (bradycardia, slow heart rate)
contra- against, opposite (contraindication, condition forbidding the use of certain treatment or medicine)
dextro- to the right (dextrocardia, location of the heart in the right hemithorax)
dys- abnormal, bad, difficult, painful, unlike (dyspnea, difficult respiration)
endo- within (endocrine, secreting within)
extra- outside of, in addition to (extrapleural, outside the pleural cavity)
hemi- half (hemiplegia, paralysis of one side of body)
hyper- above, increased, beyond (hypertension, high blood pressure)
hypo- under, decreased (hypotension, low blood pressure)
infra- below, beneath (infrasternal, below the sternum)
inter- between (interdental, between the teeth)
intra- within (intraperitoneal, within the sac of the peritoneum)
intro- in, within, into (introvert, one whose thoughts are turned inward)
mal- bad, poor (malnutrition, poor nutrition)
micro- small (microorganism, small organism)
multi- many (multipara, woman having two or more pregnancies)
ortho- straight, normal (orthodontia, dentistry dealing with straightening of teeth and prevention of deformities)
pachy- thick (pachyderma, thickening of skin)
patho- disease (pathology, science dealing with causes of and changes caused by disease)
per- through (percutaneous, through the skin)
peri- around (perinephric, the tissue surrounding the kidney)
poly- much, many (polydipsia, excessive thirst)
post- after (postoperative, after operation)
pre- before (preoperative, before operation)
pro- before (prognosis, forecast of the probable course or outcome of disease)
pseudo- false (pseudocrisis, temporary fall in temperature mistakenly taken for true crisis)
psycho- the mind (psychiatry, branch of medicine dealing with study, treatment, and prevention of mental illness)
pyo- pus (pyuria, pus in urine)
retro- backward (retroperitoneal, behind the peritoneum)
sclero- hard, hardening (scleroderma, hardening of the connective tissues)
septic- poison, putrefaction (septicemia, poison in blood)
steno- narrow, constricted (aortic stenosis, narrowing of valve from ventricle to aorta)
sub- under, beneath (subclavian, below or beneath the clavicle)
supra- above (suprarenal, above the kidney)
tachy- fast (tachycardia, fast heart rate)
thermo- heat (thermometer, instrument for measuring heat)
tox- poison (toxemia, poisons or toxins in blood)

SUFFIXES

-algia pain (neuralgia, pain in nerve)
-cele tumor, swelling (rectocele, rectum protruding into vaginal wall)
-cide destructive, killing (germicide, substance capable of killing germs)
-clysis injection (proctoclysis, introduction of fluid into rectum)
-ectasis dilation, extension (bronchiectasis, dilation of bronchi)
-ectomy surgical removal of (appendectomy, removal of appendix)
-emia blood (uremia, blood in urine)
-iatric practice of healing (geriatric, branch of medicine dealing with aged)
-itis inflammation of (appendicitis, inflammation of appendix)
-logy science of, study of (dermatology, study of diseases of skin)
-oma tumor (myoma, tumor of muscle tissue)
-osis disease, condition, excess (neurosis, emotional disorder)
-ostomy to form an opening or outlet (gastrostomy, opening into stomach)
-pathy disease (neuropathy, disease of the nervous system)
-phobia fear (claustrophobia, fear of being confined)
-phylaxis protection (prophylaxis, protection from disease)
-plegia paralysis (hemiplegia, paralysis of one side of body)
-rhea flow (diarrhea, excessive discharge from bowels)
-sclerosis hardening (arteriosclerosis, hardening of arteries)
-scope instrument for visual examination (bronchoscope, instrument for examining bronchi)
-tomy incision of (nephrotomy, incision into renal pelvis)

VOCABULARY

abnormal deviation from the normal
abortion explusion of the fetus from the uterus before the twenty-eighth week of pregnancy
abrasion scraping off of skin
abrasive sustance used for abrasion
abscess collection of pus in a cavity; it is often distinguished according to location, such as brain abscess or breast abscess, or by causative organism, such as tuberculous abscess
absorb to take up or suck up, as with a sponge
absorbent medicine or dressing that absorbs or promotes taking up of fluid
acceleration increase or quickening of rate, as in the respiration or pulse
accreditation attainment of certain standards with approval granted by recognized authority
acid class of chemical compounds that have a sour taste, turn blue litmus red, and unite with bases to form salts
acidosis increased acidity of the blood
acquired developed after birth in contrast to congenital
acuity clearness or sharpness; it is usually applied to vision, such as visual acuity
acute sudden; acute illness often have severe symptoms and is of short duration
addiction strong emotional and physiologic dependence on alcohol or a drug, which has progressed beyond voluntary control
adenitis inflammation of a gland
adhesion abnormal growing together of tissues in the body; it is usually the result of inflammation or injury
adolescence age between puberty and maturity
aerosol solution or medication that can be atomized, that is, given in spray form
affect general feeling, tone, or emotion
afterbirth placenta, umbilical cord, and fetal and maternal membranes that are expelled from the uterus after the child is born
albumin protein found in nearly every animal tissue and fluid
algae a group of plants living in the water ranging from microscopic cells to large fronds
allergens various substances to which some individuals are hypersensitive
allergy sensitivity to certain substances that do not normally elicit a hypersensitive reaction
alleviate to make easier, to lighten, or to lessen
alopecia loss of hair
ambulatory able to walk; it refers to a patient not confined to bed
amenorrhea unusual absence of menstruation
amnesia loss of memory
amputation surgical removal of any part of the body
analgesia loss of sensitivity to pain, without loss of consciousness
anaphylaxis severe, generalized reaction, resulting from hypersensitivity; it may result from injection of substances containing horse serum or from penicillin
anastomosis a union in which two parts are joined together surgically
anemia condition caused by reduction in the red blood cells, deficiency in the hemoglobin content of the red blood cells, or both
anesthesia loss of sensation or sensibility to pain
anesthetic drug used to induce anesthesia
aneurysm saclike bulge of a blood vessel
ankylosis abnormal stiffness of a joint that usually moves freely
anorexia lack of appetite for food
antagonism opposition or resistance
anterior toward the front
anthelmintic medicine that destroys or removes worms
antibody specific substance in the blood that overcomes or neutralizes foreign bodies
antidepressant a drug that modifies or relieves the state of depression

antidote medicine used to counteract poisions
antiemetic medicine used to prevent or relieve nausea and vomiting
antigen substance that stimulates the body to produce antibodies against an allergen
antihistaminic drug that relieves the symptoms of a histamine reaction
antipyretic medicine used to reduce fever
anuria failure of kidneys to secrete urine
anxiety apprehension, tension, or uneasiness associated with anticipation of danger
aortitis inflammation of the aorta
apathy a state of indifference in a situation that would ordinarily arouse some response
aperture orifice or opening
aphagia inability to swallow
aphasia inability to express oneself in speech or writing
aphonia inability to produce voice sounds
apnea lack of breathing
apoplexy stroke or paralysis
apprehension anxiety or fear
areola dark area around a central point, such as the nipple
arrhythmia abnormality in rhythm of the heart
ascites accumulation of fluid in the peritoneal cavity
aseptic freedom from bacteria or microorganisms
asphyxia suffocation
aspirate withdrawing of liquids, suction, or breathing in
assimilative that which causes absorption
asthmatic one suffering from asthma
astigmatism an error or refraction caused by abnormality in the curvature of the cornea or lens
ataxia lack of muscle coordination
atherosclerosis formation of fibrous tissue along the walls of the arteries, causing them to harden
atonic lack of strength or tone, usually applied to muscles
atresia narrowing or lack of a normal opening
atrophy wasting away or decrease in the size of any part
attitude feeling or opinion; position of the body
auscultation listening for body sounds; it is used in diagnosis
autopsy examination of a body after death
auxiliary helping, assisting, or aiding
azotemia presence of excessive nitrogen compounds in the blood
bacteremia presence of bacteria in the blood
bacteria one-cell organism (germ)
bacteriuria presence of bacteria in the urine
benign not malignant or not recurrent
bilateral appearing on both sides of the body
biliary pertaining to the liver, gallbladder, and vessels that carry their secretions
biopsy removal of a piece of tissue from the body for microscopic examination
booster an additional dose of an immunologic agent to potentiate initial immunization
bradycardia unusually slow heart rate
Braxton Hicks' contractions intermittent uterine contractions during pregnancy
bronchoscope an instrument for examining the bronchi
bronchoscopy examination of bronchi by way of the bronchoscope
buccal referring to the cheek
bursitis inflammation of the bursa; subdeltoid is most commonly affected
calculus stone formed in any part of the body
callus thickening and hardening of the skin
calorie unit of heat required to raise 1 kg of water by 1°C
cancer abnormal growth of body cells
carcinoma type of cancer; a malignant epithelial tumor
cardiac pertaining to the heart
cathartic medicine to produce bowel movement
cerumen ear wax
Chadwick's sign violet color of the vaginal mucous membrane during pregnancy
chalazion a cyst or tumor on the eyelid caused by an infection of a sebaceous gland
chancre the primary lesion of syphilis
cheilosis a fissured condition of the lips and corners of the mouth
chemotherapy treatment of diseases by chemical compounds
chestmobile mobile chest clinic for taking x-ray films, which travels from one community to another
chill severe shivering or shaking; often first symptom of infection
chiropodist *see* podiatrist
cholecystitis inflammation of the gallbladder
chorea disease with frequent, involuntary, purposeless movements
cirrhosis degeneration and chronic inflammation of the tissue of an organ
climacteric menopause
coma extreme unconsciousness from which the patient cannot be aroused
comedones blackheads
commitment legal assignment of mentally ill patient to a facility for care and treatment
communicable infections or diseases that can be passed from one person to another
condyloma an elevated, wartlike skin lesion
congenital condition present at birth
constipation condition in which defecation takes place infrequently and with difficulty
contamination soiling with infected material or with anything that may carry a potential infection
contraception birth control; means of regulating conception
contraindication condition that forbids particular course of treatment
convalescence period of recovery after an illness
coryza acute inflammation of the nasal membrane

counterirritant medicine that produces irritation to relieve inflammation
crisis turning point in a disease or paroxysmal intensification of symptoms during a disease course
cyanosis blueness of the skin as a result of lack of oxygen in the blood
cystitis inflammation of the bladder
cytoscopy examination of the bladder with aid of a cystoscope (a hollow telescopic instrument)
debility loss of strength; weakness
debridement procedure of removing infected or necrotic tissue from a wound, such as in burns before skin grafting
decubitus bedsore or pressure sore
defecation expulsion of feces, or bowel movement
defect imperfection
deformity physical malformation; disfigurement
degeneration falling or deteriorating to a lower level
dehydration removal of water; dehydration results in the body when fluid losses are greater than fluid intake
delirium a state of mental disturbance characterized by confusion, disordered speech, and often hallucinations
delirium tremens delirium induced by prolonged and excessive use of alcohol
delusion false belief that cannot be corrected by argument or appeal to reason
dementia state characterized by serious mental impairment and deterioration
demulcent medicine with soothing effect on skin or mucous membrane
dental pertaining to the teeth
denture artificial set of teeth
deodorant substance that conceals or destroys odors
depressant medicine that diminishes activity
dermatitis inflammation of the skin
dermatology branch of medicine specializing in the diagnosis and treatment of skin diseases
detergent cleansing solution or lotion
dextrocardia congenital heart condition in which heart is in right instead of left side of chest
diagnosis art and science of differentiating one disease from another
dialysis separation of certain substances from the blood or urine; use of artificial kidney is one form of dialysis
diapedesis the passage of blood corpuscles through intact vessel walls
diaphoresis profuse perspiration
diarrhea watery, unformed stools at frequent periods
diastole refilling phase of the heart cycle, occurring alternately with systole or discharging phase
digitalization administration of digitalis until a therapeutic effect has been obtained
dilation stretching or enlargement of a cavity or opening
discharge unusual or pathologic secretion from any of the body openings or from a wound
disease any abnormality of the structure or function of the body
disinfect to destroy disease-producing organisms or to prevent their growth
disorientation loss of awareness in relation to time, place, or person
dissection separation of tissue, usually for study or investigation
distal farthest from the point of attachment
distention enlargement
diuresis increased secretion of urine
diversional amusing or relaxing
donor individual who furnishes blood or other kinds of tissues to another person
dorsal toward the back
douche stream of water or fluid directed against the surface of the body or into a body cavity
drastic a powerful cathartic
droplet nuclei very small particles containing disease-producing organisms that dry and remain in the air to be carried by air movement
dropsy unusualy collection of fluid in the body tissues or cavities; edema
dyscrasias term applied to a group of blood diseases including anemia and leukemia
dysfunction unusual functioning of an organ
dysmenorrhea painful menstruation
dyspareunia painful intercourse
dyspepsia difficulty with digestion
dyspnea shortness of breath
dystrophy defective development, usually referring to the muscles
dysuria painful or difficult urination
ecchymosis escape of a large amount of blood into the tissue; it may result from a bruise or from some types of surgery
eclampsia convulsions that appear toward the end of pregnancy caused by toxemia of pregnancy
edema abnormal collection of fluid in the tissue
effacement thinning and shortening of the cervix during labor
electrocardiograph instrument that records electrical current in the heart, used in the diagnosis of cardiac disorders
electroencephalograph apparatus for recording brain waves
electrolytes mineral salts normally present in solution in the body; in case of loss, as in severe diarrhea or prolonged vomiting, electrolytes may be replaced artifically by intravenous infusion
emaciation loss of weight; it usually refers to the wasting away in certain diseases
embolus substance in the blood that plugs a blood vessel; a moving blood clot
emmenagogue medicine used to induce menstruation
emphysema swelling caused by air accumulated in the tissues, particularly the lungs
empyema collection of pus in a cavity

encephalitis inflammation of the brain
endocrine referring to the glands of internal secretion
enteritis inflammation of the intestines
enucleation surgical removal of the eyeball
enuresis incontinence of urine, usually at night
environment all that surrounds the individual; milieu
epidemic contagious disease spreading to many individuals in a community
epilepsy neurologic disease characterized by convulsions and loss of consciousness, which is caused by disturbance in electrical activity of the brain
epistaxis nosebleed
eructation forced expulsion of air from the stomach (belching)
eruption any skin rash
erythema unusual redness of the skin
escharotic a corrosive or caustic agent
esophagoscope lighted instrument for examining the esophagus
esthetic pertaining to beauty
ethics study of conduct, including moral standards and evaluation of right from wrong
etiology study of the causes of disease
euphoria exaggerated feeling of physical and emotional well-being
euthanasia death without suffering, ''mercy killing''
evacuation defecation, or emptying of the bowels
exacerbation increase in severity of a disease or its symptoms
excoriated removal of pieces of the skin; scraped or scratched
excoriation any superficial loss of substance
excreta waste materials discharged from intestine
expectorate to spit
expiration exhaling; sometimes used to refer to death
exudate discharge through tissues or pores
facies pertaining to the face or a specific surface of a body part
febrile pertaining to a fever
feces waste material from the bowels
fester sore with pus; to produce pus
fetus unborn child after the beginning of the second month of pregnancy
fever unusually high body temperature
fibrous composed of or containing fibers
flaccid flabby or limp
flatulence distention of intestines or stomach by gas
flatus gas or air in the digestive tract
fluoroscope x-ray instrument consisting of a screen, which is used to examine the body internally
fluoroscopy examination by means of a fluoroscope
formula prescription or recipe; it often refers to feeding of infants
foster home home in which a child is placed for care
fracture break in the continuity of a bone caused by trauma, twisting, or disease resulting in loss of calcium in the bone
- **closed (simple)** one in which there is no wound or break in the skin
- **Colles'** break in the lower end of the radius
- **comminuted** one in which two or more communicating breaks divide the bone into two or more fragments
- **compound** open fracture; bone protrudes through skin
- **greenstick** incomplete fracture of a long bone, splitting the shaft
- **pathologic** occurring in diseased bone with slight or no trauma
- **Pott's** fracture of the lower part of the fibula

frontal pertaining to the upper, anterior surface
fumigation destruction of microorganisms, insects, or animals by gases
functional referring to or affecting a function, as contrasted to a structure
functional disorder a disorder in which organic change is not apparent
fungus spongy plant growth
fusion joining together to make solid, as in spinal fusion
gait typical characteristic method of walking; certain diseases leave an individual with a certain gait, such as hemiplegic and tabetic
gangrene destruction or death of tissues in the body
gargle solution used for rinsing or cleaning out the mouth and throat
gastric relating to the stomach
gastritis inflammation of the stomach
gastroscope instrument for examining the interior of the stomach
gastroscopy examination of the stomach using the gastroscope
gavage feeding through a tube into the stomach
Geiger counter device used to measure amount of radioactivity; it may be used when radioactive isotopes are used for diagnosis or treatment
general paresis a psychosis associated with organic disease of the central nervous sytem, resulting from chronic syphilitic infection
geriatrics specialized branch of medicine dealing with older persons and their diseases
germicide physical or chemical agent that destroys microorganisms
gestation development of the individual in the uterus from the time of fertilization to birth; length of time for human beings is 9 months
gingivitis inflammation of the gums
glossitis inflammation of the tongue
glycosuria presence of excessive amounts of glucose in the urine
graft piece of skin or any other tissue transplanted to a different part of the body

granulation tissue that develops in a wound when it is healing
gynecology specialized branch of medicine dealing with diseases of women
hallucination an imaginary sense perception when there has been no external stimulus, such as seeing objects that do not exist
heartburn (pyrosis) feeling of fullness and burning in the esophagus and stomach, usually accompanied by the belching of gas
heliotherapy healing of disease by exposing to the sun's rays
hematemesis vomiting of blood
hematocrit examination of blood to measure the volume of erythrocytes and plasma
hematuria presence of blood in the urine
hemiplegia paralysis of one side of the body
hemoptysis spitting of blood
hemorrhage abnormal escape of blood from blood vessels
hemorrhoid varicosity in the rectum, sometimes referred to as a pile
hemothorax presence of blood in the pleural cavity
heredity passing of physical and mental characteristics from parents to children
hernia protrusion of an organ or part of an organ through an abnormal opening; it usually refers to the passage of part of the intestines through a weak place in the abdominal muscles
hiccough uncontrolled spasmodic contraction of the diaphragm, caused by irritation of the phrenic nerve
humidity amount of moisture in the air
hydrops abnormal accumulation of serious fluid in the tissues or body cavity
hydrotherapy the external use of water as a form of therapy
hydrothorax accumulation of fluid in the pleural cavity
hyperalgesia unusual sensitivity to pain
hyperemia excessive blood associated with vasodilation caused by inflammation of any part of the body
hyperopia farsightedness
hyperthyroidism disease caused by excessive amount of thyroid secretion
hypertrophy unusual enlargement or growth of an organ or part of the body
hypnosis altered state of conscious awareness induced in a suggestible subject
hypochondriac individual who is unusually concerned about his or her health
hypodermic administered under the skin; subcutaneous
hypodermoclysis injection of fluid into the subcutaneous tissue
hypoglycemia unusually low blood glucose
hypothermia procedure for lowering the body temperature; it is used as an adjunct in anesthesia for certain kinds of surgery
hypothyroidism disease caused by deficient amount of secretion from the thyroid gland
hypoxia decrease of oxygen in the tissues
hysterectomy removal of the uterus
icterus jaundice
illusion misinterpretation of an external stimulus
immune protection against disease by immunization or vaccination
immunity the ability to overcome and resist infection
incise to cut
incontinent unable to control natural excretion of urine and feces
incubation time that elapses between exposure to an infectious disease and the onset of the disease
infection invasion of the body or part of the body by microorganisms or parasites so that a disease condition results
inferior toward the lower aspect
infusion injection of solution into vein for therapeutic purpose
inflammation reaction of tissue to infection or injury, usually characterized by pain, swelling, and heat
inhalation breathing in
inherent existing inseparably in something else; innate; implanted by nature
inhibition checking or restraining an act or function
injection fluid forced into the body or a body cavity
inoculate transfer, into the body, of viruses or bacteria that cause disease
insanity legal term implying inability to know right from wrong (denotes mental incompetence)
insight self-understanding; a reasonably accurate self-judgment
insomnia inability to sleep
inspection when used during patient examination, it includes visual examination by the physician or nurse
intermittent having periods of cessation of activity
intubation inserting a tube
inunction rubbing an ointment or lotion on the skin
involuntary not controlled consciously
irradiation treating of disease by applying various rays—x rays, radium rays, or ultraviolet rays
irrigation washing of body cavity with a medicated solution or with water
irritant anything that causes increased activity or sensitiveness of any part of the body
isolation separation of individuals from others; it usually refers to individuals with contagious diseases
jaundice accumulation of bile pigments in the blood, resulting in yellow coloring of the skin and the sclera of the eyes
keratitis inflammation of the cornea
laceration wound caused by tearing of the tissues
lacrimal referring to tears
lactation secretion of milk
laryngectomy removal of the larynx
laryngoscope instrument for examining the larynx

laryngoscopy examination of the larynx by means of the laryngoscope
latent referring to a disease that is inactive but still present
lateral pertaining to the side of the body
lavage washing out of a cavity; it usually refers to the stomach
lesion evidence of change in structure or function of an organ or part of the body because of disease
lethargy sleepiness or inactivity of mental origin
leukemia malignant blood disease that is often fatal; possible cure may be near because of scientific research
leukocytes white blood cells
leukorrhea yellowish or whitish discharge from the vagina
license to permit to practice an occupation or profession
lie relationship of the long axis of the fetus to the long axis of the mother
ligature various kinds of suture material used to tie blood vessels during a surgical procedure
lipoma tumor of fatty tissue
lochia vaginal discharge after childbirth
lymphoma malignant tumor in lymphoid gland
macule a discolored lesion of the skin that is not elevated
malignancy any condition that is likely to become worse and cause death; it often refers to cancer
malingering deliberate pretense of an illness that does not exist
malpractice professional negligence or treating a patient in such a way that he or she is injured, usually by treating in contradiction to accepted rules
mania a feeling state in which one is extremely overactive
manic-depressive psychosis a class of mental disorders in which the most dramatic symptoms occur in mood disturbances
massage physiotherapy characterized by manipulation of the tissues
mastitis inflammation of the tissues of the breast
masturbation stimulation of the genitals, resulting in excitement similar to that of coitus
maturation process of maturing
meatus an opening or passage
meconium first fecal matter discharged by newborns
medial toward the midline of the body
mediastinum space in the thoracic cavity between the lungs, containing the heart
menarche first menstrual period
meningitis inflammation of the meninges, that is, the membrane covering the brain and spinal cord
menopause time in women when menstruation ceases; other terms are "climacteric" and "change of life"
menorrhagia excessive menstrual bleeding
menstruation normal periodic discharge of blood from the uterus beginning at puberty and ending in the menopause
metabolism all of the processes involved in the body in building up and destroying the living protoplasm
metastasis transfer of disease from one part of the body to another; it usually refers to cancer
metrorrhagia irregular bleeding from the uterus
microbe pathologic bacterium
microorganism any organism, plant, or animal that can be studied only with the aid of a microscope
micturition discharge of urine from the bladder
midsagittal plane that divides the body into equal left and right portions
migraine severe headaches often associated with stomach and mental disturbances
milieu the total environment, emotional and physical
miscarriage expulsion of fetus from the uterus before it is capable of living outside the uterus
mores fixed customs
mucus fluid secreted by the mucous glands
mutism lack of ability to speak
myopia nearsightedness
negativism a generalized resistance to any outside suggestions or requests
neuralgia paroxysms of pain along the course of nerves
neurosis (psychoneurosis) functional disorder in which the patient feels anxiety; loss of contact with reality is rare
nocturia excessive urination at night
nystagmus continuous involuntary movement of the eyeball
obesity condition in which there is an excessive amount of fat in the body
occupational therapy treating a patient by use of mental and physical activities chosen for their therapeutic value
ointment fatty medicated mixture for external use
oliguria lessened urinary output
ophthalmia inflammation of the eye
opiate drug derived from opium, such as codeine, heroin, and morphine
optimal best or favorable
organic pertaining to, composed of, containing, or produced by organs
orthopedics specialized branch of medicine dealing with the treatment of diseases of bones, muscles, and joints
orthopnea difficulty in breathing, relieved only by sitting in an upright position
palliative providing only temporary relief
pallor paleness or absence of normal skin color
palpation feeling the surface of the body with the hand or fingertips; it is used in physical examination
palpitation rapid heartbeat occurring in cardiac diseases or after vigorous exercise
Papanicolaou's smear test (Pap test) cytologic test to detect cancer cells
papule a solid, elevated skin lesion
paracentesis removal of fluid from a body cavity for diagnostic or therapeutic reasons
paralysis impairment or loss of muscle function or feeling

paraplegia paralysis of both legs or the lower part of the body
parasite an organism that lives in or on another organism
paroxysm sudden attack that may recur at periodic intervals
passive suffering without resistance; submissive
pasteurization destroying or inhibiting the growth of disease-causing microorganisms; in liquids, this is done by using heat for a given period of time
patency freely open to allow passage through
pathogenic ability to cause disease
pathology science dealing with the causes of disease and the changes in the structure and function of the body as a result of disease
pediatrician physician specializing in diseases of children
pediculosis infestation with lice
percussion tapping parts of body in order to determine their condition by the sound obtained (whether filled with air, fluid, etc.)
pessary device to support the uterus in a normal position
petechia small, pinpoint hemorrhage into the skin
phagocytosis the engulfment of solid particles by tissue cells
pharmacology science dealing with drugs and their action
phimosis atresia of the prepuce so that the foreskin cannot be retracted
phlegm mucus secreted by the nose and throat
phobia persistent, unrealistic fear of an object, situation, or act
physical therapy treatment of disease by physical means, such as massage or baths or both
placebo substance that has no medicinal effect but is given as if it were a medicine in order to please the patient
pneumothorax presence of air in the pleural cavity
podiatrist one specializing in care of the feet; formerly referred to as a chiropodist
pollinosis allergic reaction caused by pollen
polydipsia excessive thirst
polymenorrhea abnormally frequent menstruation
polyphagia abnormal craving for food
polyuria passing abnormally large quantities of urine
position manner of arrangement; in obstetrics refers to situation (occiput, chin, sacrum) of fetus in the pelvis
posterior toward the back
predisposition increased susceptibility to disease
premature appearing before the regular or appointed time
presbyopia impaired vision as a result of the body's aging process
presentation part of the fetus that enters the pelvis first; it can be cephalic, breech, or shoulder
proctoclysis (Murphy drip) giving fluid by rectum
proctoscope instrument for examining the inside of the rectum
proctoscopy examination of the rectum by proctoscope
prognosis probable outcome of a disease
prone lying face down
prophylaxis preventing disease
prosthesis artificial replacement of a body part, such as artificial limb or dentures
proximal nearest the point of attachment
pruritus itching of the skin that accompanies some diseases
psychiatry branch of medicine dealing with the area of mental health and mental illness
psychosis a mental disorder in which the patient has marked disturbance of personality functioning. Patient usually has some loss of contact with reality
psychotherapy the planned measures undertaken to restore a patient to mental health
psychotic suffering from a psychosis
ptosis falling down of an organ from its normal position
puberty age when the individual matures sexually
puerpera woman who has recently been delivered
puerperium time after labor; it usually refers to the period from the end of labor to the involution of the uterus, usually about 6 weeks
purulent producing or containing pus
pus serous matter produced as a result of inflammation
pustulant an agent capable of causing pustulation
pustule a skin lesion containing pus
pyelitis inflammation of the pelvis of the kidney
pyemia presence of bacteria in blood
pyogenic pus-forming or capable of forming pus
pyuria presence of pus in the urine
quarantine limiting of the movement of persons who have been exposed to contagious diseases
quickening sensation produced by movement of the fetus in the uterus, usually felt first at the end of the fifth month of pregnancy
radiate to send out as rays
radiology branch of medicine dealing with diagnostic and treatment use of radium and x-ray radiation
radiopaque cannot be penetrated by radiation
rapport sympathetic and harmonious relationship with another individual
recumbent lying down
recuperation act of recovering from an illness
recurrence return of symptoms after improvement
referred pain pain from an affected organ felt in another part of the body
reflex action unconscious movements one makes
regurgitation abnormal backflow of fluids, such as the return of stomach contents into the oral cavity
rehabilitation retraining or reeducation of a patient to all the ability he or she has
reinfection being infected by the same organism during the convalescent period or after recovery
remission temporary disappearance of symptoms of a disease
resection partial surgical removal of an organ
residual part which remains
retention failure to eliminate fluid or other substances; it is most commonly used when referring to urine

rhythm normal contraction of heart, bladder, or other organs; also refers to method of birth control
rickets disease of bones caused by lack of vitamin D that is most common in infants and children
rickettsia rod-shaped or round microorganism found in tissue cells of lice, fleas, ticks, and mites
rigidity stiffness; it usually refers to stiffness of muscles
rigor severe chill
rigor mortis rigidity of the muscles after death
rubefacient ointment or lotion that causes reddening of the skin
rumination regurgitation of food into the mouth where it is swallowed again
rupture forcible tearing or breaking down of the tissue; it usually refers to a hernia
salivation secretion of saliva
salpingitis inflammation of the fallopian tube
sanatorium institution or hospital for the treatment of patients suffering from chronic diseases, usually mental illness or tuberculosis
sarcoma type of tumor developing from bone and connective tissue
sclerosis hardening of the tissue
scoliosis lateral curvature of the spine
seborrhea unusually oily skin
sebum fatty secretion of the sebaceous glands
secretion substance having different properties from the tissue from which it is derived
sedative drug capable of inducing calmness, rest, and relaxation
seizure convulsion
semen fluid discharged by the male at ejaculation, which consists of spermatazoa and other glandular secretions
senescence process of aging
senile referring to senility
senility old age
sensation conscious awareness of stimuli affecting the sensory organs
sepsis presence of pathogenic organisms or toxins in the blood or tissues
septicemia presence in the bloodstream of toxins causing general poisoning
septum bridge dividing two cavities
serology branch of medicine dealing with the examination of serum
serum fluid resulting when blood coagulates
silicosis disease of the lungs caused by inhalation of dust, sand, and so on
sinus cavity or space within certain bones
skin grafts skin replacing damaged skin that has been destroyed by injury or disease
solute substance that is dissolved in a liquid to form a solution
solvent the liquid in which another substance is dissolved to form a solution
somnambulism sleepwalking
soporific drug that produces sleep
sordes accumulation of secretion about the teeth and mouth
spasm involuntary contraction of the muscles
specimen sample of urine, blood, or sputum taken for examination
sphygmomanometer instrument for measuring blood pressure
stasis slowing of the normal flow
station during labor, the depth to which the presenting part has descended into the pelvis
sterilization process of rendering sterile
stethoscope instrument for conveying sounds to the ear, usually used in the examination of heart and lungs
stillbirth birth of a dead fetus
stoma opening into the skin; it may be artificial or normal
strabismus eye disorder in which the optic axes cannot be directed to the same point
strangury slow and painful urination
stricture narrowing of canal or duct, such as the esophagus
stroke popular name given to cerebral hemorrhage or apoplexy
stupor loss of consciousness or marked reduction in consciousness
subacute somewhat acute; between acute and chronic
superior toward the top or head
suppository solid medicated substance for insertion into certain body openings
suppuration formation of pus
surgery branch of medicine dealing with treatment of conditions by operative means
symptom abnormal function or sensation indicating the presence of disease
syncope (fainting) temporary loss of consciousness
syndrome a group of symptoms characteristic of certain diseases
synthetic artificially produced
systole discharging or contracting phase of the heart cycle; it occurs alternately with the diastole, the relaxing or refilling phrase
tachycardia unusually high pulse rate
technician one who is specifically trained to carry out certain duties
technique method of carrying out a procedure, test, or operation
tension mental stress or pressure often accompanied by muscle tenseness
therapeutic referring to treatment activities
therapeutics special branch of medicine dealing with the treatment of disease
therapy treatment of disease
thoracoscope instrument for visual examination of the pneumothorax
thrombosis partial or complete closing of a blood vessel by a blood clot

thrombus blood clot forming within a blood vessel
tourniquet device for constricting blood vessels in order to control bleeding; usually a strip of material or rubber tubing is used
toxemia poisonous substances present in the blood
toxicology branch of medicine dealing with poisons: their sources, action, and treatment
toxin any poisonous substance
toxoid material used to immunize persons against a certain disease
tranquilizer (tranquilizing drug) a drug producing a calming effect by relieving anxiety, tension, and agitation
transfusion transfer of blood from one person to another
transverse a plane that divides the body into superior and inferior portions
trauma wound or injury
tumor any swelling developing from the tissue by growing independently of it and serving no useful purpose
tympanous distention of the abdominal cavity or the intestines by gas
ulcer local destruction of tissue
uremia disease resulting from the failure of the kidney to excrete normal urinary contents, which collect in the body and cause a toxic condition
urinalysis examination of the urine
urination (voiding) discharge of urine from the bladder
urology branch of medicine that deals with diseases of the urinary system
urticaria (hives) irritation of the skin, usually caused by allergy
vaccination innoculation for the purpose of developing active immunization against disease
varicosity dilated vein
venereal refers to diseases transmitted as a result of direct sexual contact
venesection (phlebotomy) opening of a vein to obtain blood
venipuncture puncture of a vein with a needle
ventral pertaining to the abdominal surface
vertigo feeling of movement of self or objects when no movement is present
vesicant an agent capable of producing blisters
vesicle an elevated skin lesion containing pus
virulence power of an organism to produce disease
virus minute microorganism too small to be seen under an ordinary microscope
vitamins chemical substances present in food and essential for normal growth and development
vocalize to form into voice or to utter
voiding passing of urine from the bladdder
volatile oil oil that evaporates quickly
vomiting forced explusion of material from the stomach
vomitus material forced from the stomach by vomiting
weaning changing infant feeding from the breast or bottle to cup
wen a saclike cyst
Young's rule formula for calculating dosages for children:

$$\frac{\text{age in years}}{\text{age} + 12} \times \text{Adult dose}$$

COMMON ABBREVIATIONS

$\overline{\text{aa}}$ of each
a.c. before meals
ad lib. as desired, at pleasure
alt. dieb. every other day
alt. hor. every other hour
alt. noc. every other night
amp. ampule
amt. amount
Aq. water
b.i.d. twice a day
BP blood pressure
C or cent centigrade, Celsius
c̄ with
cap. capsule
cc cubic centimeter
cm centimeter
cont. continuously
dos. a dose
dr or ʒ dram, drams
ECG electrocardiogram
EEG electroencephalogram
EKG electrocardiogram
elix. elixir
ext. extract
F or Fahr Fahrenheit
fl dr fluid dram
fl oz fluid ounce
g or gm gram
gr grain
gtt drop
gtts drops
h or hr hour
H or hypo. hypodermic
h.s. before sleep; at bedtime
IM intramuscular
IV intravenous
kg kilogram
m or ♏ minim
mg milligram
ml milliliter
noct. night
NPO nothing by mouth
o.d. every day
o.m. every morning
o.n. every night
oz or ℥ ounce
p.c. after meals

PO by mouth
p.r.n. whenever necessary
PSP phenolsulfonphthalein test
pulv. powder
q.d. every day
q.h. every hour
q. hr. every hour
q. 2hr. every 2 hours
q. 3hr. every 3 hours
q.i.d. four times a day
q.o.d. every other day
q.o.n. every other night
q.s. as much as will suffice
℞ take
Sol. solution
S.O.S. one dose only
ss or $\overline{\text{ss}}$ one half
Stat immediately
subq. subcutaneously
tab. tablet
tbsp tablespoon
t.i.d. three times a day
t.i.n. three times a night
TPR temperature, pulse, respirations
tr. or tinct. tincture
tsp teaspoon
ung. ointment
USP The United States Pharmacopeia

APPENDIX

TABLES OF WEIGHTS AND MEASURES, DIET, AND DISEASE

Table 1 □ *Tables of weights and measures*

Metric system

Length		*Weight*		*Volume*	
meter (m) basic unit		gram (g or gm) basic unit		liter (L) basic unit	
1 micrometer (μm)	= 0.000001 meter	1 microgram (mgc or μg)	= 0.000001 gram	1 milliliter* (ml)	= 0.001 liter
1 millimeter (mm)	= 0.001 meter	1 milligram (mg	= 0.001 gram	1 centiliter (cl)	= 0.01 liter
1 centimeter (cm	= 0.01 meter	1 centigram (cg)	= 0.01 gram	1 deciliter (dl)	= 0.1 liter
1 decimeter (dm)	= 0.1 meter	1 decigram (dg)	= 0.1 gram	1 dekaliter (Dl)	= 10 liters
1 dekameter (Dm)	= 10 meters	1 dekagram (Dg)	= 10 grams	1 hektoliter (Hl)	= 100 liters
1 hectometer (Hm)	= 100 meters	1 hektogram (Hg)	= 100 grams	1 kiloliter (kl)	= 1000 liters
1 kilometer (km)	= 1000 meters	1 kilogram (kg)	= 1000 grams		

Apothecaries' system

Weight		*Volume*	
20 grains (gr)	= 1 scruple (℈)	60 minims (♏)	= 1 fluidram (fʒ or ʒ)
3 scruples (℈)	= 1 dram (ʒ)	8 fluidrams (fʒ)	= 1 fluidounce (f℥ or ℥)
8 drams (ʒ)	= 1 ounce (℥)	16 fluidounces (f℥)	= 1 pint (O or pt)
12 ounces (℥)	= 1 pound (℔)	2 pints (O)	= 1 quart (qt)
		4 quarts (qt)	= 1 gallon (C, Cong, or gal)

Household equivalents

1 teaspoonful (tsp)	= 5 milliliters (ml)
1 dessertspoonful	= 10 milliliters (ml)
1 tablespoonful (tbsp)	= 15 milliliters (ml) or 1/2 ounce (ʒ)
1 teacupful	= 120 milliliters (ml) or 4 ounces (ʒ)
1 cupful	= 240 milliliters (ml) or 8 ounces (ʒ)

Other commonly used equivalents (approximate)

Weight		*Volume*	
1 grain (gr)	= 60 to 65 milligrams (mg)	1 minim (♏)	= 0.06 milliliter (ml)
		16 minims (♏)	= 1 milliliter (ml)
15 grains (gr)	= 1 gram (g)	1 fluidram (fʒ)	= 1 teaspoonful (tsp)†
1 kilogram (kg)	= 2.2 pounds (lb)	1 fluidounce (f℥)	= 30 milliliters (ml)
		1 pint (pt)	= 500 milliliters
		1 quart (qt)	= 1000 milliliters (ml)

*1 ml is considered equivalent to 1 cubic centimeter (cc).
†In medication orders, ʒi is commonly used to designate 1 tsp (5 ml).

Table 2 □ *Food and Nutrition Board, National Academy of Sciences—National Research Council Recommended Daily Dietary Allowances, Revised 1979 Designed for the Maintenance of Good Nutrition of Practically All Healthy People in the USA Mean Heights and Weights and Recommended Energy Intake*

Category	Age (years)	Weight		Height		Energy needs (with range)	
		kg	lb	cm	in	kcal	MJ
Infants	0.0-0.5	6	13	60	24	kg × 115 (95 − 145)	kg × .48
	0.5-1.0	9	20	71	28	kg × 105 (80 − 135)	kg × .44
Children	1-3	13	29	90	35	1300 (900-1800)	5.5
	4-6	20	44	112	44	1700 (1300-2300)	7.1
	7-10	28	62	132	52	2400 (1650-3300)	10.1
Males	11-14	45	99	157	62	2700 (2000-3700)	11.3
	15-18	66	145	176	69	2800 (2100-3900)	11.8
	19-22	70	154	177	70	2900 (2500-3300)	12.2
	23-50	70	154	178	70	2700 (2300-3100)	11.3
	51-75	70	154	178	70	2400 (2000-2800)	10.1
	76+	70	154	178	70	2050 (1650-2450)	8.6
Females	11-14	46	101	157	62	2200 (1500-3000)	9.2
	15-18	55	120	163	64	2100 (1200-3000)	8.8
	19-22	55	120	163	64	2100 (1700-2500)	8.8
	23-50	55	120	163	64	2000 (1600-2400)	8.4
	51-75	55	120	163	64	1800 (1400-2200)	7.6
	76+	55	120	163	64	1600 (1200-2000)	6.7
Pregnancy						+300	
Lactation						+500	

From Recommended Dietary Allowances, Revised 1979. Food and Nutrition Board, National Academy of Sciences—National Research Council, Washington, D.C.

The data in this table have been assembled from the observed median heights and weights of children . . . together with desirable weights for adults . . . for the mean heights of men (178 cm) and women (163 cm) between the ages of 18 and 34 years as surveyed in the U.S. population (HEW/NCHS data).

The energy allowances for the young adults are for men and women doing light work. The allowances for the two older age groups represent mean energy needs over these age spans, allowing for a 2% decrease in basal (resting) metabolic rate per decade and a reduction in activity of 200 kcal/day for men and women between 51 and 75 years, 500 kcal for men over 75 years and 400 kcal for women over 75 (see original text). The customary range of daily energy output is shown for adults in parentheses, and is based on a variation in energy needs of ±400 kcal at any one age (see original text and Garrow, 1978), emphasizing the range of energy intakes appropriate for any group of people.

Energy allowances for children through age 18 are based on median energy intakes of children these ages followed in longitudinal growth studies. The values in parentheses are 10th and 90th percentiles of energy intake, to indicate the range of energy consumption among children of these ages (see original text).

Table 3 □ *Best known vitamins*

Vitamin	Function	Deficiency	Sources
Fat-soluble			
A	Is essential for growth Helps eyes to adjust from light to dark Ensures healthy skin and mucous membranes	Retarded growth Night blindness Dry skin and mucous membranes	Fish-liver oils Yellow vegetables and fruits Cream and fortified margarine
D	Is needed for normal growth Regulates absorption and use of calcium by body	Soft bones Poor tooth and bone formation Rickets	Fish-liver oils Sunlight Fortified and irradiated foods
E	Normal growth Normal reproduction	Unknown	Seed-germ oils, such as wheat Vegetable greens
K	Normal clotting of blood Normal liver function	Hemorrhages	Green vegetables Medication if grave deficiency
Water-soluble			
C	Normal growth Normal cell activity Blood vessels' strength Healthy gums	Scurvy Sore and bleeding gums; bleed easily	Citrus fruits, tomatoes, potatoes, raw vegetables, and melons
B_1 (thiamine)	Normal growth Carbohydrate metabolism Heart, nerve, and muscle function	Retarded growth Loss of appetite Impaired digestion Neuritis (nerve disorders)	Pork liver, milk, green vegetables, eggs, and whole-grain and enriched cereals
B_2 (riboflavin)	Carbohydrate metabolism Healthy eyes, skin, and mouth	Retarded growth Lesions at corner of mouth and on skin Cataract-like symptoms	Meat, eggs, and milk Whole-grain cereal Vegetables
B_{12}	Is essential for normal blood formation Aids function of nerves Is necessary for normal growth and maintenance	Pernicious anemia Nervous disturbance Retarded growth	Liver, kidney, and various seafoods
Niacin	Protein and carbohydrate metabolism Function of nerves Normal growth	Pellagra Dermatitis Gastrointestinal disturbance Nervous disturbance	Milk, liver, and meat Whole-grain cereal Peanut butter

Table 4 □ *Recommended Daily Dietary Allowances,[a] Revised 1979*

	Age (years)	Weight		Height		Protein (g)	Fat-soluble vitamins		
		kg	lb	cm	in		Vitamin A (μg R.E.)[b]	Vitamin D (μg)[c]	Vitamin E (mg α T.E.)[d]
Infants	0.0-0.5	6	13	60	24	kg × 2.2	420	10	3
	0.5-1.0	9	20	71	28	kg × 2.0	400	10	4
Children	1-3	13	29	90	35	23	400	10	5
	4-6	20	44	112	44	30	500	10	6
	7-10	28	62	132	52	34	700	10	7
Males	11-14	45	99	157	62	45	1000	10	8
	15-18	66	145	176	69	56	1000	10	10
	19-22	70	154	177	70	56	1000	7.5	10
	23-50	70	154	178	70	56	1000	5	10
	51+	70	154	178	70	56	1000	5	10
Females	11-14	46	101	157	62	46	800	10	8
	15-18	55	120	163	64	46	800	10	8
	19-22	55	120	163	64	44	800	7.5	8
	23-50	55	120	163	64	44	800	5	8
	51+	55	120	163	64	44	800	5	8
Pregnant						+30	+200	+5	+2
Lactating						+20	+400	+5	+3

[a]The allowances are intended to provide for individual variations among most normal persons living in the United States under usual environmental stresses. Diets should be based on a variety of common foods in order to provide other nutrients for which human requirements have been less well defined. See original text for detailed discussion of allowances and of nutrients not tabulated.
[b]Retinol equivalents. 1 Retinol equivalent = 1 μg retinol or 6 μg β parotene. See original text for calculation of vitamin A activity of diets as retinol equivalents.
[c]As cholecalciferol. 10 μg cholecalciferol = 400 I.U. vitamin D.
[d]α tocopherol equivalents (T.E.), 1 mg d-α-tocopherol = 1 α T.E. See original text for variation in allowances and calculation of vitamin E activity of the diet as α tocopherol equivalents.
[e]1 NE (niacin equivalent) is equal to 1 mg of niacin or 0 mg of dietary tryptophan.

Water-soluble vitamins							Minerals						
Vitamin C (mg)	Thiamin (mg)	Riboflavin (mg)	Niacin (mg N.E.)[e]	Vitamin B_6 (mg)	Folacin[f] (μg)	Vitamin B_{12} (μg)	Calcium (mg)	Phosphorus (mg)	Magnesium (mg)	Iron (mg)	Zinc (mg)	Iodine (μg)
35	0.3	0.4	6	0.3	30	0.5[g]	360	240	50	10	3	40
35	0.5	0.6	8	0.6	45	1.5	540	360	70	15	5	50
45	0.7	0.8	9	0.9	100	2.0	800	800	150	15	10	70
45	0.9	1.0	11	1.3	200	2.5	800	800	200	10	10	90
45	1.2	1.4	16	1.6	300	3.0	800	800	250	10	10	120
50	1.4	1.6	18	1.8	400	3.0	1200	1200	350	18	15	150
60	1.4	1.7	18	2.0	400	3.0	1200	1200	400	18	15	150
60	1.5	1.7	19	2.2	400	3.0	800	800	350	10	15	150
60	1.4	1.6	18	2.2	400	3.0	800	800	350	10	15	150
60	1.2	1.4	16	2.2	400	3.0	800	800	350	10	15	150
50	1.1	1.3	15	1.8	400	3.0	1200	1200	300	18	15	150
60	1.1	1.3	14	2.0	400	3.0	1200	1200	300	18	15	150
60	1.1	1.3	14	2.0	400	3.0	800	800	300	18	15	150
60	1.0	1.2	13	2.0	400	3.0	800	800	300	18	15	150
60	1.0	1.2	13	2.0	400	3.0	800	800	300	10	15	150
+20	+0.4	+0.3	+2	+0.6	+400	+1.0	+400	+400	+150	[h]	+ 5	+ 25
+40	+0.5	+0.5	+5	+0.5	+100	+1.0	+400	+400	+150	[h]	+10	+ 50

[f]The folacin allowances refer to dietary sources as determined by *Lactobacillus casei* assay after treatment with enzymes ("conjugases") to make polyglutamyl forms of the vitamin available to the test organism.

[g]The RDA for vitamin B_{12} in infants is based on average concentration of the vitamin in human milk. The allowances after weaning are based on energy intake (as recommended by the American Academy of Pediatrics) and consideration of other factors such as intestinal absorption; see original text.

[h]The increased requirement during pregnancy cannot be met by the iron content of habitual American diets nor by the existing iron stores of many women; therefore the use of 30 to 60 mg of supplemental iron is recommended. Iron needs during lactation are not substantially different from those of nonpregnant women, but continued supplementation of the mother for two to three months after parturition is advisable in order to replenish stores depleted by pregnancy.

Table 5 □ *Exchange list for menu planning*

List 1. Milk exchange

Contains 12 g of carbohydrates; 8 g of protein; 10 g of fat.

Whole milk (plain or homogenized;	1 cup
Skim milk*	1 cup
Evaporated milk	1/2 cup
Powdered whole milk	1/4 cup
Powdered skim milk*	1/4 cup
Buttermilk (made with whole milk)	1 cup
Buttermilk (made with skim milk)*	1 cup

List 2. Vegetable exchange

Vegetables A

Contain little carbohydrate, protein, or fat; you may eat as much of these vegetables as you wish, except limit raw tomatoes to 1/2 cup; if cooked, use 1 cup for serving.

Asparagus	Greens	Lettuce
Broccoli	Beet	Mushroom
Brussels sprouts	Chard	Okra
Cabbage	Collard	Pepper
Cauliflower	Dandelion	Radishes
Celery	Kale	Sauerkraut
Chicory	Mustard	Stringbeans (young)
Cucumbers	Turnip	Summer squash
Escarole	Spinach	Tomatoes
Eggplant		Watercress

Vegetables B

Contains 7 grams of carbohydrate, 2 grams of protein; 1/2 cup is 1 exchange.

Beets	Pumpkin
Carrots	Rutabagas
Onions	Squash, winter
Peas, green	Turnips

List 3. Fruit exchange

Contains 10 g of carbohydrate; fruit may be fresh, dried, canned, or frozen as long as no sugar has been added.

	Amounts to use		Amounts to use
Apple (2-in. diameter)	1 small	Grapes	12
Applesauce	1/2 cup	Grape juice	1/4 cup
Apricot, fresh	2 medium	Honeydew melon	1/8 medium
Apricot, dried	4 halves	Mango	1/2 small
Banana	1/2 small	Orange	1 small
Blackberries	1 cup	Orange juice	1/2 cup
Raspberries	1 cup	Papaya	1/3 medium
Strawberries	1 cup	Peach	1 medium
Blueberries	2/3 cup	Pear	1 small
Cantaloupe (6-in. diameter)	1/4	Pineapple	1/2 cup
Cherries	10 large	Pineapple juice	1/3 cup
Dates	2	Plums	2 medium
Figs, fresh	2 large	Prunes, dried	2 medium
Figs, dried	1 small	Raisins	2 tablespoons
Grapefruit	1/2 small	Tangerine	1 large
Grapefruit juice	1/2 cup	Watermelon	1 cup

Based on material in *Meal Planning With Exchange Lists,* prepared by Committees of the American Diabetes Association, Inc., and the American Dietetic Association in cooperation with the Chronic Disease Program, Public Health Service, U.S. Department of Health and Human Services.

*Add 2 fat exchanges to meal when 1 cup is used.

†Limit to 1 exchange.

Table 5 □ *Exchange list for menu planning—cont'd*

List 4. Bread exchange

Contains 15 g of carbohydrates, 2 g of protein.

	Amounts to use		Amounts to use
Bread	1 slice	Flour	2 1/2 tablespoons
Biscuit, roll (2-in. diameter)	1	Vegetables	
Muffin (2-in. diameter)	1	Beans, peas, dried and cooked	1/2 cup
Cornbread (1 1/2-in. cube)	1	Baked beans, no pork	1/4 cup
Cereals, cooked	1/2 cup	Corn	1/3 cup
Dry, flake, and puffed types	3/4 cup	Popcorn	1 cup
Rice, grits, cooked	1/2 cup	Parsnips	2/3 cup
Spaghetti, noodles, cooked	1/2 cup	Potatoes	
Macaroni, etc., cooked	1/2 cup	White	1 small
Crackers, graham (2-in. square)	2	Mashed	1/2 cup
Crackers, oyster	20	Sweet	1/4 cup
Saltines (2-in. square)	5	Sponge cake, plain, plain (1 1/2-in. cube)	1
Soda (2 1/2-in. square)	3		
Round, thin (1 1/2-in. diameter)	6	Ice cream (omit 2 fat exchanges)	1/2 cup

List 5. Meat exchange

Contains 7 g of protein, 5 g of fat.

Meat and poultry (medium fat), e.g., beef, lamb, pork liver	1 ounce	Fish	
		Haddock, etc.	1 ounce
Cold cuts (4 1/2-in. × 1/8-in.)	1 slice	Salmon, tuna, crab, lobster	1/4 cup
Frankfurter, 8 to 9 per pound	1	Oysters	5 small
Egg	1	Sardines	3 medium
		Cheese	
		Cheddar type	1 ounce
		Cottage	1/4 cup
		Peanut butter†	2 tablespoons

List 6. Fat exchange

Contains 5 g of fat.

Butter or margarine	1 teaspoon	French dressing	1 tablespoon
Bacon, crisp	1 slice	Mayonnaise	1 teaspoon
Cream, light	2 tablespoons	Oil or cooking fat	1 teaspoon
Cream, heavy	1 tablespoon	Nuts	6 small
Cream cheese	1 tablespoon	Olives	5 small
Avocado (4-in. diameter)	1/8		

Table 6 □ *Common communicable diseases*

To prevent the spread of infection, any person suspected of having a communicable disease should be kept away from others. these may vary, practical nurses should keep in touch with local health authorities and be responsible for cooperating with them

Disease	How spread	Prevention	How long from exposure to onset
Chickenpox	Directly from person to person; indirectly through articles freshly soiled by discharges from skin and mucous membrane of infected persons	No immunization available; avoid exposure; one attack usually gives immunity	2 to 3 weeks
Common cold	Contact with discharges from nose and throat; directly from person to person; indirectly through articles freshly soiled by discharges	No specific prevention; maintain body resistance and avoid chilling and exposure to illness	12 to 72 hours
Diphtheria	Contact with discharges from nose and throat or other infected membranes; by carriers as well as by sick persons; milk may carry germs of disease	Immunization in infancy, with reinforcing doses periodically; adults exposed to infection should be given Schick test to determine susceptibility before immunization; second attacks possible	2 to 5 days, sometimes longer
Dysentery	Contact with discharges from bowels of infected persons; contaminated food and water; flies	No immunization; avoidance of known sources; personal cleanliness; proper sanitation; periodic examination of food handlers	1 to 7 days or 3 to 4 weeks
Encephalitis (sleeping sickness)	Mosquitoes; ticks	Personal cleanliness; strict isolation of patient; spray mosquitoes' breeding places; window screens; insect repellents	4 to 15 days
German measles (rubella)	Contact with discharges from throat and mouth; easily communicable	Immunization available; second attacks rare; especially important to guard women in early pregnancy against exposure	5 to 21 days
Gonorrhea	Contact with fresh discharges from genital tract of infected persons or from other infcted areas such as eyes; most frequently through sexual intercourse	No immunization; avoidance of contact; medicine put in eyes of new born babies; one attack does not confer immunity; case-finding; early diagnosis and treatment	1 to 14 days; usually 3 to 5 days
Infectious hepatitis	Contact with infected feces, serum, and contaminated food and water	Passive immunity with gamma globulin; avoid contact with infected feces, food, water, and blood serum	2 to 6 weeks
Serum hepatitis	Contact with contaminated needle or solution containing blood serum	Cleanliness and sterilization of syringes and needles; careful history of blood donors	$1\frac{1}{2}$ to 6 months

*Not communicable. Infection that has preceded this disease is communicable but has usually subsided by time symptoms of rheumatic fever

†Bacteria causing scarlet fever (hemolytic streptococci) may also cause other diseases such as streptococcal sore throat, erysipelas, and "childbed

Measures for control of communicable diseases are established either by law or regulation in various states and communities. As
in preventing the spread of disease.

Common symptoms	How long communicable	Some possible complications
Small reddish pimples or blisters, usually more abundant on covered than exposed parts of body, which become itchy; slight fever; headache	Probably not more than 1 day before or more than 6 days after pimples first appear; highly communicable during early stages	Rarely, skin eruptions may become infected
Tickling, dry sensation in throat; slight fever; chilliness; sick feeling; cough and running nose	Usually limited to early stage of disease	Bronchitis; laryngitis; pneumonia; middle ear infection in children
Inflammation of tonsils, throat, and nose, with grayish-white patches; fever	Until germs have disappeared as shown by tests, usually 2 weeks or less	Damage to heart and throat muscles; otitis media; bronchial pneumonia; peripheral neuritis
Diarrhea; fever; stools may contain mucus or blood; abdominal cramps	As long as stools contain infecting agent as checked by laboratory tests, sometimes weeks	Often recurs
Slow or sudden onset of fever, headache, vertigo, joint pains, confusion, drowsiness, and paralysis; nausea, vomiting; convulsions; hiccoughs; cranial nerve involvement	Unknown	Disturbed mental and physical functions for some time after infection
Slight cold followed by red rash on face and body; slight fever (frequently confused with scarlet fever)	From onset and for at least 4 days, possibly 7	None usually; serious for women during early pregnancy as may result in defect of baby if mother contracts measles during first trimester
Pus discharge from mucous membrane of genital tract or of eyes; pain and burning on urination	As long as germs appears in discharges, as checked by laboratory tests	Arthritis; sterility, infection of eyes of newborn infants; salpingitis or epididymitis
Anorexia; upper abdominal distress; sudden onset of chills, headache, fever, and jaundice; constipation or diarrhea; pain in or about the eyes; pruritus	As long as the virus is in the feces and blood	Liver damage; changes in mental state; bleeding from a body orifice; mild case can suddenly become serious, leading to death
Slow onset; afebrile; weakness; easily fatigued; anorexia; nausea; jaundice	As long as the virus is in the blood serum	Liver damage

Continued.

appear.
fever'' (puerperal fever).

Table 6 □ *Common communicable diseases—cont'd*

Disease	How spread	Prevention	How long from exposure to onset
Impetigo	Contact with moist discharges from sores on skin; possible nose and throat discharges	No immunization; reinfection possible; personal cleanliness; prevention of excessive scratching in such conditions as chickenpox and scabies	Perhaps 2 to 5 days
Infantile paralysis (poliomyelitis)	Contact with nose and throat and bowel discharges of infected persons or carriers	Salk and Sabin (oral) vaccines; adults have more immunity than children; one attack usually confers immunity; good sanitation and personal hygiene	Usually 7 to 14 days (may be from 3 to 35 days)
Influenza	Contact with discharges from nose and mouth and articles freshly soiled with discharges	Immunization available; repeated attacks are possible	24 to 72 hours
Measles (rubeola)	Contact with discharges of nose and throat; easily spread	Immunization available; attack may be lightened or prevented in children exposed to measles if immune serum globulin given; babies of immune mothers usually immune for first few months of life; one attack usually confers immunity	Usually about 10 days from exposure to onset of fever; 13 to 15 days to the appearance of rash; as long as 21 days if immune serum globulin has been given
Epidemic meningitis	Contact with discharges of nose and throat; carriers	No immunization; avoid contact, droplet infection, and overcrowding; stress personal cleanliness	2 to 10 days; usually 7 days
Mumps	Contact with saliva of infected persons	Immunization; second attacks have been know but are rare	12 to 26 days; usually 18 days
Rheumatic fever*	Unknown	No immunization; disease recurs; immediate and proper care of "strep" infections	Unknown; it may be several days to 8 weeks after infection before symptoms appear; average is 3 weeks
Ringworm	Contact with sores, discharges from sores, or clothing in contact with sores; contact with infected cats or dogs	No immunization; repeated attacks common; cleanliness; proper sanitation	Not known
Salmonellosis (food poisoning)	Improper refrigeration of foods; foods contaminated by excreta of infected rodents; pet turtles may be carriers	Clean, well-preserved, and well-cooked foods; examination of left-over food for foul odor and color or decomposition; examination of food handlers	6 to 48 hours

Common symptoms	How long communicable	Some possible complications
Running sores on face and hands or body, later showing crusts	As long as sores are unhealed	Occasional infection of sores; may result in death in infants
Many cases not recognized; fever, headache, drowsiness, stiff neck and back, and irritability	Not exactly known, probably latter part of incubation period and first week of acute illness; virus may be found in feces for months	Paralysis of affected parts of body
Sudden onset; fever, aching limbs and back, running nose, sore throat, bronchitis, and prostration; fatigue; sweating	Uncertain	Pneumonia
Fever, running eyes and nose, eruption in mouth, followed by rash; branny peeling of skin during convalescence	During period of running eyes and nose, usually about 9 days (from 4 days before to 5 days after rash appears)	Inflammation of middle ear; pneumonia; encephalitis
Usually sudden onset; fever, headache, nausea, and vomiting; rash occasionally; dizziness, stiff neck, and delirium	Until germs disappear from discharges, as checked by laboratory tests	Spread of infection to tissue of brain; eye and ear infections; hydrocephalus
Fever and swelling of salivary glands in cheeks and under tongue	From 1 to 2 days before the symptoms appear until swelling of glands has disappeared	Inflammation of ovaries or testicles in persons past puberty
Slow onset; fever, joint, and muscle pains; nosebleed and petechiae; rapid pulse out of proportion to temperature; loss of appetite, irritability; profuse irritating perspiration; listlessness	See footnote*	Serious damage to heart; chorea
Round, scaly patches on scalp or body; likely to appear on feet, and between toes as well; itching	As long as fungus or spores remain around sores	Occasional secondary infection of sores
Abrupt onset of nausea and vomiting; diarrhea with offensive odor; abdominal cramps and tenderness; may or may not have fever, dizziness, apprehension, delirium, and coma	Not communicable	Prostration; death

Continued.

Table 6 □ *Common communicable diseases—cont'd*

Disease	How spread	Prevention	How long from exposure to onset
Scabies	Contact with an infected person or articles in contact with an infected person	Avoid contact; repeated infestation common; cleanliness; proper sanitation	24 to 48 hours
Scarlet fever†	Contact with discharges of nose, throat, or ears of infected person; carriers; contaminated milk or other foods	No immunization; pasteurization of milk; avoidance of contact with ill persons	1 to 5 days
Smallpox (variola)	Contact with nose and throat discharges and sores on bodies of patients	Vaccination gives protection if rules are followed; one attack usually prevents another	7 to 16 days, occasionally longer; commonly 12 days
Staphylococcal infections	Contact with infected blood, exudates, sputum, stool, etc.; air-borne carriers	Asepsis and isolation; reevaluation and enforcement of basic hospital procedures and techniques	2 to 3 days
Syphilis	Contact with discharge from known sores or those hidden on mucous membrane and skin; usually contracted through sexual intercourse; blood of infected persons	No immunization; one attack does not prevent another; case-finding; recognition and treatment of early cases; health education	10 days to 3 weeks or longer
Tetanus	Infected soil, street dust, and animal feces introduced through break in skin, especially through puncture wounds such as those made by nails	Tetanus toxoid—requires enforcing at certain intervals; one attack does not protect; antitoxin given in presence of suspected wound	4 days to 3 weeks
Tuberculosis, pulmonary	Contact with discharges of nose and throat from "active" tuberculous case; occasionally by milk from tuberculous cattle	BCG vaccine given to tuberculin nonreactors; one attack does not prevent another; pasteurization of milk; killing of tuberculous cattle	Variable; probably not less than 1 month and possible longer
Typhoid fever	Contact with infected feces and urine; contaminated water or food, especially milk	Typhoid vaccine gives immunity for about 2 years; one attack usually prevents another	3 to 38 days; usually 7 to 14 days
Undulant fever (brucellosis)	Contact with infected animals; milk of infected animals	No immunization; boiling or pasteurization of milk	6 to 30 days or more
Whooping cough	Contact with infected discharges of nose and throat	Immunization giving considerable protection available; one attack usually prevents another; reinforcing doses of vaccine may be advisable within year and at 2 or 3 years of age	7 to 21 days

Common symptoms	How long communicable	Some possible complications
"Burrows" or lines of sores (row of black dots); severe itching, particularly between fingers	Until itch mite and eggs destroyed	Occasional infection of sores
Sore, inflamed throat; strawberry tongue; fever, nausea, and vomiting; later rash, usually beginning on neck and chest	Not known; 2 weeks at least	Inflammation of middle ear; damage to heart and kidneys; rheumatic fever
Abrupt onset of high fever, vomiting, headache, severe backache, delirium, convulsions, or chills, followed by eruption 1 to 5 days later; crusts fall off in 10 to 40 days; the disease may vary from mild to very severe, with high death rate	From first symptom to disappearance of crusts of eruption; most communicable in early stages of illness	Pitting of skin; occasional blindness; bronchitis; ear infection; abscesses on skin
Depends on location of infection	As long as staphylococcus can be cultured	Depends on location of infection
Sore at point of contact, which will heal but may recur during next 5 years after infection; rash, sore throat, headache; in congenital syphilis, only late manifestations, such as those listed under complications, occur	From onset and, if untreated, up to 5 years	Damage to heart and central nervous system including brain, unless treated early
Restlessness and irritability; unreasonable disposition; severe headache; difficulty in urination; profuse sweating; painful muscular movements; pain in cheek or neck muscles on chewing or swallowing; infection of umbilical cord in newborn infant	Not passed on to another person	Rare under proper treatment and prevention—highly fatal if not treated promptly; serum sickness; urticaria
Usually no noticeable symptoms until disease moderately advanced; then fatigue, loss of weight, chronic cough, loss of appetite, and afternoon rise in temperature; night sweats	For duration of active state of disease as shown by tests and x-ray study	Meningitis; miliary (general) tuberculosis; laryngitis; bronchiectasis; hemoptysis; spontaneous pneumothorax
Fever, headache, diarrhea, and stomachache; later rose spots on trunk; mouth and tongue coated with thick "fur"; pulse rapid, out of proportion to temperature	As long as typhoid germs appear in discharges from bowels as checked by laboratory tests	Hemorrhage; bronchitis; pneumonia; perforation and hemorrhage of intestine
Slow onset; irregular fever, sweating, chills, and pain in joints and muscles	Not communicable from human to human	Disease may be prolonged through months and years
Typical "whooping" cough develops from ordinary cough in 1 to 2 weeks; suspect any cough when disease known to be present in neighborhood	From onset to 3 weeks	Bronchitis; bronchial penumonia; frequently fatal to young babies; convulsions

Index

U

V

W

ANSWER SHEETS

INTRODUCTION

Review questions 1-10, pp. 3-4

NAME ____________________ (LAST FIRST MIDDLE) GRADE ________ SEX ______ (M OR F) DATE OF BIRTH ____________ (YEAR MONTH DAY)

DATE ____________ (YEAR MONTH DAY) AGE ______ SCHOOL ________________ CITY ________________

INSTRUCTOR ________________________

NAME OF TEST ________________________

BE SURE TO MAKE YOUR MARKS HEAVY AND BLACK

ERASE COMPLETELY ANY ANSWERS YOU WISH TO CHANGE

IDENTIFICATION NUMBER

	0	1	2	3	4	5	6	7	8	9
	0	1	2	3	4	5	6	7	8	9
	0	1	2	3	4	5	6	7	8	9
	0	1	2	3	4	5	6	7	8	9
	0	1	2	3	4	5	6	7	8	9
	0	1	2	3	4	5	6	7	8	9
	0	1	2	3	4	5	6	7	8	9
	0	1	2	3	4	5	6	7	8	9
	0	1	2	3	4	5	6	7	8	9
	0	1	2	3	4	5	6	7	8	9

1	1 2 3 4	2	1 2 3 4	3	1 2 3 4	4	1 2 3 4
5	1 2 3 4	6	1 2 3 4	7	1 2 3 4	8	1 2 3 4
9	1 2 3 4	10	1 2 3 4	11	1 2 3 4	12	1 2 3 4
13	1 2 3 4	14	1 2 3 4	15	1 2 3 4	16	1 2 3 4
17	1 2 3 4	18	1 2 3 4	19	1 2 3 4	20	1 2 3 4
21	1 2 3 4	22	1 2 3 4	23	1 2 3 4	24	1 2 3 4
25	1 2 3 4	26	1 2 3 4	27	1 2 3 4	28	1 2 3 4
29	1 2 3 4	30	1 2 3 4	31	1 2 3 4	32	1 2 3 4
33	1 2 3 4	34	1 2 3 4	35	1 2 3 4	36	1 2 3 4
37	1 2 3 4	38	1 2 3 4	39	1 2 3 4	40	1 2 3 4
41	1 2 3 4	42	1 2 3 4	43	1 2 3 4	44	1 2 3 4
45	1 2 3 4	46	1 2 3 4	47	1 2 3 4	48	1 2 3 4
49	1 2 3 4	50	1 2 3 4	51	1 2 3 4	52	1 2 3 4
53	1 2 3 4	54	1 2 3 4	55	1 2 3 4	56	1 2 3 4
57	1 2 3 4	58	1 2 3 4	59	1 2 3 4	60	1 2 3 4
61	1 2 3 4	62	1 2 3 4	63	1 2 3 4	64	1 2 3 4
65	1 2 3 4	66	1 2 3 4	67	1 2 3 4	68	1 2 3 4
69	1 2 3 4	70	1 2 3 4	71	1 2 3 4	72	1 2 3 4
73	1 2 3 4	74	1 2 3 4	75	1 2 3 4	76	1 2 3 4
77	1 2 3 4	78	1 2 3 4	79	1 2 3 4	80	1 2 3 4
81	1 2 3 4	82	1 2 3 4	83	1 2 3 4	84	1 2 3 4
85	1 2 3 4	86	1 2 3 4	87	1 2 3 4	88	1 2 3 4
89	1 2 3 4	90	1 2 3 4	91	1 2 3 4	92	1 2 3 4
93	1 2 3 4	94	1 2 3 4	95	1 2 3 4	96	1 2 3 4
97	1 2 3 4	98	1 2 3 4	99	1 2 3 4	100	1 2 3 4
101	1 2 3 4	102	1 2 3 4	103	1 2 3 4	104	1 2 3 4
105	1 2 3 4	106	1 2 3 4	107	1 2 3 4	108	1 2 3 4
109	1 2 3 4	110	1 2 3 4	111	1 2 3 4	112	1 2 3 4
113	1 2 3 4	114	1 2 3 4	115	1 2 3 4	116	1 2 3 4
117	1 2 3 4	118	1 2 3 4	119	1 2 3 4	120	1 2 3 4
121	1 2 3 4	122	1 2 3 4	123	1 2 3 4	124	1 2 3 4
125	1 2 3 4	126	1 2 3 4	127	1 2 3 4	128	1 2 3 4
129	1 2 3 4	130	1 2 3 4	131	1 2 3 4	132	1 2 3 4
133	1 2 3 4	134	1 2 3 4	135	1 2 3 4	136	1 2 3 4
137	1 2 3 4	138	1 2 3 4	139	1 2 3 4	140	1 2 3 4
141	1 2 3 4	142	1 2 3 4	143	1 2 3 4	144	1 2 3 4
145	1 2 3 4	146	1 2 3 4	147	1 2 3 4	148	1 2 3 4
149	1 2 3 4	150	1 2 3 4	151	1 2 3 4	152	1 2 3 4
153	1 2 3 4	154	1 2 3 4	155	1 2 3 4	156	1 2 3 4
157	1 2 3 4	158	1 2 3 4	159	1 2 3 4	160	1 2 3 4

THE PRACTICAL NURSE

Review questions 1-35, pp. 9-11

NAME ______________ (LAST FIRST MIDDLE) GRADE ________ SEX ________ (M OR F) DATE OF BIRTH ______________ (YEAR MONTH DAY)

DATE ______________ (YEAR MONTH DAY) AGE ______ SCHOOL ______________ CITY ______________

INSTRUCTOR ______________

NAME OF TEST ______________

BE SURE TO MAKE YOUR MARKS HEAVY AND BLACK

ERASE COMPLETELY ANY ANSWERS YOU WISH TO CHANGE

IDENTIFICATION NUMBER

☐	0	1	2	3	4	5	6	7	8	9
☐	0	1	2	3	4	5	6	7	8	9
☐	0	1	2	3	4	5	6	7	8	9
☐	0	1	2	3	4	5	6	7	8	9
☐	0	1	2	3	4	5	6	7	8	9
☐	0	1	2	3	4	5	6	7	8	9
☐	0	1	2	3	4	5	6	7	8	9
☐	0	1	2	3	4	5	6	7	8	9
☐	0	1	2	3	4	5	6	7	8	9
☐	0	1	2	3	4	5	6	7	8	9

1	1 2 3 4	2	1 2 3 4	3	1 2 3 4	4	1 2 3 4
5	1 2 3 4	6	1 2 3 4	7	1 2 3 4	8	1 2 3 4
9	1 2 3 4	10	1 2 3 4	11	1 2 3 4	12	1 2 3 4
13	1 2 3 4	14	1 2 3 4	15	1 2 3 4	16	1 2 3 4
17	1 2 3 4	18	1 2 3 4	19	1 2 3 4	20	1 2 3 4
21	1 2 3 4	22	1 2 3 4	23	1 2 3 4	24	1 2 3 4
25	1 2 3 4	26	1 2 3 4	27	1 2 3 4	28	1 2 3 4
29	1 2 3 4	30	1 2 3 4	31	1 2 3 4	32	1 2 3 4
33	1 2 3 4	34	1 2 3 4	35	1 2 3 4	36	1 2 3 4
37	1 2 3 4	38	1 2 3 4	39	1 2 3 4	40	1 2 3 4
41	1 2 3 4	42	1 2 3 4	43	1 2 3 4	44	1 2 3 4
45	1 2 3 4	46	1 2 3 4	47	1 2 3 4	48	1 2 3 4
49	1 2 3 4	50	1 2 3 4	51	1 2 3 4	52	1 2 3 4
53	1 2 3 4	54	1 2 3 4	55	1 2 3 4	56	1 2 3 4
57	1 2 3 4	58	1 2 3 4	59	1 2 3 4	60	1 2 3 4
61	1 2 3 4	62	1 2 3 4	63	1 2 3 4	64	1 2 3 4
65	1 2 3 4	66	1 2 3 4	67	1 2 3 4	68	1 2 3 4
69	1 2 3 4	70	1 2 3 4	71	1 2 3 4	72	1 2 3 4
73	1 2 3 4	74	1 2 3 4	75	1 2 3 4	76	1 2 3 4
77	1 2 3 4	78	1 2 3 4	79	1 2 3 4	80	1 2 3 4
81	1 2 3 4	82	1 2 3 4	83	1 2 3 4	84	1 2 3 4
85	1 2 3 4	86	1 2 3 4	87	1 2 3 4	88	1 2 3 4
89	1 2 3 4	90	1 2 3 4	91	1 2 3 4	92	1 2 3 4
93	1 2 3 4	94	1 2 3 4	95	1 2 3 4	96	1 2 3 4
97	1 2 3 4	98	1 2 3 4	99	1 2 3 4	100	1 2 3 4
101	1 2 3 4	102	1 2 3 4	103	1 2 3 4	104	1 2 3 4
105	1 2 3 4	106	1 2 3 4	107	1 2 3 4	108	1 2 3 4
109	1 2 3 4	110	1 2 3 4	111	1 2 3 4	112	1 2 3 4
113	1 2 3 4	114	1 2 3 4	115	1 2 3 4	116	1 2 3 4
117	1 2 3 4	118	1 2 3 4	119	1 2 3 4	120	1 2 3 4
121	1 2 3 4	122	1 2 3 4	123	1 2 3 4	124	1 2 3 4
125	1 2 3 4	126	1 2 3 4	127	1 2 3 4	128	1 2 3 4
129	1 2 3 4	130	1 2 3 4	131	1 2 3 4	132	1 2 3 4
133	1 2 3 4	134	1 2 3 4	135	1 2 3 4	136	1 2 3 4
137	1 2 3 4	138	1 2 3 4	139	1 2 3 4	140	1 2 3 4
141	1 2 3 4	142	1 2 3 4	143	1 2 3 4	144	1 2 3 4
145	1 2 3 4	146	1 2 3 4	147	1 2 3 4	148	1 2 3 4
149	1 2 3 4	150	1 2 3 4	151	1 2 3 4	152	1 2 3 4
153	1 2 3 4	154	1 2 3 4	155	1 2 3 4	156	1 2 3 4
157	1 2 3 4	158	1 2 3 4	159	1 2 3 4	160	1 2 3 4

BASIC SCIENCE

Review questions 1-154, pp. 53-63

NAME ______ LAST FIRST MIDDLE GRADE ______ SEX ______ M OR F DATE OF BIRTH ______ YEAR MONTH DAY

DATE ______ YEAR MONTH DAY AGE ______ SCHOOL ______ CITY ______

INSTRUCTOR ______

IDENTIFICATION NUMBER

☐	0	1	2	3	4	5	6	7	8	9
☐	0	1	2	3	4	5	6	7	8	9
☐	0	1	2	3	4	5	6	7	8	9
☐	0	1	2	3	4	5	6	7	8	9
☐	0	1	2	3	4	5	6	7	8	9
☐	0	1	2	3	4	5	6	7	8	9
☐	0	1	2	3	4	5	6	7	8	9
☐	0	1	2	3	4	5	6	7	8	9
☐	0	1	2	3	4	5	6	7	8	9
☐	0	1	2	3	4	5	6	7	8	9

NAME OF TEST ______

BE SURE TO MAKE YOUR MARKS HEAVY AND BLACK

ERASE COMPLETELY ANY ANSWERS YOU WISH TO CHANGE

1	1 2 3 4	2	1 2 3 4	3	1 2 3 4	4	1 2 3 4
5	1 2 3 4	6	1 2 3 4	7	1 2 3 4	8	1 2 3 4
9	1 2 3 4	10	1 2 3 4	11	1 2 3 4	12	1 2 3 4
13	1 2 3 4	14	1 2 3 4	15	1 2 3 4	16	1 2 3 4
17	1 2 3 4	18	1 2 3 4	19	1 2 3 4	20	1 2 3 4
21	1 2 3 4	22	1 2 3 4	23	1 2 3 4	24	1 2 3 4
25	1 2 3 4	26	1 2 3 4	27	1 2 3 4	28	1 2 3 4
29	1 2 3 4	30	1 2 3 4	31	1 2 3 4	32	1 2 3 4
33	1 2 3 4	34	1 2 3 4	35	1 2 3 4	36	1 2 3 4
37	1 2 3 4	38	1 2 3 4	39	1 2 3 4	40	1 2 3 4
41	1 2 3 4	42	1 2 3 4	43	1 2 3 4	44	1 2 3 4
45	1 2 3 4	46	1 2 3 4	47	1 2 3 4	48	1 2 3 4
49	1 2 3 4	50	1 2 3 4	51	1 2 3 4	52	1 2 3 4
53	1 2 3 4	54	1 2 3 4	55	1 2 3 4	56	1 2 3 4
57	1 2 3 4	58	1 2 3 4	59	1 2 3 4	60	1 2 3 4
61	1 2 3 4	62	1 2 3 4	63	1 2 3 4	64	1 2 3 4
65	1 2 3 4	66	1 2 3 4	67	1 2 3 4	68	1 2 3 4
69	1 2 3 4	70	1 2 3 4	71	1 2 3 4	72	1 2 3 4
73	1 2 3 4	74	1 2 3 4	75	1 2 3 4	76	1 2 3 4
77	1 2 3 4	78	1 2 3 4	79	1 2 3 4	80	1 2 3 4
81	1 2 3 4	82	1 2 3 4	83	1 2 3 4	84	1 2 3 4
85	1 2 3 4	86	1 2 3 4	87	1 2 3 4	88	1 2 3 4
89	1 2 3 4	90	1 2 3 4	91	1 2 3 4	92	1 2 3 4
93	1 2 3 4	94	1 2 3 4	95	1 2 3 4	96	1 2 3 4
97	1 2 3 4	98	1 2 3 4	99	1 2 3 4	100	1 2 3 4
101	1 2 3 4	102	1 2 3 4	103	1 2 3 4	104	1 2 3 4
105	1 2 3 4	106	1 2 3 4	107	1 2 3 4	108	1 2 3 4
109	1 2 3 4	110	1 2 3 4	111	1 2 3 4	112	1 2 3 4
113	1 2 3 4	114	1 2 3 4	115	1 2 3 4	116	1 2 3 4
117	1 2 3 4	118	1 2 3 4	119	1 2 3 4	120	1 2 3 4
121	1 2 3 4	122	1 2 3 4	123	1 2 3 4	124	1 2 3 4
125	1 2 3 4	126	1 2 3 4	127	1 2 3 4	128	1 2 3 4
129	1 2 3 4	130	1 2 3 4	131	1 2 3 4	132	1 2 3 4
133	1 2 3 4	134	1 2 3 4	135	1 2 3 4	136	1 2 3 4
137	1 2 3 4	138	1 2 3 4	139	1 2 3 4	140	1 2 3 4
141	1 2 3 4	142	1 2 3 4	143	1 2 3 4	144	1 2 3 4
145	1 2 3 4	146	1 2 3 4	147	1 2 3 4	148	1 2 3 4
149	1 2 3 4	150	1 2 3 4	151	1 2 3 4	152	1 2 3 4
153	1 2 3 4	154	1 2 3 4	155	1 2 3 4	156	1 2 3 4
157	1 2 3 4	158	1 2 3 4	159	1 2 3 4	160	1 2 3 4

FUNDAMENTALS OF NURSING

Review questions 1-100, pp. 91-99

NAME ____________ LAST FIRST MIDDLE GRADE ______ SEX ______ M OR F DATE OF BIRTH ______ YEAR MONTH DAY

DATE ____________ YEAR MONTH DAY AGE ______ SCHOOL ____________ CITY ____________

INSTRUCTOR ____________

NAME OF TEST ____________

IDENTIFICATION NUMBER

0 1 2 3 4 5 6 7 8 9
0 1 2 3 4 5 6 7 8 9
0 1 2 3 4 5 6 7 8 9
0 1 2 3 4 5 6 7 8 9
0 1 2 3 4 5 6 7 8 9
0 1 2 3 4 5 6 7 8 9
0 1 2 3 4 5 6 7 8 9
0 1 2 3 4 5 6 7 8 9
0 1 2 3 4 5 6 7 8 9
0 1 2 3 4 5 6 7 8 9

BE SURE TO MAKE YOUR MARKS HEAVY AND BLACK

ERASE COMPLETELY ANY ANSWERS YOU WISH TO CHANGE

1 1 2 3 4	2 1 2 3 4	3 1 2 3 4	4 1 2 3 4
5 1 2 3 4	6 1 2 3 4	7 1 2 3 4	8 1 2 3 4
9 1 2 3 4	10 1 2 3 4	11 1 2 3 4	12 1 2 3 4
13 1 2 3 4	14 1 2 3 4	15 1 2 3 4	16 1 2 3 4
17 1 2 3 4	18 1 2 3 4	19 1 2 3 4	20 1 2 3 4
21 1 2 3 4	22 1 2 3 4	23 1 2 3 4	24 1 2 3 4
25 1 2 3 4	26 1 2 3 4	27 1 2 3 4	28 1 2 3 4
29 1 2 3 4	30 1 2 3 4	31 1 2 3 4	32 1 2 3 4
33 1 2 3 4	34 1 2 3 4	35 1 2 3 4	36 1 2 3 4
37 1 2 3 4	38 1 2 3 4	39 1 2 3 4	40 1 2 3 4
41 1 2 3 4	42 1 2 3 4	43 1 2 3 4	44 1 2 3 4
45 1 2 3 4	46 1 2 3 4	47 1 2 3 4	48 1 2 3 4
49 1 2 3 4	50 1 2 3 4	51 1 2 3 4	52 1 2 3 4
53 1 2 3 4	54 1 2 3 4	55 1 2 3 4	56 1 2 3 4
57 1 2 3 4	58 1 2 3 4	59 1 2 3 4	60 1 2 3 4
61 1 2 3 4	62 1 2 3 4	63 1 2 3 4	64 1 2 3 4
65 1 2 3 4	66 1 2 3 4	67 1 2 3 4	68 1 2 3 4
69 1 2 3 4	70 1 2 3 4	71 1 2 3 4	72 1 2 3 4
73 1 2 3 4	74 1 2 3 4	75 1 2 3 4	76 1 2 3 4
77 1 2 3 4	78 1 2 3 4	79 1 2 3 4	80 1 2 3 4
81 1 2 3 4	82 1 2 3 4	83 1 2 3 4	84 1 2 3 4
85 1 2 3 4	86 1 2 3 4	87 1 2 3 4	88 1 2 3 4
89 1 2 3 4	90 1 2 3 4	91 1 2 3 4	92 1 2 3 4
93 1 2 3 4	94 1 2 3 4	95 1 2 3 4	96 1 2 3 4
97 1 2 3 4	98 1 2 3 4	99 1 2 3 4	100 1 2 3 4
101 1 2 3 4	102 1 2 3 4	103 1 2 3 4	104 1 2 3 4
105 1 2 3 4	106 1 2 3 4	107 1 2 3 4	108 1 2 3 4
109 1 2 3 4	110 1 2 3 4	111 1 2 3 4	112 1 2 3 4
113 1 2 3 4	114 1 2 3 4	115 1 2 3 4	116 1 2 3 4
117 1 2 3 4	118 1 2 3 4	119 1 2 3 4	120 1 2 3 4
121 1 2 3 4	122 1 2 3 4	123 1 2 3 4	124 1 2 3 4
125 1 2 3 4	126 1 2 3 4	127 1 2 3 4	128 1 2 3 4
129 1 2 3 4	130 1 2 3 4	131 1 2 3 4	132 1 2 3 4
133 1 2 3 4	134 1 2 3 4	135 1 2 3 4	136 1 2 3 4
137 1 2 3 4	138 1 2 3 4	139 1 2 3 4	140 1 2 3 4
141 1 2 3 4	142 1 2 3 4	143 1 2 3 4	144 1 2 3 4
145 1 2 3 4	146 1 2 3 4	147 1 2 3 4	148 1 2 3 4
149 1 2 3 4	150 1 2 3 4	151 1 2 3 4	152 1 2 3 4
153 1 2 3 4	154 1 2 3 4	155 1 2 3 4	156 1 2 3 4
157 1 2 3 4	158 1 2 3 4	159 1 2 3 4	160 1 2 3 4

NURSING THE ADULT PATIENT

Review questions 1-160, pp. 148-160

NAME ______ LAST FIRST MIDDLE GRADE ______ SEX ______ M OR F DATE OF BIRTH ______ YEAR MONTH DAY

DATE ______ YEAR MONTH DAY AGE ______ SCHOOL ______ CITY ______

INSTRUCTOR ______

NAME OF TEST ______

IDENTIFICATION NUMBER

0	1	2	3	4	5	6	7	8	9
0	1	2	3	4	5	6	7	8	9
0	1	2	3	4	5	6	7	8	9
0	1	2	3	4	5	6	7	8	9
0	1	2	3	4	5	6	7	8	9
0	1	2	3	4	5	6	7	8	9
0	1	2	3	4	5	6	7	8	9
0	1	2	3	4	5	6	7	8	9
0	1	2	3	4	5	6	7	8	9
0	1	2	3	4	5	6	7	8	9

BE SURE TO MAKE YOUR MARKS HEAVY AND BLACK

ERASE COMPLETELY ANY ANSWERS YOU WISH TO CHANGE

1 1 2 3 4	2 1 2 3 4	3 1 2 3 4	4 1 2 3 4
5 1 2 3 4	6 1 2 3 4	7 1 2 3 4	8 1 2 3 4
9 1 2 3 4	10 1 2 3 4	11 1 2 3 4	12 1 2 3 4
13 1 2 3 4	14 1 2 3 4	15 1 2 3 4	16 1 2 3 4
17 1 2 3 4	18 1 2 3 4	19 1 2 3 4	20 1 2 3 4
21 1 2 3 4	22 1 2 3 4	23 1 2 3 4	24 1 2 3 4
25 1 2 3 4	26 1 2 3 4	27 1 2 3 4	28 1 2 3 4
29 1 2 3 4	30 1 2 3 4	31 1 2 3 4	32 1 2 3 4
33 1 2 3 4	34 1 2 3 4	35 1 2 3 4	36 1 2 3 4
37 1 2 3 4	38 1 2 3 4	39 1 2 3 4	40 1 2 3 4
41 1 2 3 4	42 1 2 3 4	43 1 2 3 4	44 1 2 3 4
45 1 2 3 4	46 1 2 3 4	47 1 2 3 4	48 1 2 3 4
49 1 2 3 4	50 1 2 3 4	51 1 2 3 4	52 1 2 3 4
53 1 2 3 4	54 1 2 3 4	55 1 2 3 4	56 1 2 3 4
57 1 2 3 4	58 1 2 3 4	59 1 2 3 4	60 1 2 3 4
61 1 2 3 4	62 1 2 3 4	63 1 2 3 4	64 1 2 3 4
65 1 2 3 4	66 1 2 3 4	67 1 2 3 4	68 1 2 3 4
69 1 2 3 4	70 1 2 3 4	71 1 2 3 4	72 1 2 3 4
73 1 2 3 4	74 1 2 3 4	75 1 2 3 4	76 1 2 3 4
77 1 2 3 4	78 1 2 3 4	79 1 2 3 4	80 1 2 3 4
81 1 2 3 4	82 1 2 3 4	83 1 2 3 4	84 1 2 3 4
85 1 2 3 4	86 1 2 3 4	87 1 2 3 4	88 1 2 3 4
89 1 2 3 4	90 1 2 3 4	91 1 2 3 4	92 1 2 3 4
93 1 2 3 4	94 1 2 3 4	95 1 2 3 4	96 1 2 3 4
97 1 2 3 4	98 1 2 3 4	99 1 2 3 4	100 1 2 3 4
101 1 2 3 4	102 1 2 3 4	103 1 2 3 4	104 1 2 3 4
105 1 2 3 4	106 1 2 3 4	107 1 2 3 4	108 1 2 3 4
109 1 2 3 4	110 1 2 3 4	111 1 2 3 4	112 1 2 3 4
113 1 2 3 4	114 1 2 3 4	115 1 2 3 4	116 1 2 3 4
117 1 2 3 4	118 1 2 3 4	119 1 2 3 4	120 1 2 3 4
121 1 2 3 4	122 1 2 3 4	123 1 2 3 4	124 1 2 3 4
125 1 2 3 4	126 1 2 3 4	127 1 2 3 4	128 1 2 3 4
129 1 2 3 4	130 1 2 3 4	131 1 2 3 4	132 1 2 3 4
133 1 2 3 4	134 1 2 3 4	135 1 2 3 4	136 1 2 3 4
137 1 2 3 4	138 1 2 3 4	139 1 2 3 4	140 1 2 3 4
141 1 2 3 4	142 1 2 3 4	143 1 2 3 4	144 1 2 3 4
145 1 2 3 4	146 1 2 3 4	147 1 2 3 4	148 1 2 3 4
149 1 2 3 4	150 1 2 3 4	151 1 2 3 4	152 1 2 3 4
153 1 2 3 4	154 1 2 3 4	155 1 2 3 4	156 1 2 3 4
157 1 2 3 4	158 1 2 3 4	159 1 2 3 4	160 1 2 3 4

Continued.

NURSING THE ADULT PATIENT—cont'd

Review questions 161-272, pp. 160-168

NAME ______ (LAST FIRST MIDDLE) GRADE ______ SEX ______ (M OR F) DATE OF BIRTH ______ (YEAR MONTH DAY)

DATE ______ (YEAR MONTH DAY) AGE ______ SCHOOL ______ CITY ______

INSTRUCTOR ______

NAME OF TEST ______

IDENTIFICATION NUMBER

0	1	2	3	4	5	6	7	8	9
0	1	2	3	4	5	6	7	8	9
0	1	2	3	4	5	6	7	8	9
0	1	2	3	4	5	6	7	8	9
0	1	2	3	4	5	6	7	8	9
0	1	2	3	4	5	6	7	8	9
0	1	2	3	4	5	6	7	8	9
0	1	2	3	4	5	6	7	8	9
0	1	2	3	4	5	6	7	8	9
0	1	2	3	4	5	6	7	8	9

BE SURE TO MAKE YOUR MARKS HEAVY AND BLACK

ERASE COMPLETELY ANY ANSWERS YOU WISH TO CHANGE

161 1 2 3 4	162 1 2 3 4	163 1 2 3 4	164 1 2 3 4
165 1 2 3 4	166 1 2 3 4	167 1 2 3 4	168 1 2 3 4
169 1 2 3 4	170 1 2 3 4	171 1 2 3 4	172 1 2 3 4
173 1 2 3 4	174 1 2 3 4	175 1 2 3 4	176 1 2 3 4
177 1 2 3 4	178 1 2 3 4	179 1 2 3 4	180 1 2 3 4
181 1 2 3 4	182 1 2 3 4	183 1 2 3 4	184 1 2 3 4
185 1 2 3 4	186 1 2 3 4	187 1 2 3 4	188 1 2 3 4
189 1 2 3 4	190 1 2 3 4	191 1 2 3 4	192 1 2 3 4
193 1 2 3 4	194 1 2 3 4	195 1 2 3 4	196 1 2 3 4
197 1 2 3 4	198 1 2 3 4	199 1 2 3 4	200 1 2 3 4
201 1 2 3 4	202 1 2 3 4	203 1 2 3 4	204 1 2 3 4
205 1 2 3 4	206 1 2 3 4	207 1 2 3 4	208 1 2 3 4
209 1 2 3 4	210 1 2 3 4	211 1 2 3 4	212 1 2 3 4
213 1 2 3 4	214 1 2 3 4	215 1 2 3 4	216 1 2 3 4
217 1 2 3 4	218 1 2 3 4	219 1 2 3 4	220 1 2 3 4
221 1 2 3 4	222 1 2 3 4	223 1 2 3 4	224 1 2 3 4
225 1 2 3 4	226 1 2 3 4	227 1 2 3 4	228 1 2 3 4
229 1 2 3 4	230 1 2 3 4	231 1 2 3 4	232 1 2 3 4
233 1 2 3 4	234 1 2 3 4	235 1 2 3 4	236 1 2 3 4
237 1 2 3 4	238 1 2 3 4	239 1 2 3 4	240 1 2 3 4
241 1 2 3 4	242 1 2 3 4	243 1 2 3 4	244 1 2 3 4
245 1 2 3 4	246 1 2 3 4	247 1 2 3 4	248 1 2 3 4
249 1 2 3 4	250 1 2 3 4	251 1 2 3 4	252 1 2 3 4
253 1 2 3 4	254 1 2 3 4	255 1 2 3 4	256 1 2 3 4
257 1 2 3 4	258 1 2 3 4	259 1 2 3 4	260 1 2 3 4
261 1 2 3 4	262 1 2 3 4	263 1 2 3 4	264 1 2 3 4
265 1 2 3 4	266 1 2 3 4	267 1 2 3 4	268 1 2 3 4
269 1 2 3 4	270 1 2 3 4	271 1 2 3 4	272 1 2 3 4
273 1 2 3 4	274 1 2 3 4	275 1 2 3 4	276 1 2 3 4
277 1 2 3 4	278 1 2 3 4	279 1 2 3 4	280 1 2 3 4
281 1 2 3 4	282 1 2 3 4	283 1 2 3 4	284 1 2 3 4
285 1 2 3 4	286 1 2 3 4	287 1 2 3 4	288 1 2 3 4
289 1 2 3 4	290 1 2 3 4	291 1 2 3 4	292 1 2 3 4
293 1 2 3 4	294 1 2 3 4	295 1 2 3 4	296 1 2 3 4
297 1 2 3 4	298 1 2 3 4	299 1 2 3 4	300 1 2 3 4
301 1 2 3 4	302 1 2 3 4	303 1 2 3 4	304 1 2 3 4
305 1 2 3 4	306 1 2 3 4	307 1 2 3 4	308 1 2 3 4
309 1 2 3 4	310 1 2 3 4	311 1 2 3 4	312 1 2 3 4
313 1 2 3 4	314 1 2 3 4	315 1 2 3 4	316 1 2 3 4
317 1 2 3 4	318 1 2 3 4	319 1 2 3 4	320 1 2 3 4

MATERNAL AND CHILD HEALTH

Review questions 1-148, pp. 209-219

NAME ________ LAST ________ FIRST ________ MIDDLE ________ GRADE ________ SEX ________ M OR F ________ DATE OF BIRTH ________ YEAR MONTH DAY

DATE ________ YEAR MONTH DAY ________ AGE ________ SCHOOL ________ CITY ________

INSTRUCTOR ________

NAME OF TEST ________

BE SURE TO MAKE YOUR MARKS HEAVY AND BLACK

ERASE COMPLETELY ANY ANSWERS YOU WISH TO CHANGE

IDENTIFICATION NUMBER

0	1	2	3	4	5	6	7	8	9
0	1	2	3	4	5	6	7	8	9
0	1	2	3	4	5	6	7	8	9
0	1	2	3	4	5	6	7	8	9
0	1	2	3	4	5	6	7	8	9
0	1	2	3	4	5	6	7	8	9
0	1	2	3	4	5	6	7	8	9
0	1	2	3	4	5	6	7	8	9
0	1	2	3	4	5	6	7	8	9
0	1	2	3	4	5	6	7	8	9

1 — 1 2 3 4	2 — 1 2 3 4	3 — 1 2 3 4	4 — 1 2 3 4
5 — 1 2 3 4	6 — 1 2 3 4	7 — 1 2 3 4	8 — 1 2 3 4
9 — 1 2 3 4	10 — 1 2 3 4	11 — 1 2 3 4	12 — 1 2 3 4
13 — 1 2 3 4	14 — 1 2 3 4	15 — 1 2 3 4	16 — 1 2 3 4
17 — 1 2 3 4	18 — 1 2 3 4	19 — 1 2 3 4	20 — 1 2 3 4
21 — 1 2 3 4	22 — 1 2 3 4	23 — 1 2 3 4	24 — 1 2 3 4
25 — 1 2 3 4	26 — 1 2 3 4	27 — 1 2 3 4	28 — 1 2 3 4
29 — 1 2 3 4	30 — 1 2 3 4	31 — 1 2 3 4	32 — 1 2 3 4
33 — 1 2 3 4	34 — 1 2 3 4	35 — 1 2 3 4	36 — 1 2 3 4
37 — 1 2 3 4	38 — 1 2 3 4	39 — 1 2 3 4	40 — 1 2 3 4
41 — 1 2 3 4	42 — 1 2 3 4	43 — 1 2 3 4	44 — 1 2 3 4
45 — 1 2 3 4	46 — 1 2 3 4	47 — 1 2 3 4	48 — 1 2 3 4
49 — 1 2 3 4	50 — 1 2 3 4	51 — 1 2 3 4	52 — 1 2 3 4
53 — 1 2 3 4	54 — 1 2 3 4	55 — 1 2 3 4	56 — 1 2 3 4
57 — 1 2 3 4	58 — 1 2 3 4	59 — 1 2 3 4	60 — 1 2 3 4
61 — 1 2 3 4	62 — 1 2 3 4	63 — 1 2 3 4	64 — 1 2 3 4
65 — 1 2 3 4	66 — 1 2 3 4	67 — 1 2 3 4	68 — 1 2 3 4
69 — 1 2 3 4	70 — 1 2 3 4	71 — 1 2 3 4	72 — 1 2 3 4
73 — 1 2 3 4	74 — 1 2 3 4	75 — 1 2 3 4	76 — 1 2 3 4
77 — 1 2 3 4	78 — 1 2 3 4	79 — 1 2 3 4	80 — 1 2 3 4
81 — 1 2 3 4	82 — 1 2 3 4	83 — 1 2 3 4	84 — 1 2 3 4
85 — 1 2 3 4	86 — 1 2 3 4	87 — 1 2 3 4	88 — 1 2 3 4
89 — 1 2 3 4	90 — 1 2 3 4	91 — 1 2 3 4	92 — 1 2 3 4
93 — 1 2 3 4	94 — 1 2 3 4	95 — 1 2 3 4	96 — 1 2 3 4
97 — 1 2 3 4	98 — 1 2 3 4	99 — 1 2 3 4	100 — 1 2 3 4
101 — 1 2 3 4	102 — 1 2 3 4	103 — 1 2 3 4	104 — 1 2 3 4
105 — 1 2 3 4	106 — 1 2 3 4	107 — 1 2 3 4	108 — 1 2 3 4
109 — 1 2 3 4	110 — 1 2 3 4	111 — 1 2 3 4	112 — 1 2 3 4
113 — 1 2 3 4	114 — 1 2 3 4	115 — 1 2 3 4	116 — 1 2 3 4
117 — 1 2 3 4	118 — 1 2 3 4	119 — 1 2 3 4	120 — 1 2 3 4
121 — 1 2 3 4	122 — 1 2 3 4	123 — 1 2 3 4	124 — 1 2 3 4
125 — 1 2 3 4	126 — 1 2 3 4	127 — 1 2 3 4	128 — 1 2 3 4
129 — 1 2 3 4	130 — 1 2 3 4	131 — 1 2 3 4	132 — 1 2 3 4
133 — 1 2 3 4	134 — 1 2 3 4	135 — 1 2 3 4	136 — 1 2 3 4
137 — 1 2 3 4	138 — 1 2 3 4	139 — 1 2 3 4	140 — 1 2 3 4
141 — 1 2 3 4	142 — 1 2 3 4	143 — 1 2 3 4	144 — 1 2 3 4
145 — 1 2 3 4	146 — 1 2 3 4	147 — 1 2 3 4	148 — 1 2 3 4
149 — 1 2 3 4	150 — 1 2 3 4	151 — 1 2 3 4	152 — 1 2 3 4
153 — 1 2 3 4	154 — 1 2 3 4	155 — 1 2 3 4	156 — 1 2 3 4
157 — 1 2 3 4	158 — 1 2 3 4	159 — 1 2 3 4	160 — 1 2 3 4

MENTAL HEALTH NURSING

Review questions 1-53, pp. 236-240

NAME ______ LAST FIRST MIDDLE GRADE ______ SEX ______ M OR F DATE OF BIRTH ______ YEAR MONTH DAY

DATE ______ YEAR MONTH DAY AGE ______ SCHOOL ______ CITY ______

INSTRUCTOR ______

NAME OF TEST ______

BE SURE TO MAKE YOUR MARKS HEAVY AND BLACK

ERASE COMPLETELY ANY ANSWERS YOU WISH TO CHANGE

IDENTIFICATION NUMBER

	0 1 2 3 4 5 6 7 8 9
	0 1 2 3 4 5 6 7 8 9
	0 1 2 3 4 5 6 7 8 9
	0 1 2 3 4 5 6 7 8 9
	0 1 2 3 4 5 6 7 8 9
	0 1 2 3 4 5 6 7 8 9
	0 1 2 3 4 5 6 7 8 9
	0 1 2 3 4 5 6 7 8 9
	0 1 2 3 4 5 6 7 8 9
	0 1 2 3 4 5 6 7 8 9

1 — 1 2 3 4	2 — 1 2 3 4	3 — 1 2 3 4	4 — 1 2 3 4
5 — 1 2 3 4	6 — 1 2 3 4	7 — 1 2 3 4	8 — 1 2 3 4
9 — 1 2 3 4	10 — 1 2 3 4	11 — 1 2 3 4	12 — 1 2 3 4
13 — 1 2 3 4	14 — 1 2 3 4	15 — 1 2 3 4	16 — 1 2 3 4
17 — 1 2 3 4	18 — 1 2 3 4	19 — 1 2 3 4	20 — 1 2 3 4
21 — 1 2 3 4	22 — 1 2 3 4	23 — 1 2 3 4	24 — 1 2 3 4
25 — 1 2 3 4	26 — 1 2 3 4	27 — 1 2 3 4	28 — 1 2 3 4
29 — 1 2 3 4	30 — 1 2 3 4	31 — 1 2 3 4	32 — 1 2 3 4
33 — 1 2 3 4	34 — 1 2 3 4	35 — 1 2 3 4	36 — 1 2 3 4
37 — 1 2 3 4	38 — 1 2 3 4	39 — 1 2 3 4	40 — 1 2 3 4
41 — 1 2 3 4	42 — 1 2 3 4	43 — 1 2 3 4	44 — 1 2 3 4
45 — 1 2 3 4	46 — 1 2 3 4	47 — 1 2 3 4	48 — 1 2 3 4
49 — 1 2 3 4	50 — 1 2 3 4	51 — 1 2 3 4	52 — 1 2 3 4
53 — 1 2 3 4	54 — 1 2 3 4	55 — 1 2 3 4	56 — 1 2 3 4
57 — 1 2 3 4	58 — 1 2 3 4	59 — 1 2 3 4	60 — 1 2 3 4
61 — 1 2 3 4	62 — 1 2 3 4	63 — 1 2 3 4	64 — 1 2 3 4
65 — 1 2 3 4	66 — 1 2 3 4	67 — 1 2 3 4	68 — 1 2 3 4
69 — 1 2 3 4	70 — 1 2 3 4	71 — 1 2 3 4	72 — 1 2 3 4
73 — 1 2 3 4	74 — 1 2 3 4	75 — 1 2 3 4	76 — 1 2 3 4
77 — 1 2 3 4	78 — 1 2 3 4	79 — 1 2 3 4	80 — 1 2 3 4
81 — 1 2 3 4	82 — 1 2 3 4	83 — 1 2 3 4	84 — 1 2 3 4
85 — 1 2 3 4	86 — 1 2 3 4	87 — 1 2 3 4	88 — 1 2 3 4
89 — 1 2 3 4	90 — 1 2 3 4	91 — 1 2 3 4	92 — 1 2 3 4
93 — 1 2 3 4	94 — 1 2 3 4	95 — 1 2 3 4	96 — 1 2 3 4
97 — 1 2 3 4	98 — 1 2 3 4	99 — 1 2 3 4	100 — 1 2 3 4
101 — 1 2 3 4	102 — 1 2 3 4	103 — 1 2 3 4	104 — 1 2 3 4
105 — 1 2 3 4	106 — 1 2 3 4	107 — 1 2 3 4	108 — 1 2 3 4
109 — 1 2 3 4	110 — 1 2 3 4	111 — 1 2 3 4	112 — 1 2 3 4
113 — 1 2 3 4	114 — 1 2 3 4	115 — 1 2 3 4	116 — 1 2 3 4
117 — 1 2 3 4	118 — 1 2 3 4	119 — 1 2 3 4	120 — 1 2 3 4
121 — 1 2 3 4	122 — 1 2 3 4	123 — 1 2 3 4	124 — 1 2 3 4
125 — 1 2 3 4	126 — 1 2 3 4	127 — 1 2 3 4	128 — 1 2 3 4
129 — 1 2 3 4	130 — 1 2 3 4	131 — 1 2 3 4	132 — 1 2 3 4
133 — 1 2 3 4	134 — 1 2 3 4	135 — 1 2 3 4	136 — 1 2 3 4
137 — 1 2 3 4	138 — 1 2 3 4	139 — 1 2 3 4	140 — 1 2 3 4
141 — 1 2 3 4	142 — 1 2 3 4	143 — 1 2 3 4	144 — 1 2 3 4
145 — 1 2 3 4	146 — 1 2 3 4	147 — 1 2 3 4	148 — 1 2 3 4
149 — 1 2 3 4	150 — 1 2 3 4	151 — 1 2 3 4	152 — 1 2 3 4
153 — 1 2 3 4	154 — 1 2 3 4	155 — 1 2 3 4	156 — 1 2 3 4
157 — 1 2 3 4	158 — 1 2 3 4	159 — 1 2 3 4	160 — 1 2 3 4

VOCATIONAL ASPECTS

Review questions 1-45, pp. 247-250

NAME ______________________ (LAST FIRST MIDDLE) GRADE __________ SEX ______ (M OR F) DATE OF BIRTH ______________ (YEAR MONTH DAY)

DATE ______________ (YEAR MONTH DAY) AGE ______ SCHOOL ______________________ CITY ______________

INSTRUCTOR ______________________

NAME OF TEST ______________________

IDENTIFICATION NUMBER

☐	0	1	2	3	4	5	6	7	8	9
☐	0	1	2	3	4	5	6	7	8	9
☐	0	1	2	3	4	5	6	7	8	9
☐	0	1	2	3	4	5	6	7	8	9
☐	0	1	2	3	4	5	6	7	8	9
☐	0	1	2	3	4	5	6	7	8	9
☐	0	1	2	3	4	5	6	7	8	9
☐	0	1	2	3	4	5	6	7	8	9
☐	0	1	2	3	4	5	6	7	8	9
☐	0	1	2	3	4	5	6	7	8	9

BE SURE TO MAKE YOUR MARKS HEAVY AND BLACK

ERASE COMPLETELY ANY ANSWERS YOU WISH TO CHANGE

1 — 1 2 3 4	2 — 1 2 3 4	3 — 1 2 3 4	4 — 1 2 3 4
5 — 1 2 3 4	6 — 1 2 3 4	7 — 1 2 3 4	8 — 1 2 3 4
9 — 1 2 3 4	10 — 1 2 3 4	11 — 1 2 3 4	12 — 1 2 3 4
13 — 1 2 3 4	14 — 1 2 3 4	15 — 1 2 3 4	16 — 1 2 3 4
17 — 1 2 3 4	18 — 1 2 3 4	19 — 1 2 3 4	20 — 1 2 3 4
21 — 1 2 3 4	22 — 1 2 3 4	23 — 1 2 3 4	24 — 1 2 3 4
25 — 1 2 3 4	26 — 1 2 3 4	27 — 1 2 3 4	28 — 1 2 3 4
29 — 1 2 3 4	30 — 1 2 3 4	31 — 1 2 3 4	32 — 1 2 3 4
33 — 1 2 3 4	34 — 1 2 3 4	35 — 1 2 3 4	36 — 1 2 3 4
37 — 1 2 3 4	38 — 1 2 3 4	39 — 1 2 3 4	40 — 1 2 3 4
41 — 1 2 3 4	42 — 1 2 3 4	43 — 1 2 3 4	44 — 1 2 3 4
45 — 1 2 3 4	46 — 1 2 3 4	47 — 1 2 3 4	48 — 1 2 3 4
49 — 1 2 3 4	50 — 1 2 3 4	51 — 1 2 3 4	52 — 1 2 3 4
53 — 1 2 3 4	54 — 1 2 3 4	55 — 1 2 3 4	56 — 1 2 3 4
57 — 1 2 3 4	58 — 1 2 3 4	59 — 1 2 3 4	60 — 1 2 3 4
61 — 1 2 3 4	62 — 1 2 3 4	63 — 1 2 3 4	64 — 1 2 3 4
65 — 1 2 3 4	66 — 1 2 3 4	67 — 1 2 3 4	68 — 1 2 3 4
69 — 1 2 3 4	70 — 1 2 3 4	71 — 1 2 3 4	72 — 1 2 3 4
73 — 1 2 3 4	74 — 1 2 3 4	75 — 1 2 3 4	76 — 1 2 3 4
77 — 1 2 3 4	78 — 1 2 3 4	79 — 1 2 3 4	80 — 1 2 3 4
81 — 1 2 3 4	82 — 1 2 3 4	83 — 1 2 3 4	84 — 1 2 3 4
85 — 1 2 3 4	86 — 1 2 3 4	87 — 1 2 3 4	88 — 1 2 3 4
89 — 1 2 3 4	90 — 1 2 3 4	91 — 1 2 3 4	92 — 1 2 3 4
93 — 1 2 3 4	94 — 1 2 3 4	95 — 1 2 3 4	96 — 1 2 3 4
97 — 1 2 3 4	98 — 1 2 3 4	99 — 1 2 3 4	100 — 1 2 3 4
101 — 1 2 3 4	102 — 1 2 3 4	103 — 1 2 3 4	104 — 1 2 3 4
105 — 1 2 3 4	106 — 1 2 3 4	107 — 1 2 3 4	108 — 1 2 3 4
109 — 1 2 3 4	110 — 1 2 3 4	111 — 1 2 3 4	112 — 1 2 3 4
113 — 1 2 3 4	114 — 1 2 3 4	115 — 1 2 3 4	116 — 1 2 3 4
117 — 1 2 3 4	118 — 1 2 3 4	119 — 1 2 3 4	120 — 1 2 3 4
121 — 1 2 3 4	122 — 1 2 3 4	123 — 1 2 3 4	124 — 1 2 3 4
125 — 1 2 3 4	126 — 1 2 3 4	127 — 1 2 3 4	128 — 1 2 3 4
129 — 1 2 3 4	130 — 1 2 3 4	131 — 1 2 3 4	132 — 1 2 3 4
133 — 1 2 3 4	134 — 1 2 3 4	135 — 1 2 3 4	136 — 1 2 3 4
137 — 1 2 3 4	138 — 1 2 3 4	139 — 1 2 3 4	140 — 1 2 3 4
141 — 1 2 3 4	142 — 1 2 3 4	143 — 1 2 3 4	144 — 1 2 3 4
145 — 1 2 3 4	146 — 1 2 3 4	147 — 1 2 3 4	148 — 1 2 3 4
149 — 1 2 3 4	150 — 1 2 3 4	151 — 1 2 3 4	152 — 1 2 3 4
153 — 1 2 3 4	154 — 1 2 3 4	155 — 1 2 3 4	156 — 1 2 3 4
157 — 1 2 3 4	158 — 1 2 3 4	159 — 1 2 3 4	160 — 1 2 3 4

SAMPLE EXAMINATION 1

Questions 1-122, pp. 251-263

NAME ______ LAST FIRST MIDDLE GRADE ______ SEX ______ M OR F DATE OF BIRTH ______ YEAR MONTH DAY

DATE ______ YEAR MONTH DAY AGE ______ SCHOOL ______ CITY ______

INSTRUCTOR ______

NAME OF TEST ______

BE SURE TO MAKE YOUR MARKS HEAVY AND BLACK

ERASE COMPLETELY ANY ANSWERS YOU WISH TO CHANGE

IDENTIFICATION NUMBER

	0	1	2	3	4	5	6	7	8	9
	0	1	2	3	4	5	6	7	8	9
	0	1	2	3	4	5	6	7	8	9
	0	1	2	3	4	5	6	7	8	9
	0	1	2	3	4	5	6	7	8	9
	0	1	2	3	4	5	6	7	8	9
	0	1	2	3	4	5	6	7	8	9
	0	1	2	3	4	5	6	7	8	9
	0	1	2	3	4	5	6	7	8	9
	0	1	2	3	4	5	6	7	8	9

1 1 2 3 4	2 1 2 3 4	3 1 2 3 4	4 1 2 3 4
5 1 2 3 4	6 1 2 3 4	7 1 2 3 4	8 1 2 3 4
9 1 2 3 4	10 1 2 3 4	11 1 2 3 4	12 1 2 3 4
13 1 2 3 4	14 1 2 3 4	15 1 2 3 4	16 1 2 3 4
17 1 2 3 4	18 1 2 3 4	19 1 2 3 4	20 1 2 3 4
21 1 2 3 4	22 1 2 3 4	23 1 2 3 4	24 1 2 3 4
25 1 2 3 4	26 1 2 3 4	27 1 2 3 4	28 1 2 3 4
29 1 2 3 4	30 1 2 3 4	31 1 2 3 4	32 1 2 3 4
33 1 2 3 4	34 1 2 3 4	35 1 2 3 4	36 1 2 3 4
37 1 2 3 4	38 1 2 3 4	39 1 2 3 4	40 1 2 3 4
41 1 2 3 4	42 1 2 3 4	43 1 2 3 4	44 1 2 3 4
45 1 2 3 4	46 1 2 3 4	47 1 2 3 4	48 1 2 3 4
49 1 2 3 4	50 1 2 3 4	51 1 2 3 4	52 1 2 3 4
53 1 2 3 4	54 1 2 3 4	55 1 2 3 4	56 1 2 3 4
57 1 2 3 4	58 1 2 3 4	59 1 2 3 4	60 1 2 3 4
61 1 2 3 4	62 1 2 3 4	63 1 2 3 4	64 1 2 3 4
65 1 2 3 4	66 1 2 3 4	67 1 2 3 4	68 1 2 3 4
69 1 2 3 4	70 1 2 3 4	71 1 2 3 4	72 1 2 3 4
73 1 2 3 4	74 1 2 3 4	75 1 2 3 4	76 1 2 3 4
77 1 2 3 4	78 1 2 3 4	79 1 2 3 4	80 1 2 3 4
81 1 2 3 4	82 1 2 3 4	83 1 2 3 4	84 1 2 3 4
85 1 2 3 4	86 1 2 3 4	87 1 2 3 4	88 1 2 3 4
89 1 2 3 4	90 1 2 3 4	91 1 2 3 4	92 1 2 3 4
93 1 2 3 4	94 1 2 3 4	95 1 2 3 4	96 1 2 3 4
97 1 2 3 4	98 1 2 3 4	99 1 2 3 4	100 1 2 3 4
101 1 2 3 4	102 1 2 3 4	103 1 2 3 4	104 1 2 3 4
105 1 2 3 4	106 1 2 3 4	107 1 2 3 4	108 1 2 3 4
109 1 2 3 4	110 1 2 3 4	111 1 2 3 4	112 1 2 3 4
113 1 2 3 4	114 1 2 3 4	115 1 2 3 4	116 1 2 3 4
117 1 2 3 4	118 1 2 3 4	119 1 2 3 4	120 1 2 3 4
121 1 2 3 4	122 1 2 3 4	123 1 2 3 4	124 1 2 3 4
125 1 2 3 4	126 1 2 3 4	127 1 2 3 4	128 1 2 3 4
129 1 2 3 4	130 1 2 3 4	131 1 2 3 4	132 1 2 3 4
133 1 2 3 4	134 1 2 3 4	135 1 2 3 4	136 1 2 3 4
137 1 2 3 4	138 1 2 3 4	139 1 2 3 4	140 1 2 3 4
141 1 2 3 4	142 1 2 3 4	143 1 2 3 4	144 1 2 3 4
145 1 2 3 4	146 1 2 3 4	147 1 2 3 4	148 1 2 3 4
149 1 2 3 4	150 1 2 3 4	151 1 2 3 4	152 1 2 3 4
153 1 2 3 4	154 1 2 3 4	155 1 2 3 4	156 1 2 3 4
157 1 2 3 4	158 1 2 3 4	159 1 2 3 4	160 1 2 3 4

SAMPLE EXAMINATION 2

Questions 1-120, pp. 264-275

NAME ______________ (LAST FIRST MIDDLE) GRADE ______ SEX ______ (M OR F) DATE OF BIRTH ______ (YEAR MONTH DAY)

DATE ______ (YEAR MONTH DAY) AGE ______ SCHOOL ______ CITY ______

INSTRUCTOR ______

NAME OF TEST ______

IDENTIFICATION NUMBER

☐	0	1	2	3	4	5	6	7	8	9
☐	0	1	2	3	4	5	6	7	8	9
☐	0	1	2	3	4	5	6	7	8	9
☐	0	1	2	3	4	5	6	7	8	9
☐	0	1	2	3	4	5	6	7	8	9
☐	0	1	2	3	4	5	6	7	8	9
☐	0	1	2	3	4	5	6	7	8	9
☐	0	1	2	3	4	5	6	7	8	9
☐	0	1	2	3	4	5	6	7	8	9
☐	0	1	2	3	4	5	6	7	8	9

BE SURE TO MAKE YOUR MARKS HEAVY AND BLACK

ERASE COMPLETELY ANY ANSWERS YOU WISH TO CHANGE

1 — 1 2 3 4	2 — 1 2 3 4	3 — 1 2 3 4	4 — 1 2 3 4
5 — 1 2 3 4	6 — 1 2 3 4	7 — 1 2 3 4	8 — 1 2 3 4
9 — 1 2 3 4	10 — 1 2 3 4	11 — 1 2 3 4	12 — 1 2 3 4
13 — 1 2 3 4	14 — 1 2 3 4	15 — 1 2 3 4	16 — 1 2 3 4
17 — 1 2 3 4	18 — 1 2 3 4	19 — 1 2 3 4	20 — 1 2 3 4
21 — 1 2 3 4	22 — 1 2 3 4	23 — 1 2 3 4	24 — 1 2 3 4
25 — 1 2 3 4	26 — 1 2 3 4	27 — 1 2 3 4	28 — 1 2 3 4
29 — 1 2 3 4	30 — 1 2 3 4	31 — 1 2 3 4	32 — 1 2 3 4
33 — 1 2 3 4	34 — 1 2 3 4	35 — 1 2 3 4	36 — 1 2 3 4
37 — 1 2 3 4	38 — 1 2 3 4	39 — 1 2 3 4	40 — 1 2 3 4
41 — 1 2 3 4	42 — 1 2 3 4	43 — 1 2 3 4	44 — 1 2 3 4
45 — 1 2 3 4	46 — 1 2 3 4	47 — 1 2 3 4	48 — 1 2 3 4
49 — 1 2 3 4	50 — 1 2 3 4	51 — 1 2 3 4	52 — 1 2 3 4
53 — 1 2 3 4	54 — 1 2 3 4	55 — 1 2 3 4	56 — 1 2 3 4
57 — 1 2 3 4	58 — 1 2 3 4	59 — 1 2 3 4	60 — 1 2 3 4
61 — 1 2 3 4	62 — 1 2 3 4	63 — 1 2 3 4	64 — 1 2 3 4
65 — 1 2 3 4	66 — 1 2 3 4	67 — 1 2 3 4	68 — 1 2 3 4
69 — 1 2 3 4	70 — 1 2 3 4	71 — 1 2 3 4	72 — 1 2 3 4
73 — 1 2 3 4	74 — 1 2 3 4	75 — 1 2 3 4	76 — 1 2 3 4
77 — 1 2 3 4	78 — 1 2 3 4	79 — 1 2 3 4	80 — 1 2 3 4
81 — 1 2 3 4	82 — 1 2 3 4	83 — 1 2 3 4	84 — 1 2 3 4
85 — 1 2 3 4	86 — 1 2 3 4	87 — 1 2 3 4	88 — 1 2 3 4
89 — 1 2 3 4	90 — 1 2 3 4	91 — 1 2 3 4	92 — 1 2 3 4
93 — 1 2 3 4	94 — 1 2 3 4	95 — 1 2 3 4	96 — 1 2 3 4
97 — 1 2 3 4	98 — 1 2 3 4	99 — 1 2 3 4	100 — 1 2 3 4
101 — 1 2 3 4	102 — 1 2 3 4	103 — 1 2 3 4	104 — 1 2 3 4
105 — 1 2 3 4	106 — 1 2 3 4	107 — 1 2 3 4	108 — 1 2 3 4
109 — 1 2 3 4	110 — 1 2 3 4	111 — 1 2 3 4	112 — 1 2 3 4
113 — 1 2 3 4	114 — 1 2 3 4	115 — 1 2 3 4	116 — 1 2 3 4
117 — 1 2 3 4	118 — 1 2 3 4	119 — 1 2 3 4	120 — 1 2 3 4
121 — 1 2 3 4	122 — 1 2 3 4	123 — 1 2 3 4	124 — 1 2 3 4
125 — 1 2 3 4	126 — 1 2 3 4	127 — 1 2 3 4	128 — 1 2 3 4
129 — 1 2 3 4	130 — 1 2 3 4	131 — 1 2 3 4	132 — 1 2 3 4
133 — 1 2 3 4	134 — 1 2 3 4	135 — 1 2 3 4	136 — 1 2 3 4
137 — 1 2 3 4	138 — 1 2 3 4	139 — 1 2 3 4	140 — 1 2 3 4
141 — 1 2 3 4	142 — 1 2 3 4	143 — 1 2 3 4	144 — 1 2 3 4
145 — 1 2 3 4	146 — 1 2 3 4	147 — 1 2 3 4	148 — 1 2 3 4
149 — 1 2 3 4	150 — 1 2 3 4	151 — 1 2 3 4	152 — 1 2 3 4
153 — 1 2 3 4	154 — 1 2 3 4	155 — 1 2 3 4	156 — 1 2 3 4
157 — 1 2 3 4	158 — 1 2 3 4	159 — 1 2 3 4	160 — 1 2 3 4

SAMPLE EXAMINATION 3

Questions 1-121, pp. 276-288

NAME ____________ LAST FIRST MIDDLE GRADE ________ SEX ____ M OR F DATE OF BIRTH ____________ YEAR MONTH DAY

DATE ____________ YEAR MONTH DAY AGE ______ SCHOOL ____________________ CITY ____________

INSTRUCTOR ________________________

NAME OF TEST ______________________

BE SURE TO MAKE YOUR MARKS HEAVY AND BLACK

ERASE COMPLETELY ANY ANSWERS YOU WISH TO CHANGE

IDENTIFICATION NUMBER

	0	1	2	3	4	5	6	7	8	9
	0	1	2	3	4	5	6	7	8	9
	0	1	2	3	4	5	6	7	8	9
	0	1	2	3	4	5	6	7	8	9
	0	1	2	3	4	5	6	7	8	9
	0	1	2	3	4	5	6	7	8	9
	0	1	2	3	4	5	6	7	8	9
	0	1	2	3	4	5	6	7	8	9
	0	1	2	3	4	5	6	7	8	9
	0	1	2	3	4	5	6	7	8	9

1 — 1 2 3 4	2 — 1 2 3 4	3 — 1 2 3 4	4 — 1 2 3 4
5 — 1 2 3 4	6 — 1 2 3 4	7 — 1 2 3 4	8 — 1 2 3 4
9 — 1 2 3 4	10 — 1 2 3 4	11 — 1 2 3 4	12 — 1 2 3 4
13 — 1 2 3 4	14 — 1 2 3 4	15 — 1 2 3 4	16 — 1 2 3 4
17 — 1 2 3 4	18 — 1 2 3 4	19 — 1 2 3 4	20 — 1 2 3 4
21 — 1 2 3 4	22 — 1 2 3 4	23 — 1 2 3 4	24 — 1 2 3 4
25 — 1 2 3 4	26 — 1 2 3 4	27 — 1 2 3 4	28 — 1 2 3 4
29 — 1 2 3 4	30 — 1 2 3 4	31 — 1 2 3 4	32 — 1 2 3 4
33 — 1 2 3 4	34 — 1 2 3 4	35 — 1 2 3 4	36 — 1 2 3 4
37 — 1 2 3 4	38 — 1 2 3 4	39 — 1 2 3 4	40 — 1 2 3 4
41 — 1 2 3 4	42 — 1 2 3 4	43 — 1 2 3 4	44 — 1 2 3 4
45 — 1 2 3 4	46 — 1 2 3 4	47 — 1 2 3 4	48 — 1 2 3 4
49 — 1 2 3 4	50 — 1 2 3 4	51 — 1 2 3 4	52 — 1 2 3 4
53 — 1 2 3 4	54 — 1 2 3 4	55 — 1 2 3 4	56 — 1 2 3 4
57 — 1 2 3 4	58 — 1 2 3 4	59 — 1 2 3 4	60 — 1 2 3 4
61 — 1 2 3 4	62 — 1 2 3 4	63 — 1 2 3 4	64 — 1 2 3 4
65 — 1 2 3 4	66 — 1 2 3 4	67 — 1 2 3 4	68 — 1 2 3 4
69 — 1 2 3 4	70 — 1 2 3 4	71 — 1 2 3 4	72 — 1 2 3 4
73 — 1 2 3 4	74 — 1 2 3 4	75 — 1 2 3 4	76 — 1 2 3 4
77 — 1 2 3 4	78 — 1 2 3 4	79 — 1 2 3 4	80 — 1 2 3 4
81 — 1 2 3 4	82 — 1 2 3 4	83 — 1 2 3 4	84 — 1 2 3 4
85 — 1 2 3 4	86 — 1 2 3 4	87 — 1 2 3 4	88 — 1 2 3 4
89 — 1 2 3 4	90 — 1 2 3 4	91 — 1 2 3 4	92 — 1 2 3 4
93 — 1 2 3 4	94 — 1 2 3 4	95 — 1 2 3 4	96 — 1 2 3 4
97 — 1 2 3 4	98 — 1 2 3 4	99 — 1 2 3 4	100 — 1 2 3 4
101 — 1 2 3 4	102 — 1 2 3 4	103 — 1 2 3 4	104 — 1 2 3 4
105 — 1 2 3 4	106 — 1 2 3 4	107 — 1 2 3 4	108 — 1 2 3 4
109 — 1 2 3 4	110 — 1 2 3 4	111 — 1 2 3 4	112 — 1 2 3 4
113 — 1 2 3 4	114 — 1 2 3 4	115 — 1 2 3 4	116 — 1 2 3 4
117 — 1 2 3 4	118 — 1 2 3 4	119 — 1 2 3 4	120 — 1 2 3 4
121 — 1 2 3 4	122 — 1 2 3 4	123 — 1 2 3 4	124 — 1 2 3 4
125 — 1 2 3 4	126 — 1 2 3 4	127 — 1 2 3 4	128 — 1 2 3 4
129 — 1 2 3 4	130 — 1 2 3 4	131 — 1 2 3 4	132 — 1 2 3 4
133 — 1 2 3 4	134 — 1 2 3 4	135 — 1 2 3 4	136 — 1 2 3 4
137 — 1 2 3 4	138 — 1 2 3 4	139 — 1 2 3 4	140 — 1 2 3 4
141 — 1 2 3 4	142 — 1 2 3 4	143 — 1 2 3 4	144 — 1 2 3 4
145 — 1 2 3 4	146 — 1 2 3 4	147 — 1 2 3 4	148 — 1 2 3 4
149 — 1 2 3 4	150 — 1 2 3 4	151 — 1 2 3 4	152 — 1 2 3 4
153 — 1 2 3 4	154 — 1 2 3 4	155 — 1 2 3 4	156 — 1 2 3 4
157 — 1 2 3 4	158 — 1 2 3 4	159 — 1 2 3 4	160 — 1 2 3 4

SAMPLE EXAMINATION 4

Questions 1-120, pp. 289-299

NAME ______________ LAST FIRST MIDDLE GRADE ________ SEX ________ M OR F DATE OF BIRTH ________ YEAR MONTH DAY

DATE ______________ YEAR MONTH DAY AGE ______ SCHOOL ______________ CITY ______________

INSTRUCTOR ______________________

NAME OF TEST ______________________

BE SURE TO MAKE YOUR MARKS HEAVY AND BLACK

ERASE COMPLETELY ANY ANSWERS YOU WISH TO CHANGE

IDENTIFICATION NUMBER

	0 1 2 3 4 5 6 7 8 9
	0 1 2 3 4 5 6 7 8 9
	0 1 2 3 4 5 6 7 8 9
	0 1 2 3 4 5 6 7 8 9
	0 1 2 3 4 5 6 7 8 9
	0 1 2 3 4 5 6 7 8 9
	0 1 2 3 4 5 6 7 8 9
	0 1 2 3 4 5 6 7 8 9
	0 1 2 3 4 5 6 7 8 9
	0 1 2 3 4 5 6 7 8 9

1 1 2 3 4	2 1 2 3 4	3 1 2 3 4	4 1 2 3 4
5 1 2 3 4	6 1 2 3 4	7 1 2 3 4	8 1 2 3 4
9 1 2 3 4	10 1 2 3 4	11 1 2 3 4	12 1 2 3 4
13 1 2 3 4	14 1 2 3 4	15 1 2 3 4	16 1 2 3 4
17 1 2 3 4	18 1 2 3 4	19 1 2 3 4	20 1 2 3 4
21 1 2 3 4	22 1 2 3 4	23 1 2 3 4	24 1 2 3 4
25 1 2 3 4	26 1 2 3 4	27 1 2 3 4	28 1 2 3 4
29 1 2 3 4	30 1 2 3 4	31 1 2 3 4	32 1 2 3 4
33 1 2 3 4	34 1 2 3 4	35 1 2 3 4	36 1 2 3 4
37 1 2 3 4	38 1 2 3 4	39 1 2 3 4	40 1 2 3 4
41 1 2 3 4	42 1 2 3 4	43 1 2 3 4	44 1 2 3 4
45 1 2 3 4	46 1 2 3 4	47 1 2 3 4	48 1 2 3 4
49 1 2 3 4	50 1 2 3 4	51 1 2 3 4	52 1 2 3 4
53 1 2 3 4	54 1 2 3 4	55 1 2 3 4	56 1 2 3 4
57 1 2 3 4	58 1 2 3 4	59 1 2 3 4	60 1 2 3 4
61 1 2 3 4	62 1 2 3 4	63 1 2 3 4	64 1 2 3 4
65 1 2 3 4	66 1 2 3 4	67 1 2 3 4	68 1 2 3 4
69 1 2 3 4	70 1 2 3 4	71 1 2 3 4	72 1 2 3 4
73 1 2 3 4	74 1 2 3 4	75 1 2 3 4	76 1 2 3 4
77 1 2 3 4	78 1 2 3 4	79 1 2 3 4	80 1 2 3 4
81 1 2 3 4	82 1 2 3 4	83 1 2 3 4	84 1 2 3 4
85 1 2 3 4	86 1 2 3 4	87 1 2 3 4	88 1 2 3 4
89 1 2 3 4	90 1 2 3 4	91 1 2 3 4	92 1 2 3 4
93 1 2 3 4	94 1 2 3 4	95 1 2 3 4	96 1 2 3 4
97 1 2 3 4	98 1 2 3 4	99 1 2 3 4	100 1 2 3 4
101 1 2 3 4	102 1 2 3 4	103 1 2 3 4	104 1 2 3 4
105 1 2 3 4	106 1 2 3 4	107 1 2 3 4	108 1 2 3 4
109 1 2 3 4	110 1 2 3 4	111 1 2 3 4	112 1 2 3 4
113 1 2 3 4	114 1 2 3 4	115 1 2 3 4	116 1 2 3 4
117 1 2 3 4	118 1 2 3 4	119 1 2 3 4	120 1 2 3 4
121 1 2 3 4	122 1 2 3 4	123 1 2 3 4	124 1 2 3 4
125 1 2 3 4	126 1 2 3 4	127 1 2 3 4	128 1 2 3 4
129 1 2 3 4	130 1 2 3 4	131 1 2 3 4	132 1 2 3 4
133 1 2 3 4	134 1 2 3 4	135 1 2 3 4	136 1 2 3 4
137 1 2 3 4	138 1 2 3 4	139 1 2 3 4	140 1 2 3 4
141 1 2 3 4	142 1 2 3 4	143 1 2 3 4	144 1 2 3 4
145 1 2 3 4	146 1 2 3 4	147 1 2 3 4	148 1 2 3 4
149 1 2 3 4	150 1 2 3 4	151 1 2 3 4	152 1 2 3 4
153 1 2 3 4	154 1 2 3 4	155 1 2 3 4	156 1 2 3 4
157 1 2 3 4	158 1 2 3 4	159 1 2 3 4	160 1 2 3 4